Recent Progress in Gastrointestinal Surgery

Recent Progress in Gastrointestinal Surgery

Editor: Diana Pollard

AMERICAN
MEDICAL PUBLISHERS
www.americanmedicalpublishers.com

AMERICAN
MEDICAL PUBLISHERS
www.americanmedicalpublishers.com

Cataloging-in-Publication Data

Recent progress in gastrointestinal surgery / edited by Diana Pollard.
p. cm.
Includes bibliographical references and index.
ISBN 978-1-63927-498-7
1. Gastrointestinal system--Surgery. 2. Gastroenterology. 3. Surgery. I. Pollard, Diana.
RD540 .R43 2022
61743--dc23

American Medical Publishers,
41 Flatbush Avenue,
1st Floor, New York,
NY 11217, USA

ISBN 978-1-63927-498-7 (Hardback)

Contents

Preface

This book aims to highlight the current researches and provides a platform to further the scope of innovations in this area. This book is a product of the combined efforts of many researchers and scientists, after going through thorough studies and analysis from different parts of the world. The objective of this book is to provide the readers with the latest information of the field.

The gastrointestinal (GI) tract is the organ system comprising of the mouth, esophagus, stomach and intestines as well as the liver, pancreas and gallbladder. This system is responsible for the ingestion, digestion and absorption of food and its nutrients. Various disorders and conditions affect the gastrointestinal tract such as inflammations, infections and cancer. Many of these conditions require surgery. Gastrointestinal surgery can be upper or lower GI surgery. Upper GI surgery is characterized by its complexity and may include procedures such as liver resection, pancreaticoduodenectomy and esophagectomy. Lower GI surgery is performed on the lower GI tract, and includes surgical procedures performed on the small intestine, rectum, anus and colon. Some of the common procedures included in lower GI surgery are colectomy and colorectal surgery. This book contains some path-breaking studies in gastrointestinal surgery. Also included herein is a detailed explanation of the various surgical techniques and procedures employed in the management of GI disorders. The topics covered herein offer the readers new insights in gastroenterology and gastrointestinal surgery.

I would like to express my sincere thanks to the authors for their dedicated efforts in the completion of this book. I acknowledge the efforts of the publisher for providing constant support. Lastly, I would like to thank my family for their support in all academic endeavors.

Editor

1

Pneumatosis intestinalis leading to perioperative hypovolemic shock

Yukako Takami*, Toshimori Koh, Minoru Nishio and Noboru Nakagawa

Abstract

Pneumatosis intestinalis (PI) is an uncommon disorder defined as multiple foci of gas within the intestinal wall. Despite recognition of an increasing number of cases of PI, the optimal management strategy, whether through surgical or other means, remains controversial. The present report describes the case of a patient with PI who underwent exploratory laparotomy without specific findings and who ultimately died due to extensive intestinal hemorrhage that was possibly triggered by surgery.

Keywords: pneumatosis intestinalis surgical management, death, hemorrhage, autopsy

Background

Pneumatosis intestinalis (PI) is an uncommon and poorly understood disorder defined by the presence of multiple gas foci within the intestinal wall. In adult patients, PI may be associated with a good prognosis in response to conservative management, but severe cases require surgical management and sometimes result in death. The surgical indications and surgical risks associated with PI have not been definitively established, despite an increasing number of cases. The present report describes the case of a patient with PI who underwent exploratory laparotomy without specific findings and who ultimately developed fulminant intramural intestinal hemorrhage that was possibly triggered by surgery.

Case presentation

Case report

An 81-year-old female nursing home resident presented to our Emergency Department with hematochezia. Past medical history included appendectomy, atrial fibrillation treated with cibenzoline, an 11-year history of rheumatoid arthritis treated with prednisone at 5 mg/day, prior cerebral infarction with ongoing treatment with cilostazol at 200 mg/day, and a percutaneous endoscopic gastrostomy (PEG) established 1 year previously. On arrival, the patient did not show severe status on physical examination and vital signs were within normal limits, including a blood pressure of 130/80 mmHg. Abdominal examination only revealed abdominal distention and mild tenderness in the right upper quadrant, without guarding or rebound tenderness. Bloody stools were observed in her diaper. Noteworthy findings from laboratory evaluation comprised only an elevated white blood cell count (WBC) of 10.6 $\times 10^3/\mu L$ and mildly elevated C-reactive protein of 1.6 mg/dL. No anemia was apparent, hematocrit was 41.9% and hemoglobin level was 13.5 g/dL. However, computed tomography (CT) revealed diffuse intramural gas from the ascending colon to the transverse colon and a large amount of free air in the abdominal cavity without portal venous air, extraluminal fluid collections or any specific signs indicating ileus or mesenteric artery occlusion (Figure 1). Upper gastrointestinal (GI) endoscopy showed no evidence of perforation in the upper GI tract. Arterial blood gas analysis showed: pH, 7.38; bicarbonate, 24.3 mmol/L; and WBC increased to 11.8 $\times 10^3/\mu L$.

Persistence of abdominal symptoms, absence of upper GI perforation, and results from CT strongly suggested lower intestinal perforation and consequent intestinal necrosis. We therefore decided to perform emergent laparotomy. At the beginning of the operation, vital signs remained stable. Observation of the abdominal cavity found no hydroperitoneum, but intraabdominal tissues appeared friable and hemorrhagic. Although the intestine was explored very carefully from the ligament of Treitz to the pouch of Douglas, no indications of

* Correspondence: yukakotakami@yahoo.co.jp
Department of Surgery, Social Insurance Kobe Central Hospital, 2-1-1, Sohyama-cho, Kita-ku, Kobe City 651-1145, Japan

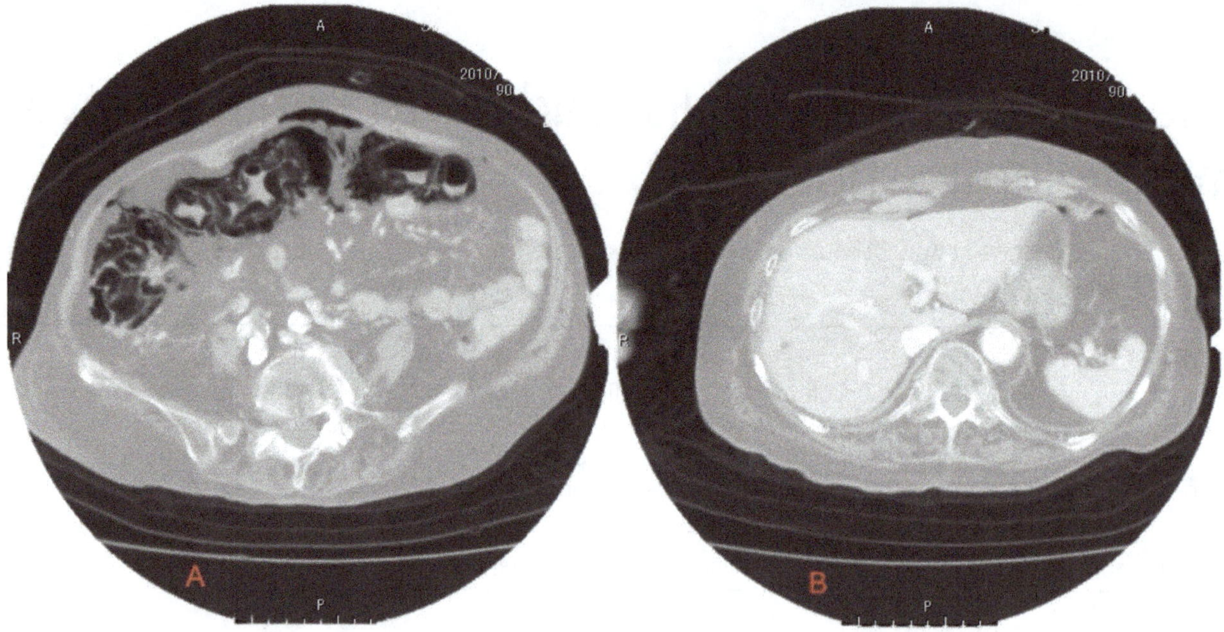

Figure 1 CT. Abdominal CT reveals diffuse intramural gas from the ascending colon to the transverse colon and a large amount of free air in the abdominal cavity without portal venous air or extraluminal fluid collections. This study shows diffuse pneumoperitoneum, which led us to suspect the presence of gastrointestinal perforation. Portal venous gas, which frequently follows severe pneumatosis intestinalis, is also absent.

gross perforation, ischemia, or tumor were identified. However, multiple subserosal bubbles (diameter, 1-2 mm) were observed, mainly around the transverse colon (Figure 2). During these procedures, the spleen was slightly injured. Although the injury itself was only slight and easy to repair immediately using pressure with oxidized cellulose (Surgicel), bleeding appeared to continue and total blood loss was estimated at 730 mL. Blood pressure decreased to 65/43 mmHg. Hemoglobin and hematocrit decreased markedly to 4.8 g/dL and 15.3%, respectively. Without any gross detection of intestinal perforation, exploratory laparotomy was completed with placement of two Penrose drains within the abdominal cavity, at which point total blood loss was estimated at 1100 mL. Blood pressure was 58/33 mmHg, heart rate was 67 beats/min, and body temperature was 32.9°C. Despite all resuscitation measures including transfusion, the patient died of hypovolemic shock 3 h after closure of the incision. The total amount of blood produced by the drains was 220 mL.

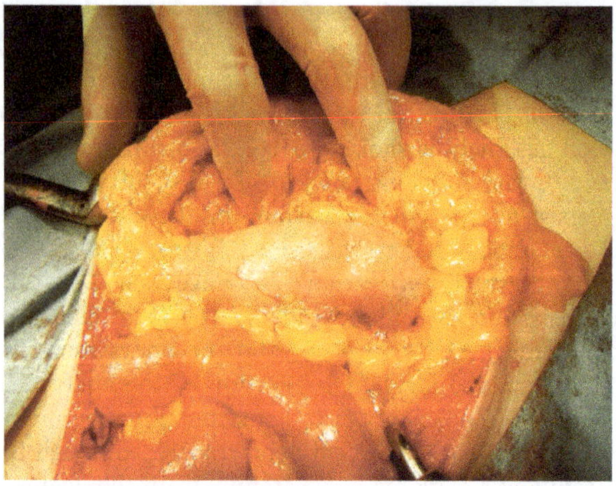

Figure 2 Intraoperative findings. Intraoperatively, macroscopic examination of the abdominal cavity shows multiple subserosal bubbles with a diameter of 1-2 mm, mainly around the transverse colon. The appearance of these cystic bubbles is compatible with the characteristics of pneumatosis intestinalis.

Autopsy

Autopsy was performed at 20 h 25 min after death. A total of 150 mL of hemorrhagic ascites was observed within the abdomen. Diffuse bleeding was apparent around the left diaphragm, and multiple nodular hemorrhages were detected on the greater omentum. The spleen weighed 50 g, with no specific gross abnormalities other than a small amount of bleeding, and the liver weighed 820 g. The PEG tube was without abnormality. No specific findings were noted from the duodenum to the terminal ileum. Multiple emphysematous foci were detected on the serosa and mucosa from the terminal ileum to the descending colon (Figure 3), and a 3-cm hematoma was present on the serosa of the ascending colon. Blood was grossly detected intratubally from the terminal ileum to the descending colon. Diffuse hemorrhagic changes were present

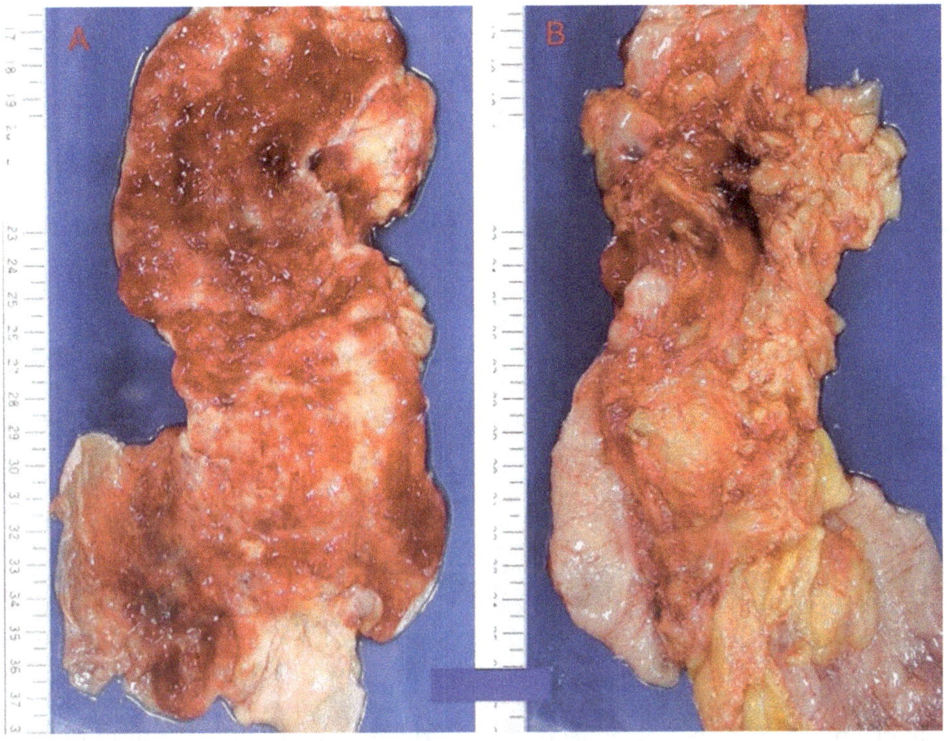

Figure 3 Macroscopic appearance of the ascending colon. These pictures show two sides of a specimen of the ascending colon dissected at autopsy (A: mucosal side; B: serous side). The macroscopic appearance of the specimen shows diffuse hemorrhage on both serous and mucosal sides, but a lack of any necrotic feature, consistent with a finding of intraluminal bleeding.

horizontally on the mucosal side and to a lesser degree on the serous side, consistent with a finding of intraluminal bleeding. Numerous cystic bubbles, each 1-2 mm in diameter, were present within several layers in vertical specimens of the mucosal layer. No signs of obvious necrotic change or coagulant necrosis were seen within the intestine. On the basis of the autopsy findings, cause of death was determined as hypovolemic shock due to intraluminal hemorrhage from the terminal ileum to the descending colon, with fulminant onset in the perioperative period.

Discussion

PI is an uncommon condition characterized by the presence of multiple cystic or linear gas deposits within the intestinal wall. In adult patients, PI is frequently asymptomatic and detected only incidentally. DuVernoi first described the condition in 1783. Despite increasing recognition of PI with more prevalent use of CT and colonoscopy, the pathogenesis remains poorly understood, even though the majority of the literature on PI has placed an emphasis on explaining its etiology.

PI is frequently asymptomatic in adults and does not require specific therapy unless abdominal pain, emesis, fever, diarrhea or hematochezia is present. Pneumoperitoneum and pneumoretroperitoneum can be present, but are generally considered as complications rather than causes of PI [1]. Peritonitis may occur, but is uncommon, and perforation is typically absent when only mild clinical symptoms are present [1]. Most reported cases of adult PI detail a benign course in response to conservative management with hyperbaric oxygenation or metronidazole. Death may occur in rare cases, typically associated with severe comorbid conditions (e.g., cancer, immunosuppressed status due to chemotherapy, diabetes mellitus, or portal venous air embolism) [2-5], or acute abdomen followed by bowel ischemia, bowel obstruction, and portal venous gas (PVG) [6]. The cause of death described in fatal PI cases ranges from sepsis to concomitant malignancies, as well as air embolus in the portal vein or colon perforation [2,5,7,8]. To the best of our knowledge, no previous reports have described life-threatening hemorrhage simply due to PI in adults in either the perioperative or non-perioperative period.

Surgical management of PI, usually consisting of urgent laparotomy in patients with acute abdomen, remains controversial. While surgery is probably necessary in severe cases, routine utilization of surgical management may be associated with poor prognosis. This determination is complicated by the fact that most studies of PI have described etiology or radiographic findings, but few have addressed clinical management, particularly from a surgical perspective [9-11]. Knechtle evaluated 27 patients with PI and reported the highest mortality rate among PI patients with bowel ischemia who underwent surgery, demonstrating associations of low pH (<7.3), low serum bicarbonate (<20 mmol/L) and elevated serum lactic acid (LA) (>2 mmol/L) with ischemic bowel and mortality [9]. Hawn et al. assessed 86 patients showing PI on CT and reported a mortality rate of 73% among patients with complicated ischemic bowel and 83% in patients with hepatic failure [10]. These investigators identified elevated serum LA (>2.0 mmol/L) as a predictor of mortality and recommended urgent surgical intervention in patients with elevated LA [9,10]. Further, they reported that cystic emphysema was associated with favorable prognosis, while linear emphysema was associated with poor prognosis [9,10], and described CT findings of focal thickening, dilated or fluid-filled bowel segments, portal or mesenteric venous gas, and thrombi in the superior mesenteric artery [10]. Greenstein suggested that indications for surgical management include WBC $>12\times10^3/\mu L$, and/or emesis, particularly in patients >60 years old [11]. He also reported that patients with sepsis at the time of PI diagnosis were at high risk for mortality regardless of whether surgical management was performed [11]. Interestingly, although the combination of PI and PVG has previously been reported to show a high mortality rate, surgically treated PI patients with PVG showed a slightly decreased risk of death in that report [11].

In the present case, intestinal perforation was suspected due to the presence of pneumoperitoneum on CT. Laparotomy revealed gross PI without any macroscopic intestinal perforation. In retrospect, the present case satisfied the surgical indications detailed in previous studies, although LA was not assessed in our patient. Of note, metabolic acidosis was not present preoperatively, explaining the absence of bowel ischemia and consequent sepsis.

In terms of the relationship between PI and hemorrhage, some reports have described adult PI presenting with hematochezia. However, most of those reports described a benign course, and the present case appears to represent the first report of an adult patient with PI who developed intraluminal hemorrhage resulting in hypovolemic shock and death in the perioperative period. Discussion of the factors that may have contributed to bleeding is important in this case. For example, cilostazol can increase the risk of bleeding, and prednisone can cause disruption of gastrointestinal tissues, both of which may have increased the risk of GI compromise. However, weights of the spleen and liver were within normal limits, and hemorrhage was localized to the described areas of the colon, suggesting that bleeding was not due to splenic and/or endoceliac bleeding caused by splenic injury or other complications during the laparotomy. To discuss the origin of the hemorrhage in greater detail, body weight of the patient was approximately 40 kg, preoperative hematocrit was 41.9% and hematocrit after the rapid hemorrhage was 15.3%. According to the Gross formula, acute blood loss = blood volume × [Hct(i) - Hct(f)]/Hct(m), where Hct(i), Hct(f) and Hct(m) were the initial, final and mean (of initial and final values) hematocrits, respectively. In the current case, acute blood loss was calculated as approximately 2600 mL. Intraoperatively assessed blood loss from the abdominal cavity was 1100 mL, including the splenic bleeding. Postoperatively, platelets decreased to $80\times10^3/\mu L$ from the preoperative level of $182\times10^3/\mu L$. The postoperative platelet level may indicate occurrence of disseminated intravascular coagulation (DIC), but because postoperative laboratory data obtained before death only examined complete blood cell count, our ability to evaluate the existence of DIC was limited. Furthermore, the patient presented with hematochezia from admission, at which point she presented with neither abnormal vital signs nor anemia. Spontaneous intestinal bleeding could be assumed to have continued during the whole clinical course from admission until death. Furthermore, given the lack of intraoperative colonoscopy, it is difficult to completely exclude the possibility of rough manipulation of the bowel causing the severe hemorrhage. In addition to the etiology of PI remaining unclear, clear explanation for the intestinal bleeding in the current case is difficult to provide. However, the previously stable blood pressure, hemoglobin and hematocrit all rapidly and substantially decreased only right after the slight injury to the spleen, 2 h after the incision and lysis of adhesions of the whole lower intestine had already been finished without encountering any problems. On the basis of this fact, we concluded that intestinal hemorrhage leading to hypovolemic shock was due to the rupture of pneumatosis accelerated by some molecular factors released following splenic injury, rather than simply the splenic bleeding itself. Although the pathophysiological process underlying PI remains poorly understood, we speculate that some molecular factors released during surgical intervention, particularly after partial injury of the spleen, accelerated rupture of the submucosal emphysema followed by intraluminal hemorrhage.

Conclusion

This represents a rare case of PI that initially presented in benign fashion before progressing rapidly to a fulminant and fatal course. Had the bleeding lesion been clearly identified, complete resection could have been performed during laparotomy and may have resulted in a different outcome.

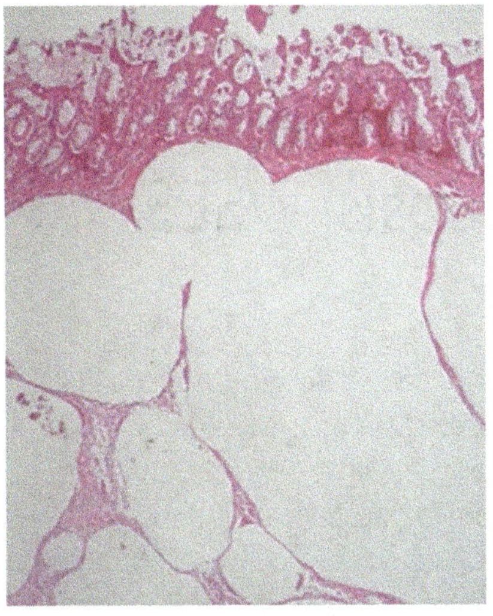

Figure 4 Microscopic histological appearance of the ascending colon. Microscopic histological appearance of the specimen of the ascending colon shows multiple foci of pneumatosis, which are compatible with pneumatosis cystoides intestinalis. This study also shows hemorrhage within the mucosa without any necrotic features.

PI is frequently asymptomatic in adults and detected incidentally. The true incidence of PI is thus likely much higher than appreciated. The present case serves as an illustrative example of the risk of surgical management in patients with PI. Surgeons should recognize that surgery may induce rupture of intestinal pneumatosis.

Consent

Written informed consent for publication of this case report and all accompanying images was obtained from the patient's next of kin. A copy of the written informed consent is available for review.

Abbreviations

PI: pneumatosis intestinalis; PEG: percutaneous endoscopic gastrostomy; WBC: white blood cell; CT: computed tomography; GI: gastrointestinal; PVG: portal venous gas; LA: lactic acid; DIC: disseminated intravascular coagulation.

Acknowledgements

We would like to thank Dr. Toshihiko Miyake, who performed the autopsy and provided pathological commentary and photographs for Figures 3 and 4.

Authors' contributions

YT participated in the care of this patient and observed the autopsy, conducted a search of the literature, and authored this manuscript. TK participated in the care of this patient and provided editorial commentary. MN participated in the care of this patient. NN is the chief director of the Department of Surgery and oversaw the editing process.
All authors have read and approved the submitted version of the manuscript.

Competing interests

The authors declare that they have no competing interests.

References

1. Portolani N, Baiocchi GL, Gadaldi S, Fisogni S, Villanacci V: **Dysplasia in perforated intestinal pneumatosis complicating a previous jejuno-ileal bypass: a cautionary note.** *World J Gastroenterol* 2009, **15(33)**:4189-4192.
2. Eimoto T: **Pneumatosis cystoides intestinalis. Autopsy study of two fatal cases in adults.** *Acta Pathol Jpn* 1978, **28(3)**:481-490.
3. Tato F, Mack M, Meissner O, Schlondorff D: **A severe case of pneumatosis cystoides intestinalis with massive accumulation of gas outside the gastrointestinum.** *Z Gastroenterol* 2001, **39(9)**:797-800.
4. Maeda Y, Inaba N, Aoyagi M, Kaneda E, Shiigai T: **Fulminant pneumatosis intestinalis in a patient with diabetes mellitus and minimal change nephritic syndrome.** *Intern Med* 2007, **46(1)**:41-44, Epub 2007 Jan 1.
5. Bonnell H, French SW: **Fatal air embolus associated with pneumatosis cystoides intestinalis.** *Am J Forensic Med Pathol* 1982, **3(1)**:69-72.
6. Khalil PN, Huber-Wagner S, Ladurner R, Kleespies A, Siebeck M, Mutschler W, Hallfeldt K, Kanz KG: **Natural history, clinical pattern, and surgical considerations of pneumatosis intestinalis.** *Eur J Med Res* 2009, **14(6)**:231-239.
7. Suzuki H, Murata K, Sakamoto A: **An autopsy case of fulminant sepsis due to pneumatosis cystoides intestinalis.** *Leg Med (Tokyo)* 2009, **11(Suppl 1)**: S528-530, Epub 2009 Mar 4.
8. Rosenbaum HD: **Pneumatosis cystoides intestinalis; report of the first case complicated by fatal rupture of the colon.** *Am J Roentgenol Radium Ther Nucl Med* 1957, **78(4)**:681-684.
9. Knechtle SJ, Davidoff AM, Rice PR: **Pneumatosis intestinalis. Surgical management and clinical outcome.** *Ann Surg* 1990, **212(2)**:160-165.
10. Hawn MT, Canon CL, Lockhart ME, Gonzalez QH, Shore G, Bondora A, Vickers SM: **Serum lactic acid determines the outcomes of CT diagnosis of pneumatosis of the gastrointestinal tract.** *Am Surg* 2004, **70(1)**:19-23, discussion 23-24.
11. Greenstein AJ, Nguyen SQ, Berlin A, Corona J, Lee J, Wong E, Factor SH, Divino CM: **Pneumatosis intestinalis in adults: management, surgical indications, and risk factors for mortality.** *J Gastrointest Surg* 2007, **11(10)**:1268-1274, Epub 2007 Aug 9.

2

The role of the open abdomen procedure in managing severe abdominal sepsis: WSES position paper

Massimo Sartelli[1*], Fikri M. Abu-Zidan[2], Luca Ansaloni[3], Miklosh Bala[4], Marcelo A. Beltrán[5], Walter L. Biffl[6], Fausto Catena[7], Osvaldo Chiara[8], Federico Coccolini[3], Raul Coimbra[9], Zaza Demetrashvili[10], Demetrios Demetriades[11], Jose J. Diaz[12], Salomone Di Saverio[13], Gustavo P. Fraga[14], Wagih Ghnnam[15], Ewen A. Griffiths[16], Sanjay Gupta[17], Andreas Hecker[18], Aleksandar Karamarkovic[19], Victor Y. Kong[20], Reinhold Kafka-Ritsch[21], Yoram Kluger[22], Rifat Latifi[23], Ari Leppaniemi[24], Jae Gil Lee[25], Michael McFarlane[26], Sanjay Marwah[27], Frederick A. Moore[28], Carlos A. Ordonez[29], Gerson Alves Pereira[30], Haralds Plaudis[31], Vishal G. Shelat[32], Jan Ulrych[33], Sanoop K. Zachariah[34], Martin D. Zielinski[35], Maria Paula Garcia[36] and Ernest E. Moore[6]

Abstract

The open abdomen (OA) procedure is a significant surgical advance, as part of damage control techniques in severe abdominal trauma. Its application can be adapted to the advantage of patients with severe abdominal sepsis, however its precise role in these patients is still not clear.

In severe abdominal sepsis the OA may allow early identification and draining of any residual infection, control any persistent source of infection, and remove more effectively infected or cytokine-loaded peritoneal fluid, preventing abdominal compartment syndrome and deferring definitive intervention and anastomosis until the patient is appropriately resuscitated and hemodynamically stable and thus better able to heal.

However, the OA may require multiple returns to the operating room and may be associated with significant complications, including enteroatmospheric fistulas, loss of abdominal wall domain and large hernias.

Surgeons should be aware of the pathophysiology of severe intra-abdominal sepsis and always keep in mind the option of using open abdomen to be able to use it in the right patient at the right time.

Introduction

The open abdomen (OA) procedure is one of the greatest surgical advances in recent times and may have enormous application in the daily management of critically ill surgical patients. The OA may be a useful option for treating patients with abdominal sepsis. However its precise role in these patients is still not clear.

On the basis of the source and nature of the microbial contamination, peritonitis can be classified into primary, secondary and tertiary [1].

* Correspondence: massimosartelli@gmail.com
[1]Department of Surgery, Macerata Hospital, Via Santa Lucia 2, 62100 Macerata, Italy
Full list of author information is available at the end of the article

Primary peritonitis is a diffuse bacterial infection without loss of integrity of the gastrointestinal tract. It is a rare condition occurring mainly in infancy, early childhood and in cirrhotic patients.

Secondary peritonitis is the most common form of peritonitis and results from loss of integrity of the gastrointestinal tract due to perforation (e.g. perforated duodenal ulcer) or by direct invasion from infected intra-abdominal viscera (e.g. gangrenous appendicitis) [2].

Tertiary peritonitis is defined as a severe recurrent or persistent intra-abdominal infection >48 h after apparently successful and adequate surgical source control of secondary peritonitis [3]. Although it is less common, it may comprise of a severe systemic inflammation response [4]. Tertiary peritonitis is associated with microbial shift towards nosocomial flora including *Staphylococci coagulase-negative*, *Candida*, *Enterococci*, *Pseudomonas*, *Enterobacter* and other opportunistic bacteria and fungi [3, 4]. Mortality rate in tertiary peritonitis is very high, ranging from 30 to 64 % [4].

Abdominal sepsis is the host's systemic inflammatory response to bacterial or yeast peritonitis [5].

Sepsis from an abdominal origin is initiated by the outer membrane component of gram-negative organisms (e.g., lipopolysaccharide [LPS], lipid A, endotoxin) or gram-positive organisms (e.g., lipoteichoic acid, peptidoglycan), as well toxins from anaerobic bacteria [6]. This leads to the release of proinflammatory cytokines such as tumor necrosis factor α (TNF-α), and interleukins 1 and 6 (IL-1, IL-6). TNF-α and interleukins lead to the production of toxic mediators [6], which may cause a complex, multifactorial syndrome that may evolve into conditions of varying severity and may lead to the functional impairment of one or more vital organs or systems [7].

Severe sepsis is defined as sepsis associated with organ dysfunction or tissue hypoperfusion [8]. Whereas, septic shock is defined as severe sepsis associated with refractory hypotension despite adequate fluid resuscitation [8]. Previous studies have demonstrated that mortality rates increase dramatically in patients with severe sepsis and septic shock [9] and that aggressive treatment of these patients may improve outcomes [10]. Mortality rates have recently stabilized due to advances in treatment options that manage the underlying infection and supports failing organs, however they remain high [11].

In 2014 the definitive data from the CIAOW study (Complicated intra-abdominal infections worldwide observational study) were published [12]. The study describes the epidemiological, clinical, and treatment profiles of complicated intra-abdominal infections in a worldwide context. The overall mortality rate was 10.5 %. Analyzing the subgroups of patients with severe sepsis and septic shock at hospital admission the mortality rate reached 36.5 %.

There are many risk factors that most commonly may precipitate severe sepsis and septic shock, including advanced age, acquired immunodeficiency syndrome, and use of immunosuppressive agents [11]. However, organ failure risk factors generally include the causative organism and the patient's genetic composition, underlying health status, and pre-existing organ function [11].

It has been observed that in some patients, peritonitis may trigger an excessive immune response and sepsis may quickly and progressively evolve into severe sepsis, septic shock, and finally to multi organ failure [13].

These patients may benefit from aggressive surgical treatment and source control following an initial emergency laparotomy to control the local inflammatory response.

Three strategies in the management of these difficult patients have been reported [2, 14]:

- Relaparotomy on demand (when required by the patient's clinical condition)
- Planned relaparotomy in the 36-48-h post-operative period (when relaparotomy is planned after first operation)
- Open abdomen procedure

Choosing the best option is not a simple task. In 2007, van Ruler et al., published a randomized clinical trial comparing on-demand vs. planned relaparotomy strategy in patients with severe peritonitis. Patients in the on-demand relaparotomy group did not have a significantly lower mortality rate or major peritonitis-related morbidity compared with the planned relaparotomy group but they had a substantial reduction in re-laparotomies, health care utilization, and medical costs [15]. However accurate and timely identification of patients who need a relaparotomy is a very difficult decision-making process. At present there are no clinical criteria to select patients for a relaparotomy [14].

Open abdomen procedure (OA), is defined as intentionally leaving the fascial edges of the abdomen un-approximated (laparostomy). The abdominal contents are exposed and protected with a temporary coverage [16]. The OA technique, when used appropriately, may be useful in the management of surgical patients with severe abdominal sepsis (severe sepsis/septic shock) [17]. However, the role of the OA in the management of severe peritonitis is still being debated [18].

Robledo et al. compared open versus closed abdomen procedures in 40 patients with severe secondary peritonitis [18]. They found no significant difference in mortality rates (55 % open versus 30 % closed), nevertheless, the relative risk and odds ratio for death in the open group (1.83 and 2.85, respectively) led to termination of the study at the first interim analysis. However, in that study, the temporary abdominal closure was accomplished by a sandwich technique with non-absorbable mesh sutured to the fascia.

Although current clinical guidelines suggest that OA technique should not be used routinely, but individualized for each patient with abdominal sepsis [19], OA may be an important option in surgical management of severe peritonitis [20].

The management of the OA can be safely achieved with acceptable outcomes but it remains expensive [21]. Its overuse may potentially lead to increased morbidity, of which enteroatmospheric fistulas are the most serious complication [22]. Compared with trauma patients,

patients with abdominal sepsis have been described to have worse outcomes after OA, with increased incidence of fistula formation, intra abdominal abscesses, and a higher delayed primary closure rate [12]. A correct management of the OA procedure is crucial to reduce the associated complications.

Due to patients heterogeneity included within individual studies, an OA classification system was proposed by Bjorck et al. in 2009 [23] and updated by Kirkpatrick et al. [19] (Appendix 1).

Decision making process for leaving the abdomen open in patients with abdominal sepsis

Outcomes of patients with severe sepsis/septic shock due to abdominal source are related to early aggressive hemodynamic support, prompt surgical source control and early and adequate antimicrobial therapy.

Sepsis source control is based on three principles: drainage and lavage of the infected fluid or other collections, debridement of infected/necrotic tissue and definitive or temporary measures to correct anatomic derangements (for example closure of perforated viscus) and to restore optimal function [24]. In critically ill patients with severe sepsis these principles can be applied at different times in the same patient.

Deciding whether to complete the initial operation or perform an abbreviated surgery in critically ill patients is an important and complex decision. The OA concept is closely linked to damage control surgery, and may be easily adapted to patients with advanced sepsis and can incorporate the principles of the Surviving Sepsis Campaign [8]. In these patients an OA approach may be required for different reasons including: controlling any persistent source of infection, preventing abdominal compartment syndrome and deferring definitive intervention and anastomosis.

Damage control surgery in patients with severe sepsis

The origins of damage control surgery was initially developed in the 1980s by Stone at the Grady General Hospital (Atlanta, GA, USA) [25], and detailed by Burch at the Ben Taub General Hospital (Houston, TX, USA) in the early 1990s [26]. The abbreviated laparotomy for trauma patients was defined as the initial control of surgical bleeding by simple operative techniques such as packing etc. for life saving techniques. The patient was taken to ICU where subsequent resuscitation corrected hypothermia, acidosis, and coagulopathy. Once the patient had regained their physiologic reserve, definitive re-exploration and reconstructive surgery was performed with or without final abdominal closure. This type of management can be successfully applied for severe abdominal sepsis including OA technique.

Patients may progress to severe sepsis and septic shock having progressive organ dysfunction, hypotension, myocardial depression and then coagulopathy. These patients are hemodynamically unstable and clearly not optimal candidates for immediate complex operative interventions [27]. After initial surgery, the patient is rapidly taken to the ICU for physiologic optimization. Early treatment with aggressive hemodynamic support can limit the damage of sepsis-induced tissue hypoxia and may limit the over stimulation of endothelial activity [8]. Following the early hemodynamic support, in principle after 24–48 h, reoperation may be performed with or without final abdominal closure.

Relaparotomy and 'relook'

OA facilitates repeated abdominal exploration in the patients with peritonitis and severe sepsis/septic shock. Reoperations, in managing patients with severe sepsis/septic shock due to severe peritonitis, are common and may be useful in attenuating the inflammatory response of patients with ongoing infections.

In some patients, peritoneal infection may quickly lead to an excessive inflammatory response, causing organ failure. In these patients, an early reintervention with surgical lavage of the peritoneal cavity and evacuation of toxic content and inflammatory cytokines may be crucial for stopping the septic cascade. This allows better control of the local inflammatory response and improved outcomes.

Several studies have evaluated clinical variables that may be associated with the need for relaparotomy in the immediate post-operative period [28–31]. In a retrospective study of 219 consecutive patients who underwent emergency laparotomy for secondary peritonitis, van Ruler et al. [28] showed that both the origin of secondary peritonitis and findings at emergency laparotomy were poor indicators for an early relaparotomy. Signs of progressive or persistent organ failure during early postoperative period were the best indicators for ongoing infection.

In a retrospective study involving 523 consecutive patients with secondary peritonitis, Koperna et al. [29] evaluated outcomes of 105 patients in whom standard surgical treatment of secondary peritonitis failed and who had to undergo relaparotomy for persisting abdominal sepsis (study group). While there were no differences in mortality between "planned relaparotomy" and "relaparotomy on demand", re-exploration performed more than 48 h after the initial operation resulted in a significantly higher mortality rate (76.5 % versus 28 %; $p = 0.0001$). The lowest mortality rate (9 %) was achieved in patients who underwent reoperation within 48 h. The results of this study showed that timely relaparotomy should be done early and within 48 h.

The final decision to perform a re-operation on a patient in the on-demand setting is complex and generally it is based on the patient generalized septic response and on the lack of clinical improvement during early postoperative period [5, 28]. The on-demand strategy implies a vigilant observation of the patient and includes reoperation when patients show clinical deterioration or do not improve [32]. However, these conditions are not well defined [33] and often relaparotomy may be performed too late. In patients with severe sepsis and septic shock, OA allows easy second-look to control the source of infection and evacuate inflamed and toxic content, reducing the load of peritoneal cytokines and other inflammatory substances and preventing their production by removing the source itself.

Prevention of abdominal compartment syndrome

The systemic inflammatory response syndrome, increased vascular permeability and aggressive crystalloid resuscitation predispose to fluid sequestration with formation of peritoneal fluid. Patients with advanced sepsis commonly develop shock bowel resulting in excessive bowel oedema. These changes and associated forced closure of the abdominal wall may result in increased intra-abdominal pressure (IAP) ultimately leading to intra-abdominal hypertension (IAH) [34]. Although recognized over 150 years ago, the pathophysiologic implications of elevated IAP have essentially been rediscovered only within the last two decades [35, 36]. In 2013, the World Society of the Abdominal Compartment Syndrome has published practice guidelines for the management of intra-abdominal hypertension [19]. IAP was classified into four grades:

Grade I IAP	12–15 mmHg
Grade II IAP	16–20 mmHg
Grade III IAP	21–25 mmHg
Grade IV IAP	> 25 mmHg

Elevated IAP commonly causes marked deficits in both regional and global perfusion that may result in significant organ failure. An uncontrolled IAH, with an IAP exceeding 20 mmHg and a new organ failure onset leads to abdominal compartment syndrome (ACS) [19]. This in turn has further effects on intra-abdominal organs, as well as indirect effects on remote organ(s) and system(s). ACS is a potentially lethal complication characterized by effects on splanchnic, cardiovascular, pulmonary, renal, and central nervous systems [19]. Ventricular filling is reduced as a result of decreased venous return caused by the compression of the inferior vena cava or portal vein. Preload measurements such as central venous pressure (CVP) and pulmonary artery occlusion pressure (PAOP) may be falsely elevated. Critical clinical conditions play an important role in aggravating the effects of elevated IAP and may reduce the threshold of IAH that causes the clinical manifestations of ACS. The combination of IAH and the physiological effects of severe sepsis and septic shock may result in high morbidity and mortality rates [16]. Especially in the case of severe peritonitis the physiological effect of ACS to gastrointestinal tract may aggravate the abdominal sepsis. Specifically the mucosal-barrier function is altered causing increased permeability and bacterial translocation [37].

The earliest and potentially most effective means of treating ACS in high-risk patient is its recognition and prompt intervention. Presumptive decompression should be considered at the time of laparotomy in patients who demonstrate risk factors for IAH/ACS [37]. The decision to perform a laparostomy in patients with abdominal sepsis is usually based on the intraoperative judgment of the surgeon without IAP measurements during the operation.

Delayed intestinal anastomosis

An additional advantage of the OA strategy in abdominal sepsis is to delay the bowel anastomosis [38] and the potential to avoid stoma formation.

The staged laparotomy was initially described in trauma setting with resection of injured bowel without anastomosis and returning to complete GI reconstruction once the patient is stable [39].

In patients with severe secondary peritonitis and significant hemodynamic instability and compromised tissue perfusion, primary anastomosis is at high risk for anastomotic leakage resulting in increased mortality. In these patients, consideration should be given to initially control the source of peritoneal contamination and delay the bowel anastomosis. In a retrospective study by Ordonez et al., 112 patients with secondary peritonitis requiring bowel resection who were managed with staged laparotomy were analyzed [40]. Deferred primary anastomosis was performed in 34 patients where the bowel ends were closed at first operation. Definitive anastomosis were reconstructed at the subsequent operation after physiological stabilization in the intensive care unit (ICU) and repeated peritoneal washes until the septic source was controlled. In contrast, 78 patients underwent small bowel or colonic diversion followed by similar ICU stabilization and peritoneal washes. In both groups, the abdomens were left open at the initial operation and a Velcro system or vacuum pack was used for temporary abdominal closure. The mean number of laparotomies was four in both groups. There were more patients with colon resections in the diversion group (80 % vs. 47 %). There was no significant difference in hospital mortality (12 % for deferred anastomosis vs. 17 % for diversion), frequency of anastomotic leaks or fistulas (9 % vs. 5 %), or ARDS (18 % vs. 31 %). The authors concluded that in critically ill patients with severe secondary peritonitis managed with staged laparotomies, deferred primary anastomosis can be performed safely as long as adequate control of the septic foci and restoration of deranged physiology is achieved prior to reconstruction.

A high rate of intestinal reconstruction and a low mortality rate was demonstrated in a prospective study by Kafka et al. [41] in patients with generalized peritonitis (Hinchey III and IV) treated with initial damage control surgery and vacuum assisted abdominal closure.

Among 51 patients, bowel continuity was restored in 38 patients, in four protected by a loop ileostomy. Five anastomotic leaks (13 %) were encountered requiring loop ileostomy (two patients) or Hartmann's procedure (three patients). Postoperative abscesses were seen in four patients, abdominal wall dehiscence in one and relaparotomy for drain-related small bowel perforation in one. The overall mortality rate was 10 %. 35/46 (76 %) of the surviving patients left the hospital with reconstructed colon continuity. Fascial closure was achieved in all patients.

In patients with advanced sepsis, open abdomen allows surgeons to abbreviate initial surgery in the face of severe physiological compromise, relook surgery in patients with ongoing sepsis, preventing abdominal compartment syndrome and delay intestinal anastomosis until the patient is appropriately resuscitated and hemodynamically stable. OA may be a useful surgical option in those patients having severe sepsis and septic shock. An "on demand" strategy may be reserved for more stable patients.

Management of patients with open abdomen

Source control

The first stage of open abdomen procedure in managing abdominal sepsis is an adequate and prompt source control. The primary objectives of surgical intervention include:

a) determining the cause of peritonitis;
b) draining fluid collections;
c) controlling the origin of the abdominal sepsis.

Once an OA strategy is decided, the optimal method chosen for laparostomy should allow an easy re-entry to the abdominal cavity, and allow for expansion in order to prevent ACS.

Resuscitation and antimicrobial therapy

The second stage of open abdomen procedures involves resuscitation, which should include fluid administration, vasopressive agents and adequate antimicrobial therapy.

Aggressive hemodynamic support can limit sepsis-induced tissue damage and prevent the over stimulation of endothelial activity. Current Surviving Sepsis guidelines emphasize the importance of traditional mean arterial pressure (MAP) >65 mmHg, central venous pressure (CVP) of 8–12 mmHg in combination with a central venous oxygen saturation (ScvO2) >70 % and Urine output >0.5 mL/kg/h [8].

Empiric antimicrobial therapy should be started as soon as possible in patients with severe sepsis with or without septic shock [8]. An inadequate antimicrobial regimen is associated with unfavorable outcomes in critical ill patients [42]. For these patients, a de-escalated approach may be the most appropriate strategy. A broad-spectrum antimicrobial regimen should be started in the initial stages of treatment. Subsequent modification (de-escalation) of the initial regimen becomes possible later, when culture results are available and clinical status can be better assessed. This is usually achieved 48–72 h after initiation of empiric therapy [42].

Antimicrobial therapy should be reassessed daily, because the pathophysiological changes may significantly affect antibiotics pharmacokinetics in the critically ill patients [42].

In these patients *Candida* species infection may be clinically significant and is usually associated with poor prognosis. Although appropriate antifungal therapy is essential for controlling invasive *Candida* infections and improving outcome, early diagnosis of invasive candidiasis remains a challenge because criteria for starting empirical antifungal therapy in critically ill patients are poorly defined [43].

Antifungal empirical treatment depends on the identification of patients at increased risk for invasive candidiasis such as patients with *candida* colonization and on the positive predictive value of risk assessment strategies, such as the colonization index, candida score, and predictive rules based on combinations of risk factors [44].

Returning to the operating room

In principle, following 24 to 48 h after the initial surgery the patient should be taken back to the operating room for re-operation. Re-operation should be performed within 24–48 h after the initial surgery because exploration of peritoneal cavity with lavage, drainage and source control is feasible. The abdominal exploration may be more difficult later due to the intraperitoneal adhesions and risks enteric injury.

Fascial closure

Following re-exploration, the goal is early and definitive closure of the abdomen, in order to reduce the complications associated with an open abdomen [45], such as enteroatmospheric fistulas, fascial retraction with loss of abdominal wall domain, and development of massive incisional hernias.

Early definitive closure is the basis of preventing or reducing the risk of these complications [45, 46].

The literature suggests a bimodal distribution of primary closure rates, with early closure depending on post-operative intensive care management and delayed closure depending on the choice of the temporary abdominal closure technique [47].

A systematic review and meta-analysis to evaluate whether early fascial abdominal closure had advantages over delayed approach was published in 2014 [48]. Mortality, complications, and length of stay were compared between early and delayed fascial closure. In total, 3125 patients were included for the final analysis, and 1942 (62 %) patients successfully achieved early fascial closure. Compared with delayed abdominal closure, early fascial closure was associated with reduced mortality (12.3 % versus 24.8 %, RR, 0.53, $P < 0.0001$) and complication rate (RR, 0.68, $P < 0.0001$). The study confirmed the clinical advantages of early fascial closure compared with delayed closure in treatment of patients with open abdomen.

Early fascial closure is commonly performed within 4–7 days days of the initial laparostomy [40]. Primary fascial closure can be achieved in many cases within few days from the initial operation without technical difficulties. Patients having abdominal sepsis are less likely to achieve an early fascial closure [49] it should be performed as soon as possible after severe abdominal sepsis is controlled [50].

Ideally, the fascia should be closed in patients whose adequate source control is performed with no further planned surgical intervention, severe sepsis is controlled and fascial closure is feasible without relevant increase of IAP.

However, patients undergoing primary fascial closure need strict monitor of their status to assess the possibility of a definitive operation. An early fascia-to-fascia closure can not be successful if early surgical source control fails [51].

Restrictive fluid resuscitation may be suggested for the hemodynamic support of critically ill patients with abdominal sepsis [5]. Some evidence exists to support implementing restrictive fluid therapy protocols in critically ill patients with abdominal sepsis and IAH [52].

In these patients, fluid resuscitation should be controlled to avoid fluids overload, which may aggravate gut oedema and lead to increased intra-abdominal pressure [5]. Reduction of bowel oedema with a conservative fluid resuscitation may increase the chances for early definitive abdominal closure. Intra-vesical measurements of IAP should be frequently performed in patients with severe sepsis or septic shock of abdominal origin, to monitor the trend of IAP and decide the timing of fascial closure.

It has been proposed that leaving patients with open abdomen on continuous neuromuscular blockade (NMB) can improve closure rates. However, the current evidence comparing continuous NMB to simple sedation is equivocal [53, 54]. Active diuresis is often used to decrease bowel and abdominal wall oedema and facilitate fascial closure. Yet, there is no convincing data to suggest that use of diuretics improves the rate or time to closure [19].

Delayed fascial closure is defined as fascial abdominal closure achieved 7 or more days after the initial OA procedure [47]. The delayed abdominal wall closure may be often problematic because of fascial edges lateralization leading to unfavourably high tensile midline forces. Abdominal wall closure should be performed by approximating the fascial edges progressively and incrementally, each time the patient undergoes surgery until it is completely closed.

Temporary abdominal closure

The ideal temporary abdominal closure (TAC) method should protect the abdominal contents, prevent evisceration, allow removal of infected or toxic fluid from the peritoneal cavity, prevent the formation of fistulas, avoid damage to the fascia, preserve the abdominal wall domain, make re-operation easy, safe and facilitate definitive closure [55].

Many different techniques of TAC have been introduced during the past 10 years [56]. Numerous reports exist on all these techniques, but patient groups remain small, with a high heterogeneity, making comparison of techniques and outcomes difficult [56]. Various advantages and disadvantages of different forms of TAC are shown in Table 1. Although numerous TAC techniques have been applied in the setting of abdominal sepsis, many of those modalities are not primarily intended to close the infected abdomen, (e.g. skin only, meshes, or zipper)

The first and easiest method to perform a laparostomy was the application of a plastic silo (the 'Bogota bag'). This system is inexpensive, readily available and preserves the intact fascia when sutured to the skin edges. However, it does not provide sufficient traction to the wound edges and allows the fascial edges to retract laterally, resulting in difficult fascial closure under significant tension, especially if the closure is delayed [16].

Table 1 Advantages and disadvantages of different types of temporary abdominal closure (TAC) techniques

Technique	Equipment	Advantages	Disadvantages
Skin only closure	Skin staples, towel clips or sutures	Cheap, available, minimises heat and fluid loss	Damage to the skin, risk of evisceration, no control of fluid loss, incidence of ACS
'Bogota' bag	Sterile 3 litre Saline bag cut and shaped and sutured to fascial edges	Cheap, available, minimises heat and fluid loss	Damage to the fascial edges, risk of evisceration, no control of fluid loss. Allows some assessment of intestinal viability.
Opsite Sandwich technique	Polyethylene sheet, Opsite dressings, abdominal packs, 2 suction drains and wall suction.	Cheap, available, minimises heat and fluid loss is controlled and measurable	Incomplete fluid control and need for available wall suction.
Absorbable mesh	Vicryl or similar MESH	Absorbable mesh, infection resistance, protects from evisceration, can be skin grafted.	High rate of subsequent incisional herniation
Non-absorbable mesh or commercial 'Zipper'	Commerical Whittman patch	Abdominal re-exploration is easy, maintains abdominal domain, gradual abdominal closure possible	Commercial equipment required and multiple trips to the operating theatre usually required for closure.
Vacuum Assisted Closure (VAC)	Commercial equipment	Prevents loss of abdominal domain, collects and monitors fluid loss, decreases ACS, no damage to skin or abdominal fascia.	Expensive commercial equipment required. Usually requires GA to change VAC system

Negative pressure therapy (NPT)

Negative pressure therapy techniques have become the most extensively used methods for temporary abdominal wall closure.

It is an easy method and uses a fenestrated polyethylene sheet between the abdominal viscera and parietal peritoneum, followed by a moist towel, kerlix gauze bandage rolls with closed suction drains or a sponge covered with an occlusive adhesive drape and is known as the "vacuum pack technique" or the opsite sandwich technique [57]. This method is inexpensive, easily applied and changed, protects the viscera, prevents adhesions, removes exudate and prevents some loss of domain [58, 59]. Commercially prepared negative pressure dressings are available and the initial dressing may be changed to commercial dressing, if early closure is impossible.

NPT actively drains toxin or bacteria-rich intraperitoneal fluid and has resulted in a high rate of fascial and abdominal wall closure [60]. Animal studies suggested that OA techniques using constant negative pressure to the peritoneal cavity may remove inflammatory ascites, reduce the systemic inflammatory response and improve organ injury [61]. NPT is still associated with high morbidity and high incidence of ventral hernia formation in surviving patients. This is caused by difficulties in definitive closure of the abdominal wall, especially after prolonged application of NPT. However, it is a highly promising method of temporary abdominal closure in the management of critically ill patients with abdominal sepsis [62, 63].

Enteroatmospheric fistulas formation is one of the most devastating complications of OA procedure and NPT. The development of fistulae correlates to duration of NPT and frequency of changing the dressing [64].

Nevertheless, recently published articles indicate that NPT can be applied for the successful treatment of enteroatmospheric fistulas [65] provided an adequate isolation and external drainage of the EAF is obtained. The rationale of obtaining an effective control and diversion of the fistula output is essential for a clean granulation of the exposed bowel and epithelization of the abdomen [66].

A practical algorithm for EAF management based on size, location, output and number of EAF's (single or multiple), has been recently proposed [67].

The combination of NPT with fascial-approximation techniques using dynamic closure procedures to approximate fascial edges is safe and can facilitate delayed closure of open abdomen in septic patients [68, 69].

A systematic review and meta-analysis of the open abdomen and temporary abdominal closure techniques in non-trauma patients was recently published [70]. The search identified 74 studies describing 78 patient series, comprising 4,358 patients of which 3,461 (79 %) had peritonitis. The best results in terms of achieving delayed fascial closure and reducing the risk of enteroatmospheric fistula were shown for NPT with continuous fascial traction. Despite that the authors concluded that the overall quality of the available evidence was poor, and uniform recommendations cannot be made.

In 2012 a retrospective analysis evaluating the use of vacuum-assisted closure and mesh-mediated fascial traction (VACM) as temporary abdominal closure was published. The study compared 50 patients treated with VACM and 54 using non-traction techniques (control group). VACM resulted in a higher fascial closure rate and lower planned hernia rate compared with methods that did not provide fascial traction [71].

Recently a prospective study of 108 patients with diffuse peritonitis and open abdomen enrolled from January 2006 to December 2013 was published. Sixty-nine patients were treated with mesh-foil laparostomy without negative pressure and 49 with vacuum-assisted closure (VAC) [72].

The results clearly suggested the advantage of negative pressure therapy in comparison to the temporary abdominal closure with mesh-foil laparostomy in the cases with severe diffuse peritonitis.

While VAC was associated with low incidence of enteroatmospheric fistula, the fascial approximation techniques (mesh mediated fascial traction and dynamic retention sutures) were associated with less lateral fascial retraction and significant increase of fascial closure. Even if there is lack of good quality of evidence, the combination of NPT and fascial approximation technique is the most promising TAC method [65].

Nutrition support

Nutrition is known to be a key component in the recovery of patients following severe injury or abdominal sepsis. The open abdomen is a significant source of protein and nitrogen loss (up to 2 g per day) [73], failure to account for this may lead to malnutrition with overall poor outcome. Enteral feeding does not increase the risk of ACS [74].

Whilst, there is no strong evidence of enteral nutrition policy in patients with OA, multiple retrospective reviews and one prospective study demonstrate that enteral nutrition is safe within 36 h to 4 days of damage control laparotomy [75–78]. These studies have demonstrated increased rates of fascial closure and demonstrated decreased infectious complications with early enteral nutrition.

Delayed abdominal wall reconstruction

Primary fascial closure of the abdomen is occasionally not possible. A plan must be made to prevent a ventral hernia development in this scenario.

Delayed repair by bridging biological meshes has been proposed [79]. The role of biological mesh in the management of open abdomen has not been completely clarified and may result in bulging or recurrences [80]. In 2012 the Italian Biological Prosthesis Working Group (IBPWG) proposed a decisional algorithm in using biological meshes to restore abdominal wall defects [81]. Well-controlled prospective investigations are necessary to better define the role of biological meshes.

If definitive fascial closure is not possible another option may be skin only closure to cover the exposed viscera and protect it, minimizing further injury to the exposed bowel. Ostomies should be placed as lateral as possible to be adequate [82].

The open abdomen may result in late development of large, debilitating hernias of the abdominal wall which require delayed repair with synthetic meshes after hospital discharge.

A useful technique for the repair of large midline abdominal wall hernias as consequence of open is abdomen component separation technique (CST).

This technique for reconstructing abdominal wall defects without the use of prosthetic material was described in 1990, by Ramirez et al. [83, 84].

The technique is based on enlargement of the abdominal wall surface by mobilisation of the muscular layers without severing the innervation and blood supply of the muscles [85, 86].

In a prospective randomized trial comparing component separation technique with bridging the defect with prosthetic material, CST was found to be superior to the insertion of prosthetic material. Nevertheless a similar reherniation rate was found after a after a 24 months follow-up [87]. The scars or ostomies in the anterolateral part of abdominal wall can make separation of abdominal layers difficult and can limit the feasibility of CST.

Enteroatmospheric fistula

The development of enteroatmospheric fistula is the most serious local complication in patients with OA. The exposed bowel is at risk of fistulisation, especially in long standing OA and in the presence of synthetic meshes and residual infection [88].

The formation of an enteroatmospheric fistulas in an OA is a challenge for surgeons. Spontaneous closure is rare, because of they have no well-vascularized overlying tissue and no true fistula tract [89, 90].

Key components of management enteroatmospheric fistulas include adequate delivery of nutrition, electrolyte/fluid deficit correction and adequate broader spectrum antimicrobial therapy. A useful acronym to apply to the management of such patients is "SNAP," representing management of Sepsis and Skin care, Nutritional support, definition of intestinal Anatomy, and development of a surgical Procedure to deal with the fistula [91].

In literature several methods to manage such fistulas have been described.

The most common strategies for enteroatmospheric fistulas management are:

(a) control and divert the fistula output, using systems such as nipple or ring with negative pressure therapy applied over tissue around to allow granulation;
(b) skin grafting over granulation tissue around the fistula, to apply a colostomy bag;

(c) definitive surgical treatment of fistula when the patient is fully recovered, without sepsis and in good nutritional status, usually after 6 to 12 months.

However, whenever possible or technically feasible, the most effective therapy of enteroatmospheric fistula is prevention and closure of open abdomen as soon as possible.

The open abdomen procedure, although a lifesaving technique, presents a clinical challenge because it may be associated with significant morbidity.

Ideally, the fascia should be closed in patients whose adequate source control is performed with no further planned surgical intervention, severe sepsis is controlled and fascial closure is feasible without relevant increase of IAP.

Fascia should be definitively closed as soon as possible (early facial closure).

Negative pressure wound therapy techniques in combination with fascial approximation techniques should be used for delayed closure.

Conclusions

OA as part of a damage control strategy may be a lifesaving strategy in a well-selected group of surgical patients with severe abdominal sepsis. Once severe sepsis has been controlled, definitive surgical reconstruction should be performed within 48 h.

Rapid closure by negative pressure and dynamic retention sutures of the fascia should be the primary objective in the management of these patients, in order to prevent severe morbidity such as fistulae, loss of domain and massive incisional hernias. The open abdomen strategy presents a clinical challenge that is associated with significant morbidity and OA should be used in the right patients at the right time. Even with the lack of strong evidence in international literature, OA may be an important option in the surgeon's strategy for the treatment of severe abdominal sepsis. Well-designed prospective and randomised studies are required to adequately define the role of OA and negative pressure in managing patients with abdominal sepsis.

Surgeons should be aware of physiopathology of sepsis and always keep in mind the rationale of open abdomen to be able to use it in the right patient at the correct time. A correct management is crucial to avoid severe complications.

Despite lack of high quality data, OA may be an important option in the surgeon's armamentarium for the treatment of severe peritonitis.

Well-designed prospective studies are required *to better define the role of OA in managing patients with abdominal sepsis.*

Appendix

Appendix 1. OA classification system [19]

1. No fixation
   - 1 A Clean, no fixation
   - 1 B Contaminated, no fixation
   - 1 C Enteric leak, no fixation
2. Developing fixation
   - 2 A Clean, developing fixation
   - 2 B Contaminated, developing fixation
   - 2 C Enteric leak, developing fixation
3. Frozen abdomen
   - 3 A Clean, frozen abdomen
   - 3 B Contaminated, frozen abdomen
4. Established enteroatmospheric fistula, frozen abdomen

Competing interests
The authors declare that there is no conflict of interests regarding the publication of this paper.

Authors' contributions
MS wrote the manuscript. All authors reviewed and approved the final manuscript.

Author details
[1]Department of Surgery, Macerata Hospital, Via Santa Lucia 2, 62100 Macerata, Italy. [2]Department of Surgery, College of Medicine and Health Sciences, UAE University, Al-Ain, United Arab Emirates. [3]General Surgery I, Papa Giovanni XXIII Hospital, Bergamo, Italy. [4]Trauma and Acute Care Surgery Unit, Hadassah Hebrew University Medical Center, Jerusalem, Israel. [5]Department of Surgery, Hospital San Juan de Dios, La Serena, Chile. [6]Department of Surgery, University of Colorado, Denver Health Medical Center, Denver, USA. [7]Emergency Surgery Department, Maggiore Parma Hospital, Parma, Italy. [8]Emergency Department, Niguarda Ca' Granda Hospital, Milan, Italy. [9]Division of Trauma, Surgical Critical Care, Burns, and Acute Care Surgery, University of California San Diego Health Science, San Diego, USA. [10]Department of Surgery, Tbilisi State Medical University, Kipshidze Central University Hospital, Tbilisi, Georgia. [11]Trauma, Emergency Surgery, Surgical Critical Care, University of Southern California, Los Angeles, USA. [12]Shock Trauma Center, University of Maryland School of Medicine, Baltimore, USA. [13]Trauma Surgery Unit, Maggiore Hospital, Bologna, Italy. [14]Division of Trauma Surgery, Hospital de Clinicas, School of Medical Sciences, University of Campinas, Campinas, Brazil. [15]Department of Surgery Mansoura, Faculty of Medicine, Mansoura University, Mansoura, Egypt. [16]Department of Surgery, Queen Elizabeth Hospital, Birmingham, UK. [17]Department of Surgery Government Medical College and Hospital, Chandigarh, India. [18]Department of General and Thoracic Surgery, University Hospital of Giessen, Giessen, Germany. [19]Clinic for Emergency Surgery, Faculty of Medicine, University of Belgrade, Belgrade, Serbia. [20]Department of Surgery, Edendale Hospital, Pietermaritzburg, Republic of South Africa. [21]Department of Visceral, Thorax and Transplant Surgery, University of Innsbruck, Innsbruck, Austria. [22]Department of General Surgery, Rambam Health Care Campus, Haifa, Israel. [23]Department of Surgery, Trauma Research Institute, University of Arizona, Tucson, AZ, USA. [24]Abdominal Center, University Hospital Meilahti, Helsinki, Finland. [25]Department of Surgery, Yonsei University College of Medicine, Seoul, South Korea. [26]Department of Surgery, University Hospital of the West Indies, Kingston, Jamaica. [27]Department of Surgery, Post-Graduate Institute of Medical Sciences, Rohtak, India. [28]Department of Surgery, University of Florida, Gainesville, FL, USA. [29]Department of Surgery, Fundación Valle del Lili, Hospital Universitario del Valle, Universidad del Valle, Cali, Colombia. [30]Division of Emergency and Trauma Surgery, Ribeirão Preto Medical School, Ribeirão Preto, Brazil. [31]Department of General and Emergency Surgery, Riga East Clinical University Hospital "Gailezers", Riga, Latvia. [32]Department of Surgery, Tan Tock Seng Hospital, Singapore, Singapore. [33]1st Surgical

Department of First Faculty of Medicine, General University Hospital, Prague Charles University, Prague, Czech Republic. [34]Department of Surgery, MOSC Medical College Kolenchery, Cochin, India. [35]Department of Surgery, Mayo Clinic, Rochester, MN, USA. [36]Centro de investigaciones clínicas, Fundación Valle del Lili, Cali, Colombia.

References

1. Gupta S, Kaushik R. Peritonitis - the Eastern experience. World J Emerg Surg. 2006;1:13.
2. Sartelli M. A focus on intra-abdominal infections. World J Emerg Surg. 2010;5:9. doi:10.1186/1749-7922-5-9.
3. Calandra T, Cohen J. International Sepsis Forum Definition of Infection in the ICU Consensus Conference. The international sepsis forum consensus conference on definitions of infection in the intensive care unit. Crit Care Med. 2005;33(7):1538–48.
4. Mishra SP, Tiwary SK, Mishra M, Gupta SK. An introduction of Tertiary Peritonitis. J Emerg Trauma Shock. 2014;7(2):121–3.
5. Sartelli M, Catena F, Di Saverio S, Ansaloni L, Malangoni M, Moore EE, et al. Current concept of abdominal sepsis: WSES position paper. World J Emerg Surg. 2014;9(1):22.
6. LaRosa SP. Sepsis: Menu of new approaches replaces one therapy for all. Cleve Clin J Med. 2002;69:65–73.
7. Levy MM, Fink MP, Marshall JC, Abraham E, Angus D, Cook D, et al. SCCM/ ESICM/ACCP/ATS/ SIS International Sepsis definitions conference. Crit Care Med. 2001;2003(31):1250–6.
8. Dellinger RP, Levy MM, Carlet JM, Bion J, Parker MM, Jaeschke R, et al. Surviving sepsis campaign: international guidelines for management of severe sepsis and septic shock: 2008. Crit Care Med. 2008;36(1):296–327.
9. Bone RC, Balk RA, Cerra FB, Dellinger RP, Fein AM, Knaus WA, et al. American College of Chest Physicians/Society of Critical Care Medicine Consensus Conference: definitions for sepsis and organ failure and guidlines for the use of innovative therapies in sepsis. Chest. 1992;101:1644–55.
10. Esteban A, Frutos-Vivar F, Ferguson ND, Peñuelas O, Lorente JA, Gordo F, et al. Sepsis incidence and outcome: contrasting the intensive care unit with the hospital ward. Crit Care Med. 2007;35(5):1284–9.
11. Angus DC, van der Poll T. Severe sepsis and septic shock. N Engl J Med. 2013;369(9):840–51.
12. Sartelli M, Catena F, Ansaloni L, Coccolini F, Corbella D, Moore EE, et al. Complicated intra-abdominal infections worldwide: the definitive data of the CIAOW Study. World J Emerg Surg. 2014;9:37.
13. Koperna T, Semmler D, Marian F. Risk stratification in emergency surgical patients: is the APACHE II score a reliable marker of physiological impairment? Arch Surg. 2001;136(1):55–9.
14. Kiewiet JJ, van Ruler O, Boermeester MA, Reitsma JB. A decision rule to aid selection of patients with abdominal sepsis requiring a relaparotomy. BMC Surg. 2013;13:28.
15. Van Ruler O, Mahler CW, Boer KR, Reuland EA, Gooszen HG, Opmeer BC, et al. Comparison of on-demand vs planned relaparotomy strategy in patients with severe peritonitis: a randomized trial. JAMA. 2007;298:865–72.
16. Leppäniemi AK. Laparostomy: why and when? Crit Care. 2010;14(2):216. doi:10.1186/cc8857. Epub 2010 Mar 9.
17. Ivatury RR. Update on open abdomen management: achievements and challenges. World J Surg. 2009;33:1150–3.
18. Robledo FA, Luque-de-León E, Suárez R, Sánchez P, de-la-Fuente M, Vargas A, et al. Open versus closed management of the abdomen in the surgical treatment of severe secondary peritonitis: a randomized clinical trial. Surg Infect (Larchmt). 2007;8:63–72.
19. Kirkpatrick AW, Roberts DJ, De Waele J, Jaeschke R, Malbrain ML, De Keulenaer B, et al. Pediatric Guidelines Sub-Committee for the World Society of the Abdominal Compartment Syndrome. Intra-abdominal hypertension and the abdominal compartment syndrome: updated consensus definitions and clinical practice guidelines from the World Society of the Abdominal Compartment Syndrome. Intensive Care Med. 2013;39(7):1190–206.
20. Schein M. Surgical management of intra-abdominal infection: is there any evidence? Langenbecks Arch Surg. 2002;387(1):1–7.
21. De Siqueira J, Tawfiq O, Garner J. Managing the open abdomen in a district general hospital. Ann R Coll Surg Engl. 2014;96(3):194–8.
22. Yuan Y, Ren J, He Y. Current status of the open abdomen treatment for intra-abdominal infection. Gastroenterol Res Pract. 2013;2013:532013. Epub 2013 Oct 2.
23. Bjorck M, Bruhin A, Cheatham M, et al. Classification – important step to improve management of patients with an open abdomen. World J Surg. 2009;33(6):1154–7.
24. Marshall JC, al Naqbi A. Principles of source control in the management of sepsis. Crit Care Clin. 2009;25(4):753–68.
25. Stone HH, Strom PR, Mullins RJ. Management of the major coagulopathy with onset during laparotomy. Ann Surg. 1983;197(5):532–5.
26. Burch JM, Ortiz VB, Richardson RJ, Martin RR, Mattox KL, Jordan Jr GL. Abbreviated laparotomy and planned reoperation for critically injured patients. Ann Surg. 1992;215(5):476–83.
27. Moore LJ, Moore FA. Epidemiology of sepsis in surgical patients. Surg Clin North Am. 2012;92(6):1425–43.
28. van Ruler O, Lamme B, Gouma DJ, Reitsma JB, Boermeester MA. Variables associated with positive findings at relaparotomy in patients with secondary peritonitis. Crit Care Med. 2007;35(2):468–76.
29. Koperna T, Schulz F. Relaparotomy in peritonitis: prognosis and treatment of patients with persisting intraabdominal infection. World J Surg. 2000;24(1):32–7. 92.
30. Lamme B, Mahler CW, van Ruler O, Gouma DJ, Reitsma JB, Boermeester MA. Clinical predictors of ongoing infection in secondary peritonitis: systematic review. World J Surg. 2006;30(12):2170–81. 94.
31. Hinsdale JG, Jaffe BM. Re-operation for intra-abdominal sepsis. Indications and results in modern critical care setting. Ann Surg. 1984;199(1):31–6.
32. van Ruler O, Kiewiet JJ, Boer KR, Lamme B, Gouma DJ, Boermeester MA, et al. Failure of available scoring systems to predict ongoing infection in patients with abdominal sepsis after their initial emergency laparotomy. BMC Surg. 2011;11:38.
33. van Ruler O, Lamme B, de Vos R, Obertop H, Reitsma JB, Boermeester MA. Decision making for relaparotomy in secondary peritonitis. Dig Surg. 2008;25(5):339–46.
34. Bailey J, Shapiro MJ. Abdominal compartment syndrome. Crit Care. 2000;4(1):23–9.
35. Van Hee R. Historical highlights in concept and treatment of abdominal compartment syndrome. Acta Clin Belg Suppl. 2007;1:9–15.
36. Demetriades D. Total management of the open abdomen. Int Wound J. 2012;9 Suppl 1:17–24.
37. Papavramidis TS, Marinis AD, Pliakos I, Kesisoglou I, Papavramidou N. Abdominal compartment syndrome - Intra-abdominal hypertension: Defining, diagnosing, and managing. J Emerg Trauma Shock. 2011;4(2):279–91.
38. Ordoñez CA, Pino LF, Badiel M, Sánchez AI, Loaiza J, Ballestas L, et al. Safety of performing a delayed anastomosis during damage control laparotomy in patients with destructive colon injuries. J Trauma. 2011;71(6):1512–7.
39. Morris Jr JA, Eddy VA, Blinman TA, Rutherford EJ, Sharp KW. The staged celiotomy for trauma. Issues in unpacking and reconstruction. Ann Surg. 1993;217(5):576–84. discussion 584–6.
40. Ordonez CA, Sanchez AI, Pineda JA, et al. Deferred primary anastomosis versus diversion in patients with severe secondary peritonitis managed with staged laparotomies. World J Surg. 2010;34:169–76.
41. Kafka-Ritsch R, Birkfellner F, Perathoner A, Raab H, Nehoda H, Pratschke J, et al. Damage control surgery with abdominal vacuum and delayed bowel reconstruction in patients with perforated diverticulitis Hinchey III/IV. J Gastroenterol Surg. 2012;16:1915–22.
42. Sartelli M, Viale P, Catena F, Ansaloni L, Moore E, Malangoni M, et al. 2013 WSES guidelines for management of intra-abdominal infections. World J Emerg Surg. 2013;8:3.
43. Leroy G, Lambiotte F, Thévenin D, Lemaire C, Parmentier E, Devos P, et al. Evaluation of "Candida score" in critically ill patients: a prospective, multicenter, observational, cohort study. Ann Intensive Care. 2011;1(1):50.
44. Eggimann P, Que YA, Revelly JP, Pagani JL. Preventing invasive candida infections. Where could we do better? J Hosp Infect. 2015;89(4):302–8.
45. Demetriades D, Salim A. Management of the open abdomen. Surg Clin North Am. 2014;94(1):131–53.
46. Regner JL, Kobayashi L, Coimbra R. Surgical strategies for management of the open abdomen. World J Surg. 2012;36(3):497–510.
47. Godat L, Kobayashi L, Costantini T, Coimbra R. Abdominal damage control surgery and reconstruction: World society of emergency surgery position paper. World J Emerg Surg. 2013;8(1):53.

48. Chen Y, Ye J, Song W, Chen J, Yuan Y, Ren J. Comparison of outcomes between early fascial closure and delayed abdominal closure in patients with open abdomen: a systematic review and meta-analysis. Gastroenterol Res Pract. 2014;2014:784056.
49. Paul JS, Ridolfi TJ. A case study in intra-abdominal sepsis. Surg Clin North Am. 2012;92(6):1661-77.
50. Lambertz A, Mihatsch C, Röth A, Kalverkamp S, Eickhoff R, Neumann UP, et al. Fascial closure after open abdomen: Initial indication and early revisions are decisive factors - A etrospective cohort study. Int J Surg. 2015;13:12–6.
51. Padalino P, Dionigi G, Minoja G, Carcano G, Rovera F, Boni L, et al. Fascia-to-fascia closure with abdominal topical negative pressure for severe abdominal infections: preliminary results in a department of general surgery and intensive care unit. Surg Infect (Larchmt). 2010;11(6):523–8.
52. Regli A, De Keulenaer B, De Laet I, Roberts D, Dabrowski W, Malbrain ML. Fluid therapy and perfusional considerations during resuscitation in critically ill patients with intra-abdominal hypertension. Anaesthesiol Intensive Ther. 2015;47(1):45–53.
53. Teixeira PG, Salim A, Inaba K, Brown C, Browder T, Margulies D, et al. A prospective look at the current state of open abdomens. Am Surg. 2008;74:891–7.
54. Webb LH, Patel MB, Dortch MJ, Miller RS, Gunter OL, Collier BR. Use of a furosemide drip does not improve earlier primary fascial closure in the open abdomen. J Emerg Trauma Shock. 2012;5:126–30.
55. Schein M, Saadia R, Jamieson JR, Decker GA. The 'sandwich technique' in the management of the open abdomen. Br J Surg. 1986;73(5):369–70.
56. Kreis BE, de Mol van Otterloo AJ, Kreis RW. Open abdomen management: a review of its history and a proposed management algorithm. Med Sci Monit. 2013;19:524–33.
57. Brock WB, Barker DE, Burns RP. Temporary closure of open abdominal wounds: the vacuum pack. Am Surg. 1995;61(1):30–5.
58. Campbell A, Chang M, Fabian T, Franz M, Kaplan M, Moore F, et al. Management of the open abdomen: from initial operation to definitive closure. Am Surg. 2009;75:S1–S22.
59. Barker DE, Green JM, Maxwell RA, Smith PW, Mejia VA, Dart BW, et al. Experience with vacuum-pack temporary abdominal wound closure in 258 trauma and general and vascular surgical patients. J Am Coll Surg. 2007;204(5):784–92. discussion 792–3.
60. Plaudis H, Rudzats A, Melberga L, Kazaka I, Suba O, Pupelis G. Abdominal negative-pressure therapy: a new method in countering abdominal compartment and peritonitis - prospective study and critical review of literature. Ann Intensive Care. 2012;2 Suppl 1:S23.
61. Kubiak BD, Albert SP, Gatto LA, Snyder KP, Maier KG, Vieau CJ, et al. Peritoneal negative pressure therapy prevents multiple organ injury in a chronic porcine sepsis and ischemia/reperfusion model. Shock. 2010;34:525–34.
62. Rausei S, Amico F, Frattini F, Rovera F, Boni L, Dionigi G. A review on vacuum-assisted closure therapy for septic peritonitis open abdomen management. Surg Technol Int. 2014;25:68–72.
63. Boele van Hensbroek P, Wind J, Dijkgraaf MG, Busch OR, Goslings JC. Temporary closure of the open abdomen: a systematic review on delayed primary fascial closure in patients with an open abdomen. World J Surg. 2009;33(2):199–207.
64. Verdam FJ, Dolmans DE, Loos MJ, Raber MH, de Wit RJ, Charbon JA, et al. Delayed primary closure of the septic open abdomen with a dynamic closure system. World J Surg. 2011;35(10):2348–55.
65. Terzi C, Egeli T, Canda AE, Arslan NC. Management of enteroatmospheric fistulae. Int Wound J. 2014;11 Suppl 1:17–21.
66. Di Saverio S, Villani S, Biscardi A, Giorgini E, Tugnoli G. Open abdomen with concomitant enteroatmospheric fistula: validation, refinements, and adjuncts to a novel approach. J Trauma. 2011;71(3):760–2.
67. Di Saverio S, Tarasconi A, Inaba K, Navsaria P, Coccolini F, Costa Navarro D, et al. Open abdomen with concomitant enteroatmospheric fistula: attempt to rationalize the approach to a surgical nightmare and proposal of a clinical algorithm. J Am Coll Surg. 2015;220(3):e23–33.
68. Fortelny RH, Hofmann A, Gruber-Blum S, Petter-Puchner AH, Glaser KS. Delayed closure of open abdomen in septic patients is facilitated by combined negative pressure wound therapy and dynamic fascial suture. Surg Endosc. 2014;28(3):735–40.
69. Ferreira F, Barbosa E, Guerreiro E, Fraga GP, Nascimento Jr B, Rizoli S. Sequential closure of the abdominal wall with continuous fascia traction (using mesh or suture) and negative pressure therapy. Rev Col Bras Cir. 2013;40(1):85–9.
70. Atema JJ, Gans SL, Boermeester MA. Systematic review and meta-analysis of the open abdomen and temporary abdominal closure techniques in non-trauma patients. World J Surg. 2015;39:912–25.
71. Rasilainen SK, Mentula PJ, Leppäniemi AK. Vacuum and mesh-mediated fascial traction for primary closure of the open abdomen in critically ill surgical patients. Br J Surg. 2012;99(12):1725–32.
72. Mutafchiyski VM, Popivanov GI, Kjossev KT, Chipeva S. Open abdomen and VAC® in severe diffuse peritonitis. J R Army Med Corps. 2015 Feb 23. doi: 10.1136/jramc-2014-000386. [Epub ahead of print].
73. Cheatham ML, Safcsak K, Brzezinski SJ, Lube MW. Nitrogen balance, protein loss, and the open abdomen. Crit Care Med. 2007;35(1):127–31.
74. Cothren CC, Moore EE, Ciesla DJ, Johnson JL, Moore JB, Haenel JB, et al. Postinjury abdominal compartment syndrome does not preclude early enteral feeding after definitive closure. Am J Surg. 2004;188(6):653–8.
75. Collier B, Guillamondegui O, Cotton B, Donahue R, Conrad A, Groh K, et al. Feeding the open abdomen. JPEN J Parenter Enteral Nutr. 2007;31:410–5.
76. Burlew CC, Moore EE, Cuschieri J, Jurkovich GJ, Codner P, Nirula R, et al. Who should we feed? Western trauma association multi-institutional study of enteral nutrition in the open abdomen after injury. Trauma Acute Care Surg. 2012;73:1380–7. discussion 1387–1388.
77. Byrnes MC, Reicks P, Irwin E. Early enteral nutrition can be successfully implemented in trauma patients with an "open abdomen". Am J Surg. 2010;199:359–62. discussion 363.
78. Dissanaike S, Pham T, Shalhub S, Warner K, Hennessy L, Moore EE, et al. Effect of immediate enteral feeding on trauma patients with an open abdomen: protection from nosocomial infections. J Am Coll Surg. 2008;207:690–7.
79. Kissane NA, Itani KM. A decade of ventral incisional hernia repairs with biologic acellular dermal matrix: what have we learned? Plast Reconstr Surg. 2012;130(5 Suppl 2):194S–202S.
80. de Moya MA, Dunham M, Inaba K, et al. Long-term outcome of acellular dermal matrix when used for large traumatic open abdomen. J Trauma. 2008;65:349–53.
81. Coccolini F, Agresta F, Bassi A, Catena F, Crovella F, Ferrara R, et al. Proposal for a decisional model in using biological prosthesis. World J Emerg Surg. 2012;7(1):34.
82. Jernigan TW, Fabian TC, Croce MA, Moore N, Pritchard FE, Minard G, et al. Staged management of giant abdominal wall defects: acute and long-term results. Ann Surg. 2003;238(3):349–55. discussion 355–7.
83. Cheesborough JE, Park E, Souza JM, Dumanian GA. Staged management of the open abdomen and enteroatmospheric fistulae using split-thickness skin grafts. Am J Surg. 2014;207(4):504–11.
84. Ramirez OM, Ruas E, Lee Dellon A. "Components separation" method for closure of abdominal wall defects: an anatomic and clinical study. Plast Reconstr Surg. 1990;86:519–26.
85. De Vries Reilingh TS, van Goor H, Rosman C, Bemelmans MH, de Jong D, van Nieuwenhoven EJ, et al. "Components separation technique" for the repair of large abdominal wall hernias. J Am Coll Surg. 2003;196:32–7.
86. Rasilainen SK, Mentula PJ, Leppäniemi AK. Components separation technique is feasible for assisting delayed primary fascial closure of open abdomen. Scand J Surg. 2015;13.
87. DiBello JN, Moore JH. Sliding myofascial flap of the rectus abdominis muscle for the closure of recurrent ventral hernias. Plast Reconstr Surg. 1996;98:464–9.
88. de Vries Reilingh TS, van Goor H, Charbon JA, Rosman C, Hesselink EJ, van der Wilt GJ, et al. Repair of giant midline abdominal wall hernias: "components separation technique" versus prosthetic repair: interim analysis of a andomized controlled trial. World J Surg. 2007;31(4):756–63.
89. Losanoff JE, Richman BW, Jones JW. Intestinal fistulization in the open treatment of peritonitis. Am J Surg. 2003;185:394.
90. Mastboom WJ, Kuypers HH, Schoots FJ, Wobbes T. Small-bowel perforation complicating the open treatment of generalized peritonitis. Arch Surg. 1989;124:689–92.
91. Kaushal M, Carlson GL. Management of enterocutaneous fistulas. Clin Colon Rectal Surg. 2004;17(2):79–88.

3

Acute pancreatitis due to pancreatic hydatid cyst

Amin Makni*, Mohamed Jouini, Montassar Kacem and Zoubeir Ben Safta

Abstract

Hydatid disease is a major health problem worldwide. Primary hydatid disease of the pancreas is very rare and acute pancreatitis secondary to hydatid cyst has rarely been reported. We report the case of a 38-year-old man who presented acute pancreatitis. A diagnosis of hydatid cyst of the pancreas, measuring 10 cm, was established by abdominal computed tomography before surgery. The treatment consisted of a distal pancreatectomy. The postoperative period was uneventful. Additionally, a review of the literature regarding case reports of acute pancreatitis due to pancreatic hydatid cyst is presented.

Keywords: Hydatid cyst, Pancreas, Pancreatectomy, Pancreatitis

Background

Hydatid disease caused by the larval stage of the Echinococcus parasite is a public health problem in endemic countries, especially in Tunisia. Hydatid disease can involve any organ. The liver is the most common organ involved and, together with the lungs, account for 90% of cases. Other involved sites (less than 10% of cases) are muscles, bones, kidneys, brain, and spleen. Pancreatic hydatid cysts are rare, accounting for less than 1% of cases [1,2]. Isolated involvement of the pancreas is unusual, and acute pancreatitis secondary caused by primary pancreatic hydatid cyst has rarely been reported (less than 2% of cases in endemic areas) [3]. To our knowledge, 8 cases have been reported in the literature [4-11]. We reviewed and summarized the findings from reported cases of hydatid acute pancreatitis as indicated in the English literature, as well as presenting the findings from our case (see Table 1). Only one article was not available [7] and was not included in Table 1.

Case presentation

A 38-year-old man was admitted to our clinic with complaints of diffuse abdominal pain, nausea, vomiting for 7 days. The patient did not have any fever or jaundice. Moreover, he did not have any significant medical antecedents. On physical examination, vital signs were normal. Tenderness in the epigastrium was detected while examination of other systems was normal. Laboratory analyses were as follows: white blood cells were 13 000/mmc; hemoglobin was 14 g/dl; platelets were 142 000/mmc; amylase was 2100 U/l (normal value < 105); alanine aminotransferase (ALT) was 300 U/l (normal value < 40); aspartate transaminase (AST) was 120 U/l (normal value < 40); alkaline phosphatase (ALP) was 270 U/l (normal value < 290); gamma-glutamyl transpeptidase (GGT) was 130 U/l (normal value < 49); total bilirubin was 9 mg/l (normal value < 10); direct bilirubin was 3 mg/l (normal value < 8 mg/l); C-reactive protein was 20 mg/l (normal value < 5); and erythrocyte sedimentation rate was 70 mm/h. Serological tests including HBsAg, anti-HBc IgM and anti-HCV were negative. Hydatid serology, which was based on an enzyme-linked immunosorbent assay (ELISA) test for echinococcal antigens, was positive (with a value of 3,2 U/l). Lung radiography and hepatic ultrasound were normal. Abdominal computed tomography (CT) revealed a multiloculated 100 × 90 mm cystic lesion in both the corpus and the tail of the pancreas, which was also associated with an enlargement of the pancreas and with a peripancreatic edema, indicating an acute pancreatitis. Abdominal CT-scan showed also daughter cysts, some peripheral calcifications and a detachment of the hydatid membrane in the pancreatic cyst. This is evidenced by a pressure drop inside the cyst and thus, an opening of the cyst in the pancreatic duct which is dilated (Figure 1). Nothing was detected in the liver or in any other organs. Three weeks later, the patient underwent surgery for primary pancreatic

* Correspondence: aminmakni@msn.com
Department of Surgery 'A', La Rabta Hospital, Tunis, Tunisia

Table 1 Up-to-date review of cases of hydatid acute pancreatitis

Case n°	Source	Year	Age (sex)	Location	Size (mm)	Type of the pancreatitis	Pathogenesis ¥	Surgical treatment	Follow-up (months)
1	Augustin et al. [4]	1984	30 (male)	Body	...	...	Opening	Left pancreatectomy +splenectomy	...
2	Papadimitriou [5]	1987	35 (male)	Head	50	Edematous	Opening	cyst fenestration	12
4	Ozmen et al. [7]	2005	18 (female)	Head	43	Necrotizing	Compression	Total cystectomy	16
5	Pouget et al. [8]	2009	29 (male)	Body	30	Edematous	Opening	Left pancreatectomy +splenectomy	3
6	Diop et al. [9]	2010	29 (male)	Tail	80	Edematous	Opening	Left pancreatectomy	48
7	Karakas et al. [10]	2010	18 (male)	Body	70	Edematous	Opening	cyst fenestration	4
8	Chammakhi et al. [11]	2010	32 (Female)	Tail	80	Necrotizing	Opening	Left pancreatectomy +splenectomy	6
9	Present case	2011	38 (male)	Body	100	Edematous	Opening	Left pancreatectomy +splenectomy	3

¥ Pathogenesis: Opening of the hydatid cyst in the main pancreatic duct or compression of the main pancreatic duct by the pancreatic hydatid cyst
Missing data

hydatid disease. Intraoperatively, following the dissection of the pancreatic tail including the cyst, a distal pancreatectomy with splenectomy was performed (Figure 2). The main pancreatic duct was disobstructed from the scolices. Histopathological examination revealed a hydatid cyst in the corpus of the pancreas opening in the main pancreatic duct (Figure 3). The region was drained and the abdomen closed. Postoperative evolution was without complication. The patient was discharged on day 6 post-operative. A 800 mg/day Albendazole therapy lasting 3 months after surgery was started on the patient. After an eight months follow-up, the patient is currently well with neither diabetes nor any signs of recurrence.

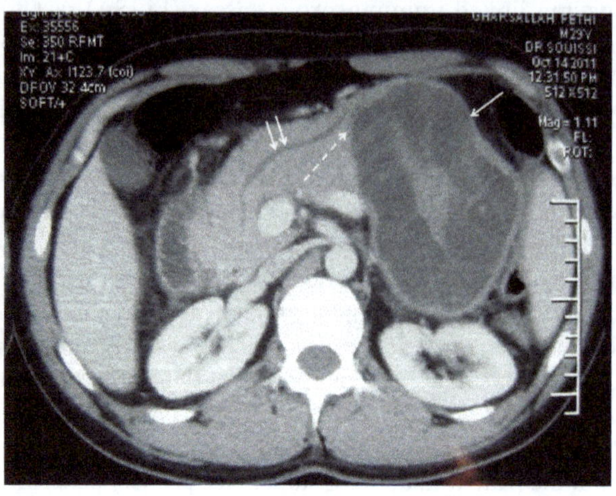

Figure 1 Abdominal CT-scan shows a pancreatic cystic mass of 10 cm, with a clean and calcified wall and containing daughter cysts (one arrow). The main pancreatic duct is dilated (two arrows). Between the main pancreatic duct and the cyst, abdominal CT-scan shows a detachement of the hydatid membrane in the pancreatic cyst (dotted arrow).

Discussion

Pancreatic location of hydatid disease is rare (less than 1%) compared to the other sites of hydatid disease [1,2]. The mode of infestation is either hematogenous, when there is a failure of trapping oncospherse by the liver and lung filters, or more rarely through lymphatic

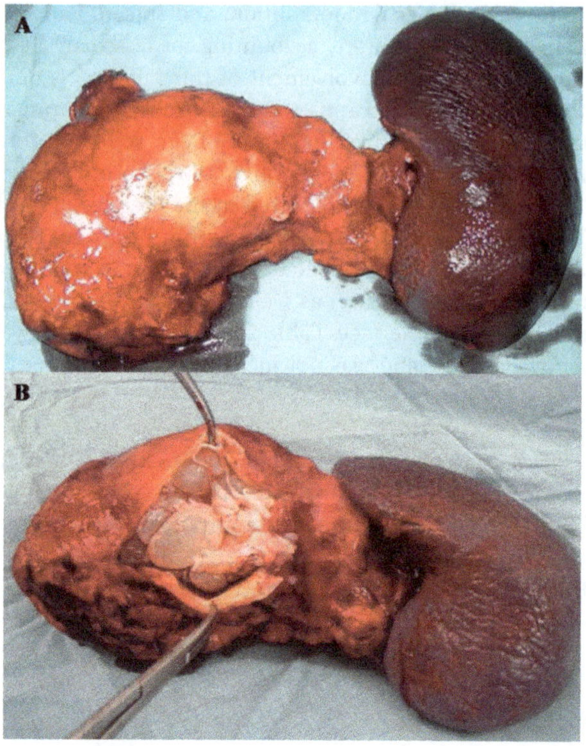

Figure 2 Specimen's photograph. A- A specimen of the left pancreatectomy with splenectomy, with a tumor in the corpus of the pancreas. **B-** At the opening of the cyst, we see its own wall and daughter cysts.

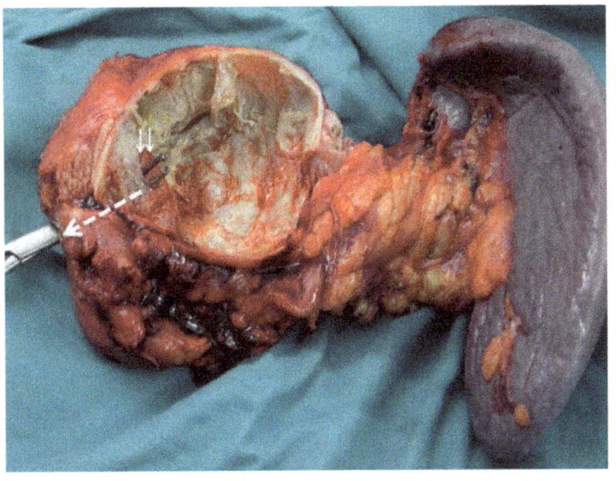

Figure 3 Specimen's photograph shows a fistula between the pancreatic hydatid cyst and the main pancreatic duct (two arrows). The dotted arrow indicates the direction of the migration of hydatid scolices from pancreatic hydatid cyst into the main pancreatic duct.

spread [1]. The location is solitary in the pancreas in 90% of cases. The cyst can be found in the head in 50-57%, in the body in 24-34% or in the tail in 16-19% [3]. Clinical presentation varies according to the anatomic location and potential complications of the cyst (e.g. infection, rupture, biliary or intestinal fistula, segmental portal hypertension, vascular thrombosis, acute or chronic pancreatitis) [3]. With respect to the pathogenesis of pancreatitis, such as liver cysts [12,13], pancreatic hydatid cysts may cause acute pancreatitis [4-11]. While parasite migration into the common bile duct is advocated as the etiological mechanism to explain acute pancreatitis caused by liver hydatidosis, it remains unclear why some patients affected by pancreatic cysts develop this complication. Accordingly, two hypotheses are posited: main pancreatic duct compression caused by the cyst itself [7] and main pancreatic duct obstruction by hydatid scolices' migration from the hydatid cyst [6,8,9]. To date, and to the best of our knowledge, only 8 cases of acute pancreatitis due to pancreatic hydatid cyst have been reported [4-11].

The mean age of the patients was 28 years, with a range of 18-38 years. The ratio of men to women was 3. The cyst was found in the body (n = 4), tail (n = 2) or head (n = 2). The location was solitarily in the pancreas (n = 7), and associated with a liver hydatid cyst (n = 1) [9]. No specific complaints or signs at physical examination are known to distinguish hydatid cyst from other etiology of acute pancreatitis. Therefore, the final diagnosis was made only after either ultrasonography or computed tomography.

Ultrasonography will typically demonstrate a multivesicular cyst, limited by a clean wall, containing daughter cysts and some peripheral calcifications [2]. Computed tomographic findings, such as rounded cystic lesions with curvilinear calcification may allow to make the diagnosis in the appropriate clinical setting [14]. Computed tomography will also identify the prognostic stage of acute pancreatitis, which allows first, to establish the monitoring protocol, and second, to specify the time of surgery. Moreover, the abdominal CT scan can also provide indirect evidence indicating the opening of the cyst in the main pancreatic duct: the dilation of Wirsung's canal and the detachment of the hydatid membrane, which was the case in our patient. Regarding the direct sign, only Diop et al. had reported direct visualization of the migration of hydatid material from a hydatid cyst of the pancreas into the main pancreatic duct, based on data from magnetic resonance imaging and endoscopic ultrasound [9]. The cyst diameter ranged from 30 to 100 mm. In our patient, the mass size was 100 mm (missing value = 1).

Surgical treatment of hydatid pancreatic cysts may be challenging. Furthermore, depending on the cyst's location, several procedures have been suggested, ranging from cyst fenestration, internal derivation, to central or distal pancreatectomy [5-7,15-17]. As the presence of a cystopancreatic fistula may cause a long-lasting pancreatic leak after fenestration [5,16], a derivative/resective procedure is preferred in such cases. When conservative treatment is performed within local conditions that do not allow an internal derivation (inflammation seen in connection with acute pancreatitis), a possible postoperative pancreatic fistula can be treated using endoscopic retrogradecholangiopancreatography (ERCP) and placing a pancreatic stent [10]. Bedioui et al. [16] suggested intraoperative cholangiopancreatography to identify a fistula between the cyst and the main pancreatic duct, leading thus to the most appropriate surgical treatment. This diagnosis could be given preoperatively through magnetic resonance imaging or endoscopic ultrasound, allowing for planning the correct surgical strategy [9,16]. In this review of literature, procedures that have been performed were as following: left pancreatectomy (n = 5) from which one was with splenic preservation, cyst fenestration (n = 2) and total cystectomy (n = 1). No recurrence was diagnosed after a mean of 13 month (missing value = 1).

Conclusion

Hydatid cyst of the pancreas is an extremely rare pathology but it may be a causal factor in acute pancreatitis, especially in endemic areas. Radiological examinations may help clinicians in diagnosing cystic masses in the pancreas. In the case of acute pancreatitis due to pancreatic hydatid cyst, there is definitely a closed relationship between the main pancreatic duct and the pancreatic cyst, imposing a derivative or a resective procedure.

Consent

Written informed consent was obtained from the patient for publication of this case report and accompanying images. A copy of the written consent is available for review by the Editor-in-Chief of this journal.

Authors' contributions

AM prepared the manuscript and performed the literature review. MJ formulated and assisted in the preparation of the manuscript. AM and MK conceived and performed the technique described in this manuscript. ZBS had given final approval of the version to be published. All authors have read and approved the final manuscript.

Competing interests

The authors declare that they have no competing interests.

References

1. Dziri C: **Hydatid disease–continuing serious public health problem: introduction.** *World J Surg* 2001, **25**:1-3.
2. Khiari A, Mzali R, Ouali M, Kharrat M, Kechaou MS, Beyrouti MI: **Hydatid cyst of the pancreas. A propos of 7 cases.** *Ann Gastroenterol Hepatol* 1994, **30**:87-91.
3. Hammad A, Mentouri B: **Acute pancreatitis in Algeria. Report of 221cases.** *Am J Surg* 1985, **149**:709-711.
4. Augustin N, Gamstätter G, Neher M, Schreyer T, Störkel S: **Echinococcus cysticus of the pancreas in the clinical picture of acute pancreatitis.** *Chirurg* 1984, **55**:661-664.
5. Papadimitriou J: **Pancreatic abscess due to infected hydatid disease.** *Surgery* 1987, **102**:880-882.
6. Sebbag H, Partensky C, Roche J, Ponchon T, Martins A: **Recurrent acute pancreatitis from the rupture of a solitary pancreatic hydatid cyst into Wirsung's canal.** *Gastroenterol Clin Biol* 1999, **23**:793-794.
7. Ozmen MM, Moran M, Karakahya M, Coskun F: **Recurrent acute pancreatitis due to a hydatid cyst of the pancreatic head: a case report and review of the literature.** *JOP* 2005, **6**:354-358, review.
8. Pouget Y, Mucci S, O'Toole D, Lermite E, Aubé C, Hamy A: **Recurrent acute pancreatitis revealing a hydatid cyst of the pancreas.** *Rev Med Interne* 2009, **30**:358-360.
9. Diop SP, Costi R, Le Bian A, Carloni A, Meduri B, Smadja C: **Acute pancreatitis associated with a pancreatic hydatid cyst: understanding the mechanism by EUS.** *Gastrointest Endosc* 2010, **72**:1312-1314.
10. Karakas E, Tuna Y, Basar O, Koklu S: **Primary pancreatic hydatid disease associated with acute pancreatitis.** *Hepatobiliary Pancreat Dis Int* 2010, **9**:441-442.
11. Chammakhi-Jemli C, Mekaouer S, Miaoui A, *et al*: **Hydatid cyst of the pancreas presenting with acute pancreatitis.** *J Radiol* 2010, **91**:797-799.
12. Van Steenbergen W, Fevery J, Broeckaert L, *et al*: **Hepatic echinococcosis ruptured into the biliary tract: clinical, radiological and therapeutic features during five episodes of spontaneous biliary rupture in three patients with hepatic hydatidosis.** *J Hepatol* 1987, **4**:133-139.
13. Sáez-Royuela F, Yuguero L, López-Morante A, *et al*: **Acute pancreatitis caused by hydatid membranes in the biliary tract: treatment with endoscopic sphincterotomy.** *Gastrointest Endosc* 1999, **49**:793-796.
14. Missas S, Gouliamos A, Kourias E, Kalovidouris A: **Primary hydatid disease of the pancreas.** *Gastrointest Radiol* 1987, **12**:37-38.
15. Bayat AM, Azhough R, Hashemzadeh S, *et al*: **Hydatid cyst of pancreas presented as a pancreatic pseudocyst.** *Am J Gastroenterol* 2009, **104**:1324-1326.
16. Bedioui H, Chebbi F, Ayadi S, *et al*: **Primary hydatid cyst of the pancreas: Diagnosis and surgical procedures. Report of three cases.** *Gastroenterol Clin Biol* 2008, **32**:102-106.
17. Moosavi SR, Kermany HK: **Epigastric mass due to a hydatid cyst of the pancreas. A case report and review of the literature.** *JOP* 2007, **8**:232-234.

4

Delayed appendectomy versus early appendectomy in the treatment of acute appendicitis

Chang Sik Shin, Young Nam Roh and Jae Il Kim*

Abstract

Background: The controversy still exists about the timing of operation for appendicitis. The aim of this study was to compare the outcomes between early appendectomy and delayed appendectomy and assess the feasibility of delayed operation.

Methods: The medical records of patients with acute appendicitis who received operation between January 1, 2011 and December 31, 2011, were retrospectively reviewed. Outcome measures were white blood cell (WBC) count at postoperative first day, time to soft diet, complication rate, surgical site infection (SSI) rate, length of hospital stay, and readmission within 30 days.

Results: During the study period, a total of 478 patients underwent appendectomies, and 145 patients were excluded, leaving 333 who met inclusion criteria. Based on the time from arrival at hospital to incision, they were divided into two groups: 177 (53.2%) in group A and 156 (46.8%) in group B. There were no significant differences in preoperative demographics and clinical data between two groups. The mean WBC count at postoperative first day of group B were lower than that of group A ($p = 0.0039$). There were no significant differences in time to soft diet, length of postoperative hospital stay, complication rate, and readmission rate between two groups. SSI including intra-abdominal abscess was also shown no significant difference (Group A, 1.7% and Group B, 3.9%; $p = 0.3143$).

Conclusions: This study revealed that delayed appendectomy was safe and feasible for adult patient although the clinical outcomes of delayed appendectomy were not superior to those of early appendectomy. We suggest that surgeons would decide the appropriate timing of appendectomy with consideration other situations such as available hospital resources.

Keywords: Appendicitis, Early appendectomy, Delayed appendectomy

Introduction

Acute appendicitis has been the most common intra-abdominal condition requiring operation. Emergency appendectomy at the time of diagnosis was the standard of care for treatment of acute appendicitis during last century. Any delay in operation has been believed to increase postoperative morbidity or progress to complicated appendicitis such as perforated appendicitis or periappendiceal abscess [1,2].

However, the concept of emergency appendectomy has been recently challenged by studies which suggested that acute appendicitis could be treated medically, or delaying surgery did not show any increasing morbidity [3-7]. On the other hand, there are other studies which supported that appendicitis needed emergency surgical procedure and delay in surgery increased complication and length of hospital stay [8-10].

The controversy still exists about the timing of operation for appendicitis. The aim of this study was to compare the outcomes between early appendectomy and delayed appendectomy and assess the feasibility of delayed operation.

* Correspondence: erythrokim@paik.ac.kr
Department of Surgery, Ilsan Paik Hospital, Inje University College of Medicine, 170 Juhwaro, Ilsanseogu, Goyangsi, Gyeonggido, Republic of Korea

Materials and methods

Patients

This study was designed as a retrospective, observational study at a single institution. The medical records of patients with acute appendicitis who received operation between January 1, 2011 and December 31, 2011, were retrospectively reviewed. We excluded the following patients: (1) those who were under 16 years or over 65 years old, (2) those who underwent other surgical procedures along with appendectomy, such as cholecystectomy or oophorectomy, (3) pregnant women, and those with severe other medical disease requiring intensive care, (4) those who underwent incidental, interval, and negative appendectomies. The patients were then divided into two groups for comparison: Group A, those with a time from arrival to incision less than 8 hours and Group B, those with a time from arrival to incision longer than 8 hours.

Data collection

The data were collected from the electronic medical records (EMR). The following parameters were included: demographics, duration from onset of symptoms to visit our hospital, time from arrival to diagnosis as appendicitis, time form diagnosis to operation, initial vital signs, initial laboratory findings, method of appendectomy, combined drainage procedures, pathologic findings, postoperative laboratory findings, time to a soft diet, postoperative complications, length of hospital stay, hospital costs, and readmissions within 30 days of surgery. We analyzed preoperative, operative, and postoperative clinical data obtained from each group. Hospital costs consisted of the total costs covered by National Health Insurance (NHI) and charges for non-covered items—non-covered bed charges or materials. The data on the following items were analyzed: the total hospital costs, the total costs covered by NHI and copayment by patients.

Outcome measures

Outcome measures were white blood cell (WBC) count at postoperative first day, time to soft diet, complication rate, surgical site infection (SSI), length of hospital stay, and readmission within 30 days.

Statistical analysis

The data were analyzed using SAS enterprise ver. 5.1 statistical software (SAS Inc, Cary, NC, USA). Demographics and clinical characteristics were expressed as means for continuous variables or proportions for categorical variables. The chi-square test was used to compare differences in categorical variables. Student's t test or the Wilcoxon rank sum test was used to compare differences in continuous variables. The p value of less than 0.05 was considered statistically significant.

Results

During the study period, a total of 478 patients underwent appendectomies, and 145 patients were excluded, leaving 333 who met inclusion criteria. Demographics and clinical characteristics of included cases are shown in Table 1. The mean age of patients was 35.4 years. There were 190 males (57.1%) and 143 females (42.9%). The average time from arrival at our hospital to diagnosis was 3.0 hours. The average time from diagnosis as appendicitis to skin incision was 6.6 hours. The average time form arrival to incision was 9.6 hours. Based on the time from arrival at our hospital to incision, they were divided into two groups: 177 (53.2%) in group A and 156 (46.8%) in group B.

Comparisons of demographics and preoperative characteristics between two groups are shown in Table 2. There were significant differences in time parameter due to study design. There were no significant differences in age, sex ratio, body mass index (BMI), body temperature, initial WBC count, and comorbidities between two groups. Comparisons of operative characteristics between two groups are shown in Table 3. There were no significant differences in the ratio of laparoscopic appendectomy, operating time, the ratio of complicated appendicitis, and the ratio of accompanying external drainage procedure, and the ratio of accompanied by appendicoliths. There were significant differences between two groups in the

Table 1 Demographics and clinical characteristics

Total number of cases	333
Age (years)	35.4 ± 12.4
Male: Female	190 (57.1%): 143 (42.9%)
Body mass index (kg/m^2)	23.0 ± 3.3
Initial body temperature (°C)	37.4 ± 0.7
Initial white blood cell (WBC) count (×10^3/mm^3)	12.9 ± 3.9
Comorbidities	32 (9.6%)
Hours from onset of symptoms to hospital	24.3 ± 29.9
Hours from arrival to diagnosis	3.0 ± 2.0
Hours from diagnosis to incision	6.6 ± 4.7
Hours from arrival to incision	9.6 ± 5.0
Method of appendectomy (OA: LA)	248 (74.5%): 85 (25.5%)
Operation at night (22:00–06:00), case (%)	47 (14.1%)
Complicated appendicitis, case (%)	68 (20.4%)
Appendicoliths, case (%)	128 (38.4%)
Combined drainage, case (%)	63 (19.0%)
WBC, postoperative first day (×10^3/mm^3)	10.0 ± 3.3
Time to soft diet (day)	1.8 ± 1.0
Postoperative hospital stay (day)	4.6 ± 2.7
Complication, case (%)	11 (3.3%)
Readmission within 30 days, case (%)	2 (0.6%)

Table 2 Comparisons of demographics and preoperative characteristics between two groups

	Group A (≤ 8 hours)	Group B (> 8 hours)	*P* value
Number of cases	177 (53.2%)	156 (46.8%)	
Age (yrs)	35.9 ± 125	34.7 ± 12.1	0.3758
Sex ratio (Male: Female)	103:74	87:69	0.6592
Body mass index (kg/m^2)	23.1 ± 3.4	22.7 ± 3.1	0.2822
Body temperature (°C)	37.4 ± 0.7	37.4 ± 0.6	0.7701
Initial white blood cell count (×10^3/mm^3)	12.6 ± 3.8	13.3 ± 4.0	0.1150
Comorbidities	21 (11.9%)	11 (7.0%)	0.1915
Hours from onset of symptoms to hospital	26.4 ± 22.5	22.0 ± 16.7	0.1835
Hours from arrival to diagnosis	2.4 ± 1.1	3.6 ± 2.6	<0.0001
Hours from diagnosis to operation	3.4 ± 1.4	10.4 ± 4.3	<0.0001
Hours from arrival to operation	5.8 ± 1.5	13.9 ± 4.0	<0.0001

ratio of operation at night (Group A, 22.0% and Group B, 5.1%; $p < 0.0001$), and in the ratio of accompanying external drainage procedure (Group A, 24.9% and Group B, 12.2%; $p = 0.0033$).

Comparisons of postoperative outcomes between two groups are shown in Table 4. The mean WBC count at postoperative first day of group B were lower than that of group A (p = 0.0039). There were no significant differences in time to soft diet, length of postoperative hospital stay, complication rate, and readmission rate between two groups. Although surgical site infection (SSI) rate including intra-abdominal abscess (IA) of group B was slightly higher than that of group A, there was also no significant statistical difference (Group A, 1.7% and Group B, 3.9%; $p = 0.3143$). Table 5 shows results of hospital costs between two groups and there were no significant differences in all comparative variables.

Discussion

In Korea, the imaging modalities are so popular, and the payments are covered by national health insurance system.

Table 3 Comparisons of operative characteristics between two groups

	Group A (≤ 8 hours)	Group B (> 8 hours)	*P* value
Laparoscopic appendectomy, case (%)	42 (23.7%)	43 (27.6%)	0.4513
Operation at night (22:00–06:00), case (%)	39 (22.0%)	8 (5.1%)	<0.0001
Operating time (minute)	56.3 ± 21.8	53.5 ± 19.4	0.2236
Complicated appendicitis, case (%)	40 (22.6%)	28 (18.0%)	0.3408
Appendicoliths, case (%)	73 (41.2%)	55 (35.3%)	0.3097
Combined drainage, case (%)	44 (24.9%)	19 (12.2%)	0.0033

Table 4 Comparisons of postoperative outcomes between two groups

	Group A (≤ 8 hours)	Group B (> 8 hours)	*P* value
WBC, postoperative first day (×10^3/mm^3)	10.5 ± 3.2	9.5 ± 3.3	0.0039
Time to soft diet (day)	1.9 ± 1.1	1.7 ± 0.8	0.0806
Postoperative hospital stay (day)	4.9 ± 2.8	4.4 ± 2.7	0.0719
Complication, case (%)	3 (1.7%)	8 (5.1%)	0.1225
Surgical site infection, case (%)	3 (1.7%)	6 (3.9%)	0.3143
Readmission within 30 days, case (%)	1 (0.6%)	1 (0.6%)	1.0000

Radiologic evaluation could help surgeons to confirm the diagnosis and to recognize the location of appendix, and/or other intra-abdominal conditions requiring other procedures. All patients in this study received radiologic evaluation such as abdominal computed tomography (CT), abdominal ultrasonography and they were diagnosed with acute appendicitis.

Appendectomy has still been the most common non-elective surgical procedure performed by general surgeons [11,12]. It was usually prepared at the time of diagnosis as appendicitis and done within hours to prevent the progression of inflammation. However, the quality of antibiotics was improved in the last few decades and interval appendectomy for periappendiceal abscess was shown better outcomes than early operation. Recent studies suggested that periappendiceal abscess in selected cases could be managed by nonsurgical treatment without interval appendectomy [13,14]. Furthermore, successful results of nonsurgical antibiotics treatment for selected cases with uncomplicated appendicitis were reported in recent literatures [6,15,16]. However, at the present, we do not agree that appendicitis is medical disease.

Controversies regarding the timing of operation in patients needed operation still exist. Some studies still supported that the outcomes of immediate or prompt appendectomy were better than those of delayed appendectomy [8-10,17,18]. They advocated that delayed appendectomy produced more postoperative complication

Table 5 Comparisons of hospital costs between two groups

	Group A (≤ 8hours)	Group B (> 8 hours)	*P* value
Total hospital costs	2,682,450 ± 733,183	2,618,006 ± 727,865	0.4225
Total costs covered by NHI	1,477,012 ± 378,827	1,449,149 ± 408,321	0.5189
Copayment by a patient	479,003 ± 115,575	461,984 ± 149,649	0.2511

Values are presented as KRW (Korean won, Korean monetary unit).
1 USD = 1,108 KRW.
NHI, National Health Insurance.

such as surgical site infection. On the other hand, some studies suggested that there was no significant difference of outcomes between early and delayed appendectomy [7,19,20]. In addition, several studies showed negative impact of prolonged working hours for residents or sleep deprivation on clinical performance and cognitive abilities [21,22].

The timing of surgery was actually affected by other factors such as limited operating room availability, limited anesthesia availability, limited equipment availability, as well as decision of a surgeon like results in survey of pediatric surgeons [23]. In our hospital, all of eight surgeons preferred early appendectomy and they performed appendectomy within a few hours after diagnosis except midnight, if possible. However, number of surgical residents was reduced and diseases to need operation were increased during last decade. Therefore waiting time to appendectomy has been naturally lengthened although early appendectomy was planned.

In our study, there were no significant differences in demographics, preoperative clinical characteristics between early appendectomy and delayed appendectomy groups. It means that disease severity such as fever, WBC count either uncomplicated or complicated appendicitis did not affect the timing of surgery. In addition, there was no significant difference in the ratio of accompanied by appendicoliths between two groups. In our study, the presence of appendicoliths did not affect the timing of surgery unlike with results of recent studies [24,25].

There were no significant differences in time to soft diet and length of postoperative hospital stay between two groups. There were also no significant differences in all parameters regarding hospital costs between two groups. Especially, there was no significant difference in complication rate including surgical site infection. One patient in group A and one patient in group B readmitted due to postoperative intra-abdominal abscess within 30 days. These results were similar with previous other studies [7,19,20]. Therefore delayed appendectomy is safe similar with early appendectomy.

Moreover, mean WBC count at postoperative first day of group B was lower than that of group A. These results might be due to sufficient and effective preoperative intravenous (IV) antibiotics injection to cover aerobic and anaerobic colonic flora [26]. In our hospital, when a patient was diagnosed as uncomplicated appendicitis by clinical and radiologic evaluation, IV cephalosporin (first or second generation) was given to the patient. If a patient was diagnosed as complicated appendicitis, IV metronidazole was added. As a result, patients in group A received single dose preoperative antibiotics and patients in group B received those twice or three times.

There are several limitations of this study. Firstly, this study was retrospective observational study. As above mentioned, several situations such as lack of resident, tight operation schedule made prospective study difficult. Secondly, optimal timing of appendectomy could not be elucidated. We expect to solve these limitations through the large prospective randomized trial in the near future.

Conclusions

We still consider that appendicitis is not a medical disease but a surgical disease. This study revealed that delayed appendectomy was safe and feasible for adult patients with appendicitis although the clinical outcomes of delayed appendectomy were not superior to those of early appendectomy. Therefore, we suggest that surgeons would decide the appropriate timing of appendectomy with consideration other situations such as available hospital resources.

Competing interests
This work was supported by the 2012 Inje University research grant. We declare that we have no competing interests.

Authors' contributions
CSS, YNR, and JIK carried out study design, acquisition and analysis of data, and drafted the manuscript. JIK carried out the statistical analysis. YNR and JIK revised the manuscript. All authors read and approved the final manuscript.

References

1. Temple CL, Huchcroft SA, Temple WJ: **The natural history of appendicitis in adults. A prospective study.** *Ann Surg* 1995, **221**(3):278–281.
2. Eldar S, Nash E, Sabo E, Matter I, Kunin J, Mogilner JG, Abrahamson J: **Delay of surgery in acute appendicitis.** *Am J Surg* 1997, **173**(3):194–198.
3. Hansson J, Korner U, Khorram-Manesh A, Solberg A, Lundholm K: **Randomized clinical trial of antibiotic therapy versus appendicectomy as primary treatment of acute appendicitis in unselected patients.** *Br J Surg* 2009, **96**(5):473–481.
4. Styrud J, Eriksson S, Nilsson I, Ahlberg G, Haapaniemi S, Neovius G, Rex L, Badume I, Granstrom L: **Appendectomy versus antibiotic treatment in acute appendicitis. a prospective multicenter randomized controlled trial.** *World J Surg* 2006, **30**(6):1033–1037.
5. Varadhan KK, Humes DJ, Neal KR, Lobo DN: **Antibiotic therapy versus appendectomy for acute appendicitis: a meta-analysis.** *World J Surg* 2010, **34**(2):199–209.
6. Liu K, Fogg L: **Use of antibiotics alone for treatment of uncomplicated acute appendicitis: a systematic review and meta-analysis.** *Surgery* 2011, **150**(4):673–683.
7. Nagpal K, Udgiri N, Sharma N, Curras E, Cosgrove JM, Farkas DT: **Delaying an appendectomy: is it safe?** *Am Surg* 2012, **78**(8):897–900.
8. Udgiri N, Curras E, Kella VK, Nagpal K, Cosgrove J: **Appendicitis, is it an emergency?** *Am Surg* 2011, **77**(7):898–901.
9. Ditillo MF, Dziura JD, Rabinovici R: **Is it safe to delay appendectomy in adults with acute appendicitis?** *Ann Surg* 2006, **244**(5):656–660.
10. Earley AS, Pryor JP, Kim PK, Hedrick JH, Kurichi JE, Minogue AC, Sonnad SS, Reilly PM, Schwab CW: **An acute care surgery model improves outcomes in patients with appendicitis.** *Ann Surg* 2006, **244**(4):498–504.
11. Pittman-Waller VA, Myers JG, Stewart RM, Dent DL, Page CP, Gray GA, Pruitt BA Jr, Root HD: **Appendicitis: why so complicated? Analysis of 5755 consecutive appendectomies.** *Am Surg* 2000, **66**(6):548–554.
12. Lee HJ, Park YH, Kim JI, Choi PW, Park JH, Heo TG, Lee MS, Kim CN, Chang SH: **Comparison of clinical outcomes and hospital cost between open appendectomy and laparoscopic appendectomy.** *J Korean Surg Soc* 2011, **81**(5):321–325.

13. Andersson RE, Petzold MG: **Nonsurgical treatment of appendiceal abscess or phlegmon: a systematic review and meta-analysis.** *Ann Surg* 2007, **246**(5):741–748.
14. Lugo JZ, Avgerinos DV, Lefkowitz AJ, Seigerman ME, Zahir IS, Lo AY, Surick B, Leitman IM: **Can interval appendectomy be justified following conservative treatment of perforated acute appendicitis?** *J Surg Res* 2010, **164**(1):91–94.
15. Vons C, Barry C, Maitre S, Pautrat K, Leconte M, Costaglioli B, Karoui M, Alves A, Dousset B, Valleur P, *et al*: **Amoxicillin plus clavulanic acid versus appendicectomy for treatment of acute uncomplicated appendicitis: an open-label, non-inferiority, randomised controlled trial.** *Lancet* 2011, **377**(9777):1573–1579.
16. Sakorafas GH, Mastoraki A, Lappas C, Sampanis D, Danias N, Smyrniotis V: **Conservative treatment of acute appendicitis: heresy or an effective and acceptable alternative to surgery?** *Eur J Gastroenterol Hepatol* 2011, **23**(2):121–127.
17. Teixeira PG, Sivrikoz E, Inaba K, Talving P, Lam L, Demetriades D: **Appendectomy timing: waiting until the next morning increases the risk of surgical site infections.** *Ann Surg* 2012, **256**(3):538–543.
18. Giraudo G, Baracchi F, Pellegrino L, Dal Corso HM, Borghi F: **Prompt or delayed appendectomy? Influence of timing of surgery for acute appendicitis.** *Surg today* 2013, **43**(4):392–396.
19. Yardeni D, Hirschl RB, Drongowski RA, Teitelbaum DH, Geiger JD, Coran AG: **Delayed versus immediate surgery in acute appendicitis: do we need to operate during the night?** *J Pediatr Surg* 2004, **39**(3):464–469. discussion 464–469.
20. Stahlfeld K, Hower J, Homitsky S, Madden J: **Is acute appendicitis a surgical emergency?** *Am Surg* 2007, **73**(6):626–629. discussion 629–630.
21. Eastridge BJ, Hamilton EC, O'Keefe GE, Rege RV, Valentine RJ, Jones DJ, Tesfay S, Thal ER: **Effect of sleep deprivation on the performance of simulated laparoscopic surgical skill.** *Am J Surg* 2003, **186**(2):169–174.
22. Kahol K, Leyba MJ, Deka M, Deka V, Mayes S, Smith M, Ferrara JJ, Panchanathan S: **Effect of fatigue on psychomotor and cognitive skills.** *Am J Surg* 2008, **195**(2):195–204.
23. Dunlop JC, Meltzer JA, Silver EJ, Crain EF: **Is nonperforated pediatric appendicitis still considered a surgical emergency? A survey of pediatric surgeons.** *Acad Pediatr* 2012, **12**(6):567–571.
24. Ishiyama M, Yanase F, Taketa T, Makidono A, Suzuki K, Omata F, Saida Y: **Significance of size and location of appendicoliths as exacerbating factor of acute appendicitis.** *Emerg Radiol* 2013, **20**(2):125–130.
25. Lien WC, Wang HP, Liu KL, Chen CJ: **Appendicolith delays resolution of appendicitis following nonoperative management.** *J Gastrointest Surg* 2012, **16**(12):2274–2279.
26. Maa J, Kirkwood KS: **The Appendix.** In *Sabiston Textbook of Surgery: The Biological Basis of Modern Surgical Practice.* 19th edition. Edited by Sabiston DC, Townsend CM. Philadelphia, PA: Elsevier Saunders; 2012:1279–1293.

Current concept of abdominal sepsis: WSES position paper

Massimo Sartelli[1*], Fausto Catena[2], Salomone Di Saverio[3], Luca Ansaloni[4], Mark Malangoni[5], Ernest E Moore[6], Frederick A Moore[7], Rao Ivatury[8], Raul Coimbra[9], Ari Leppaniemi[10], Walter Biffl[6], Yoram Kluger[11], Gustavo P Fraga[12], Carlos A Ordonez[13], Sanjay Marwah[14], Igor Gerych[15], Jae Gil Lee[16], Cristian Tranà[1], Federico Coccolini[4], Francesco Corradetti[17] and James Kirkby-Bott[18]

Abstract

Although sepsis is a systemic process, the pathophysiological cascade of events may vary from region to region. Abdominal sepsis represents the host's systemic inflammatory response to bacterial peritonitis.
It is associated with significant morbidity and mortality rates, and is the second most common cause of sepsis-related mortality in the intensive care unit.
The review focuses on sepsis in the specific setting of severe peritonitis.

Introduction

Abdominal sepsis is associated with significant morbidity and mortality rates.

Results of prospective trials have often overestimated the outcomes of patients with severe peritonitis [1]. Treatment of patients who have complicated intra-abdominal infections (IAIs) by adequate management, has generally been described to produce satisfactory results; recent clinical trials have demonstrated an overall mortality of 2% to 3% among patients with complicated IAIs [1,2].

However, results from published clinical trials may not be representative of the true morbidity and mortality rates of such infections. Patients who have perforated appendicitis are usually over represented in clinical trials [1]. Furthermore patients with intra-abdominal infection enrolled in clinical trials have often an increased likelihood of cure and survival. In fact trial eligibility criteria often restrict the inclusion of patients with co-morbid diseases that would increase the death rate of patients with intra-abdominal infections.

After excluding patients with perforated appendicitis, Merlino et al. [3] found that the cure rate among patients who had intra-abdominal infections and were enrolled in clinical trials, was much higher than that of patients who were not enrolled (79% versus 41%) and that the mortality rate was much lower (10% versus 33%).

Epidemiological studies of patients with intra-abdominal infections including severely ill subjects, have demonstrated higher mortality rates [4].

In the CIAO study the overall mortality rate was 7.7% (166/2152) [5]. Analyzing the subgroup of patients with severe sepsis or septic shock at admission to hospital the mortality rate reached 32.4% (89/274). In patients with severe sepsis or septic shock in the immediate post-operative period, the mortality rate was 42.3% (110/266).

Abdominal sepsis represents the host's systemic inflammatory response to bacterial or yeast peritonitis.

In the event of peritonitis gram-negative, gram-positive, as well as anaerobic bacteria, including common gut flora, such as *Escherichia coli, Klebsiella pneumoniae, Streptococcus spp.* and *Bacteroides fragilis*, enter the peritoneal cavity. Sepsis from an abdominal origin is initiated by the outer membrane component of gram-negative organisms (e.g., lipopolysaccharide [LPS], lipid A, endotoxin) or gram-positive organisms (e.g., lipoteichoic acid, peptidoglycan), as well anaerobe toxins. This lead to the release of proinflammatory cytokines such as tumor necrosis factor α (TNF-α), and interleukins 1 and 6 (IL-1, IL-6). TNF-α and interleukins lead to the production of toxic mediators, including prostaglandins, leukotrienes, platelet-activating factor, and phospholipase A2, that damage the endothelial lining, leading to increased capillary leakage [6]. Cytokines

* Correspondence: massimosartelli@gmail.com
[1]Department of Surgery, Macerata Hospital, Macerata, Italy
Full list of author information is available at the end of the article

lead to the production of adhesion molecules on endothelial cells and neutrophils. Neutrophil-endothelial cell interaction leads to further endothelial injury through the release of neutrophil components. Activated neutrophils release nitric oxide, a potent vasodilator that leads to septic shock. Cytokines also disrupt natural modulators of coagulation and inflammation, activated protein C (APC) and antithrombin. As a result, multiple organ failure may occur.

Early detection and timely therapeutic intervention can improve the prognosis and overall clinical outcome of septic patients. However, early diagnosis of sepsis can be difficult; determining which patients presenting with signs of infection during an initial evaluation, do currently have, or will later develop a more serious illness is not an easy or straightforward task.

Sepsis is a complex, multifactorial syndrome which can evolve into conditions of varying severity. If left untreated, it may lead to the functional impairment of one or more vital organs or systems [7].

Severity of illness and the inherent mortality risk escalate from sepsis, through severe sepsis and septic shock up multi-organ failure.

Previous studies have demonstrated that mortality rates increase dramatically in the event of severe sepsis and septic shock [8]. Severe sepsis may be a reasonable approximation of the "tipping point" between stable and critical clinical conditions in the management of intra-abdominal infections. Severe sepsis is defined as sepsis associated with at least one acute organ dysfunction, hypoperfusion, or hypotension.

It is well known that hypotension is associated with an increased risk of sudden and unexpected death in patients admitted to hospital with non traumatic diseases [9]; identifying patients with severe sepsis early and correcting the underlying microvascular dysfunction may improve patient outcomes. If not corrected, microvascular dysfunction can lead to global tissue hypoxia, direct tissue damage, and ultimately, organ failure [10].

The Surviving Sepsis Campaign international guidelines for management of severe sepsis and septic shock were recently updated [11]. These guidelines are the cornerstone for the management of severe sepsis and septic shock, but they do not focus on the specific setting of intra-abdominal infections.

Although sepsis is a systemic process, the pathophysiological cascade may vary from organ to organ.

There are few data regarding systemic and local responses during peritonitis in humans and on their correlation to patients outcomes [12-14].

Based on findings of high concentrations of cytokines in the peritoneal compartment, some evidences suggested that intra-abdominal sepsis may result in a cytokine-mediated inflammatory response that is initially compartmentalized in the peritoneal cavity [15,16].

Animal models have shown that peritonitis is associated with a significant and prolonged peritoneal inflammatory response which is adversely correlated with survival outcome [17].

The levels of selected peritoneal cytokines have been reported to be significantly different between animals that survived as compared to those who died following a septic challenge [18].

Plausibility of peritoneal compartmentalization of initial inflammatory response during peritonitis was highlighted by a recent prospective cohort study of patients with secondary generalized peritonitis [19]. It confirmed that IL-1, TNFα, IL-6, IL-10 and IFNγ are present at high concentrations in the peritoneal fluid of patients with peritonitis. The results of this study showed a large gradient between peritoneal fluid and plasma concentrations of cytokines, with no correlation between peritoneal and plasma levels, suggesting that plasma levels may increase only after saturation of tissues within the abdominal compartment.

The inflammatory response in patients with sepsis depends on the causative pathogen and the host (genetic characteristics and coexisting illnesses), with differential responses at local, regional, and systemic levels [20].

The host inflammatory response probably changes over time in parallel with the clinical course. Sepsis, in the early stages of the inflammatory process, should be considered as a local/peritoneal disease. In advanced stages, severe sepsis and septic shock should be considered as a systemic disease, and patients who are extremely unstable and exhibit high rates of mortality should be managed more aggressively.

In certain patients peritonitis can quickly lead to an excessive inflammatory response, and early and aggressive mechanical peritoneal control is determinant for stopping the septic process. In those patients inability to control or interrupt the local inflammatory response is associated with poor outcomes.

In patients with ongoing sepsis, several laparotomies may be required. Under these circumstances, open abdomen allows the surgeon to perform subsequent laparotomies more efficiently and prevent the onset of abdominal compartment syndrome that may further worsen the systemic disease.

The review focuses on management of patients with severe sepsis or septic shock in the specific setting of severe peritonitis.

Diagnosis

Reducing time to diagnosis of severe sepsis is thought to be a critical component in reducing mortality from sepsis-related multiple organ dysfunction [11]. Delineating the source of infection as accurately as possible prior to surgery is the primary aim and the first step in managing intra-abdominal infections. In severe abdominal sepsis however, delays in operative management may lead to worse outcomes and early exploration is always recommended when peritonitis is suspected even if the source of infection is not recognized pre-operatively with certainty.

The diagnosis of intra-abdominal sepsis is based primarily on clinical assessment. Typically, the patient is admitted to the emergency department with abdominal pain and a systemic inflammatory response, including fever, tachycardia, and tachypnoea. Abdominal rigidity suggests the presence of peritonitis. However, clinical assessment alone is not always reliable in critically ill patients due to a variety of clinical constraints (e.g., impaired consciousness, severe underlying disease, etc.). Hypotension, oliguria, and acute altered mental status are waring signs of the patient's transition from sepsis to severe sepsis.

Plain abdominal films are often the first imaging obtained for patients presenting with peritonitis. Upright films are useful for identifying free air under the diaphragm (most often on the right side), which can result from perforated viscera. Free air may be present in most cases of anterior gastric and duodenal perforation. However it is much less frequent with perforations of the small bowel and colon and is unusual with appendiceal perforation. Abdominal plain films have low sensitivity and specificity, and have, in most cases, been replaced by abdominal computed tomography (CT). However, plain films of the abdomen remain a reasonable initial study for patients with suspected peritonitis who, on the basis of history and physical examination, are likely candidates for surgical exploration. In this case, abdominal plain films may confirm evidence of perforation in short time.

Ultrasonography and computed tomography have become essential diagnostic tools in abdominal sepsis. The diagnostic approach to confirm the source of abdominal infection in septic patients depends largely on the haemodynamic stability of the patient [21].

Critically ill patients who are haemodynamically unstable or have developed severe acute respiratory distress syndrome (ARDS) requiring high-level ventilatory support, are at significant risk during transport to the radiology department In unstable patients who do not undergo an immediate laparotomy and whose critical condition prevents them from leaving ICU for further imaging, ultrasound (US) is the best available imaging modality [22]. It is portable, it can be performed at the bed side, it is reproducible and can be easily repeated. Major drawbacks are ileus and obesity, which may significantly mask the US view. US is also strongly operator-dependent. In suspected biliary sepsis US is always the preferred initial diagnostic modality for acute cholecystitis and emphysematous cholecystitis.

In stable patients, abdominal computerized tomography (CT) is the imaging modality of choice, especially when the diagnosis is uncertain. However, in patients with severe sepsis, if the diagnosis of peritonitis is made clinically or by previous radiological examinations (plain films of the abdomen or US), additional CT scanning may be unnecessary and would only delay much-needed surgical intervention [22].

Another option in the diagnosis of critically ill patients suffering from intra-abdominal sepsis is bedside laparoscopy, as it can avoid patient transport to the radiological department or operating room is very accurate, and maintains ICU monitoring [23]. Laparoscopy provides a "minimally invasive" definitive modality to diagnose intra-abdominal sepsis. It may quickly provide the necessary information to address further management. However, the overall mortality of patients undergoing diagnostic laparoscopy in the ICU is high, regardless of diagnostic findings during this procedure. The use of diagnostic laparoscopy should be limited to patients in whom a therapeutic intervention is strongly suspected [24].

Antimicrobial therapy

A key component of the first-line management of the septic patient is the administration of IV antimicrobial therapy. Antimicrobial therapy plays a pivotal role in the management of intra-abdominal infections, especially in patients with severe sepsis who require immediate empiric antibiotic therapy.

An insufficient or otherwise inadequate antimicrobial regimen is one of the variables more strongly associated with unfavorable outcomes in critical ill patients [25]. Empiric antimicrobial therapy should be started as soon as possible in patients with severe sepsis with or without septic shock [26-28].

A prospective observational study by Riché et al. involving 180 patients with secondary generalized peritonitis, reported significantly higher mortality rates in patients presenting with septic shock (35%) compared to those presenting without it (8%) [29].

The role of the infecting pathogen on the patients response in secondary peritonitis has been poorly investigated.

Some authors support the concept of a 'generic septic response' in which an identical immune response is triggered by any type of bacteria [30,31].

Contrastingly, others suggest that different types of pathogens may elicit various inflammatory responses, despite a common pathway of activation.

Riche et al. have found that polymicrobial cultures or anaerobes in the peritoneal fluid were associated with more frequent septic shock [29].

A recent prospective cohort study showed that patients in whom anaerobes or *Enterococcus* species [19] were isolated from peritoneal fluid cultures released more TNFα in their plasma than those who were infected with other strains. The hypothesis that different types of pathogens may elicit various inflammatory responses, was already highlighted in animal models. In rats with peritonitis, Montravers *et al.* showed that adjunction of *Enterococcus faecalis* was associated with increased mortality as well as higher levels of TNFα and IL-6 in peritoneal fluid [32,33].

Evidence regarding a specific role of some pathogens on the pattern of the sepsis response is rather small, preventing any definitive conclusion from these results.

However it is well known that patients with severe sepsis or septic shock may benefit from aggressive antimicrobial treatment in order to curb the spread of the multiple organ dysfunction syndrome caused by an ongoing peritoneal trigger.

For these patients, a de-escalated approach may be the most appropriate strategy. Increasing rates of resistance and a more comprehensive understanding of the sepsis process have prompted many experts to advocate the use of broad-spectrum antimicrobial regimens in the initial stages of treatment for sepsis [34,35]. Subsequent modification (de-escalation) of the initial regimen becomes possible later, when culture results are available and clinical status can be better assessed, 48–72 hours after initiation of empiric therapy.

When treating abdominal sepsis, clinicians must be aware that drug pharmacokinetics may differ significantly between patients due to the variable pathophysiology of sepsis, and must also take into account the pathophysiological and immunological status of the patient [36].

The "dilution effect", also called the 'third spacing' phenomenon, must be considered when administering hydrophilic agents such as β-lactams, aminoglycosides, and glycopeptides, which selectively distribute to the extracellular space. Low plasma antimicrobial levels can contribute to lower than expected antimicrobial concentrations in peritoneal fluid with potentially reduced antimicrobial delivery to the target tissues. In fact, the target plasma concentration (Ct) that should be achieved with the loading dose (LD) depends solely on the volume of distribution (Vd) of the drug (LD = Ct × Vd). If the Vd is enlarged the Ct will results in a lower than expected level with the standard LD [36].

Higher than standard loading doses of β-lactams, aminoglycosides, or glycopeptides should be administered to ensure optimal drug exposure to the infection site in patients with severe sepsis or septic shock [36].

Lastly it should be kept in mind that the loading dose of lipophilic antibiotics (Macrolides, Fluoroquinolones, Tetracyclines, Chloramphenicol, Rifampicin, Linezolid) which are not influenced by the "diluition effect", should not be influenced by the severe sepsis or septic shock status [36].

Once appropriate initial loading is achieved, it is mandatory to reassess the antimicrobial regimen daily, because the pathophysiological changes that may occur, may significantly affect drug disposition in the critically ill patients. Lower than standard dosages of renally excreted drugs must be administered in the presence of impaired renal function, while higher than standard dosages of renally excreted drugs may be needed for optimal exposure in patients with glomerular hyperfiltration [36].

In Table 1 recommended dosing regimens of the most frequently used renally excreted antimicrobials according to renal function are illustrated.

Table 1 Recommended dosing regimens of the most frequently used renally excreted antimicrobials according to renal function [21]

	Renal function			
Antibiotic	**Increased**	**Normal**	**Moderately impaired**	**Severely impaired**
Piperacillin/ tazobatam	16/2 g q24 h CI or 3.375 q6 h EI over 4 hours	4/0.5 g q6 h	3/0.375 g q6 h	2/0.25 g q6 h
Imipenem	500 mg q4 h or 250 mg q3 h over 3 hours CI	500 mg q6 h	250 mg q6 h	250 mg q12 h
Meropenem	1 g q6 h over 6 hours CI	500 mg q6 h	250 mg q6 h	250 mg q12 h
Ertapenem	ND	1 g q24 h	1 g q24 h	500 mg q24 h
Gentamycin	9 to 10 mg/kg q24 h[b]	7 mg/kg q24 h	7 mg/kg q36–48 h	7 mg/kg q48–96 h
Amikacin	20 mg/kg q24 h	15 mg/kg q24 h	15 mg/kg q36–48 h[b]	15 mg/kg q48–96 h
Ciprofloxacin	600 mg q12 h or 400 mg q8 h	400 mg q12 h	400 mg q12 h	400 mg q24 h
Levofloxacin	500 mg q12 h	750 mg q24 h	500 mg q24 h	500 mg q48 h
Vancomycin	30 mg/kg q24 h CI	500 mg q6 h	500 mg q12 h	500 mg q24–72 h
Teicoplanin	LD 12 mg/kg q12 h for 3 to 4 doses; MD 6 mg/kg q12 h	LD 12 mg/kg q12 h for 3 to 4 doses; MD 4 to 6 mg/kg q12 h	LD 12 mg/kg q12 h for 3 to 4 doses; MD 2 to 4 mg/kg q12 h	LD 12 mg/kg q12 h for 3 to 4 doses; MD 2 to 4 mg/kg q24 h
Tigecycline	LD 100 mg; MD 50 mg q12 h	LD 100 mg; MD 50 mg q12 h	LD 100 mg; MD 50 mg q12 h	LD 100 mg; MD 50 mg q12 h

Regarding the administration of antibiotics, treatment efficacy against a certain microorganism can involve the specific drug concentration and/or the time when the drug is introduced to the binding site [36].

Concentration-dependent antibiotics, such as aminoglycosides and quinolones, are more effective at higher concentrations. They therefore feature a concentration-dependent post-antibiotic effect, and bactericidal action continues for a period of time after the antibiotic level falls below the minimum inhibitory concentration (MIC) [36].

Concentration-dependent agents administered in high dosage, short-course, once-a-day treatment regimens may promote more rapid and efficient bactericidal action and prevent the development of resistant strains.

There is good evidence for extended duration of aminoglycoside dosing in critically ill patients. In terms of toxicity, aminoglycosides nephrotoxicity is caused by a direct effect on the renal cortex and the uptake into the renal cortex can be saturated. Thus a dosing strategy of extended duration reduces the renal cortex exposure to aminoglycosides and reduces the risk of nephrotoxicity [37].

Time-dependent antibiotics, such as β-lactams and glycopeptides, demonstrate optimal bactericidal activity when drug concentrations are maintained above the MIC. Unlike concentration-dependent agents, they have a negligible post-antibiotic effect.

The efficacy of time-dependent antibacterial agents in severely ill patients is based on the constant maintenance of supra-inhibitory drug concentrations; as such, clinicians should consider multiple doses per day [38].

In critically ill patients, continuous infusion of β-lactam antibiotics may facilitate faster and more consistent therapeutic levels as compared to intermittent bolus dosing. Although randomized clinical trials are needed to confirm these findings, continuous infusion of β-lactam antibiotics has proven to be a useful time-dependent approach for treating critically ill patients [39].

The empirically designed antimicrobial regimen is based on the underlying severity of infection, the pathogens presumed to be involved, and the risk factors indicative of major resistance patterns.

Intra-abdominal infections in critically ill patients can be treated with either single or multiple antimicrobial regimens depending on the range requirements of antimicrobial coverage [40].

Piperacillin/tazobactam is a beta-lactam/beta-lactamase inhibitor combination with in vitro activity towards gram-positive (including Enterococci), gram-negative and anaerobic organisms [41].

Piperacillin/tazobactam retains in vitro activity against broad-spectrum beta-lactamase-producing, many extended-spectrum beta-lactamase-producing Enterobacteriaceae and many *Pseudomonas* isolates [42]. It is still a good antimicrobial agent in critically ill patients with community-acquired intra-abdominal infections.

Carbapenems have a spectrum of antimicrobial activity that includes Gram-positive (except resistant gram positive cocci) and Gram-negative aerobic and anaerobic pathogens.

Group 2 carbapenems include imipenem/cilastatin, meropenem and doripenem, sharing activity against non-fermentative gram-negative bacilli and being particularly suitable for severe intra-abdominal infections [43].

Doripenem is a new 1-ß-methyl carbapenem which, similarly to imipenem and meropenem, has a broad-spectrum activity against Gram-positive, Gram-negative, and anaerobic bacteria [44]. Doripenem seems more effective, in vitro, than meropenem and imipenem against Pseudomonas aeruginosa [44].

In the last few years carbapenem overuse has been associated with increasing rates of resistance among enterobacteriacea [45], particularly *Klebsiella pneumonia.* From an epidemiological point of view, it is necessary to control the spread of carbapenemase producing gram negative bacteria by optimization of carbepenems use. The use of carbapenems in critically ill patients is acceptable and well indicated. Tigecycline represents a valid option for complicated intra-abdominal infections due to its favorable in vitro activity against enterococci, ESBL-producing strains of *E. coli* and *Klebsiella* and anaerobic organisms. Tigecycline has showed also considerable antimicrobial activity against *Acinetobacter* spp [46,47]. It does not have in vitro activity towards *Pseudomonas aeruginosa* and *Proteus mirabilis.*

Given its in vitro activity against multidrug resistant (MDR) bacteria, tigecycline represents an interesting treatment option for intra-abdominal infections at risk for MDR [48].

Recently, an analysis of clinical trials for both approved and unapproved indications for tigecycline (including one trial on complicated intra-abdominal infections), showed an increased risk of death among patients receiving tigecycline. This observation led to a FDA recommendation against the use of tigecycline in severe infections [49].

Because of its tissue penetration in peritoneal and soft tissues [50], tigecycline is a very useful drug used in peritoneal infections. In patients with severe sepsis or septic shock of abdominal origin, in which the inflammatory process extends to the circulatory system, tigecycline should always be associated with another antimicrobial.

Although the epidemiological role of candida species in intra-abdominal infections has not yet been conclusively defined by the medical community, the clinical role of candida is nevertheless significant given that invasive candidiasis is generally associated with poor clinical prognosis. However, the presence of *Candida* in patients with no signs of infection is considered a contaminant and may not require treatment.

Fluconazole has been widely used for the treatment of candidiasis since its approval by the FDA in 1990.

The azoles act primarily by inhibiting the cytochrome P450-dependent enzyme lanosterol 14-alpha-demethylase, necessary for the conversion of lanosterol to ergosterol in the cellular membrane of fungi [51].

Most *C. albicans* isolated from invasive candidiasis infections, remain fully susceptible to fluconazole, which has been the treatment of choice for these infections in most settings including intra-abdominal infections [52]. However, epidemiological data demonstrate that the frequency of *Candida* infections is rising, with an increase in the proportion of infections caused by non-albicans *Candida* species that are intrinsically resistant or variably susceptible to fluconazole [52].

Several randomized clinical trials have demonstrated the efficacy of the echinocandins in the treatment of candidaemia and invasive candidiasis [53].

The echinocandins: anidulafungin, caspofungin, and micafungin have a broad and similar spectrum of in vitro and in vivo activity against most Candida spp. [54].

Echinocandins have several potential advantages over fluconazole for the treatment of invasive candidiasis. They have a broader spectrum of activity (encompassing fluconazole-resistant *C. glabrata* and *C. krusei*) and potent fungicidal activity against most Candida species [55].

In the specific setting of intra-abdominal infections, echinocandins are generally recommended as a first line empiric therapy for critical ill patients, while fluconazole is typically recommended for less severe cases [21].

Haemodynamic support

One of the most likely explanations for the high morbidity and mortality rates associated with severe sepsis is the development of cardiovascular insufficiency, which can lead to global tissue hypoxia.

In severe sepsis, the early haemodynamic profile is characterized by hypovolaemia, vaso-regulatory dysfunction, and myocardial depression. Increased capillary leakage and venous capacitance ultimately result in decreased venous return to the heart. Additionally, cytokines released during the patient's immune response may trigger further myocardial depression.

These haemodynamic alterations associated with the early stages of sepsis are often accompanied by an increase in systemic oxygen demand and impaired oxygen delivery, thereby inducing global tissue hypoxia. Global tissue hypoxia may overstimulate endothelial cell activity, which can subsequently lead to the systemic inflammatory cascade characteristic of sepsis [56,57].

Early treatment with aggressive haemodynamic support can limit the damage of sepsis-induced tissue hypoxia and prevent the over stimulation of endothelial activity.

Rivers et al. [58] demonstrated that early goal-directed therapy (EGDT), initiated in the emergency department, reduces the in-hospital mortality rates of patients in septic shock.

It has been established that the general prognostic value of a lactate of 4 mM/L on hospital admission is important; multiple studies have confirmed the risk stratification of this lactate level for illness severity and mortality in both the pre-hospital and in-hospital setting [59-63]. Lactate clearance has also been associated with decreased mortality in patients with severe sepsis and septic shock [64]. However, 20 to 50% of septic shock patients do not have elevated lactate levels at presentation or during their clinical course, yet still develop organ failure [65-67].

Fluid resuscitation

Fluid resuscitation should be initiated as early as possible in the course of treatment for severe sepsis regardless of a patient's lactate level.

Fluid resuscitation is a major component of cardiovascular support in early sepsis. Although the need for fluid resuscitation in sepsis is well established, the goals and components of this treatment are still a matter of debate also in patients with peritonitis.

The absence of clear benefits following the administration of colloid solutions compared to crystalloid [68], supports a high-grade recommendation for the use of crystalloid solutions in the initial resuscitation of patients with severe sepsis and septic shock [11].

Intravascular volume is the first parameter to be assessed during hemodynamic optimization.

In patients with generalized peritonitis, fluid resuscitation should be kept under control to avoid fluids overload, which may aggravate gut oedema and lead to increased intra-abdominal pressure. Increasing intra-abdominal pressure causes progressive hypoperfusion of splanchnic circulation. Pathophysiological effects include gut oedema leading to bacterial translocation and release of cytokines, therefore aggravating the sepsis cascade [69].

Several studies have already shown that a positive fluid balance in critical illness may be strongly associated with a higher severity of organ dysfunction and with worse outcomes [70].

Pathophysiological mechanisms associated with the inflammatory response lead to capillary leakage. Although crystalloids are isotonic, a significant amount of the volume given may migrate into the extra-vascular space due to increased capillary permeability and changes in oncotic pressure.

In patient with severe generalized peritonitis excessive infusion of fluids may become a counterproductive strategy.

The frequency with which intra-abdominal hypertension develops in abdominal sepsis may have other important clinical consequences in addition to its impact on sepsis resuscitation endpoints. Current surviving sepsis guidelines emphasize the importance of traditional mean arterial pressure (MAP) >65 mm Hg, central venous pressure (CVP) of 8–12 mmHg in combination with a central venous oxygen saturation (ScvO2) > 70% and Urine output >0.5 mL/kg/hr [11]. However, in patients with severe sepsis or septic shock of abdominal origin, high intra-abdominal pressure may profoundly influence commonly used septic shock resuscitation endpoints such as CVP (falsely elevated) and urine output (markedly decreased).

Repeated intravesical measurements of intra-abdominal pressure should be frequently performed in patients with severe sepsis or septic shock of abdominal origin, to identify patients at risk for intra-abdominal hypertension.

Monitoring the fluid status of critically ill patients at risk for intra-abdominal hypertension is crucial. In recent decades we have witnessed rapid advances in fluid monitoring techniques. Pulmonary artery catheters (PACs) have been widely used for more than three decades, but their usefulness in improving patient outcomes seems disappointing. Trials have consistently shown that PACs do no improve patient outcomes and may significantly increase medical costs [71]. With the declining use of PACs, there has been an increasing number of alternatives for hemodynamic monitoring.

Echocardiography is a useful noninvasive tool which can directly visualize the heart and assess cardiac function. Its use was long limited by the absence of accurate indices to diagnose hypovolemia and predict the effect of volume expansion. In the last years echocardiography has been used to develop new parameters of fluid responsiveness, taking advantage of its ability to monitor cardiac function. Echocardiography has been shown to predict fluid responsiveness accurately and is now a complete and noninvasive tool able to accurately determine hemodynamic status in circulatory failure [72,73]. It is strongly operator-dependent, and it does not allow continuous monitoring.

The PiCCO system (Pulse index Contour Continuous Cardiac Output, Pulsion Medical Systems, Germany) is another interesting alternative. It incorporates a transpulmonary thermodilution technique (TPTD) and continuous pulse contour analysis. It is minimally invasive and does not require intracardiac catheterization. It can give beat-by-beat monitoring of cardiac output, and can provide accurate information on volume status [74].

Vasopressor agents

Vasopressor agents should be administered early in patients with severe sepsis or septic shock of abdominal origin to restore organ perfusion. Their early use may prevent excessive fluid resuscitation.

Vasopressor drugs maintain adequate blood pressure and preserve perfusion pressure thus optimizing blood flow in various organs. Norepinephrine is now the first-line vasopressor agent used to correct hypotension in the event of septic shock [11]. Norepinephrine is more efficacious than dopamine and may be more effective for reversing hypotension in patients with septic shock.

In 1993, Martin et al. showed in a prospective, double-blind, randomized trial that norepinephrine was more effective and reliable than dopamine to reverse the abnormalities of hyper dynamic septic shock [75]. The Surviving Sepsis Campaign guidelines favour norepinephrine [11] and there have been studies since the 2008 update to bolster this preference. De Backer et al. investigated this question in a meta-analysis, focusing only on those patients with septic shock and again showed that dopamine was associated with greater mortality than norepinephrine [76].

It is well known that dopamine may cause more tachycardia and may be more arrhythmogenic than norepinephrine [77], and as an alternative vasopressor agent to norepinephrine, it should be used only in patients with low risk of tachyarrhythmias and absolute or relative bradycardia.

Epinephrine is a potent α-adrenergic and β-adrenergic agent that increases mean arterial pressure by increasing both, cardiac index and peripheral vascular tone. There are concerns regarding the use of epinephrine in septic patients due to its potential to decrease regional blood flow, particularly in the splanchnic circulation, and elevations in serum lactate. However, no trials have shown that epinephrine results in worse outcomes, so it may be used as an alternative to norepinephrine [78,79].

Vasopressin is a peptide hormone synthesized in the hypothalamus and subsequently transported to the pituitary gland where it is stored. It is released in response to decreased blood volume, decreased intravascular volume, and increased plasma osmolality. Vasopressin constricts vascular smooth muscle by directly activating V1 receptors and simultaneously increasing the vasculature's responsiveness to catecholamines [80].

Vasopressin (up to 0.03 U/min) can be added to norepinephrine with the intent of raising MAP to target or decreasing the norepinephrine dose [11].

Inotropic agents

Dobutamine is frequently used to treat septic shock patients as an inotropic agent increasing cardiac output, stroke index, and oxygen delivery (Do_2). However, the tendency of dobutamine to increase Do_2 to supranormal values in critically ill patients has raised serious questions regarding its safety in the treatment of septic shock. The Surviving Sepsis Campaign Guidelines recommend [11] that a dobutamine infusion should be administered in the event of myocardial dysfunction as indicated by elevated cardiac filling pressures and low cardiac output or ongoing signs of hypoperfusion, despite achieving adequate intravascular volume and adequate MAP.

Acute kidney injury in surgical sepsis

In patients with surgical sepsis, particular attention should always be paid to acute kidney injury (AKI). A prospective observational institutional study recently published, has shown that AKI frequently complicates surgical sepsis, and serves as a powerful predictor of hospital mortality in severe sepsis and septic shock. During the 36-month study period ending on December 2010, 246 patients treated for surgical sepsis were evaluated in the study. AKI occurred in 67% of all patients, and 59%, 60%, and 88% of patients had sepsis, surgical sepsis, and septic shock, respectively.

Patients with AKI had fewer ventilator-free and intensive care unit free days and a decreased likelihood of discharge to home. Morbidity and mortality increased with severity of AKI, and AKI of any severity was found to be a strong predictor of hospital mortality (odds ratio, 10.59; 95% confidence interval, 1.28Y87.35; p = 0.03) in surgical sepsis [81].

Source control

Initial operation

The timing and adequacy of source control are of outmost importance in the management of intra-abdominal sepsis, as late and/or incomplete procedures may have severely adverse consequences on outcome.

Source control encompasses all measures undertaken to eliminate the source of infection, reduce the bacterial inoculum and correct or control anatomic derangements to restore normal physiologic function [82,83].

This generally involves drainage of abscesses or infected fluid collections, debridement of necrotic or infected tissues and definitive control of the source of contamination.

It is well known that inadequate source control at the time of the initial operation has been associated with increased mortality in patients with severe intra-abdominal infections [84].

Early control of the septic source can be achieved using both operative and non-operative techniques.

An operative intervention remains the most viable therapeutic strategy for managing intra-abdominal sepsis in critical ill patients.

The initial aim of the surgical treatment of peritonitis is the elimination of bacterial contamination and inflammatory substances and prevention or reduction, if possible, of fibrin formation.

Generally, the surgical source control employed depends on the anatomical source of infection, the degree of peritoneal inflammation and generalized septic response, and the patient's pre-morbid condition.

Surgical source control entails resection or suture of a diseased or perforated viscus (e.g. diverticular perforation, gastroduodenal perforation), removal of the infected organ (e.g. appendix, gallbladder), debridement of necrotic tissue, resection of ischemic bowel and repair/resection of traumatic perforations with primary anastomosis or exteriorization of the bowel.

Laparotomies are usually performed using a midline incision.

The primary objectives of surgical intervention include a) determining the cause of peritonitis, b) draining fluid collections, c) controlling the origin of the abdominal sepsis.

Special attention should be given to areas where abscesses may form such as the pelvis, the para-colic gutters, and the subphrenic spaces. These areas should be carefully exposed and debrided, avoiding bleeding by excessive peeling of the fibrin, and drained.

In case of suspected gastro-intestinal perforation, the whole extent of the GI tract, starting from the gastroesophgeal junction to the lower rectum should be thoroughly and carefully examined. If no perforation is found, the gastrocolic omentum should always be opened to expose the lesser sac to allow visualization of the posterior wall of stomach for any hidden perforation as well as careful examination of the body and tail of pancreas.

Special attention should be paid while draining and debriding the left subphrenic space since there is high risk of splenic injury during surgical manipulation due to fibrinous adhesions with the splenic capsule. Splenic bleeding maybe difficult to control due to adhesions and might warrant splenectomy which adds to the morbidity and potential mortality in an already compromised patient.

Intra-abdominal lavage is a matter of ongoing controversy. Some authors have favoured peritoneal lavage because it helps in removal as well as in dilution of peritoneal contamination by irrigation with great volumes of saline [85]. However, its application with or without antibiotics in abdominal sepsis is largely unsubstantiated in the literature [86].

In recent years, laparoscopy has been gaining wider acceptance in the diagnosis and treatment of intra-abdominal infections.

Laparoscopic approach in the treatment of peritonitis is feasible and effective without any specific complications in experienced hands. Laparoscopy has the advantage to allow, at the same time, an adequate diagnosis and appropriate treatment with the less invasive abdominal approach [87]. However, in unstable patients laparoscopy is generally avoided because increased intra-abdominal pressure due to pneumoperitoneum seems to have a negative effect in critical ill patients leading to acid–base balance disturbances, as well as changes in cardiovascular and pulmonary physiology [88].

Relaparotomy strategy

In certain circumstances, infection not completely controlled may trigger an excessive immune response and sepsis may progressively evolve into severe sepsis, septic shock, and organ failure [89].

Such patients would benefit from immediate and aggressive surgical treatment with subsequent re-laparotomy strategies, to curb the spread of organ dysfunctions caused by ongoing sepsis.

Unfortunately, early assessment of the severity of peritonitis is difficult in emergency surgical patients and none of the existing and widely used 'severity-of-disease' scores, specifically developed for critically ill patients, were clinically useful in the identification of patients with ongoing infection needing a re-laparotomy [90]. Surgical strategies following an initial emergency laparotomy include subsequent "re-laparotomy on demand" (when required by the patient's clinical condition) as well as planned re-laparotomy in the 36-48-hour postoperative period.

On-demand laparotomy should be performed only when absolutely necessary and only for those patients who would clearly benefit from additional surgery.

Several studies have evaluated clinical variables that may be associated with the need for on-demand re-laparotomy in the immediate post-operative period [91-97].

Van Ruler et al. [92] in 2008 reported the results of a questionnaire asking surgeons to rank the importance of 21 clinical variables on their decision to re-operate in patients with secondary peritonitis. They found that diffuse extent of the abdominal contamination, localization of the infectious focus (upper gastrointestinal tract including small bowel), and both, extremely low and high leukocyte counts, independently predicted a re-laparotomy. These variables had only moderate predictive accuracy. The results of the questionnaire demonstrated that there was no consensus among surgeons about which variables are important in the decision-making process for re-laparotomy. The final decision to perform a re-operation on a patient in the on-demand setting is generally based on the patients generalized septic response and on the lack of clinical improvement.

Performing a case–control study, Koperna and Schulz [91] retrospectively reviewed 523 consecutive patients with secondary peritonitis. They focused their attention on 105 patients, in whom standard surgical treatment of secondary peritonitis failed and who had to undergo relaparotomy for persisting abdominal sepsis (study group). The authors showed that patients re-operated on after 48 hours had a significantly higher mortality rate than those operated on earlier (76.5% versus 28%; p < .001).

Planned relaparotomies, on the other hand, are performed every 36–48 hours for purposes of inspection, drainage, and peritoneal lavage of the abdominal cavity.

The concept of a planned relaparotomy for severe peritonitis has been debated for over thirty years. Reoperations are performed every 48 hours for reassessing the peritoneal inflammary process until the abdomen is free of ongoing peritonitis; then the abdomen is closed. The advantages of the planned re-laparotomy approach are optimization of resource utilization and reduction of the potential risk for gastrointestinal fistulas and delayed hernias.

The results of a clinical trial published in 2007 investigating the differences between on-demand and planned re-laparotomy strategies in patients with severe peritonitis found few advantages for the planned re-laparotomy strategy; however, the study mentioned that this later group exhibited a reduced need for additional re-laparotomies, decreased patient dependency on subsequent health care services, and decreased overall medical costs [98].

Open abdomen

An open abdomen (OA) procedure is the best way of implementing re-laparotomies. The role of the OA in the management of severe peritonitis has been a controversial issue.

In 2007, a randomised study compared open and closed abdomens for the "on demand re-laparotomy" group in the treatment of severe peritonitis. The study was prematurely terminated following the treatment of 40 subjects due to a significantly higher mortality rate in the open abdomen group compared to the temporarily closed abdomen group (55% vs. 30%). OA procedures were performed using only non-absorbable polypropylene mesh [99].

Although guidelines suggest not to routinely utilize the open abdomen approach for patients with severe intra-peritoneal contamination undergoing emergency laparotomy for intra-abdominal sepsis [100], OA has now been accepted as a strategy in treating intra-abdominal sepsis [101].

An OA approach in severe secondary peritonitis may be required for three different reasons, often used in combination: inadequate source control, severely deranged physiology (the operation is purposely abbreviated due to the severe physiological derangement and suboptimal local conditions for healing, and restoration of intestinal continuity is deferred to the second operation, i.e. the deferred anastomosis approach) [102], and prevention of abdominal compartment syndrome [103-105].

The rationale of the OA strategy in patients with severe abdominal sepsis refers to the cytokine release that is compartmentalized in the peritoneal cavity. Inability to control or interrupt the local inflammatory response is associated with higher mortality rates in these patients. The attenuation of the local inflammatory response may be best achieved with mechanical control by reducing the load of cytokines and other inflammatory substances [106] and by preventing their production, thus removing the source itself. Sometimes more laparotomies are required to complete source control and OA allows the surgeon to perform subsequent planned laparotomies more efficiently.

An interesting non-comparative descriptive case series [106] studied the inflammatory response in peritoneal exudate and plasma of patients undergoing planned re-laparotomy for severe secondary peritonitis. In septic patients undergoing re-laparotomy for severe peritonitis, endotoxin, tumour necrosis factor alpha, interleukin-1 and interleukin-6 levels, were higher in the peritoneal cavity then in plasma. When patients underwent re-laparotomy, the level of those cytokines was significantly decreased in survivors.

OA management has been described in patients with intra-abdominal sepsis when a single laparotomy failed to control local inflammatory response, or the risk of organ dysfunction increased after effective drainage and debridement [107-109].

In the event of massive fluid resuscitation, bowel oedema and the forced closure of a non-compliant abdominal wall may cause intra-abdominal hypertension (IAH). Uncontrolled IAH exceeding 25 mm Hg may cause abdominal compartment syndrome (ACS), which is a potentially lethal complication characterized by adverse effects on pulmonary, cardiovascular, renal, splanchnic, and central nervous system physiology [109].

The combination of IAH and the physiological effects of sepsis, result in high morbidity and mortality rates. At present there are no definite criteria to guide the surgeon in deciding whether to use the OA strategy [110]. The OA strategy allows surgeons to extend the concept of damage control surgery to abdominal severe sepsis.

The term damage control surgery (DCS) for trauma patients was introduced in 1993. It was defined as initial control of haemorrhage and contamination, allowing for resuscitation to normal physiology in the intensive care unit and subsequent definitive re-exploration [111,112].

The adaptation of damage control surgery for trauma to other areas generally is useful in those patients who are at risk to develop a similar loss of physiologic reserve with intolerance to the shocked physiological state [113]. Similarly to the trauma patient with the lethal triad of acidosis, hypothermia and coagulopathy, many patients with severe sepsis or septic shock may present in a similar fashion. For those patients, DCS can truly be life saving. Patients progressing from sepsis through severe sepsis with organ dysfunction into septic shock, can present with vasodilation, hypotension, and myocardial depression, combined with coagulopathy. These patients are profoundly haemodynamically unstable and are clearly not optimal candidates for complex operative interventions [114].

Abdominal closure should be temporary, and the patient is rapidly taken to the ICU for physiologic optimization. This includes optimization of volume resuscitation and mechanical ventilation, correction of coagulopathy and hypothermia, and monitoring for eventual ACS developement. Over the following 24 to 48 hours, when abnormal physiology is corrected the patient can be safely taken back to the operating room for re-operation.

An additional advantage of DCS in abdominal sepsis is the possibility to delay the bowel anastomosis [115].

The surgical strategy for the management of patients with compromised bowel in secondary peritonitis has been usually the resection of the perforated viscus followed by primary anastomosis or a diversion. In patients with severe secondary peritonitis and significant hemodynamic instability and compromised tissue perfusion, the use of primary anastomosis is limited because of the high risk of suture/anastomotic failure, leakage, and increased surgical mortality. In these patients, it is advisable to control the source of peritoneal contamination and to perform an intestinal ostomy delaying bowel anastomosis.

In a retrospective study from Colombia, 112 patients with secondary peritonitis requiring bowel resection and managed with staged laparotomy were analyzed [116]. Deferred primary anastomosis was used in 34 patients where the bowel ends were closed at first operation and definitive anastomoses were reconstructed at the subsequent operation following physiological stabilization in the ICU and repeated peritoneal washes until the septic source was controlled. In contrast, 78 patients underwent small bowel or colonic diversion followed by similar ICU stabilization and peritoneal washes. In both groups, the abdomens were left open at the initial operation and a Velcro system or vacuum pack was used for temporary abdominal closure. The mean number of laparotomies was four in both groups. There were more patients with colon resections in the diversion group (80% vs. 47%). There was no significant difference in hospital mortality (12% for deferred anastomosis vs. 17% for diversion), frequency of anastomotic leaks or fistulas (9% vs. 5%), or ARDS (18% vs. 31%). The authors concluded that in critically ill patients with severe secondary peritonitis managed with staged laparotomies, deferred primary anastomosis can be performed safely as long as adequate control of the septic foci and restoration of deranged physiology is achieved prior to reconstruction.

In a non-randomized study of 27 consecutive patients with perforated diverticulitis (Hinchey III/IV), the patients were managed either with sigmoid resection and primary anastomosis, or limited sigmoid resection or suture, open abdomen and primary anastomosis or colostomy at second operation 24–48 hours later, or Hartmann procedure; sigmoid resection and end colostomy [117]. All 6 patients with primary anastomosis survived without complications, but there was an obvious selection bias. Of the 6 patients undergoing Hartmann's procedure, one died of sepsis and 5 were discharged with stoma. In the interesting group of 15 patients with deferred anastomosis or stoma and open abdomen, 9 patients had intestinal continuity restored during the second look operation with one fatal anastomotic leakage.

In a prospective study of 51 patients with perforated diverticulitis (Hinchey III/IV) were initially managed with limited resection, lavage and TAC with vacuum-assisted closure followed by second, reconstructive operation 24–48 hours later [118]. Bowel continuity was restored in 38 patients, in 4 protected by a loop ileostomy. Five anastomotic leaks (13%) were encountered requiring loop ileostomy (2 patients) or Hartmann's procedure (3 patients). Postoperative abscesses were seen in 4 patients, abdominal wall dehiscence in one and re-laparotomy for drain-related small bowel perforation in one. The overall mortality rate was 10% and 35/46 (76%) of the surviving patients left the hospital with reconstructed colon continuity. Fascial closure was achieved in all patients.

Following stabilization of the patient, the goal is the early and definitive closure of the abdomen, in order to reduce the complications associated with an open abdomen [119].

A review of the literature suggests a bimodal distribution of primary closure rates, with early closure dependent on post operative intensive care management whilst delayed closure is more affected by the choice of the temporary abdominal closure technique [120].

Primary fascial closure can be achieved in many cases within few days from the initial operation. It would not be successful if early surgical source control failed [121,122].

Sequential fascial closure could immediately be started once abdominal sepsis is well controlled [123]. In these cases, surgeons should perform a progressive closure, where the abdomen is incrementally closed each time the patient undergoes a reoperation.

Within 10 to 14 days the fascia retracts laterally and becomes adherent to the overlying fat; this makes primary closure impossible. Therefore, it is important to prevent the retraction of the myo-fascial unit.

Several materials can be used to achieve temporary closure of the abdomen: gauze; mesh; impermeable self-adhesive membrane dressings, zippers and negative pressure therapy (NPT) techniques.

The ideal temporary abdominal closure method should be able to protect the abdominal contents, to prevent evisceration, to allow removal of infected or toxic fluid from the peritoneal cavity, to prevent the formation of fistulas, to avoid damage to the fascia, to preserve the abdominal wall domain, to make re-operation easy, safe and facilitate definitive closure [110].

The surgical options for management of the OA are now more diverse and sophisticated, but there is a lack of prospective randomized controlled trials demonstrating the superiority of any particular method.

At present, negative pressure therapy (NPT) techniques have become the most extensively used methods for temporary abdominal wall closure. NPT actively drains toxin or bacteria-rich intra peritoneal fluid and has resulted in a high rate of fascial and abdominal wall closure [110].

A systematic review conducted in 2012 [124] found only 11 comparative studies, including 2 randomized controlled trials (RCTs) and 9 cohort studies, examining the efficacy and safety of negative pressure peritoneal therapy *versus* alternate temporal abdominal closure methods among critically ill or injured adults.

However, all studies were associated with at least a moderate risk of bias and significant clinical heterogeneity, the authors concluded that there was insufficient evidence to support the preferential use of negative pressure peritoneal therapy after damage control laparotomy.

Animal data suggest that OA techniques employing constant negative pressure to the peritoneal cavity may remove inflammatory ascites, reduce the systemic inflammatory response, and improve organ injury and potentially outcomes [125].

This method is still associated with high morbidity and high incidence of ventral hernia formation in surviving patients caused by difficulties in definitive closure of the abdominal wall after prolonged application of NPT but it could be a highly promising method in the management of patients with increased IAP and severe sepsis due to severe peritonitis [126].

A systematic review published in 2009 [127] investigated which temporary abdominal closure technique is associated with the highest delayed primary fascial closure (FC) rate.

No comparative studies were identified. 51 articles were included. The techniques described were vacuum-assisted closure (VAC; 8 series), vacuum pack (15 series), artificial burr (4 series), Mesh/sheet (16 series), zipper (7 series), silo (3 series), skin closure (2 series), dynamic retention sutures (DRS), and loose packing (1 series each).

These results suggested that the artificial burr and the VAC were associated with the highest FC rates and the lowest mortality rates.

Other techniques used for progressive FC include a combination of NPT with a temporary mesh sutured to the fascial edges. The mesh is tightened every few days, until the fascial defect is small enough so the mesh can be removed and the fascia closed primarily.

In 2012, a retrospective analysis evaluating the use of vacuum-assisted closure and mesh-mediated fascial traction (VACM) as temporary abdominal closure was published [128]. The study compared 50 patients treated with (VACM) and 54 using non-traction techniques (control group). VACM resulted in a higher fascial closure rate and lower planned hernia rate than methods that did not provide fascial traction.

Occasionally, abdominal closure is only partially achieved, resulting in late development of large, debilitating hernias of the abdominal wall which will eventually require complex surgical repair. In these cases, delayed repair or use of biological meshes has been proposed [129].

Another option, if definitive fascial closure is not possible, is closure of the skin only and subsequent management of the eventration by a deferred abdominal closure with synthetic meshes after hospital discharge [127].

Adjuntive measures

Recombinant human activated protein C (rhAPC), also known as drotrecogin alfa, was included in the previous Surviving Sepsis Campaign guidelines [130] based on the PROWESS study group [131] and ENHANCE study group [132] studies.

Based on the preliminary data of the PROWESS-SHOCK study [133], showing a 28-day all-cause mortality rate of 26.4% in patients treated with rhAPC compared with 24.4% in those given placebo, the US Food and Drug Administration (FDA) has withdrawn drotrecogin alfa from the market [134] and now, rhAPC should not be used in any patients with septic shock.

Corticosteroids

The recommendations regarding the use of corticosteroids have changed over time and the clinical benefits of corticosteroids in the treatment of severe sepsis and septic shock remain controversial.

A systematic review of corticosteroids in the treatment of severe sepsis and septic shock in adult patients published in 2009 valued 17 randomized trials (2138 patients) and 3 quasi-randomized trials (n = 246) of acceptable methodological quality, and pooled the results in a subsequent meta-analysis [135]. The authors concluded that corticosteroid therapy has been used in varied doses for treating sepsis and related syndromes for more than 50 years, but its ability to reduce mortality rates has never been conclusively proven. Since 1998, studies have consistently used prolonged low-dose corticosteroid therapy, and follow-up analyses of this subgroup have found that such regimens tend to reduce short-term mortality.

In 2011 Annane published an evidenced based guide [136] regarding corticosteroids for severe sepsis. He concluded that corticosteroids should be initiated only in patients with sepsis who require 0.5 μg/kg per minute or more of norepinephrine and should be continued for 5 to 7 days except in patients with poor haemodynamic response after 2 days of corticosteroids and with a cortisol increment of more than 250 nmol/L after a standard adrenocorticotropin hormone (ACTH) test.

The Surviving Sepsis Campaign guidelines [11] recommend corticosteroids be used in patients with refractory septic shock (poorly responsive to fluids and vasopressor therapy) and do not recommend routine assessment for relative adrenal insufficiency.

Nutritional support

The effect of nutritional support in critically ill patients with sepsis has been debated in recent years. As for all critically ill patients, nutritional support, preferably via the enteral route, should be commenced in patients with severe sepsis or septic shock once initial resuscitation and adequate perfusion pressure is achieved [137].

Early enteral nutrition has theoretical advantages in maintaining the integrity of the gut mucosa and on the prevention of bacterial translocation.

Studies on different subpopulations of critically ill patients, mostly surgical patients, are not consistent and none was individually powered for mortality, with very low mortality rates. Although no consistent effect on mortality was observed, some early enteral feeding studies showed benefit on secondary outcomes such reduced length of mechanical ventilation, and reduced ICU and hospital stay [138-140].

Conclusions

The Surviving Sepsis Campaign international guidelines for management of severe sepsis and septic shock were recently updated. These guidelines are the cornerstone for the management of severe sepsis and septic shock, but they do not focus on the specific setting of intra-abdominal infections.

Although sepsis is a systemic process, the pathophysiological events differ for every organ and in the specific setting of intra-abdominal infections the management of sepsis may vary from that of sepsis of other etiologies.

Outcomes of severe intra-abdominal infections accompanied by severe sepsis are related to early diagnosis, aggressive and early optimization of physiology, early surgical management with source control and aggressive critical care management. Reoperations are common and may be useful in attenuating the inflammatory response and optimizing the immune response.

Competing interests
The authors declare that they have no competing interests.

Authors' contributions
MS wrote the manuscript. All authors reviewed and approved the final manuscript.

Author details
[1]Department of Surgery, Macerata Hospital, Macerata, Italy. [2]Department of Emergency Surgery, Maggiore Parma Hospital, Parma, Italy. [3]Trauma Surgery Unit, Maggiore Hospital, Bologna, Italy. [4]General Surgery Department, Papa Giovanni XXIII hospital, Bergamo, Italy. [5]American Board of Surgery, Philadelphia, USA. [6]Department of Surgery, Denver Health Medical Center, Denver, CO, USA. [7]Department of Surgery, University of Florida, Gainesville, Florida, USA. [8]Department of Surgery, Virginia Commonwealth University Medical Center, Richmond, VA, USA. [9]Department of Surgery, UC San Diego Health System, San Diego, USA. [10]Department of Abdominal Surgery, University Hospital Meilahti, Helsinki, Finland. [11]Department of General Surgery, Rambam Health Care Campus, Haifa, Israel. [12]Division of Trauma Surgery, Hospital de Clinicas -, School of Medical Sciences, University of Campinas, Campinas, Brazil. [13]Department of Surgery, Universidad del Valle, Fundacion Valle del Lili, Cali, Colombia. [14]Department of Surgery, Pt BDS Post-graduate Institute of Medical Sciences, Rohtak, India. [15]Department of Surgery 1, Lviv Regional Hospital, Danylo Halytsky Lviv National Medical University, Lviv, Ukraine. [16]Department of Surgery, Yonsei University College of Medicine, Seoul, Korea. [17]Department of Anesthesiology, Macerata Hospital, Macerata, Italy. [18]Department of Surgery, University Hospital Southampton, Southampton, UK.

References

1. Mazuski JE, Solomkin JS: **Intra-abdominal infections.** *Surg Clin North Am* 2009, **89**(2):421–437.
2. Babinchak T, Ellis-Grosse E, Dartois N, Rose GM, Loh E: **The efficacy and safety of tigecycline for the treatment of complicated intra-abdominal infections: analysis of pooled clinical data.** *Clin Infect Dis* 2005, **41**(Suppl 5):S354–S367.
3. Merlino JI, Malangoni MA, Smith CM, Lange RL: **Prospective randomized trials affect the outcomes of intraabdominal infection.** *Ann Surg* 2001, **233**(6):859–866.
4. Mazuski JE, Sawyer RG, Nathens AB, DiPiro JT, Schein M, Kudsk KA, Yowler C: **Therapeutic agents committee of the surgical infections society. The surgical infection society guidelines on antimicrobial therapy for intra-abdominal infections: evidence for the recommendations.** *Surg Infect (Larchmt)* 2002, **3**(3):175–233.
5. Sartelli M, Catena F, Ansaloni L, Leppaniemi A, Taviloglu K, van Goor H, Viale P, Lazzareschi DV, Coccolini F, Corbella D, de Werra C, Marrelli D, Colizza S, Scibè R, Alis H, Torer N, Navarro S, Sakakushev B, Massalou D, Augustin G, Catani M, Kauhanen S, Pletinckx P, Kenig J, di Saverio S, Jovine E, Guercioni G, Skrovina M, Diaz-Nieto R, Ferrero A, *et al*: **Complicated intra-abdominal infections in Europe: a comprehensive review of the CIAO study.** *World J Emerg Surg* 2012, **7**(1):36.
6. LaRosa SP: **Sepsis: Menu of new approaches replaces one therapy for all.** *Cleve Clin J Med* 2002, **69:**65–73.
7. Levy MM, Fink MP, Marshall JC, Abraham E, Angus D, Cook D, Cohen J, Opal SM, Vincent JL, Ramsay G: **SCCM/ESICM/ACCP/ATS/SIS international sepsis definitions conference.** *Crit Care Med* 2001, **2003**(31):1250–1256.
8. Bone RC, Balk RA, Cerra FB, Dellinger RP, Fein AM, Knaus WA, Schein RM, Sibbald WJ: **American college of chest physicians/society of critical care medicine consensus conference: definitions for sepsis and organ failure and guidlines for the use of innovative therapies in sepsis.** *Chest* 1992, **101:**1644–1655.
9. Jones AE, Yiannibas V, Johnson C, Kline JA: **Emergency department hypotension predicts sudden unexpected in-hospital mortality: a prospective cohort study.** *Chest* 2006, **130:**941–946.
10. Esteban A, Frutos-Vivar F, Ferguson ND, Peñuelas O, Lorente JA, Gordo F, Honrubia T, Algora A, Bustos A, García G, Diaz-Regañón IR, de Luna RR: **Sepsis incidence and outcome: contrasting the intensive care unit with the hospital ward.** *Crit Care Med* 2007, **35**(5):1284–1289.
11. Dellinger RP, Levy MM, Rhodes A, Annane D, Gerlach H, Opal SM, Sevransky JE, Sprung CL, Douglas IS, Jaeschke R, Osborn TM, Nunnally ME, Townsend SR, Reinhart K, Kleinpell RM, Angus DC, Deutschman CS, Machado FR, Rubenfeld GD, Webb S, Beale RJ, Vincent JL, Moreno R: **Surviving sepsis campaign guidelines committee including the pediatric subgroup. Surviving sepsis campaign: international guidelines for management of severe sepsis and septic shock, 2012.** *Intensive Care Med* 2013, **39**(2):165–228.
12. Tsukada K, Katoh H, Shiojima M, Suzuki T, Takenoshita S, Nagamachi Y: **Concentrations of cytokines in peritoneal fluid after abdominal surgery.** *Eur J Surg* 1993, **159:**475–479.
13. Patel RT, Deen KI, Youngs D, Warwick J, Keighley MR: **Interleukin 6 is a prognostic indicator of outcome in severe intra-abdominal sepsis.** *Br J Surg* 1994, **81:**1306–1308.
14. Damas P, Ledoux D, Nys M, Vrindts Y, de Groote D, Franchimont P, Lamy M: **Cytokine serum level during severe sepsis in human. Il6 as a marker of severity.** *Ann Surg* 1992, **215:**356–362.
15. Holzheimer RG, Schein M, Wittmann DH: **Inflammatory response in peritoneal exudate and plasma of patients undergoing planned relaparotomy for severe secondary peritonitis.** *Arch Surg* 1995, **130:**1314–1319.
16. Cavaillon JM, Munoz C, Fitting C, Misset B, Carlet J: **Circulating cytokines: the tip of the iceberg?** *Circ Shock* 1992, **38**(2):145–152.
17. Martineau L, Shek PN: **Peritoneal cytokine concentrations and survival outcome in an experimental bacterial infusion model of peritonitis.** *Crit Care Med* 2000, **28**(3):788–794.
18. Hendriks T, Bleichrodt RP, Lomme RM, de Man BM, van Goor H, Buyne OR: **Peritoneal cytokines predict mortality after surgical treatment of secondary peritonitis in the rat.** *J Am Coll Surg* 2010, **211:**263–270.
19. Riché F, Gayat E, Collet C, Matéo J, Laisné MJ, Launay JM, Valleur P, Payen D, Cholley BP: **Local and systemic innate immune response to secondary human peritonitis.** *Crit Care* 2013, **17**(5):R201.
20. Angus DC, van der Poll T: **Severe sepsis and septic shock.** *N Engl J Med* 2013, **369**(9):840–851.
21. Sartelli M, Viale P, Catena F, Ansaloni L, Moore E, Malangoni M, Moore FA, Velmahos G, Coimbra R, Ivatury R, Peitzman A, Koike K, Leppaniemi A, Biffl W, Burlew CC, Balogh ZJ, Boffard K, Bendinelli C, Gupta S, Kluger Y, Agresta F, di Saverio S, Wani I, Escalona A, Ordonez C, Fraga GP, Junior GA, Bala M, Cui Y, Marwah S, *et al*: **2013 WSES guidelines for management of intra-abdominal infections.** *World J Emerg Surg* 2013, **8**(1):3. doi:10.1186/1749-7922-8-3.
22. Emmi V, Sganga G: **Diagnosis of intra-abdominal infections: clinical findings and imaging.** *Infez Med* 2008, **16**(Suppl 1):19–30.
23. Jaramillo EJ, Treviño JM, Berghoff KR, Franklin ME Jr: **Bedside diagnostic laparoscopy in the intensive care unit: a 13-year experience.** *JSLS* 2006, **10**(2):155–159.
24. Ceribelli C, Adami EA, Mattia S, Benini B: **Bedside diagnostic laparoscopy for critically ill patients: a retrospective study of 62 patients.** *Surg Endosc* 2012, **26**(12):3612–5.
25. Shani V, Muchtar E, Kariv G, Robenshtok E, Leibovici L: **Systematic review and meta-analysis of the efficacy of appropriate empiric antibiotic therapy for sepsis.** *Antimicrob Agents Chemother* 2010, **54**(11):4851–4863.
26. Ferrer R, Artigas A, Suarez D, Palencia E, Levy MM, Arenzana A, Pérez XL, Sirvent JM, Edusepsis Study Group: **Edusepsis study group: effectiveness of treatments for severe sepsis: a prospective, multicenter, observational study.** *Am J Respir Crit Care Med* 2009, **180:**861–866.
27. Castellanos-Ortega A, Suberviola B, García-Astudillo LA, Holanda MS, Ortiz F, Llorca J, Delgado-Rodríguez M: **Impact of the surviving sepsis campaign protocols on hospital length of stay and mortality in septic shock patients: results of a three-year follow-up quasi-experimental study.** *Crit Care Med* 2010, **38:**1036–1043.
28. Puskarich MA, Trzeciak S, Shapiro NI, rnold RC, Horton JM, Studnek JR, Kline JA, Jones AE, Emergency Medicine Shock Research Network (EMSHOCKNET): **Emergency medicine shock research network (EMSHOCKNET): association between timing of antibiotic administration and mortality from septic shock in patients treated with a quantitative resuscitation protocol.** *Crit Care Med* 2011, **39:**2066–2071.
29. Riché FC, Dray X, Laisné MJ, Matéo J, Raskine L, Sanson-Le Pors MJ, Payen D, Valleur P, Cholley BP: **Factors associated with septic shock and mortality in generalized peritonitis: comparison between community-acquired and postoperative peritonitis.** *Crit Care* 2009, **13**(3):R99.

30. Fry D: **The generic response.** *Crit Care Med* 2008, **36:**1369–1370.
31. Tang BM, McLean AS, Dawes IW, Huang SJ, Cowley MJ, Lin RC: **Gene-expression profiling of gram-positive and gram-negative sepsis in critically ill patients.** *Crit Care Med* 2008, **36:**1125–1128.
32. Montravers P, Andremont A, Massias L, Carbon C: **Investigation of the potential role of Enterococcus faecalis in the pathophysiology of experimental peritonitis.** *J Infect Dis* 1994, **169:**821–830.
33. Montravers P, Mohler J, Saint Julien L, Carbon C: **Evidence of the proinflammatory role of enterococcus faecalis in polymicrobial peritonitis in rats.** *Infect Immun* 1997, **65:**144–149.
34. Höffken G, Niederman M: **Nosocomial pneumonia. The importance of a de-escalating strategy for antibiotic treatment of pneumonia in the ICU.** *Chest* 2002, **122:**2183–2196.
35. Rello J, Vidaur L, Sandiumenge A, Rodríguez A, Gualis B, Boque C, Diaz E: **De-escalation therapy in ventilator-associated pneumonia.** *Crit Care Med* 2004, **32:**2183–2190.
36. Pea F, Viale P: **Bench-to-bedside review: appropriate antibiotic therapy in severe sepsis and septic shock–does the dose matter?** *Crit Care* 2009, **13**(3):214.
37. Hatala R, Dinh T, Cook DJ: **Once-daily aminoglycoside dosing in immunocompetent adults: a meta-analysis.** *Ann Intern Med* 1996, **124:**717–725.
38. McKenzie C: **Antibiotic dosing in critical illness.** *J Antimicrob Chemother* 2011, **66**(Suppl 2):ii25–ii31.
39. Roberts JA, Lipman J, Blot S, Rello J: **Better outcomes through continuous infusion of time-dependent antibiotics to critically ill patients?** *Curr Opin Crit Care* 2008, **14**(4):390–396.
40. Solomkin JS, Mazuski JE, Bradley JS, Rodvold KA, Goldstein EJ, Baron EJ, O'Neill PJ, Chow AW, Dellinger EP, Eachempati SR, Gorbach S, Hilfiker M, May AK, Nathens AB, Sawyer RG, Bartlett JG: **Diagnosis and management of complicated intra-abdominal infection in adults and children: guidelines by the Surgical Infection Society and the Infectious Diseases Society of America.** *Clin Infect Dis* 2010, **50**(2):133–164.
41. Powell LL, Wilson SE: **The role of beta-lactam antimicrobials as single agents in treatment of intra-abdominal infection.** *Surg Infect (Larchmt)* 2000, **1**(1):57–63.
42. Al-Hasan MN, Lahr BD, Eckel-Passow JE, Baddour LM: **Antimicrobial resistance trends of Escherichia coli bloodstream isolates: a population-based study, 1998–2007.** *J Antimicrob Chemother* 2009, **64**(1):169–174.
43. Jones RN, Huynh HK, Biedenbach DJ, Fritsche TR, Sader HS: **Doripenem (S-4661), a novel carbapenem: comparative activity against contemporary pathogens including bactericidal action and preliminary in vitro methods evaluations.** *J Antimicrob Chemother* 2004, **54**(1):144–154.
44. Brown SD, Traczewski MM: **Comparative in vitro antimicrobial activity of a new carbapenem, doripenem: tentative disc diffusion criteria and quality control.** *J Antimicrob Chemother* 2005, **55**(6):944–949.
45. Michalopoulos AS, Karatza DC: **Multidrug-resistant Gram-negative infections: the use of colistin.** *Expert Rev Anti Infect Ther* 2010, **8**(9):1009–1017.
46. Papaparaskevas J, Tzouvelekis LS, Tsakris A, Pittaras TE, Legakis NJ: **Hellenic tigecycline study group: in vitro activity of tigecycline against 2423 clinical isolates and comparison of the available interpretation breakpoints.** *Diagn Microbiol Infect Dis* 2010, **66**(2):187–194.
47. Sekowska A, Gospodarek E: **Susceptibility of Klebsiella spp. to tigecycline and other selected antibiotics.** *Med Sci Monit* 2010, **16**(6):BR193–BR196.
48. Stein GE, Babinchak T: **Tigecycline: an update.** *Diagn Microbiol Infect Dis* 2013, **75**(4):331–336.
49. US Food and Drug Administration: **FDA drug safety communication: increased risk of death with Tygacil (tigecycline) compared to other antibiotics used to treat similar infections [online].** Available from URL: http://www.fda.gov/Drugs/DrugSafety/ucm224370.htm.
50. Stein GE, Smith CL, Missavage A, Saunders JP, Nicolau DP, Battjes SM, Kepros JP: **Tigecycline penetration into skin and soft tissue.** *Surg Infect (Larchmt)* 2011, **12**(6):465–467.
51. Zonios DI, Bennett JE: **Update on azole antifungals.** *Semin Respir Crit Care Med* 2008, **29**(2):198–210.
52. Pfaller MA, Diekema DJ: **Epidemiology of invasive candidiasis: a persistent public health problem.** *Clin Microbiol Rev* 2007, **20:**133–163.
53. Glockner A: **Treatment and prophylaxis of invasive candidiasis with anidulafungin, caspofungin and micafungin: review of the literature.** *Eur J Med Res* 2011, **16**(4):167–179.
54. Chen SC, Slavin MA, Sorrell TC: **Echinocandin antifungal drugs in fungal infections: a comparison.** *Drugs* 2011, **71**(1):11–41.
55. Ostrosky-Zeichner L, Rex JH, Pappas PG, Hamill RJ, Larsen RA, Horowitz HW, Powderly WG, Hyslop N, Kauffman CA, Cleary J, Mangino JE, Lee J: **Antifungal susceptibility survey of 2,000 bloodstream Candida isolates in the United States.** *Antimicrob Agents Chemother* 2003, **47:**3149–3154.
56. Karimova A, Pinsky DJ: **The endothelial response to oxygen eprivation: biology and clinical implications.** *Intensive Care Med* 2001, **27:**19–31.
57. Benjamin E, Leibowitz AB, Oropello J, Iberti TJ: **Systemic hypoxic and inflammatory syndrome: An alternative designation for "sepsis syndrome".** *Crit Care Med* 1992, **20:**680–682.
58. Rivers E: **Early goal-directed therapy in the treatment of severe sepsis and septic shock.** *N Eng J Med* 2001, **345:**1368–1377.
59. Aduen J, Bernstein WK, Khastgir T, Miller J, Kerzner R, Bhatiani A, Miller J, Kerzner R, Bhatiani A, Lustgarten J, Bassin AS, Davison L, Chernow B: **The use and clinical importance of a substrate-specific electrode for rapid determination of blood lactate concentrations.** *JAMA* 1994, **272:**1678–1685.
60. Mikkelsen ME, Miltiades AN, Gaieski DF, Goyal M, Fuchs BD, Shah CV, Bellamy SL, Christie JD: **Serum lactate is associated with mortality in severe sepsis independent of organ failure and shock.** *Crit Care Med* 2009, **37:**1670–1677.
61. Trzeciak S, Dellinger RP, Chansky ME, Arnold RC, Schorr C, Milcarek B, Hollenberg SM, Parrillo JE: **Serum lactate as a predictor of mortality in patients with infection.** *Intensive Care Med* 2007, **33:**970–977.
62. Shapiro NI, Howell MD, Talmor D, Nathanson LA, Lisbon A, Wolfe RE, Weiss JW: **Serum lactate as a predictor of mortality in emergency department patients with infection.** *Ann Emerg Med* 2005, **45:**524–528.
63. Pearse RM: **Extending the role of lactate measurement into the prehospital environment.** *Crit Care* 2009, **13:**115.
64. Nguyen HB, Rivers EP, Knoblich BP, Jacobsen G, Muzzin A, Ressler JA, Tomlanovich MC: **Early lactate clearance is associated with improved outcome in severe sepsis and septic shock.** *Crit Care Med* 2004, **32:**1637–1642.
65. James JH, Luchette FA, McCarter FD, Fischer JE: **Lactate is an unreliable indicator of tissue hypoxia in injury or sepsis.** *Lancet* 1999, **354:**505–508.
66. Dugas D, Mackenhauer J, Joyce N, Donnino M: **Prevalence and characteristics of nonlactate and lactate expressors in septic shock.** *Crit Care Med* 2009, **37**(Suppl):A227.
67. Cannon CM, for the Multicenter Severe S, Septic Shock Collaborative G. The GENESIS Project (GENeralization of Early Sepsis InterventionS): **A multicenter quality improvement collaborative.** *Acad Emerg Med* 2010, **17:**1258.
68. Perel P, Roberts I: **Colloids versus crystalloids for fluid resuscitation in critically ill patients.** *Cochrane Database Syst Rev* 2011, **3:**CD000567.
69. Walker J, Criddle LM: **Pathophysiology and management of abdominal compartment syndrome.** *Am J Crit Care* 2003, **12**(4):367–371.
70. Brandt S, Regueira T, Bracht H, Porta F, Djafarzadeh S, Takala J, Gorrasi J, Borotto E, Krejci V, Hiltebrand LB, Bruegger LE, Beldi G, Wilkens L, Lepper PM, Kessler U, Jakob SM: **Effect of fluid resuscitation on mortality and organ function in experimental sepsis models.** *Crit Care* 2009, **13**(6):R186.
71. Harvey S, Young D, Brampton W, Cooper AB, Doig G, Sibbald W, Rowan K: **Pulmonary artery catheters for adult patients in intensive care.** *Cochrane Database Syst Rev* 2006, **19**(3), CD003408.
72. Charron C, Caille V, Jardin F, Vieillard-Baron A: **Echocardiographic measurement of fluid responsiveness.** *Curr Opin Crit Care* 2006, **12**(3):249–254.
73. Manasia AR, Nagaraj HM, Kodali RB, Croft LB, Oropello JM, Kohli-Seth R, Leibowitz AB, DelGiudice R, Hufanda JF, Benjamin E, Goldman ME: **Feasibility and potential clinical utility of goal-directed transthoracic echocardiography performed by noncardiologist intensivists using a small hand-carried device (SonoHeart) in critically ill patients.** *J Cardiothorac Vasc Anesth* 2005, **19**(2):155–9.
74. Zhang Z, Xu X, Yao M, Chen H, Ni H, Fan H: **Use of the PiCCO system in critically ill patients with septic shock and acute respiratory distress syndrome: a study protocol for a randomized controlled trial.** *Trials* 2013, **14:**32.
75. Martin C, Papazian L, Perrin G, Saux P, Gouin F: **Norepinephrine or dopamine for the treatment of hyperdynamic septic shock?** *Chest* 1993, **103**(6):1826–1831.
76. de Backer D, Aldecoa C, Njimi H, Vincent JL: **Dopamine versus norepinephrine in the treatment of septic shock: a meta-analysis*.** *Crit Care Med* 2012, **40**(3):725–730.

77. Regnier B, Rapin M, Gory G, Lemaire F, Teisseire B, Harari A: **Haemodynamic effects of dopamine in septic shock.** *Intensive Care Med* 1977, **3**:47–53.
78. Seguin P, Bellissant E, Le Tulzo Y, Laviolle B, Lessard Y, Thomas R, Mallédant Y: **Effects of epinephrine compared with the combination of dobutamine and norepinephrine on gastric perfusion in septic shock.** *Clin Pharmacol Ther* 2002, **71**:381–388.
79. Myburgh JA, Higgins A, Jovanovska A, CAT Study investigators: **A comparison of epinephrine and norepinephrine in critically ill patients.** *Intensive Care Med* 2008, **34**:2226–2234.
80. Holmes CL, Patel BM, Russell JA, Walley KR, Walley KR: **Physiology of vasopressin relevant to management of septic shock.** *Chest* 2001, **120**:989–1002.
81. White LE, Hassoun HT, Bihorac A, Moore LJ, Sailors RM, McKinley BA, Valdivia A, Moore FA: **Acute kidney injury is surprisingly common and a powerful predictor of mortality in surgical sepsis.** *J Trauma Acute Care Surg* 2013, **75**(3):432–438.
82. Marshall JC: **Principles of source control in the early management of sepsis.** *Curr Infect Dis Rep* 2010, **12**(5):345–353.
83. Marshall JC, al Naqbi A: **Principles of source control in the management of sepsis.** *Crit Care Clin* 2009, **25**(4):753–768.
84. Wacha H, Hau T, Dittmer R, Ohmann C: **Risk factors associated with intraabdominal infections: a prospective multicenter study. Peritonitis study group.** *langenbecks Arch Surg* 1999, **384**:24–32.
85. Sugimoto K, Hirata M, Kikuno T, Takishima T, Maekawa K, Ohwada T: **Large-volume intraoperative peritoneal lavage with an assistant device for treatment of peritonitis caused by blunt traumatic rupture of the small bowel.** *J Trauma* 1995, **39**(4):689–692.
86. Lopez N, Kobayashi L, Coimbra R: **A Comprehensive review of abdominal infections.** *World J Emerg Surg* 2011, **6**:7.
87. Agresta F, Ciardo LF, Mazzarolo G, Michelet I, Orsi G, Trentin G, Bedin N: **Peritonitis: laparoscopic approach.** *World J Emerg Surg* 2006, **24**:1–9.
88. Anderson ID, Fearon KC, Grant IS: **Laparotomy for abdominal sepsis in the critically ill.** *Br J Surg* 1996, **83**(4):535–539.
89. Koperna T, Semmler D, Marian F: **Risk stratification in emergency surgical patients: is the APACHE II score a reliable marker of physiological impairment?** *Arch Surg* 2001, **136**(1):55–59.
90. van Ruler O, Kiewiet JJ, Boer KR, Lamme B, Gouma DJ, Boermeester MA, Reitsma JB: **Failure of available scoring systems to predict ongoing infection in patients with abdominal sepsis after their initial emergency laparotomy.** *BMC Surg* 2011, **23**:11–38.
91. Koperna T, Schulz F: **Relaparotomy in peritonitis: prognosis and treatment of patients with persisting intraabdominal infection.** *World J Surg* 2000, **24**(1):32–37.
92. van Ruler O, Lamme B, de Vos R, Obertop H, Reitsma JB, Boermeester MA: **Decision making for relaparotomy in secondary peritonitis.** *Dig Surg* 2008, **25**(5):339–346.
93. Lamme B, Mahler CW, van Ruler O, Gouma DJ, Reitsma JB, Boermeester MA: **Clinical predictors of ongoing infection in secondary peritonitis: systematic review.** *World J Surg* 2006, **30**(12):2170–2181.
94. Hinsdale JG, Jaffe BM: **Re-operation for intra-abdominal sepsis. Indications and results in modern critical care setting.** *Ann Surg* 1984, **199**(1):31–36.
95. Hutchins RR, Gunning MP, Lucas DN, Allen-Mersh TG, Soni NC: **Relaparotomy for suspected intraperitoneal sepsis after abdominal surgery.** *World J Surg* 2004, **28**(2):137–141.
96. van Ruler O, Lamme B, Gouma DJ, Reitsma JB, Boermeester MA: **Variables associated with positive findings at relaparotomy in patients with secondary peritonitis.** *Crit Care Med* 2007, **35**(2):468–476.
97. Holzheimer RG, Gathof B: **Re-operation for complicated secondary peritonitis-how to identify patients at risk for persistent sepsis.** *Eur J Med Res* 2003, **8**(3):125–134.
98. van Ruler O, Mahler CW, Boer KR, Reuland EA, Gooszen HG, Opmeer BC, de Graaf PW, Lamme B, Gerhards MF, Steller EP, van Till JW, de Borgie CJ, Gouma DJ, Reitsma JB, Boermeester MA: **Comparison of on-demand vs planned relaparotomy strategy in patients with severe peritonitis: a randomized trial.** *JAMA* 2007, **298**:865–872.
99. Robledo FA, Luque-de-León E, Suárez R, Sánchez P, de-la-Fuente M, Vargas A, Mier J: **Open versus closed management of the abdomen in the surgical treatment of severe secondary peritonitis: a randomized clinical trial.** *Surg Infect (Larchmt)* 2007, **8**:63–72.
100. Kirkpatrick AW, Roberts DJ, de Waele J, Jaeschke R, Malbrain ML, de Keulenaer B, Duchesne J, Bjorck M, Leppaniemi A, Ejike JC, Sugrue M, Cheatham M, Ivatury R, Ball CG, Reintam Blaser A, Regli A, Balogh ZJ, D'Amours S, Debergh D, Kaplan M, Kimball E, Olvera C: **Pediatric Guidelines Sub-Committee for the World Society of the Abdominal Compartment Syndrome. Intra-abdominal hypertension and the abdominal compartment syndrome: updated consensus definitions and clinical practice guidelines from the World Society of the Abdominal Compartment Syndrome.** *Intensive Care Med* 2013, **39**(7):1190–1206.
101. Merrell RC: **The abdomen as source of sepsis in critically ill patients.** *Crit Care Clin* 1995, **11**(2):255–272.
102. Waibel BH, Rotondo MF: **Damage control in trauma and abdominal sepsis.** *Crit Care Med* 2010, **38**(9 Suppl):S421–S430.
103. Jansen JO, Loudon MA: **Damage control surgery in a non-trauma setting.** *Br J Surg* 2007, **94**(7):789–790.
104. Amin AI, Shaikh IA: **Topical negative pressure in managing severe peritonitis: a positive contribution?** *World J Gastroenterol* 2009, **15**(27):3394–3397.
105. Schmelzle M, Alldinger I, Matthaei H, Aydin F, Wallert I, Eisenberger CF, Schulte Am Esch J 2nd, Dizdar L, Topp SA, Yang Q, Knoefel WT: **Long-term vacuum-assisted closure in open abdomen due to secondary peritonitis: a retrospective evaluation of a selected group of patients.** *Dig Surg* 2010, **27**(4):272–278.
106. Schein M: **Planned reoperations and open management in critical intra-abdominal infections: prospective experience in 52 cases.** *World J Surg* 1991, **15**:537–545.
107. Adkins AL, Robbins J, Villalba M, Bendick P, Shanley CJ: **Open abdomen management of intra-abdominal sepsis.** *Am Surg* 2004, **70**:137–140.
108. Horwood J, Akbar F, Maw A: **Initial experience of laparostomy with immediate vacuum therapy in patients with severe peritonitis.** *Ann R Coll Surg Engl* 2009, **91**(8):681–687.
109. Demetriades D: **Total management of the open abdomen.** *Int Wound J* 2012, **9**(Suppl 1):17–24.
110. Paul JS, Ridolfi TJ: **A case study in intra-abdominal sepsis.** *Surg Clin North Am* 2012, **92**(6):1661–1677.
111. Rotondo MF, Schwab CW, McGonigal MD, Phillips GR 3rd, Fruchterman TM, Kauder DR, Latenser BA, Angood PA: **'Damage control': an approach for improved survival in exsanguinating penetrating abdominal injury.** *J Trauma* 1993, **35**(3):375–382.
112. Godat L, Kobayashi L, Costantini T, Coimbra R: **Abdominal damage control surgery and reconstruction: World society of emergency surgery position paper.** *World J Emerg Surg* 2013, **8**(1):53.
113. Waibel BH, Rotondo MM: **Damage control surgery: it's evolution over the last 20 years.** *Rev Col Bras Cir* 2012, **39**(4):314–321.
114. Moore LJ, Moore FA: **Epidemiology of sepsis in surgical patients.** *Surg Clin North Am* 2012, **92**(6):1425–1443.
115. Ordoñez CA, Pino LF, Badiel M, Sánchez AI, Loaiza J, Ballestas L, Puyana JC: **Safety of performing a delayed anastomosis during damage control laparotomy in patients with destructive colon injuries.** *J Trauma* 2011, **71**(6):1512–1517.
116. Ordonez CA, Sanchez AI, Pineda JA, Badiel M, Mesa R, Cardona U, Arias R, RossoF, Granados M, Gutiérrez-Martínez MI, Ochoa JB, Peitzman A, Puyana JC: **Deferred primary anastomosis versus diversion in patients with severe secondary peritonitis managed with staged laparotomies.** *World J Surg* 2010, **34**:169–176.
117. Perathoner A, Klaus A, Muhlmann G, Oberwalder M, Margreiter R, Kafka-Ritsch, Oberwalder M, Margreiter R, Kafka-Ritsch Q: **Damage control with abdominal vacuum therapy (VAC) to manage perforated diverticulitis with advanced generalized peritonitis – a proof of concept.** *Int J Colorectal Dis* 2010, **25**:767–774.
118. Kafka-Ritsch R, Birkfellner F, Perathoner A, Raab H, Nehoda H, Pratschke J, Zitt M: **Damage control surgery with abdominal vacuum and delayed bowel reconstruction in patients with perforated diverticulitis Hinchey III/IV.** *J Gastroenterol Surg* 2012, **16**:1915–1922.
119. Yuan Y, Ren J, He Y: **Current status of the open abdomen treatment for intra-abdominal infection.** *Gastroenterol Res Pract* 2013:532013. Epub 2013 Oct 2.
120. Regner JL, Kobayashi L, Coimbra R: **Surgical strategies for management of the open abdomen.** *World J Surg* 2012, **36**(3):497–510.
121. Padalino P, Dionigi G, Minoja G, Carcano G, Rovera F, Boni L, Dionigi R: **Fascia-to-fascia closure with abdominal topical negative pressure for severe abdominal infections: preliminary results in a department of**

general surgery and intensive care unit. *Surg Infect (Larchmt)* 2010, **11**(6):523–528.

122. Tsuei BJ, Skinner JC, Bernard AC, Kearney PA, Boulanger BR: **The open peritoneal cavity: etiology correlates with the likelihood of fascial closure.** *Am Surg* 2004, **70**(7):652–656.
123. Pliakos I, Papavramidis TS, Mihalopoulos N, Koulouris H, Kesisoglou I, Sapalidis K, Deligiannidis N, Papavramidis S: **Vacuum-assisted closure in severe abdominal sepsis with or without retention sutured sequential fascial closure: a clinical trial.** *Surgery* 2010, **148**(5):947–953.
124. Roberts DJ, Zygun DA, Grendar J, Ball CG, Robertson HL, Ouellet JF, Cheatham ML, Kirkpatrick AW: **Negative-pressure wound therapy for critically ill adults with open abdominal wounds: a systematic review.** *J Trauma Acute Care Surg* 2012, **73**(3):629–639.
125. Kubiak BD, Albert SP, Gatto LA, Snyder KP, Maier KG, Vieau CJ, Roy S, Nieman GF: **Peritoneal negative pressure therapy prevents multiple organ injury in a chronic porcine sepsis and ischemia/reperfusion model.** *Shock* 2010, **34:**525–534.
126. Plaudis H, Rudzats A, Melberga L, Kazaka I, Suba O, Pupelis G: **Abdominal negative-pressure therapy: a new method in countering abdominal compartment and peritonitis - prospective study and critical review of literature.** *Ann Intensive Care* 2012, **20**(2 Suppl 1):S23.
127. Boele van Hensbroek P, Wind J, Dijkgraaf MG, Busch OR, Goslings JC: **Temporary closure of the open abdomen: a systematic review on delayed primary fascial closure in patients with an open abdomen.** *World J Surg* 2009, **33**(2):199–207.
128. Rasilainen SK, Mentula PJ, Leppäniemi AK: **Vacuum and mesh-mediated fascial traction for primary closure of the open abdomen in critically ill surgical patients.** *Br J Surg* 2012, **99**(12):1725–1732.
129. Kissane NA, Itani KM: **A decade of ventral incisional hernia repairs with biologic acellular dermal matrix: what have we learned?** *Plast Reconstr Surg* 2012, **130**(5 Suppl 2):194S–202S.
130. Dellinger RP, Levy MM, Carlet JM, Bion J, Parker MM, Jaeschke R, Reinhart K, Angus DC, Brun-Buisson C, Beale R, Calandra T, Dhainaut JF, Gerlach H, Harvey M, Marini JJ, Marshall J, Ranieri M, Ramsay G, Sevransky J, Thompson BT, Townsend S, Vender JS, Zimmerman JL, Vincent JL, International Surviving Sepsis Campaign Guidelines Committee; American Association of Critical-Care Nurses; American College of Chest Physicians; American College of Emergency Physicians; Canadian Critical Care Society; European Society of Clinical Microbiology and Infectious Diseases; European Society of Intensive Care Medicine; European Respiratory Society; International Sepsis Forum; Japanese Association for Acute Medicine; Japanese Society of Intensive Care Medicine; Society of Critical Care Medicine; Society of Hospital Medicine; Surgical Infection Society; World Federation of Societies of Intensive and Critical Care Medicine: **Surviving Sepsis Campaign: International guidelines for management of severe sepsis and septic shock.** *Crit Care Med* 2008, **36:**296–327.
131. Bernard GR, Vincent JL, Laterre PF, LaRosa SP, Dhainaut JF, Lopez-Rodriguez A, Steingrub JS, Garber GE, Helterbrand JD, Ely EW, Fisher CJ Jr: **Recombinant human protein C Worldwide Evaluation in Severe Sepsis (PROWESS) study group. Efficacy and safety of recombinant human activated protein C for severe sepsis.** *N Engl J Med* 2001, **344:**699–709.
132. Hodder RV, Hall R, Russell JA, Fisher HN, Lee B: **Early drotrecogin alpha (activated) administration in severe sepsis is associated with lower mortality: a retrospective analysis of the Canadian ENHANCE cohort.** *Crit Care* 2009, **13**(3):R78.
133. Finfer S, Ranieri VM, Thompson BT, Barie PS, Dhainaut JF, Douglas IS, Gårdlund B, Marshall JC, Rhodes A: **Design, conduct, analysis and reporting of a multi-national placebo-controlled trial of activated protein C for persistent septic shock.** *Intensive Care Med* 2008, **34**(11):1935–1947.
134. Savel RH, Munro CL: **Evidence-based backlash: the tale of drotrecogin alfa.** *Am J Crit Care* 2012, **21**(2):81–83.
135. Annane D, Bellissant E, Bollaert PE, Briegel J, Confalonieri M, de Gaudio R, Keh D, Kupfer Y, Oppert M, Meduri GU: **Corticosteroids in the treatment of severe sepsis and septic shock in adults: a systematic review.** *JAMA* 2009, **301**(22):2362–2375.
136. Annane D: **Corticosteroids for severe sepsis: an evidence-based guide for physicians.** *Ann Intensive Care* 2011, **1**(1):7.
137. Cohen J, Chin wD: **Nutrition and sepsis.** *World Rev Nutr Diet* 2013, **105:**116–125.
138. Marik PE, Zaloga GP: **Early enteral nutrition in acutely ill patients: a systematic review.** *Crit Care Med* 2001, **29:**2264–2270.
139. Heyland DK, Dhaliwal R, Drover JW, Gramlich L, Dodek P: **Canadian critical care clinical practice guidelines committee: Canadian clinical practice guidelines for nutrition support in mechanically ventilated, critically ill adult patients.** *JPEN J Parenter Enteral Nutr* 2003, **27:**355–373.
140. Doig GS, Heighes PT, Simpson F, Sweetman EA, Davies AR: **Early enteral nutrition, provided within 24 h of injury or intensive care unit admission, significantly reduces mortality in critically ill patients: a meta-analysis of randomised controlled trials.** *Intensive Care Med* 2009, **35:**2018–2027.

6

Role of clinical judgment and tissue harmonic imaging ultrasonography in diagnosis of paediatric acute appendicitis

Ossama Zakaria[1,2*], Tamer A Sultan[3], Tarek H Khalil[4] and Tamer Wahba[5]

Abstract

Background: Appendicitis is the most common surgical emergency in children; yet, diagnosis of equivocal presentations continues to challenge clinicians.

Aim: The objective of this study was to investigate the hypothesis that the use of a modified clinical practice and harmonic ultrasonographic grading scores (MCPGS) may improve the accuracy in diagnosing acute appendicitis in the pediatric population.

Patients & Methods

Main outcome measures: Sensitivity, specificity, and accuracy of the modified scoring system. Five hundred and thirty patients presented with suspected diagnosis of acute appendicitis during the period from December 2000 to December 2009 were enrolled in this study. Children's data that have already been published of those who presented with suspected diagnosis of acute appendicitis- to whom a special clinical practice grading scores (CPGS) incorporating clinical judgment and results of gray scale ultrasonography (US) was applied- were reviewed and compared to the data of 265 pediatric patients with equivocal diagnosis of acute appendicitis (AA), to whom a modified clinical practice grading scores (MCPGS) was applied. Statistical analyses were carried out using Z test for comparing 2 sample proportions and student's *t*-test to compare the quantitative data in both groups. Sensitivity and specificity for the 2 scoring systems were calculated using Epi-Info software.

Results: The Number of appendectomies declined from 200 (75.5%) in our previous CPGS to 187 (70.6%) in the MCPGS ($P > 0.05$).

Specificity was significantly higher when applying MCPGS (90.7%) in this study compared to 70.47% in our previous work when CPGS was applied ($P < 0.01$). Furthermore, the positive predictive value (PPV) was significantly higher (95.72%) than in our previous study (82.88%), ($P < 0.01$). Overall agreement (accuracy) of MCPGS was 96.98%. Kappa = 0.929 ($P < 0.001$). Negative predictive power was 100%. And the Overall agreement (accuracy) was 96.98%.

Conclusions: MCPGS tends to help in reduce the numbers of avoidable and unnecessary appendectomies in suspected cases of pediatric acute appendicitis that may help in saving hospital resources.

Keywords: Acute appendicitis in Children, Tissue Harmonic Imaging (THI), Ultrasound scan, Appendicitis clinical score

* Correspondence: ossamaz2004@yahoo.com

[1]Division of Pediatric Surgery, Departments of Surgery, Faculty of Medicine, Suez Canal University, Ismailia, Egypt

Full list of author information is available at the end of the article

Introduction

Certainty of clinical diagnosis is the most challenging task in clinical practice. It is relatively straight forward to look up the treatment once a correct diagnosis has been made. A single perfect diagnostic test for acute appendicitis does not exist [1-3].

Despite the number of algorithms and diagnostic tests available, about 20% of patients with appendicitis are misdiagnosed [3-9].

Presence of normal appendix ranges from 5-25% out of suspected cases of acute appendicitis [5,10-13]. Negative appendectomies were thought to be relatively harmless; nevertheless, they result in considerable unnecessary clinical and economic costs [14]. Even despite the uncertainty of diagnosis, appendicitis demands prompt treatment in order not to be neglected and misdiagnosed leading to progression of the disease with its associated morbidity and mortality that may include the risk of perforation which happens in approximately one third of the cases [5,15,16].

In an attempt to improve diagnosis, attention has turned to radiological imaging. The use of ultrasound scan (US) has been advocated as the readily available simple and fast imaging modality particularly in thin patients and children. A normal appendix is not frequently observed using gray-scale US [17,18]. On the other hand Harmonic imaging (HI) increases the contrast and spatial resolution resulting in artifact-free images, and has been shown to significantly improve abdominal ultrasonography. Only a handful of reports exist regarding its application in pediatric patients. Most of them do not encompass its use in acute appendicitis [19].

This work aimed to investigate and assess the hypothesis that the use of a modified clinical grading judgment and Tissue Harmonic Imaging ultrasonography (THI), as a modified score-aided diagnosis; MCPGS may improve the accuracy in the diagnosis of children with equivocal pictures of acute appendicitis and to compare these results with those of previously published data of CPGS [1,2].

Patients and Methods

This two centers study was carried out during the period from December 2000 to December 2009. Data of pediatric patients with suspected acute appendicitis who underwent the clinical judgment and US score aided CGPS were reviewed; this data was published before [1].

This was a modification of previously published scoring methods [2,3] including certain subjective clinical parameters measured as 1 point such as fever of 38, anorexia and vomiting, tachycardia of more than 120 beats/minute. Abdominal pain parameters were also measured with special emphasis on guarding or rigidity, positive per-rectal examinations, however, positive rebound tenderness was given 3 points in this score method as well as other clinical, laboratory and harmonic US measurements (Table 1).

Two hundred sixty five (265) pediatric patients were the core of our current study. In those patients; the proposed usage of THI, clinical judgment and practice as a modified score aided system MCPGS was applied.

The MCPGS with twenty five variables including harmonic ultrasound (US) examination and a marker of inflammatory response was assessed in multivariate analysis using the finding of acute appendicitis at operation as the end point were enrolled in this study (Table 2). Exclusion criteria included those who were proved to have other causes of acute abdominal pain rather than acute appendicitis.

Ultrasonography was performed using linear and curved transducers with ultrasound frequencies ranged between 2.5 and 7.5 MHz, commercially available ultrasound systems (Siemens Sonoline Elegra, Germany). The examination was performed with both conventional and THI- US. Scanning parameters were optimized for each method, and all images were obtained with use of the same focal zone. A cine playback mode was used to obtain identical images in two standard planes, longitudinal and transverse scans. Images were obtained with the two methods in random sequence to facilitate their masking for the observers. Harmonic images were acquired at a transmitting frequency of 2.0 MHz and a receiving harmonic bandwidth of 4.0 MHz. Conventional US images were obtained at a frequency of 3.5 MHz, which is the commonly used frequency at abdominal imaging in adults. The harmonic and conventional US modes were switched by means of a toggle switch on the scanner control panel. In both the previous CPGS and the current MCPGS rationale of active watchful waiting in suspected appendicitis was a prudent and safe strategy with the use of at least one time repetition of conventional US or THI- US with no increase in the risk of perforation (Figures 1,2,3). All appendices were routinely sent for histopathological examination.

Collected data were statistically analyzed using χ^2 test. Continuous variables were analyzed using student's *t*-test. $P \leq 0.5$ were considered statistically significant. Sensitivity and specificity were calculated for the CPGS. Kappa test was used to verify the specificity. All calculations were performed using SAS version 8.2.

Results

In the current studied group of patients; age and sex analysis shows that cases with and without appendectomy are similar and there is no aggregation of cases in a certain age group or in a certain sex (Table 3). In 187

Table 1 Clinical Practice Guideline Scoring System (CPGS) [1]:

			1	0	Score
Clinical data	General	- Fever	Yes	No	
		- HR	> 120/min.	< 120/min.	
		- Vomiting	Yes	No	
		- Dehydration	Yes	No	
	Abdominal	***Abd. pain***			
		- Localized	Yes	No	
		- History of similar - attacks	No	Yes	
		- Character	Constant	Intermittent	
		- Severity	Intolerable	Tolerable	
		- Course	Progressive	Regressive	
		- Relief by antispasmodic	No	Yes	
		- Bowel Habit alteration	Yes	No	
		- Rebound tenderness	Yes (3)	No	
		- Guarding or rigidity	Yes	No	
		- +ve P.R. examination	Yes	No	
Investigations	Laboratory	- WBCs leukocytosis	Yes	No	
		- Urine analysis (Findings of UTI)	Yes	No	
	Focused abdominal U.S.	- Appendicitis or mass	Yes	No	
		- +ve findings in female Adnxae	No	Yes	
		- +ve findings in liver, Gall bladder, billiary passages	No	Yes	
		- +ve findings kidneys	No	Yes	
		- Free fluid	Yes	No	
Total score					

Interpretation of results:
21 - 15 = highly suggestive of appendicitis.
14 - 8 = Patient needs repeated evaluation for conclusive result.
7 - 0 = the diagnosis of acute appendicitis in not likely.

patients (70.6%) appendectomy was performed, out of them 90 patients (48.1%) showed MCPGS between 15 and 22, those patients were kept with no oral feeding (NPO), intravenous fluid infusion (IV fluid) of appropriate type and amount according to patient's age before undergoing appendectomy. Only 8 out of the total appendectomies (4.3%) were normal at histopathological evaluation. The remaining 97 patients (36.6%) initially showed MCPGS of 8-14. On repeated evaluation every 2 hours for a maximum of 6 times and repetition of THI-US during the repeated evaluation for at least one time, their score progressed to 15 or more [61 patients (62.9%) with a MCPGS of 15-17, 11 patients (11.3%) with MCPGS of 18, and 25 patients (25.8%) with MCPGS of 19]. During the observation period, no antibiotics were given in order not to alter the clinical picture. However, antibiotics were started once the diagnosis was confirmed. No false negative cases were recorded when using MCPGS. (Tables 3, 4)

On the other hand, 78 children (29.4%) did not undergo appendectomy, 48 of them (61.5%) showed MCPGS of 8 or less at the initial examination, they were referred to the Pediatric Medical Care with no need for surgical interventions. Thirty patients (38.5%) showed MCPGS between 9 and 14 declining with repeated examinations until their score became definitely 8 or less, they were managed medically. (Tables 5, 6)

Specificity of MCPGS was higher than that of CPGS, this may be attributed to the use of harmonic US in this modified scoring system that seems to be significantly superior to the conventional grey scale US 90.69% in group I (Table 5) compared to a specificity of 70.47% in group II ($Z = 5.999$, $P < 0.01$). Also the Positive Predictive Value for group II (95.72%) was significantly higher than that of group I ($Z = 4.727$, $P < 0.01$). Applying Kappa analysis revealed the Kappa Measure for over all agreement to be (96.98%). These results show the high specificity of our finding for the MCPGS. (Figure 4)

Discussion

Acute appendicitis traditionally has been a clinical diagnosis and remains so to this day. The diagnosis can be difficult to make in many children who may present with typical symptoms or an equivocal physical examination [18].

In our current study, we evaluated the newly advocated modified clinical practice grading score (MCPGS);

Table 2 Modified clinical practice and harmonic ultrasonographic grading score (MCPGS):

			1	0	Score
Clinical data	**General**	- Fever	Yes	No	
		- HR	> 120/min.	< 120/min.	
		- Vomiting	Yes	No	
	Abdominal	***Abd. Pain***			
		- Localized	Yes	No	
		- History of similar - attacks	No	Yes	
		- Character	Constant	Intermittent	
		- Severity	Intolerable	Tolerable	
		- Course	Progressive	Regressive	
		- Relief by antispasmodic	No	Yes	
		- Bowel Habit alteration	Yes	No	
		- Tenderness	Yes	No	
		- Guarding or rigidity	Yes	No	
		- +ve P.R.	Yes	No	
		Associated intra- abdomin,. Disease	No	Yes	
Investigations	**Laboratory**	- High WBCs	Yes	No	
		- Elevated CRP	Yes	No	
		- Urine analysis (Findings of UTI)	No	Yes	
	Tissue Harmonic U.S. RLQ	-Aperistaltic non-Compressible blind ended tubular structure	Yes	No	
		-Distinct thickened appendicial wall layers	Yes	No	
		- Outer diameter > 6 mm	Yes	No	
		-Target sign appearance	Yes	No	
		-Appendicolith(s)	Yes	No	
		-Periappendiceal fluid collection	Yes	No	
		- Echogenic Prominent pericecal fat Appendicolith	Yes	No	
		- +ve findings in female Adnxae	No	Yes	
Total score					

Interpretation of results:

15 - 25 = highly suggestive of appendicitis.

8 - 14 = Patient needs repeated evaluation for conclusive result.

0 - 7 = the diagnosis of acute appendicitis in not likely.

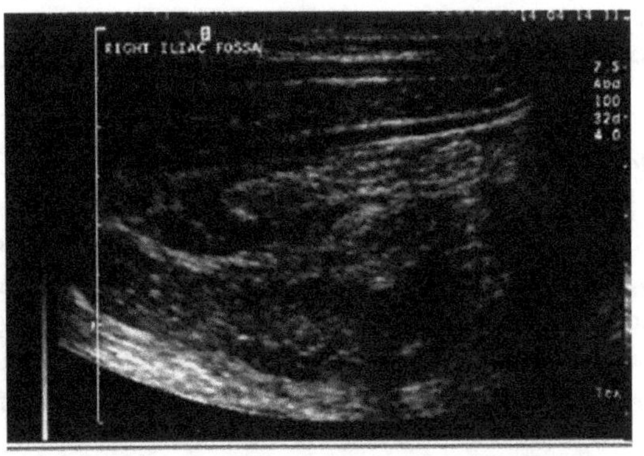

Figure 1 Acute appendicitis by conventional US in a longitudinal scan using linear transducer with 7.5 MHz frequency showing a thick walled blind ended apristaltic non compressible inflamed appendix.

based on clinical judgment, laboratory investigations for inflammatory response and THI- US examination studies in association with the strategy of active watchful waiting performing repeated clinical examinations as well as at least one time repetition of THI before the decision-making process. It was highly accurate in the diagnosis of acute appendicitis in children. The specificity of the MCPGS was 90.69% compared to a specificity of 70.47% in the children to whom CPGS and active watchful waiting strategy was applied. In addition, we observed a statistically significant decrease in the negative appendectomy rate in MCPGS compared with those in CPGS.

Our study aimed at avoiding the selection bias mentioned before in similar scoring system [19]. Age and sex analysis shows that cases with and without appendectomy

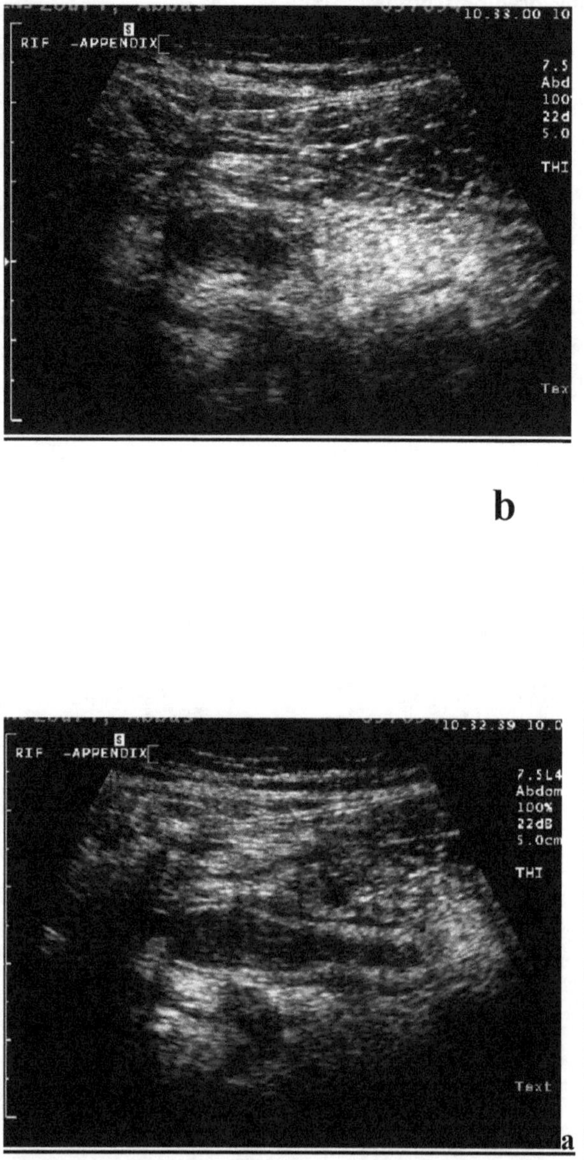

Figure 2 Acute appendicitis by tissue harmonic imaging sonography (THI) using linear transducer with 7.5 MHz revealed: A. Longitudinal scan showing aperistaltic non compressible blind ended tubular structure with distinct thickened wall layers and diameter > 6 mm. **B**. Transverse scan showing target sign appearance.

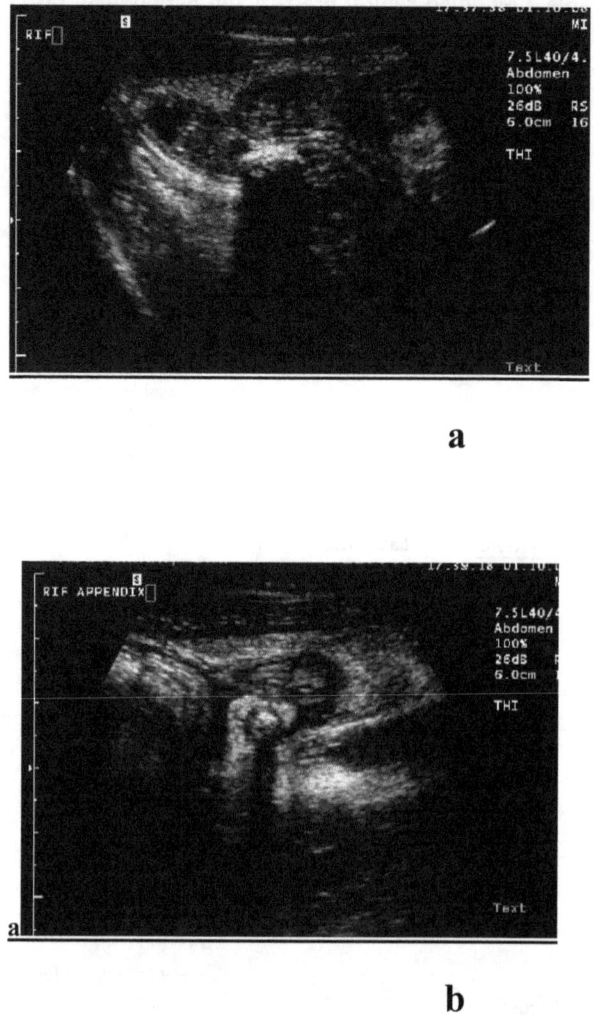

Figure 3 Acute appendicitis by tissue harmonic imaging sonography (THI) using linear transducer with 7.5 MHz revealed: A. Longitudinal scan showing a well defined adequately demarcated aperistaltic non compressible blind ended tubular structure with distinct thickened wall layers and diameter > 6 mm associated with intraluminal curvilinear calcification with posterior acoustic shadowing that reflects an appendicolith. **B**. Transverse scan showing target sign appearance with the appearance of the appendicolith with its characteristic posterior acoustic shadowing.

are similar and there is no aggregation of cases in a certain age group or in a certain sex. Therefore, the MCPGS can be used at any age and for any sex. Moreover, even those patients who were referred by pediatricians expected to be appendicitis were included as well as self referral that can be appendicitis or not. This illustrates that even if the cases are referred by pediatricians the score can still be used to differentiate cases.

The decrease in negative appendectomies occurred without a rise in the perforation rate. In fact, the perforation rate was lower under the MCPGS, although this change was not significant. Screening ultrasound scanning for pediatric appendicitis has suboptimal accuracy, particularly in obese children with a low likelihood of appendicitis who should not routinely undergo ultrasound scanning. However, when followed by a second ultrasound scanning or a clinical reassessment, it offers high diagnostic accuracy in lean children [20].

Targeted abdominal examination as well as THI constituted around 75% of our MCPGS scoring system with the aim of increasing its specificity without affecting the system sensitivity.

Table 3 Characteristics of studied children with clinically suspected appendicitis

Character	Number (%)
Age (months)	
Minimum-maximum (mean ± SD)	18-203 (140.63 ± 25.923)
Gender	
Male	159 (60.0%)
Female	106 (40.0%)
Referring site	
None (parent decision)	229 (86.4%)
Health establishment (Pediatrician)	36 (13.6%)
Duration of symptoms before admission (hours)	
Minimum-maximum (mean ± SD)	6-48 (23.15 ± 11.182)
MCPGS*	
Minimum-maximum (mean ± SD)	1-22 (11.54 ± 6.113)
Final Outcome	
No surgery	78 (29.4%)
Appendectomy with negative histopathology	8 (3.0%)
Appendectomy with positive histopathology	179 (67.6%)

MCPGS = Modified Clinical Practice Guideline Score

In our previously published data [1]; traditional clinical judgment and grey scale US score aided CPGS was performed, 200 patients (75.5%) underwent appendectomy, of them 35 appendices (17.5%) were normal at histopathological evaluation. The remaining 65 patients (24.5%) were discharged from the Pediatric Surgical Facility as not having appendicitis. Yet, out of those 65; 3 children (4.6%), (2 males and 1 female) were re-admitted. US was repeated suggesting acute appendicitis. They underwent appendectomy with positive pathological results. A total of 203 appendectomies (76.6%) were performed in this CPGS group.

Table 5 Significant predictors of acute appendicitis using forward likelihood multiple logistic models

Predictor	β coefficient	Wald test	Exp B	95% Confidence Interval	
				LL	UL
MCPGS	0.795	50.851	2.214	1.780	2.755
Duration	-0.052	3.795	0.949	0.901	1.00
Constant	-5.187	25.711			

The model succeeded to correctly diagnose 95.5% of all cases, 97.2% of the positive cases, and 91.9% of the negative cases.
LL = Lower limit of the confidence interval of the odds ratio
UP = Upper limit of the confidence interval of the odds ratio (Exp B)

Moreover, our current results showed the superiority of THI over conventional US for lesion visibility, with THI being preferred over conventional US for 65% of cases. The findings were clearer and better defined with THI which thereby improved the detection of subtle lesions. Tissue harmonic imaging theoretically improved signal-to-noise ratios by reducing noise from side lobe artifact in the near field and echo detection from multiple scattering events.

This reduced noise was most likely responsible for the superiority of THI over conventional US in the visualization of the findings and improved the confidence of diagnosis for most cases. THI was superior to conventional US in the visualization of lesions containing highly reflective tissues such as fat, calcium and air. It is therefore recommended to be used in obese patients. Better definition of the posterior acoustic shadows in calcifications and appendicolith(s) [21-28].

In our previous study the negative appendectomy rate was 17.5% compared to 4.3% in the current work. Contrary to our previous results [1] some published data expressed a negative appendectomy rate of 5.5% by applying somewhat similar scoring system [19]. The reason for such difference may be their use of computerized tomography scanning (CT) in their system. However, the difference in the negative appendectomy

Table 4 Comparing characteristics of children with and without appendicitis

Character	With Appendicitis# (n = 179)	Without Appendicitis (n = 86)	Test *(P)*
Age (mean ± SD)	141.87 ± 23.584	138.06 ± 30.206	*t* = 1.12 (0.264)
Gender			X2 = 0.413 (0.520)
Male	105 (58.7)	54 (62.8)	
Female	74 (41.3)	32 (37.2)	
Referring Agent			X2 = 0.015 (0.903)
None	155 (86.6)	74 (86.0)	
Pediatrician	24 (13.4)	12 (14.0)	
Duration (mean ± SD)	22.54 ± 11.224	24.43 ± 11.051	Z = 1.497 (0.134)
MCPGS (mean ± SD)	14.82 ± 4.185	4.72 ± 3.120	12.393* (< 0.001)

* Significant, P < 0.05.
\# include no surgery and surgery with negative histopathology

Table 6 Diagnostic screening criteria of MCPGS to detect children with acute appendicitis

MCPGS	Acute Appendicitis	Free	Total
Positive score (8+)	179 (100.0)	8 (9.3)	187 (70.6)
Negative score (< 8)	0 (0.0)	78 (90.7)	78 (29.4)
Total	179 (100.0)	86 (100.0)	265 (100.0)

Sensitivity = 100%
Specificity = 90.7%
Positive predictive power = 95.72%
Negative predictive power = 100%
Overall agreement (accuracy) = 96.98%
Kappa = 0.929 (P < 0.001)

rate does not support the use of such an expensive sophisticated and hazardous radiological tool to children. CT scanning is not always available in all centers limiting its incorporation in clinical practice guideline scoring system. A recently published study of a practice guideline found that CT scan did not improve the accuracy of diagnosis in patients with suspected appendicitis [29]. Their guideline did not specifically address the appropriate use of CT scan.

Our MCPGS results, however, did show a great decline in the rate of negative appendectomies. This goes with data of some authors who showed that an imaging protocol using US followed by CT in their patients with equivocal presentations improved the accuracy of diagnosis of appendicitis [30].

We presented our results of MCPGS which evolved from this and other studies recommending ultrasound as the imaging modality of choice in most patients. In addition the recommendation of MCPGS was not limited to imaging alone. Most clinical practice scoring guidelines encourage, but do not require complaints with recommendations [31]. Measuring complaints can be challenging because scoring guidelines can include numerous recommendations and because patients, especially children do not always match preconceived scenarios [32]. Although many barriers limit physician acceptance of scoring guidelines [33], the compliance with our MCPGS is consistent with other developed

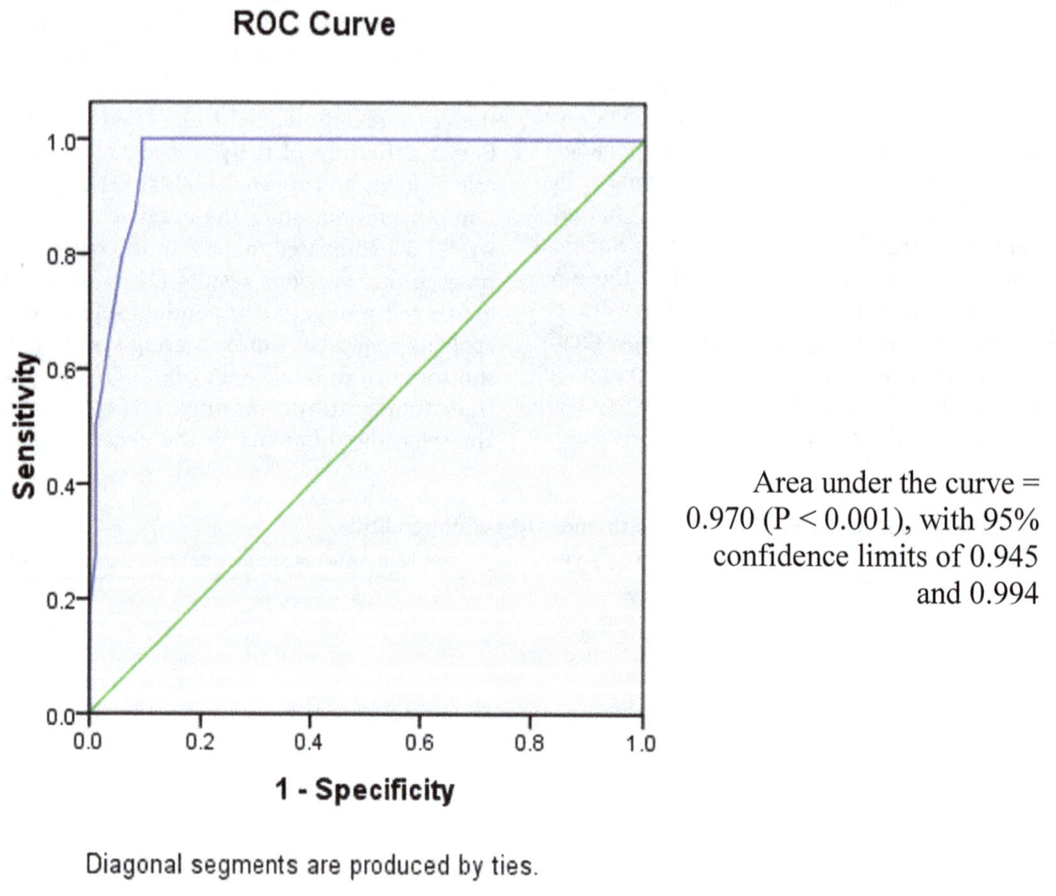

Figure 4 Receiver operating Characteristics curve of MCPGS to detect children with acute appendicitis. Area under the curve = 0.970 (P < 0.001), with 95% confidence limits of 0.945 and 0.994

practice scoring guidelines [2,3,6-9,34]. A considerable portion of the improvement seen in our study could be because of the utilization and accuracy of suitable imaging.

Practice scoring guidelines and clinical pathways have been implemented for many conditions [26], including acute appendicitis [16,30,35]. Analysis of such guidelines can focus on any combination of patient outcome, resource utilization or complaints with recommendation [16,34-38].

Although most appendicitis scoring guideline and pathways focus on decreasing postoperative treatment cost, a few concentrate diagnosis itself. One such pathway in a pediatric hospital achieved a significant reduction in the number of laboratory tests and X-rays without adversely affecting the incidence of negative appendectomies or perforation [34].

In our proposed MCPGS we included the minimum necessary laboratory investigations to measure the inflammatory response and time and effort saving tissue harmonic abdominal ultrasound scan in order to decrease the probabilities of misdiagnosing acute abdominal pain due to other reasons as acute appendicitis.

In our previous and current studies; all patients underwent the active watchful waiting strategy. This excludes that the decision-making process did result strictly from the MCPGS, and was not rather based on the repeated clinical re-evaluation that was adopted also on CPGS. This exactly shows that our proposed score is superior to the real life common clinical practice.

It may be concluded that the use of a modified clinical and THI ultrasonographic grading score (MCPGS) with the rationale of active watchful waiting in suspected appendicitis with at least one time repetition of THI-US was a prudent and safe strategy. It may improve the accuracy of diagnosing acute appendicitis in the pediatric population as it is superior to the real life common clinical practice.

It leads to fewer negative appendectomies compared with those children to whom it was not applied or other scoring systems were applied as the CPGS with the same strategy of active watchful waiting and repeated US, without a significant change in the perforation rate. Moreover, inpatient observation for serial examinations was reduced significantly. Our clinical practice grading scores can have considerable impact on the diagnosis of acute appendicitis in children. A larger cohort is necessary to validate our findings.

Acknowledgements
We would like to acknowledge Dr Essam Abd El Bari and Dr. M Yasser Ibrahim for their assistance in revising the manuscript.

Author details
[1]Division of Pediatric Surgery, Departments of Surgery, Faculty of Medicine, Suez Canal University, Ismailia, Egypt. [2]Sporting Students' Health Insurance Hospital, Alexandria, Egypt. [3]Department of Surgery Faculty of Medicine, Meoufyia University, Egypt. [4]Department of Radiology, Faculty of Medicine, Suez Canal University, Ismailia, Egypt. [5]Department of Radiology, Students' Hospital Alexandria University, Egypt.

Authors' contributions
OMZ has inspired the idea, collected the data and created the analysis and wrote most of the manuscript. TAS helped in collecting the data, analysis and writing of the manuscript. THK and TW have performed the sonography, collected the data and helped on manuscript writing. All authors read and approved the final manuscript.

Competing interests
The authors declare that they have no competing interests.

References

1. Zakaria OM, Adly OA, El-Labban GA, Khalil HT: **Acute Appendicitis In Children: A Clinical Practice Guideline Scoring System.** *Suez Canal Univ Med J* 2005, **8**:20-26.
2. François Y, Bonvoisin S, Descos L, Vignal J: **Prospective study of a predictive scoring system for the diagnosis of appendicitis in patients with right lower quadrant pain. Long-term outcome].** *Gastroenterol Clin Biol* 1991, **15**:794-799.
3. Samuel M: **Pediatric appendicitis score.** *J Pediatr Surg* 2002, **37**:877-881.
4. Rezak A, Abbas HM, Ajemian MS, Dudrick SJ, Kwasnik EM: **Decreased use of computed tomography with a modified clinical scoring system in diagnosis of pediatric acute appendicitis.** *Arch Surg* 2011, **146**:64-67.
5. Dado G, Anania G, Baccarani U, Marcotti E, Donini A, Risaliti A, Pasqualucci A, Bresadola F: **Application of a clinical score for the diagnosis of acute appendicitis in childhood: A retrospective analysis of 197 patients.** *J Pediatr Surg* 2000, **35**:1320-1322.
6. Escribá A, Gamell AM, Fernández Y, Quintillá JM, Cubells CL: **Prospective validation of two systems of classification for the diagnosis of acute appendicitis.** *Pediatr Emerg Care* 2011, **27**:165-169.
7. Shera AH, Nizami FA, Malik AA, Naikoo ZA, Wani MA: **Clinical scoring system for diagnosis of acute appendicitis in children.** *Indian J Pediatr* 2011, **78**:287-290.
8. Shreef KS, Waly AH, Abd-Elrahman S, Abd Elhafez MA: **Alvarado score as an admission criterion in children with pain in right iliac fossa.** *Afr J Paediatr Surg* 2010, **7**:163-165.
9. Bhatt M, Joseph L, Ducharme FM, Dougherty G, McGillivray D: **Prospective validation of the pediatric appendicitis score in a Canadian pediatric emergency department.** *Acad Emerg Med* 2009, **16**:591-596.
10. Neilson IR, Laberge JM, Nguyen LT, Moir C, Doody D, Sonnino RE, Youssef S, Guttman FM: **Appendicitis in children: Current therapeutic recommendations.** *J Pediatr Surg* 1990, **25**:1113-1116.
11. Pearl RH, Hale DA, Molloy M, Schutt DC, Jaques DP: **Pediatric appendectomy.** *J Pediatr Surg* 1995, **30**:173-178.
12. Körner H, Söndenaa K, Söreide JA, Andersen E, Nysted A, Lende TH, Kjellevold KH: **Incidence of acute nonperforated and perforated appendicitis: Age-specific and sex-specific analysis.** *World J Surg* 1997, **21**:313-317.
13. Stephen AE, Segev DL, Ryan DP, Mullins ME, Kim SH, Schnitzer JJ, Doody DP: **The diagnosis of acute appendicitis in a pediatric population: To CT or not to CT.** *J Pediatr Surg* 2003, **38**:367-371.
14. Partrick DA, Janik JE, Janik JS, Bensard DD, Karrer FM: **Increased CT scan utilization does not improve the diagnostic accuracy of appendicitis in children.** *J Pediatr Surg* 2003, **38**:659-662.
15. Flum DR, Koepsell T: **The clinical and economic correlates of misdiagnosed appendicitis: Nationwide analysis.** *Arch Surg* 2002, **137**:799-804.
16. Putnam TC, Gagliano N, Emmens RW: **Appendicitis in children.** *Surg Gynecol Obstet* 1990, **170**:527-532.

17. Emil S, Laberge JM, Mikhail P, Baican L, Flageole H, Nguyen L, Shaw K: **Appendicitis in Children: A Ten-Year Update of Therapeutic Recommendations.** *J Pediatr Surg* 2003, **38**:236-242.
18. Zielke A, Sitter H, Rampp T, Bohrer T, Rothmund M: **Clinical decision-making, ultrasonography, and scores for evaluation of suspected acute appendicitis.** *World J Surg* 2001, **25**:578-584.
19. Emil S, Mikhail P, Laberge JM, Flageole H, Nguyen LT, Shaw KS, Baican L, Oudjhane K: **Clinical versus sonographic evaluation of acute appendicitis in children: A comparison of patient characteristics and outcomes.** *J Pediatr Surg* 2001, **36**:780-783.
20. Schuh S, Man C, Cheng A, Murphy A, Mohanta A, Moineddin R, Tomlinson G, Langer JC, Doria AS: **Predictors of non-diagnostic ultrasound scanning in children with suspected appendicitis.** *J Pediatr* 2011, **158**:112-118.
21. Smink DS, Finkelstein JA, Garcia Peña BM, Shannon MW, Taylor GA, Fishman SJ: **Diagnosis of Acute Appendicitis in Children Using a Clinical Practice Guideline.** *J Pediatr Surg* 2004, **39**:458-463.
22. Perez J, Barone JE, Wilbanks TO, Jorgensson D, Corvo PR: **Liberal use of computed tomography scanning does not improve diagnostic accuracy in appendicitis.** *Am J Surg* 2003, **185**:194-197.
23. Peña BM, Taylor GA, Fishman SJ, Mandl KD: **Effect of an imaging protocol on clinical outcomes among pediatric patients with appendicitis.** *Pediatrics* 2002, **110**:1088-1093.
24. Grossman RG, Homer C, Goldman DA: **Case 2: Establishing and running a clinical practice guideline program at Children's Hospital, Boston.** In *Implementing Clinical Practice Guidelines.* Edited by: Margolis CZ, Cretin S. Chicago, IL, AHA Press; 1999:151-175.
25. Cretin S: **Evaluating and monitoring clinical practice guidelines.** In *Implementing Clinical Practice Guidelines.* Edited by: Margolis CZ, Cretin S. Chicago, IL, AHA Press; 1999:121-138.
26. Cabana MD, Rand CS, Powe NR, Wu AW, Wilson MH, Abboud PA, Rubin HR: **Why don't physicians follow clinical practice guidelines? A framework for improvement.** *JAMA* 1999, **282**:1458-1465.
27. Grimshaw JM, Russell IT: **Effect of clinical guidelines on medical practice: A systematic review of rigorous evaluations.** *Lancet* 1993, **342**:1317-1322.
28. Warner BW, Kulick RM, Stoops MM, Mehta S, Stephan M, Kotagal UR: **An evidenced-based clinical pathway for acute appendicitis decreases hospital duration and cost.** *J Pediatr Surg* 1998, **33**:1371-1375.
29. Firilas AM, Higginbotham PH, Johnson DD, Jackson RJ, Wagner CW, Smith SD: **A new economic benchmark for surgical treatment of appendicitis.** *Am Surg* 1999, **65**:769-773.
30. Choudhry S, Gorman B, Charboneau JW, Tradup DJ, Beck RJ, Kofler JM, Groth DS: **Comparison of Tissue Harmonic Imaging with Conventional US in Abdominal Disease.** *RadioGraphics* 2000, **20**:1127-1135.
31. Ward B, Baker AC, Humphrey VF: **Nonlinear propagation applied to the improvement of resolution in diagnostic medical ultrasound.** *J Acoust Soc Am* 1997, **101**:143-154.
32. Starritt HC, Duck FA, Hawkins AJ, Humphrey VF: **The development of harmonic distortion in pulsed finite-amplitude ultrasound passing through liver.** *Phys Med Biol* 1986, **31**:1401-1409.
33. Starritt HC, Perkins MA, Duck FA, Humphrey VF: **Evidence for ultrasonic finite-amplitude distortion in muscle using medical equipment.** *J Acoust Soc Am* 1985, **77**:302-306.
34. Muir TG: **Nonlinear effects in acoustic imaging.** *Acoust Imag* 1980, **9**:93-109.
35. Ragavendra N, Chen H, Powers JE, Nilawat C, Robert JM, Carangi C, Laifer-Narin SL: **Harmonic imaging of porcine intraovarian arteries using sonographic contrast medium: initial findings.** *Ultrasound Obstet Gynecol* 1997, **9**:266-270.
36. Wu JY, Shung KK: **Nonlinear energy exchange among harmonic modes and its applications to nonlinear imaging.** *J Acoust Soc Am* 1990, **88**:2852-2858.
37. Siegel S: **Nonparametric statistics for the behavioral sciences.** New York, NY: McGraw-Hill; 1956, 68-75.
38. Shapiro RS, Wagreich J, Parsons RB, Stancato-Pasik A, Yeh HC, Lao R: **Tissue harmonic imaging sonography: evaluation of image quality compared with conventional sonography.** *AJR Am J Roentgenol* 1998, **171**:1203-1206.

7

International normalized ratio and serum C-reactive protein are feasible markers to predict complicated appendicitis

Maru Kim, Sung-Jeep Kim and Hang Joo Cho*

Abstract

Background: Diagnostic approach for complicated appendicitis is still controversial. We planned this study to analyze preoperative laboratory markers that may predict complications of appendicitis.

Methods: Patients who underwent appendectomy were retrospectively recruited. They were divided into complicated appendicitis and non-complicated appendicitis groups and their preoperative laboratory results were reviewed.

Results: A total of 234 patients were included. Elevated international normalized ratio (INR) and serum C-reactive protein (CRP) were associated with complicated appendicitis ($p = 0.001$). On ROC curve analysis, area under the curve (AUC) of CRP and INR were 0.796 and 0.723, respectively.

Conclusions: INR and CRP increased significantly in patients with complicated appendicitis. Further studies evaluating INR and CRP in patients undergoing conservative management for appendicitis are required.

Keywords: Appendicitis, Complication, C-reactive protein, International normalized ratio, Diagnosis

Background

Appendicitis is a common disease. Lifetime risk for having appendicitis is reported to be about 7 to 10 % [1, 2]. Usual management of appendicitis is laparoscopic appendectomy, which has lower complication rate, length of hospital stay, and mortality than open appendectomy [3–5]. However, morbidity or mortality after laparoscopic appendectomy could be happened [6–8].

Many studies analyzing the conservative management of appendicitis have been published. Almost all of these studies looked at managing uncomplicated appendicitis [9–11], including the use of antibiotics in conservative management. No definite method is currently available to distinguish complicated from uncomplicated appendicitis preoperatively, despite the fact that several studies about predicting complicated appendicitis were published [3, 12–15]. In this study, we tried to utilize preoperative laboratory markers to predict whether appendicitis was complicated or not.

* Correspondence: surgeryman@catholic.ac.kr
Department of Trauma Surgery, College of Medicine, The Catholic University of Korea, Seoul, Republic of Korea

Methods

Institutional review board of Uijeongbu St. Mary's hospital approved this retrospective study and informed consent was waived. Medical records of patients who underwent appendectomy between February 2014 and September 2014 were reviewed. The following data were collected; general characteristics as sex, and age; initial laboratory results including white blood cell counts (WBC), neutrophil percent, serum total bilirubin (TB), serum C-reactive protein (CRP) and international normalized ratio (INR); and perioperative data as operation record, pathologic report, initial body temperature (BT). Hospital stay, and wound complications—defined as pus-like discharge from wound—were checked, as secondary outcomes, to analyze post-operative outcomes. Pathological confirmation of appendicitis was mandatory for inclusion in the study. Patients with other inflammatory conditions such as diverticulitis, pelvic inflammatory disease, torsion of ovary, small bowel perforation and intussusceptions were excluded. Additionally, patients with missing values or after incidental appendectomy were excluded.

Based on patients' records, perforated appendicitis, periappendiceal abscess, and peritonitis were regarded as complicated appendicitis (CA), whereas other findings were regarded as non-complicated appendicitis (NA). Upper limits for normal WBC, CRP, TB, and INR were specified at 10×10^9/L, 0.3 mg/dL, 1.2 mg/dL and 1.22, respectively. Body temperature higher than 37.2 °C was regarded as fever. Type of appendicitis and clinical outcomes were correlated to laboratory results.

Independent t-test was used for quantitative analysis and Chi-square and Fisher's exact test were used for qualitative analysis. P-value of less than 0.05 was regarded as statistically significant. Additionally, receiver operating characteristic (ROC) curve analysis was used to evaluate each marker's accuracy. SPSS version 17.0 (SPSS Inc. Chicago, IL) was used for statistical analysis.

Results

The medical records of 258 who underwent appendectomy during the period from February 2014 to September 2014 were reviewed. Only 234 patients were eligible for enrollment in the study. Mean age of the patients was 35.8 ± 18.9 years and number of male patients was 126. Fifty-four patients had complicated appendicitis and 180 patients had uncomplicated appendicitis.

Results of laboratory markers and other basic characteristics were analyzed according to the type of appendicitis. Statistically significant elevations in CRP and INR were identified in CA patients ($p = 0.001$). In addition, they were associated with a high relative risk (relative risk [95 % confidence interval]: 1.291 [1.149–1.452], and 2.059 [1.032–4.108], respectively). On the contrary, no other associations between type of appendicitis and preoperative WBC, neutrophil percent, or TB were identified. Similarly, BT showed no statistically significant association with the type of appendicitis. These results are shown in Table 1.

ROC curve analysis was performed to examine the feasibility of each parameter. Area under curve (AUC) of CRP and INR was 0.796 and 0.723, respectively, which showed their feasibility as useful CA predictors. However, AUC of TB was only 0.576, and the other parameters showed similar AUCs that were much lower than those of CRP and INR. Results of ROC curve analysis are summarized in Table 2 and Fig. 1.

Additional analyses of post-operative outcomes, namely hospital stay and wound complications, are summarized in Table 3. Elevated CRP and INR were associated with longer hospital stay (3.20 vs. 3.94 days, $p < 0.001$; 3.70 vs. 4.85 days, $p = 0.001$, respectively). However, they did not show a statistically significant association with wound complication.

Discussion

Several approaches were proposed to diagnose acute appendicitis. There were many studies about computed tomography (CT) scan in evaluation of acute appendicitis that showed its feasibility as a diagnostic method [16, 17]. However, other studies highlighted the risk from radiation exposure after CT scan [18, 19]. Although the risk of malignancy arising after CT scan is

Table 1 Characteristics and analysis of patients according to type of appendicitis

		Non-complicated appendicitis (*n* = 180)	Complicated appendicitis (*n* = 54)	p-value
Gender	Male	92 (51.1 %)	34 (63.0 %)	0.125
	Female	88 (48.9 %)	20 (38.0 %)	
Age in years (mean ± SD)		34.7 ± 17.9	39.5 ± 21.7	0.144
WBC	Normal	44 (24.4 %)	11 (20.4 %)	0.536
	Elevated	136 (75.6 %)	43 (79.6 %)	
Neutrophil percent	Normal	70 (38.9 %)	15 (27.8 %)	0.136
	Elevated	110 (61.1 %)	39 (72.2 %)	
C-reactive protein	Normal	52 (28.9 %)	4 (7.4 %)	0.001
	Elevated	128 (71.1 %)	50 (92.6 %)	
Total bilirubin	Normal	138 (76.7 %)	37 (68.5 %)	0.227
	Elevated	42 (23.3 %)	17 (31.5 %)	
Body temperature	Normal	163 (90.6 %)	50 (92.6 %)	0.79
	Elevated	17 (9.4 %)	4 (7.4 %)	
INR	Normal	175 (97.2 %)	46 (85.2 %)	0.001
	Elevated	5 (2.8 %)	8 (14.8 %)	

WBC white blood cell counts, *INR* international normalized ratio, *SD* standard deviation, *n* number of patients

Table 2 Area under curve from receiver operating curve analysis of each parameter

	Area under curve
WBC	0.594
Neutrophil percent	0.577
C-reactive protein	0.796
Total bilirubin	0.576
Body temperature	0.552
INR	0.723

WBC white blood cell counts, *INR* international normalized ratio

rare and low, however; incorporating CT scan as a routine diagnostic method for appendicitis should be decided carefully, considering the benign nature of the disease.

Many studies looking at the power of CRP in predicting complications of appendicitis have been published recently showing positive results [20, 21]. Similarly, in the present study, elevated CRP was associated with CA and its AUC was the highest among the tested parameters. The results of the present study support the use of CRP as a predictor for complicated appendicitis.

Interestingly, our study focused on the association between INR and type of appendicitis. To the best of our knowledge, this study was the first to look at this association. Our results showed a statistically significant association between INR and both CA as well as postoperative outcome.

Clotting pathway is activated by inflammatory mediators following exposure to infectious agents like viruses and bacteria, or inflammatory cytokines like interleukin-1, interleukin-6, tissue necrosis factors, etc. [22]. Therefore in severe inflammatory conditions as sepsis, patients are prone to have bleeding tendency, known as disseminated intravascular coagulopathy, caused by excessive consumption of coagulation factors [23]. Prothrombin time is the general test used to check bleeding tendency, especially for the extrinsic pathway, and INR represents a mathematical modification of prothrombin time to allow for standardized reporting between different laboratories. We focused on the association between INR and acute appendicitis as we postulated that CA may be associated with bleeding tendency, despite rarely aggravating to sepsis. For preoperative evaluation, INR is a mandatory parameter to check, while CRP is helpful but not essential.

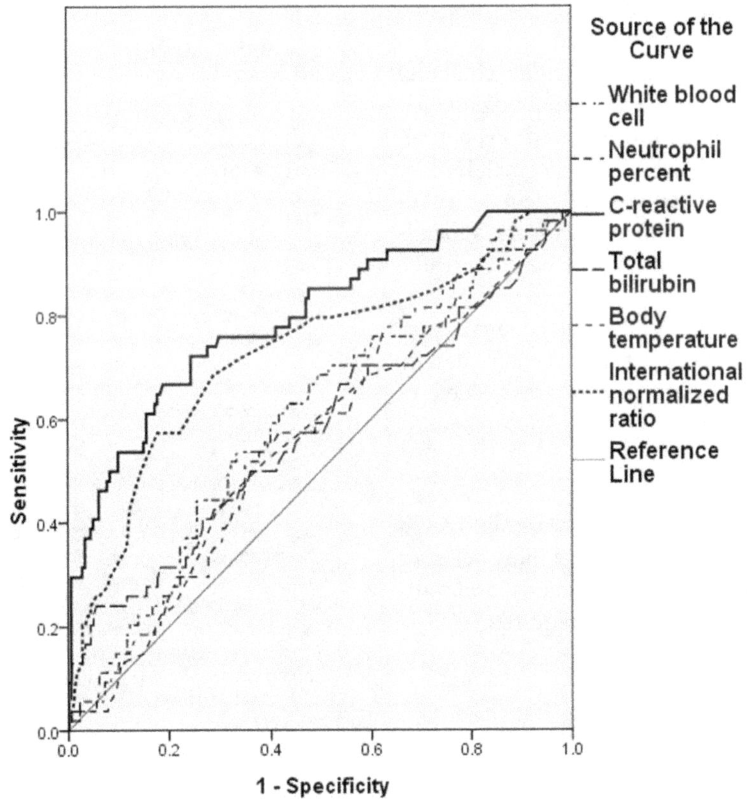

Fig. 1 Receiver operating characteristic (ROC) curve for initial laboratory parameters. The area under the ROC curve of CRP and INR was 0.796 and 0.723, respectively

Table 3 Analysis of clinical outcomes and laboratory findings

		Normal CRP ($n = 56$)	Elevated CRP ($n = 178$)	p-value
Hospital stay (days)		3.20 ± 0.84	3.94 ± 1.29	<0.001
Wound complication	No	47 (83.9 %)	164 (92.1 %)	0.072
	Yes	9 (16.1 %)	14 (7.9 %)	
		Normal INR ($n = 221$)	Elevated INR ($n = 13$)	p-value
Hospital stay (days)		3.70 ± 1.18	4.85 ± 1.68	0.001
Wound complication	No	200 (90.5 %)	11 (84.6 %)	0.072
	Yes	21 (9.5 %)	2 (15.4 %)	

CRP serum C-reactive protein, *INR* international normalized ratio, *n* number of patients

One more point to consider is the cost of each marker. INR costs 2.03 $ per test which is much cheaper than CRP (7.82 $ per test), as per the national health insurance system. Although CRP showed better AUC value, cost-effectiveness should be evaluated in further studies.

We also analyzed post-operative outcomes. Previous studies showed that CA was associated with poorer post-postoperative outcomes [24–26]. Elevated INR and CRP were associated with longer hospital stay; however, no statistical correlation with wound complication was identified. To clarify this association, further studies analyzing postoperative outcome are required.

Additionally, further studies looking at the choice of the management strategy for acute appendicitis according to laboratory findings are required. Proper selection of patients with NA who have normal INR or CRP for conservative management will help to validate conservation, hence avoiding unnecessary appendectomies. Our study may serve as the base for these future studies.

Other limitations of our study include the small sample size and the retrospective single center design. Large-scaled, multicenter-based studies are needed to further elucidate our findings.

Conclusions

In conclusion, elevated INR and CRP were associated with complicated appendicitis and longer hospital stay. Further studies relating laboratory findings and outcomes of conservative management are required.

Abbreviations

BT, body temperature; CA, complicated appendicitis; CRP, serum C-reactive protein; INR, international normalized ratio; NA, non-complicated appendicitis; TB, total bilirubin; WBC, white blood cell counts.

Acknowledgement

Not applicable.

Funding

There was no financial or other type of support.

Authors' contributions

MK was involved in study conception, design, analysis, interpretation, and writing of the manuscript; SK was involved in study conception, acquisition of data, interpretation, and revision; HC was involved in study conception, acquisition of data, design, analysis, interpretation, and writing of the manuscript. All authors read and approved the final manuscript.

Competing interests

The authors declare that they have no competing interests.

References

1. Lee JH, Park YS, Choi JS. The epidemiology of appendicitis and appendectomy in South Korea: national registry data. J Epidemiol. 2010;20:97–105.
2. D'Souza N. Appendicitis. BMJ Clin Evid. 2011;2011.
3. Noh H, Chang SJ, Han A. The diagnostic values of preoperative laboratory markers in children with complicated appendicitis. J Korean Surg Soc. 2012;83:237–41.
4. Li X, Zhang J, Sang L, Zhang W, Chu Z, Li X, et al. Laparoscopic versus conventional appendectomy–a meta-analysis of randomized controlled trials. BMC Gastroenterol. 2010;10:129.
5. Masoomi H, Nguyen NT, Dolich MO, Mills S, Carmichael JC, Stamos MJ. Laparoscopic appendectomy trends and outcomes in the United States: data from the Nationwide Inpatient Sample (NIS), 2004–2011. Am Surg. 2014;80:1074–7.
6. Grande M, Lisi G, Bianchi D, Bove P, Miano R, Esser A, et al. Bilateral ureteral obstruction in children after appendectomy. Case Rep Surg. 2015;2015:740795.
7. Rajan M, Dip F, Szomstein S, Zanghi A, Cavallaro A, Di Vita M, et al. Staple line as a cause of unusual early internal hernia after appendectomy. Int J Surg. 2014;12 Suppl 1:S159–61.
8. Andersson MN, Andersson RE. Causes of short-term mortality after appendectomy: a population-based case-controlled study. Ann Surg. 2011;254:103–7.
9. Rocha LL, Rossi FM, Pessoa CM, Campos FN, Pires CE, Steinman M. Antibiotics alone versus appendectomy to treat uncomplicated acute appendicitis in adults: what do meta-analyses say? World J Emerg Surg. 2015;10:51.
10. Tanaka Y, Uchida H, Kawashima H, Fujiogi M, Takazawa S, Deie K, et al. Long-term outcomes of operative versus nonoperative treatment for uncomplicated appendicitis. J Pediatr Surg. 2015;50:1893–7.
11. Kelly ME, Khan A, Ur Rehman J, Waldron RM, Khan W, Barry K, et al. A national evaluation of the conservative management of uncomplicated acute appendicitis: how common is this and what are the issues. Dig Surg. 2015;32:325–30.
12. Kim TH, Cho BS, Jung JH, Lee MS, Jang JH, Kim CN. Predictive factors to distinguish between patients with noncomplicated appendicitis and those with complicated appendicitis. Ann Coloproctol. 2015;31:192–7.
13. Sandstrom A, Grieve DA. Hyperbilirubinaemia: its utility in non-perforated appendicitis. ANZ J Surg. 2015. doi:10.1111/ans.13373.
14. Adams HL, Jaunoo SS. Hyperbilirubinaemia in appendicitis: the diagnostic value for prediction of appendicitis and appendiceal perforation. Eur J Trauma Emerg Surg. 2015. doi:10.1007/s00068-015-0540-x.
15. Atema JJ, van Rossem CC, Leeuwenburgh MM, Stoker J, Boermeester MA. Scoring system to distinguish uncomplicated from complicated acute appendicitis. Br J Surg. 2015;102:979–90.
16. Tsukada K, Miyazaki T, Katoh H, Masuda N, Ojima H, Fukuchi M, et al. CT is useful for identifying patients with complicated appendicitis. Dig Liver Dis. 2004;36:195–8.
17. Foley TA, Earnest 4th F, Nathan MA, Hough DM, Schiller HJ, Hoskin TL. Differentiation of nonperforated from perforated appendicitis: accuracy of CT diagnosis and relationship of CT findings to length of hospital stay. Radiology. 2005;235:89–96.

18. Griffey RT, Sodickson A. Cumulative radiation exposure and cancer risk estimates in emergency department patients undergoing repeat or multiple CT. AJR Am J Roentgenol. 2009;192:887–92.
19. Shah KH, Slovis BH, Runde D, Godbout B, Newman DH, Lee J. Radiation exposure among patients with the highest CT scan utilization in the emergency department. Emerg Radiol. 2013;20:485–91.
20. Panagiotopoulou IG, Parashar D, Lin R, Antonowicz S, Wells AD, Bajwa FM, et al. The diagnostic value of white cell count, C-reactive protein and bilirubin in acute appendicitis and its complications. Ann R Coll Surg Engl. 2013;95:215–21.
21. McGowan DR, Sims HM, Zia K, Uheba M, Shaikh IA. The value of biochemical markers in predicting a perforation in acute appendicitis. ANZ J Surg. 2013;83:79–83.
22. Grignani G, Maiolo A. Cytokines and hemostasis. Haematologica. 2000;85:967–72.
23. Levi M, Toh CH, Thachil J, Watson HG. Guidelines for the diagnosis and management of disseminated intravascular coagulation. British Committee for Standards in Haematology. Br J Haematol. 2009;145:24–33.
24. Kelly ME, Khan A, Riaz M, Bolger JC, Bennani F, Khan W, et al. The utility of neutrophil-to-lymphocyte ratio as a severity predictor of acute appendicitis, length of hospital stay and postoperative complication rates. Dig Surg. 2015;32:459–63.
25. Chen CC, Ting CT, Tsai MJ, Hsu WC, Chen PC, Lee MD, et al. Appendectomy timing: Will delayed surgery increase the complications? J Chin Med Assoc. 2015;78:395–9.
26. Kim MS, Park HW, Park JY, Park HJ, Lee SY, Hong HP, et al. Differentiation of early perforated from nonperforated appendicitis: MDCT findings, MDCT diagnostic performance, and clinical outcome. Abdom Imaging. 2014;39:459–66.

8

Position paper: timely interventions in severe acute pancreatitis are crucial for survival

Panu Mentula and Ari Leppäniemi*

Abstract

Severe acute pancreatitis has high mortality, but multiple and timely interventions can improve survival. Early in the course of the disease aggressive fluid resuscitation is needed for the prevention and treatment of shock. In conjunction with leaking capillaries this results in increased tissue edema, which may lead to intra-abdominal hypertension and abdominal compartment syndrome. Invasive hemodynamic monitoring is essential for optimizing fluid therapy while monitoring of intra-abdominal pressure is necessary for identification patients at risk of developing abdominal compartment syndrome. Abdominal compartment syndrome develops usually within the first days after hospitalization. Conservative treatment modalities are useful in prevention but also in the treatment of abdominal compartment syndrome. If conservative management fails surgical decompression of abdomen may be needed. Multiple organ dysfunction syndrome and increased intra-abdominal pressure predispose patients with severe pancreatitis to secondary infections. Extrapancreatic infections predominate during the first week of the disease, whereas infection of pancreatic necrosis usually develops later. Early enteral nutrition reduces the risk of infections whereas advantage of prophylactic antibiotics is lacking evidence. Surgery for infected pancreatic necrosis is associated with high mortality when performed within the first two weeks of the disease. Therefore surgery should be postponed as late as possible, preferably later than four weeks after disease onset.

Introduction

In the majority of patients acute pancreatitis is a mild self-limiting disease. About fifteen percent of the patients develop severe disease defined by development of persistent organ failure [1]. The mortality in acute pancreatitis is mainly associated with multiple organ failure [2] whereas the risk of dying is minimal in patients with no or transient organ dysfunction [3,4]. In acute pancreatitis, multiple organ failure is a consequence of excessive activation of a systemic inflammatory response cascade [5]. Inflammatory mediators induce end-organ endothelial cell activation leading to increased permeability [6]. Leaking microvessels cause a loss of intravascular fluid and in conjunction with vasodilatation lead to hypotension and shock. Accumulation of inflammatory cells in tissues, increased interstitial fluid and activation of coagulation with microvascular thrombosis further impair oxygen supply of tissues. Clinical manifestation of all this is a multiple organ dysfunction syndrome (MODS), which develops early during the course of acute pancreatitis. Over half of the patients with severe pancreatitis have signs of organ dysfunction on hospital admission [3] and most of the organ dysfunctions develop within the first four days after admission [7]. Over half of the deaths occur within the first week from onset of the disease, and deaths usually occurred within a week after manifestation of MODS [8].

Treatment modalities of MODS are supportive including fluid replacement therapy, vasopressors, mechanical ventilation and renal replacement therapy when necessary. In patients with acute pancreatitis, abdominal compartment syndrome (ACS) may aggravate MODS, and therefore, monitoring of intra-abdominal pressure (IAP) is crucial for identification of patients at risk of ACS [9]. Development of ACS should be prevented, if possible, by conservative methods. Surgical decompression is the last but the most effective way to decrease IAP and should not be postponed too late if patient has developed ACS [10].

Patients with acute pancreatitis have a considerable risk for developing secondary infections including bacteremia, pneumonia and infection of pancreatic or peripancreatic necrosis. Extrapancreatic infections occur predominantly during the first week of illness, whereas pancreatic necrosis

* Correspondence: ari.leppaniemi@hus.fi
Meilahti hospital, Department of Abdominal Surgery, University of Helsinki, Haartmaninkatu 4, PO Box 340, 00029 Helsinki, HUS, Finland

becomes infected later [11]. The mortality is very high in patients with persistent organ failure complicated with infected pancreatic necrosis [12]. Development of bacteremia and infected pancreatic necrosis are associated with MODS. Intestinal dysfunction plays an important role and bacterial translocation from intestine is considered the main mechanism of infection. Impaired host response systems may also predispose to clinical infections. Early enteral nutrition has been shown to reduce systemic infections [13], whereas the results from randomized trials with prophylactic antibiotics have been inconclusive [14]. Surgery is considered necessary for adequate source control when pancreatic or peripancreatic infection develops. However, because surgery for pancreatic necrosis within the first 2–3 weeks from disease onset is associated with high mortality, surgery should be postponed as late as possible [15]. Sometimes percutaneous drainage of fluid from infected acute necrotic collection may be helpful and is preferable first-line treatment for infected pancreatic necrosis during the first three weeks of illness [16].

Fluid resuscitation and abdominal compartment syndrome

Aggressive fluid therapy during the early phase of acute pancreatitis has been traditionally the cornerstone of treatment [17]. The rationale of fluid therapy is to correct hypovolemia caused by third space fluid loss. High admission hematocrit (above normal reference limits) may serve as a marker of hemoconcentration, and it is present up to 60% of patients who develop organ failure [18], but the marker is too unspecific for predictive purposes [19]. Fluid resuscitation decreases hematocrit, which could be used as resuscitation end-point. Too aggressive resuscitation may lead to inappropriate hemodilution and very low hematocrit values (<30%) may be harmful for the patients by increasing the risk of sepsis and death [20]. Moreover, excess volume loading may increase IAP and lead to development of intra-abdominal hypertension (IAH) and abdominal compartment syndrome [21]. In patients with acute pancreatitis, hematocrit and central venous pressure as resuscitation end-points are poor indicators of volume depletion [22]. Urine output (≥0.5 ml/kg/h) may serve as another resuscitation end-point, but other modalities are needed for volume management if oliguria persists after initial volume loading. According to recent systematic review there is little evidence concerning the rate of infusion, optimal resuscitation end-point and the type of fluid in patients with acute pancreatitis [23].

In those patients with pancreatitis who develop shock the same management guidelines as for septic shock patients can be applied. These include initial fluid challenge with crystalloids (rate 1000 ml/ hour) with minimum of 30 ml/kg and administration of vasopressor epinephrine to maintain adequate blood pressure [24]. Principles of early goal directed resuscitation with monitoring of CVP, MAP and either central venous oxygen saturation or mixed venous oxygen saturation [25] can be used also in acute pancreatitis. Frequently elevated IAP should be monitored and taken into account when considering resuscitation end-points [26]. Abdominal perfusion pressure (APP) could serve as a good resuscitation end-point in patients with IAH [27]. Maintaining APP above 50–60 mmHg is recommended in order to provide sufficient perfusion to abdominal organs [28]. Lactate level should be monitored and resuscitation should be targeted to normalizing the lactate level. As soon as resuscitation end-points are reached, the infusion rate should be slowed down in order to avoid fluid overloading.

Although the use of colloids can reduce overall volume needed for resuscitation, and thus, could decrease the risk of developing IAH, the use of colloids is not recommended in the guidelines of severe sepsis and septic shock [24]. Hydroxyethyl starch (HES) does not provide any benefit compared with normal saline and its use is associated with increased need for renal replacement therapy [29].

In severe pancreatitis IAH develops as a result of fluid resuscitation and capillary leakage. Fluid accumulates into retroperitoneal space, ascites may form and tissues edema develops. In addition, paralytic bowel can contain substantial amounts of fluid and air. All this takes space in the abdominal cavity, which causes distension of the abdominal wall. Abdomen can tolerate increased volume to some extent, but when abdominal wall becomes distended increasing intra-abdominal volume cause elevation in IAP. When IAH (IAP ≥12 mmHg) develops conservative methods should be applied to prevent development of ACS. These include restriction of intravenous fluids if possible, gastrointestinal decompression with nasogastric tube, and drainage of ascites fluid [30]. Abdominal wall compliance can be increased with adequate pain management; intubation and sedation usually decreases IAP and sometimes even neuromuscular blockade can be used for this purpose. An effective way to correct positive fluid balance and prevent development of ACS is early introducing of hemofiltration [31].

Renal function is impaired already at IAP level as low as 12 mmHg [32]. In patients with established IAH, IAP and APP should be monitored. A patient with shock can easily have inappropriately low APP (<50 - 60 mmHg) even with moderate IAH. Poor perfusion increases bowel mucosal injury [33], which is associated with infectious complications and organ failure in patients with pancreatitis [34]. IAH may play significant role in ischemic bowel complications [35]. Colonic necrosis [36] but also ischemic small bowel [37] can sometimes complicate to course of severe pancreatitis, but the role of IAH in these complications has not been studied. ACS probably plays a major role in early mortality caused by multiple organ failure in acute pancreatitis. Our own observation supports this: Pancreatitis patients with ACS had severe multi organ failure early during the course of the disease and early surgical decompression was associated with reduced mortality and none of the patients treated with decompression died during the first week [10].

In most cases adequate and timely conservative management including ascites drainage [30] is successful, but if ACS develops despite these interventions, surgical decompression should be done without a delay. Midline laparostomy that allows inspection of bowel viability is recommended in order to diagnose possible ischemic lesions. In acute pancreatitis surgical decompression usually leads to open abdomen of several weeks duration [10]. Vacuum assisted closure with mesh mediated fascial traction is a superior temporary abdominal closure method with low frequency of giant hernias [38,39].

Nutrition

There are no indications for fasting in pancreatitis. Although pancreatitis patient may have nausea and vomiting early during the course, these symptoms usually resolve rapidly. In patients with mild acute pancreatitis oral feeding can be started as soon as patient tolerates food; early oral feeding has been associated with faster recovery and shorter hospital stay [40]. In pancreatitis enteral feeding is superior to parenteral feeding. Enteral nutrition prevents bacterial overgrowth in the intestine and reduces bacterial translocation [41]. In pancreatitis enteral nutrition reduces significantly systemic infections, organ dysfunction and mortality [13,42]. Critically ill patients are typically at risk of malnutrition [43] and therefore nutrition of patients with acute pancreatitis should be initiated as soon as possible. Initiation of enteral feeding seems to be critical in pancreatitis; if delayed for more than 48 hours, the benefits from enteral feeding are lost [44,45]. The route of enteral feeding can be either gastric or post pyloric. Gastric feeding succeeds in most of the patients, and therefore feeding can be initiated by using a nasogastric tube [46]. Delayed gastric emptying may cause problems, and therefore gastric residual volume should be monitored every six hours. It is recommended that tube feeding is started with low infusion rate (10 ml/h) and increased by 10 ml/h until every six hours providing that gastric residual volume is below 250 ml [43]. This should be continued until target volume of enteral nutrition is achieved. If gastric emptying is problem prokinetics may help but better option is to place nasojejunal feeding tube, which usually resolves the problem. If patient does not tolerate required volume of enteral nutrition, parenteral nutrition can be combined with enteral so that caloric needs are fulfilled.

Infections and the use of antibiotics

A quarter of patients with acute pancreatitis develop infectious complication [11]. Patients with severe acute pancreatitis are more susceptible to develop infections [11]. Patients with organ dysfunctions have higher incidence of bacterial translocation [34]. They also have impaired immune system [7]. The majority of infections are extrapancreatic such as bacteremia and pneumonia. The half of these infections develop within the first week post admission [11]. Diagnosis of infected pancreatic necrosis is usually done significantly later, the peak incidence is between the third and fourth week from the onset of symptoms [11,47]. However, the actual contamination of necrosis happens probably much earlier [48]. Organ failure, early bacteremia and the extent of pancreatic necrosis are associated with increased risk of infected necrosis [11]. Diagnosis of infected pancreatic necrosis is challenging. Clinical signs of sepsis are too unspecific for definitive diagnosis and CT-scan shows gas bubbles in the necrotic collection in less than ten percent of patients [49]. Fine needle aspiration with bacterial culture has a substantial rate (20-25%) of false negative results, and thus, is not reliable to rule out infection [50].

Prophylactic antibiotics have been studied in many randomized trials with conflicting results and according to several meta-analyses and systematic reviews there is no evidence that patients benefit from prophylactic antibiotics [14,51,52]. However, there has been a nonsignificant trend for lower mortality and reduced number of infections, especially extrapancreatic infections in patients treated with prophylactic antibiotics. The randomized trials have been conducted with small samples sizes and some studies included a substantial number of patients with mild pancreatitis [53] with minimal risk of mortality and low risk of infectious complications. Although trials have not provided evidence that prophylactic antibiotic are effective they have not proved that they are not effective [54]. Taken together the limitations of the trials and the fact that patients with organ failure are susceptible to infections, we believe that the use of prophylactic antibiotic in patients with severe pancreatitis is justified. High incidence of infections in patients with severe pancreatitis and worse survival in patients who develop infection supports this policy. Indication for initiation of prophylactic antibiotics should be based on clinical judgment. Systemic inflammatory response syndrome (SIRS) [4], signs of organ dysfunction, presence of IAH [55], hyperglycemia, low plasma calcium or high creatinine [56] could be helpful in predicting severe disease.

If prophylactic antibiotics are not given, empiric use of antibiotics is encouraged in patients who develop organ dysfunctions, because there is high risk of bacteremia during the first week. Patients with severe pancreatitis fulfill the criteria of severe sepsis in case of infection and there is no rapid and reliable diagnostic method available to rule out infection. Delayed administration of antibiotics has been shown to worsen survival in patients with severe sepsis with or without septic shock [57]. After the end of the second week, empiric antibiotics may be needed for treatment of infected pancreatic necrosis if sepsis continues or the patient does not recover. Empiric antibiotics at this stage should cover potential pathogens including gram negative rods and gram positive cocci [47]. The role of empiric antifungals is not clear. Fine needle aspiration for microbiological samples should be taken if infected necrosis is suspected, although negative samples do not rule out infection [50]. Positive samples help in selection of antimicrobials and initiation of possible antifungal therapy. Prophylactic or empiric antibiotic should be discontinued when the patient recovers from organ dysfunctions and there is no evidence of infection.

Surgery for infected necrosis

Infected pancreatic or peripancreatic necrosis has traditionally been considered an indisputable indication for surgical debridement [58]. Infected necrosis is a significant source of sepsis and removal of devitalized tissue is believed to be necessary for control of sepsis. However, infection usually continues after necrosectomy, especially if necrotic tissue is left in place. Before demarcation of necrosis develops, usually after 4 weeks from disease onset, it is impossible to remove all necrotic tissue without causing hemorrhage. Early surgical debridement has been associated with high risk of hemorrhage leading to increased organ dysfunction and death. If necrosectomy for infected pancreatic necrosis is done within the first two weeks the mortality rate is 75%, but gradually decreases to 5% when done later than four weeks after the onset of symptoms [15,50,59]. Multiple organ dysfunction increases mortality risk considerably in patients with infected necrosis. The mortality rate increases in proportion to the number of failed organs [50]. Infected pancreatic necrosis does not cause significant risk of death in absence of organ dysfunction [12,50]. Because high mortality is associated with early surgery and multiple organ dysfunction, it is recommended that surgery for infected necrosis should be postponed as late as possible, preferable later than four week from disease onset. Percutaneus drainage of the liquid component of the infected acute necrotic collection may serve as a bridge to surgery [16]. Sterile collections do not need drainage. Placement of a drain into a sterile necrotic collection can result in secondary infection, and a prolonged drainage may increase the risk further [60,61].

Infected pancreatic necrosis may cause worsening of multiple organ failure between the second and fourth week of the disease. Although delayed operative treatment is associated with lower mortality rate [62], it is not always possible to postpone surgery, if the condition of the patient deteriorates. Indeed, patients operated on between days 14 and 29 from admission have significantly higher prevalence of organ failure than patients operated on later than day 29 from admission [62], which may partly explain differences in mortality. There are no randomized studies comparing operative treatment and catheter drainage in this subgroup of patients with worsening multiple organ failure after two weeks from disease onset. The only randomized trial comparing open necrosectomy and minimally invasive step-up approach included only 28 (32%) patients with multiple organ failure and the median time of interventions was 30 days from disease onset [63]. In this study, the mortality rate was the same between the groups. Unfortunately, no data of subgroup analysis of patients with multiple organ failure was shown [63]. Although the use mini-invasive techniques are increasingly used for infected pancreatic necrosis, the lowest published mortality rate in patients operated on for infected necrosis is with open debridement and closed packing with 15% mortality [50]. In patients without preoperative organ failure, minimally invasive necrosectomy is associated with fewer new-onset organ failure than open surgery [63]. However, a considerable number of patients are not suitable for mini-invasive surgery either because of localization of the necrotic collection or because intraabdominal catastrophe needs to be excluded [64].

Recommendations

The management of patients with acute pancreatitis depends on duration of the disease. The following guidelines are provided for specific time frames.

A. On admission

1. Diagnosis of acute pancreatitis is completed. Use CT-scan without contrast in case of diagnostic uncertainty.
2. Initiate fluid resuscitation with crystalloids for correction of hypovolemia with simultaneous monitoring of vital organ functions including IAP monitoring.
3. Assess severity based on clinical judgment and initiate prophylactic antibiotics in patients with probable severe pancreatitis.
4. If patient has any signs of organ dysfunction consider intensive care admission.

B. Within the first 48 hours from admission

1. Re-assess the severity daily and discontinue prophylactic antibiotics in patients with mild or moderate pancreatitis.
2. Continue monitoring of vital organ functions and IAP in accordance with fluid therapy. Optimize fluid

therapy. Reduce the infusion of crystalloids, if a patient is hemodynamically stable and does not show signs of dehydration.
3. If the patient has signs of deteriorating organ functions consider intensive care admission in order to start invasive hemodynamic monitoring and critical care.
4. In patients with IAH, calculate APP and use conservative efforts to prevent development of ACS.
5. In case ACS develops or the patient has low APP, use all possible conservative efforts to reduce IAP and correct APP, but if not effective perform surgical decompression with midline laparostomy.
6. Take blood cultures and plain chest radiographs for detection of infections.
7. Initiate enteral nutrition.

C. Within the first week from disease onset

1. Same as B1 – B6.
2. Continue enteral nutrition, target for total caloric needs through enteral route.
3. Perform contrast enhanced CT-scan on days 5–7 after disease onset in patients with normal renal function. The amount and localization of necrosis may help in predicting the need of follow-up for late complications.

D. During the second week from disease onset

1. Continue supportive care; try to get rid of excessive third space fluids if possible.
2. If the patient is septic at end of the second week or later, consider repeat CT-scan with image guided FNA and after that consider empiric antibiotics for possible infected pancreatic necrosis.
3. If infected necrosis is diagnosed, image guided percutaneous drainage of collection should be done.
4. An alternative to FNA is to put a percutaneous drain directly into the collection and take samples, however, if cultures are negative the drain should be removed as prolonged drainage may cause increased risk for infection.
5. Surgery for infected pancreatic necrosis should be avoided during the first two weeks, because necrosis is not well demarcated and surgery it is associated with high risk of hemorrhage and high mortality.

E. After the second week from disease onset

1. Same as D1 – D4, repeat CT-scan if patient deteriorates; repeat CT-scan weekly if the patient is not recovering.
2. Percutaneus drainage of infected pancreatic necrosis can be continued if the patient shows signs of recovery, some patients may even avoid surgical treatment.
3. If the patient is deteriorating despite of setting of percutaneous drainage, proceed to surgical necrosectomy, whether there is proven infection or not.
4. In patients who do not recover but are stable, surgery for pancreatic necrosis is possible, but should be postponed as late as possible, preferably later than 4 weeks after disease onset. CT-scan before surgery is recommended for localization of necrosis and to confirm the demarcation of necrosis.

Competing interests
The authors declare that they have no competing interests.

Authors' contribution
PM wrote the initial draft. AL made critical revisions, both authors read and approved the manuscript.

References
1. Banks PA, Bollen TL, Dervenis C, Gooszen HG, Johnson CD, Sarr MG, *et al*: **Classification of acute pancreatitis–2012: revision of the Atlanta classification and definitions by international consensus.** *Gut* 2013, **62**(1):102–111.
2. Halonen KI, Pettila V, Leppäniemi AK, Kemppainen EA, Puolakkainen PA, Haapiainen RK: **Multiple organ dysfunction associated with severe acute pancreatitis.** *Crit Care Med* 2002, **30**(6):1274–1279.
3. Buter A, Imrie CW, Carter CR, Evans S, McKay CJ: **Dynamic nature of early organ dysfunction determines outcome in acute pancreatitis.** *Br J Surg* 2002, **89**(3):298–302.
4. Mofidi R, Duff MD, Wigmore SJ, Madhavan KK, Garden OJ, Parks RW: **Association between early systemic inflammatory response, severity of multiorgan dysfunction and death in acute pancreatitis.** *Br J Surg* 2006, **93**(6):738–744.
5. Mayer J, Rau B, Gansauge F, Beger HG: **Inflammatory mediators in human acute pancreatitis: clinical and pathophysiological implications.** *Gut* 2000, **47**(4):546–552.
6. Hack CE, Zeerleder S: **The endothelium in sepsis: source of and a target for inflammation.** *Crit Care Med* 2001, **29**(7 Suppl):S21–S27.
7. Mentula P, Kylänpää-Bäck M-L, Kemppainen E, Takala A, Jansson S-E, Kautiainen H, *et al*: **Decreased HLA (human leucocyte antigen)-DR expression on peripheral blood monocytes predicts the development of organ failure in patients with acute pancreatitis.** *Clin Sci* 2003, **105**(4):409–417.
8. Mole DJ, Olabi B, Robinson V, Garden OJ, Parks RW: **Incidence of individual organ dysfunction in fatal acute pancreatitis: analysis of 1024 death records.** *MHPB* 2009, **11**(2):166–170.
9. De Waele JJ, Leppäniemi AK: **Intra-abdominal hypertension in acute pancreatitis.** *World J Surg* 2009, **33**(6):1128–1133.
10. Mentula P, Hienonen P, Kemppainen E, Puolakkainen P, Leppäniemi A: **Surgical decompression for abdominal compartment syndrome in severe acute pancreatitis.** *Arch Surg (Chicago, Ill: 1960)* 2010, **145**(8):764–769.
11. Besselink MG, van Santvoort HC, Boermeester MA, Nieuwenhuijs VB, Van Goor H, Dejong CHC, *et al*: **Timing and impact of infections in acute pancreatitis.** *Br J Surg* 2009, **96**(3):267–273.
12. Petrov MS, Shanbhag S, Chakraborty M, Phillips ARJ, Windsor JA: **Organ failure and infection of pancreatic necrosis as determinants of mortality in patients with acute pancreatitis.** *Gastroenterology* 2010, **139**(3):813–820.
13. Al-Omran M, Albalawi ZH, Tashkandi MF, Al-Ansary LA: **Enteral versus parenteral nutrition for acute pancreatitis.** *Cochrane Database Syst Rev* 2010, **1**:CD002837.
14. Villatoro E, Mulla M, Larvin M: **Antibiotic therapy for prophylaxis against infection of pancreatic necrosis in acute pancreatitis.** *Cochrane Database Syst Rev* 2010, **5**:CD002941.

15. Besselink MGH, Verwer TJ, Schoenmaeckers EJP, Buskens E, Ridwan BU, Visser MR, *et al*: **Timing of surgical intervention in necrotizing pancreatitis.** *Arch Surg (Chicago, Ill: 1960)* 2007, **142**(12):1194–1201.
16. van Baal MC, van Santvoort HC, Bollen TL, Bakker OJ, Besselink MG, Gooszen HG, *et al*: **Systematic review of percutaneous catheter drainage as primary treatment for necrotizing pancreatitis.** *Br J Surg* 2011, **98**(1):18–27.
17. Beger HG, Rau BM: **Severe acute pancreatitis: clinical course and management.** *World J Gastroenterol* 2007, **13**(38):5043–5051.
18. Brown A, Orav J, Banks PA: **Hemoconcentration is an early marker for organ failure and necrotizing pancreatitis.** *Pancreas* 2000, **20**(4):367–372.
19. Lankisch PG, Mahlke R, Blum T, Bruns A, Bruns D, Maisonneuve P, *et al*: **Hemoconcentration: an early marker of severe and/or necrotizing pancreatitis? A critical appraisal.** *Am J Gastroenterol* 2001, **96**(7):2081–2085.
20. Mao E-Q, Fei J, Peng Y-B, Huang J, Tang Y-Q, Zhang S-D: **Rapid hemodilution is associated with increased sepsis and mortality among patients with severe acute pancreatitis.** *Chin Med J* 2010, **123**(13):1639–1644.
21. An G, West MA: **Abdominal compartment syndrome: a concise clinical review.** *Crit Care Med* 2008, **36**(4):1304–1310.
22. Huber W, Umgelter A, Reindl W, Franzen M, Schmidt C, von Delius S, *et al*: **Volume assessment in patients with necrotizing pancreatitis: a comparison of intrathoracic blood volume index, central venous pressure, and hematocrit, and their correlation to cardiac index and extravascular lung water index.** *Crit Care Med* 2008, **36**(8):2348–2354.
23. Haydock MD, Mittal A, Wilms HR, Phillips A, Petrov MS, Windsor JA: **Fluid therapy in acute pancreatitis: anybody's guess.** *Ann Surg* 2013, **257**(2):182–188.
24. Dellinger RP, Levy MM, Rhodes A, Annane D, Gerlach H, Opal SM, *et al*: **Surviving sepsis campaign: international guidelines for management of severe sepsis and septic shock: 2012.** *Crit Care Med* 2013, **41**:580–637.
25. Rivers E, Nguyen B, Havstad S, Ressler J, Muzzin A, Knoblich B, *et al*: **Early goal-directed therapy in the treatment of severe sepsis and septic shock.** *N Engl J Med* 2001, **345**(19):1368–1377.
26. Malbrain MLNG, Ameloot K, Gillebert C, Cheatham ML: **Cardiopulmonary monitoring in intra-abdominal hypertension.** *Am Surgeon* 2011, **77**(Suppl 1):S23–S30.
27. Cheatham ML, White MW, Sagraves SG, Johnson JL, Block EF: **Abdominal perfusion pressure: a superior parameter in the assessment of intra-abdominal hypertension.** *J Trauma* 2000, **49**(4):621–626. discussion626–7.
28. Cheatham ML, Malbrain MLNG, Kirkpatrick A, Sugrue M, Parr M, De Waele J, *et al*: **Results from the international conference of experts on intra-abdominal hypertension and abdominal compartment syndrome. II. Recommendations.** *Intensive Care Med* 2007, **33**(6):951–962.
29. Myburgh JA, Finfer S, Bellomo R, Billot L, Cass A, Gattas D, *et al*: **Hydroxyethyl starch or saline for fluid resuscitation in intensive care.** *N Engl J Med* 2012, **367**(20):1901–1911.
30. Cheatham ML, Safcsak K: **Percutaneous catheter decompression in the treatment of elevated intraabdominal pressure.** *Chest* 2011, **140**(6):1428–1435.
31. Pupelis G, Plaudis H, Zeiza K, Drozdova N, Mukans M, Kazaka I: **Early continuous veno-venous haemofiltration in the management of severe acute pancreatitis complicated with intra-abdominal hypertension: retrospective review of 10 years' experience.** *Ann Intensive Care* 2012, **2**(Suppl 1):S21.
32. Dalfino L, Tullo L, Donadio I, Malcangi V, Brienza N: **Intra-abdominal hypertension and acute renal failure in critically ill patients.** *Intensive Care Med* 2008, **34**(4):707–713.
33. Rahman SH, Ammori BJ, Holmfield J, Larvin M, McMahon MJ: **Intestinal hypoperfusion contributes to gut barrier failure in severe acute pancreatitis.** *J Gastrointest Surg* 2003, **7**(1):26–35. discussion35–6.
34. Besselink MG, van Santvoort HC, Renooij W, de Smet MB, Boermeester MA, Fischer K, *et al*: **Intestinal barrier dysfunction in a randomized trial of a specific probiotic composition in acute pancreatitis.** *Ann Surg* 2009, **250**(5):712–719.
35. Björck M, Wanhainen A: **Nonocclusive mesenteric hypoperfusion syndromes: recognition and treatment.** *Semin Vasc Surg* 2010, **23**(1):54–64.
36. Mohamed SR, Siriwardena AK: **Understanding the colonic complications of pancreatitis.** *Pancreatology* 2008, **8**(2):153–158.
37. Hirota M, Inoue K, Kimura Y, Mizumoto T, Kuwata K, Ohmuraya M, *et al*: **Non-occlusive mesenteric ischemia and its associated intestinal gangrene in acute pancreatitis.** *Pancreatology* 2003, **3**(4):316–322.
38. Petersson U, Acosta S, Björck M: **Vacuum-assisted wound closure and mesh-mediated fascial traction–a novel technique for late closure of the open abdomen.** *World J Surg* 2007, **31**(11):2133–2137.
39. Rasilainen SK, Mentula PJ, Leppäniemi AK: **Vacuum and mesh-mediated fascial traction for primary closure of the open abdomen in critically ill surgical patients.** *Br J Surg* 2012, **99**(12):1725–1732.
40. Eckerwall GE, Tingstedt BBA, Bergenzaun PE, Andersson RG: **Immediate oral feeding in patients with mild acute pancreatitis is safe and may accelerate recovery–a randomized clinical study.** *Clin Nutr (Edinburgh, Scotland)* 2007, **26**(6):758–763.
41. Deitch EA: **Gut-origin sepsis: evolution of a concept.** *Surgeon* 2012, **10**(6):350–356.
42. Petrov MS, van Santvoort HC, Besselink MGH, van der Heijden GJMG, Windsor JA, Gooszen HG: **Enteral nutrition and the risk of mortality and infectious complications in patients with severe acute pancreatitis: a meta-analysis of randomized trials.** *Arch Surg (Chicago, Ill: 1960)* 2008, **143**(11):1111–1117.
43. Kiss CM, Byham-Gray L, Denmark R, Loetscher R, Brody RA: **The impact of implementation of a nutrition support algorithm on nutrition care outcomes in an intensive care unit.** *Nutr Clin Pract* 2012, **27**(6):793–801.
44. Petrov MS, Pylypchuk RD, Uchugina AF: **A systematic review on the timing of artificial nutrition in acute pancreatitis.** *Br J Nutr* 2009, **101**(6):787–793.
45. Wereszczynska-Siemiatkowska U, Swidnicka-Siergiejko A, Siemiatkowski A, Dabrowski A: **Early enteral nutrition is superior to delayed enteral nutrition for the prevention of infected necrosis and mortality in acute pancreatitis.** *Pancreas* 2013, **42**(4):640–646.
46. Eatock FC, Chong P, Menezes N, Murray L, McKay CJ, Carter CR, *et al*: **A randomized study of early Nasogastric versus nasojejunal feeding in severe acute pancreatitis.** *Am J Gastroenterol* 2005, **100**(2):432–439.
47. Beger HG, Rau B, Isenmann R, Schwarz M, Gansauge F, Poch B: **Antibiotic prophylaxis in severe acute pancreatitis.** *Pancreatology* 2005, **5**(1):10–19.
48. Gerzof SG, Banks PA, Robbins AH, Johnson WC, Spechler SJ, Wetzner SM, *et al*: **Early diagnosis of pancreatic infection by computed tomography-guided aspiration.** *Gastroenterology* 1987, **93**(6):1315–1320.
49. Besselink MG, de Bruijn MT, Rutten JP, Boermeester MA, Hofker HS, Gooszen HG, *et al*: **Surgical intervention in patients with necrotizing pancreatitis.** *Br J Surg* 2006, **93**(5):593–599.
50. Rodriguez JR, Razo AO, Targarona J, Thayer SP, Rattner DW, Warshaw AL, *et al*: **Debridement and closed packing for sterile or infected necrotizing pancreatitis: insights into indications and outcomes in 167 patients.** *Ann Surg* 2008, **247**(2):294–299.
51. Jafri NS, Mahid SS, Idstein SR, Hornung CA, Galandiuk S: **Antibiotic prophylaxis is not protective in severe acute pancreatitis: a systematic review and meta-analysis.** *Am J Surg* 2009, **197**(6):806–813.
52. Wittau M, Mayer B, Scheele J, Henne-Bruns D, Dellinger EP, Isenmann R: **Systematic review and meta-analysis of antibiotic prophylaxis in severe acute pancreatitis.** *Scand J Gastroenterol* 2011, **46**(3):261–270.
53. Isenmann R, Rünzi M, Kron M, Kahl S, Kraus D, Jung N, *et al*: **Prophylactic antibiotic treatment in patients with predicted severe acute pancreatitis: a placebo-controlled, double-blind trial.** *Gastroenterology* 2004, **126**(4):997–1004.
54. Imrey PB, Law R: **Antibiotic prophylaxis for severe acute pancreatitis.** *Am J Surg* 2010, **203**(4):556–557.
55. Dambrauskas Z, Parseliunas A, Gulbinas A, Pundzius J, Barauskas G: **Early recognition of abdominal compartment syndrome in patients with acute pancreatitis.** *World J Gastroenterol* 2009, **15**(6):717–721.
56. Mentula P, Kylänpää M-L, Kemppainen E, Jansson S-E, Sarna S, Puolakkainen P, *et al*: **Early prediction of organ failure by combined markers in patients with acute pancreatitis.** *Br J Surg* 2005, **92**(1):68–75.
57. Dellinger EP, Forsmark CE, Layer P, Levy P, Maraví-Poma E, Petrov MS, *et al*: **Determinant-based classification of acute pancreatitis severity: an International multidisciplinary consultation.** *Ann Surg* 2012, **256**(6):875–880.
58. Hartwig W, Werner J, Müller CA, Uhl W, Büchler MW: **Surgical management of severe pancreatitis including sterile necrosis.** *J Hepato-biliary-pancreatic Surg* 2002, **9**(4):429–435.
59. Götzinger P, Wamser P, Exner R, Schwanzer E, Jakesz R, Függer R, *et al*: **Surgical treatment of severe acute pancreatitis: timing of operation is crucial for survival.** *Surg Infect (Larchmt)* 2003, **4**(2):205–211.
60. Walser EM, Nealon WH, Marroquin S, Raza S, Hernandez JA, Vasek J: **Sterile fluid collections in acute pancreatitis: catheter drainage versus simple aspiration.** *Cardiovasc Intervent Radiol* 2006, **29**(1):102–107.
61. Zerem E, Imamovic G, Omerović S, Imširović B: **Randomized controlled trial on sterile fluid collections management in acute pancreatitis: should they be removed?** *Surg Endoscopy* 2009, **23**(12):2770–2777.

9

Antimicrobials: a global alliance for optimizing their rational use in intra-abdominal infections (AGORA)

Massimo Sartelli[1*], Dieter G. Weber[2], Etienne Ruppé[3], Matteo Bassetti[4], Brian J. Wright[5], Luca Ansaloni[6], Fausto Catena[7], Federico Coccolini[8], Fikri M. Abu-Zidan[9], Raul Coimbra[10], Ernest E. Moore[11], Frederick A. Moore[12], Ronald V. Maier[13], Jan J. De Waele[14], Andrew W. Kirkpatrick[15], Ewen A. Griffiths[16], Christian Eckmann[17], Adrian J. Brink[18], John E. Mazuski[19], Addison K. May[20], Rob G. Sawyer[21], Dominik Mertz[22], Philippe Montravers[23], Anand Kumar[24], Jason A. Roberts[25], Jean-Louis Vincent[26], Richard R. Watkins[27], Warren Lowman[28], Brad Spellberg[29], Iain J. Abbott[30], Abdulrashid Kayode Adesunkanmi[31], Sara Al-Dahir[32], Majdi N. Al-Hasan[33], Ferdinando Agresta[34], Asma A. Althani[35], Shamshul Ansari[36], Rashid Ansumana[37], Goran Augustin[38], Miklosh Bala[39], Zsolt J. Balogh[40], Oussama Baraket[41], Aneel Bhangu[42], Marcelo A. Beltrán[43], Michael Bernhard[44], Walter L. Biffl[45], Marja A. Boermeester[46], Stephen M. Brecher[47], Jill R. Cherry-Bukowiec[48], Otmar R. Buyne[49], Miguel A. Cainzos[50], Kelly A. Cairns[51], Adrian Camacho-Ortiz[52], Sujith J. Chandy[53], Asri Che Jusoh[54], Alain Chichom-Mefire[55], Caroline Colijn[56], Francesco Corcione[57], Yunfeng Cui[58], Daniel Curcio[59], Samir Delibegovic[60], Zaza Demetrashvili[61], Belinda De Simone[62], Sameer Dhingra[63], José J. Diaz[64], Isidoro Di Carlo[65], Angel Dillip[66], Salomone Di Saverio[67], Michael P. Doyle[68], Gereltuya Dorj[69], Agron Dogjani[70], Hervé Dupont[71], Soumitra R. Eachempati[72], Mushira Abdulaziz Enani[73], Valery N. Egiev[74], Mutasim M. Elmangory[75], Paula Ferrada[76], Joseph R. Fitchett[77], Gustavo P. Fraga[78], Nathalie Guessennd[79], Helen Giamarellou[80], Wagih Ghnnam[81], George Gkiokas[82], Staphanie R. Goldberg[76], Carlos Augusto Gomes[83], Harumi Gomi[84], Manuel Guzmán-Blanco[85], Mainul Haque[86], Sonja Hansen[87], Andreas Hecker[88], Wolfgang R. Heizmann[89], Torsten Herzog[90], Adrien Montcho Hodonou[91], Suk-Kyung Hong[92], Reinhold Kafka-Ritsch[93], Lewis J. Kaplan[94], Garima Kapoor[95], Aleksandar Karamarkovic[96], Martin G. Kees[97], Jakub Kenig[98], Ronald Kiguba[99], Peter K. Kim[100], Yoram Kluger[101], Vladimir Khokha[102], Kaoru Koike[103], Kenneth Y. Y. Kok[104], Victory Kong[105], Matthew C. Knox[106], Kenji Inaba[107], Arda Isik[108], Katia Iskandar[109], Rao R. Ivatury[76], Maurizio Labbate[110], Francesco M. Labricciosa[111], Pierre-François Laterre[112], Rifat Latifi[113], Jae Gil Lee[114], Young Ran Lee[115], Marc Leone[116], Ari Leppaniemi[117], Yousheng Li[118], Stephen Y. Liang[119], Tonny Loho[120], Marc Maegele[121], Sydney Malama[122], Hany E. Marei[35], Ignacio Martin-Loeches[123], Sanjay Marwah[124], Amos Massele[125], Michael McFarlane[126], Renato Bessa Melo[127], Ionut Negoi[128], David P. Nicolau[129], Carl Erik Nord[130], Richard Ofori-Asenso[131], AbdelKarim H. Omari[132], Carlos A. Ordonez[133], Mouaqit Ouadii[134], Gerson Alves Pereira Júnior[135], Diego Piazza[136], Guntars Pupelis[137], Timothy Miles Rawson[138], Miran Rems[139], Sandro Rizoli[140], Claudio Rocha[141], Boris Sakakhushev[142], Miguel Sanchez-Garcia[143], Norio Sato[103], Helmut A. Segovia Lohse[144], Gabriele Sganga[145], Boonying Siribumrungwong[146], Vishal G. Shelat[147], Kjetil Soreide[148], Rodolfo Soto[149], Peep Talving[150], Jonathan V. Tilsed[151], Jean-Francois Timsit[152], Gabriel Trueba[153], Ngo Tat Trung[154], Jan Ulrych[155], Harry van Goor[49], Andras Vereczkei[156], Ravinder S. Vohra[157], Imtiaz Wani[158], Waldemar Uhl[90], Yonghong Xiao[159], Kuo-Ching Yuan[160], Sanoop K. Zachariah[161], Jean-Ralph Zahar[162], Tanya L. Zakrison[163], Antonio Corcione[164], Rita M. Melotti[165], Claudio Viscoli[166] and Perluigi Viale[167]

* Correspondence: massimosartelli@gmail.com; m.sartelli@virgilio.it
[1]Department of Surgery, Macerata Hospital, Via Santa Lucia 2, 62100 Macerata, Italy
Full list of author information is available at the end of the article

Abstract

Intra-abdominal infections (IAI) are an important cause of morbidity and are frequently associated with poor prognosis, particularly in high-risk patients.

The cornerstones in the management of complicated IAIs are timely effective source control with appropriate antimicrobial therapy. Empiric antimicrobial therapy is important in the management of intra-abdominal infections and must be broad enough to cover all likely organisms because inappropriate initial antimicrobial therapy is associated with poor patient outcomes and the development of bacterial resistance.

The overuse of antimicrobials is widely accepted as a major driver of some emerging infections (such as *C. difficile*), the selection of resistant pathogens in individual patients, and for the continued development of antimicrobial resistance globally. The growing emergence of multi-drug resistant organisms and the limited development of new agents available to counteract them have caused an impending crisis with alarming implications, especially with regards to Gram-negative bacteria.

An international task force from 79 different countries has joined this project by sharing a document on the rational use of antimicrobials for patients with IAIs. The project has been termed AGORA (Antimicrobials: A Global Alliance for Optimizing their Rational Use in Intra-Abdominal Infections). The authors hope that AGORA, involving many of the world's leading experts, can actively raise awareness in health workers and can improve prescribing behavior in treating IAIs.

Background

Judicious, careful and rational use of antimicrobials is an integral part of good clinical practice. This attitude maximizes the utility and therapeutic efficacy of treatment, and minimizes the risks associated with emerging infections and the selection of resistant pathogens. The indiscriminate and excess use of antimicrobial drugs appears the most significant factor in the emergence of resistant microorganisms in recent years.

We propose that clinical leaders drive antimicrobial stewardship and education programs to help standardize and improve prescribing behaviors. Furthermore, we argue that endorsement and guidance on the appropriate use of antimicrobials from leading scientific societies and clinical leaders within a specialty are vital to address the global threat of antimicrobial resistance and to provide support to policy makers.

AGORA, (Antimicrobials: A Global Alliance for Optimizing their Rational Use in Intra-Abdominal Infections) was conceived to actively raise the awareness of the rational and judicious use of antimicrobial medications in the treatment of intra-abdominal infections, in modern health care. This collaboration involves an international multidisciplinary task force, promoted by the World Society of Emergency Surgery (WSES), and endorsed by: the Surgical Infection Society (SIS), the American Association for the Surgery of Trauma (AAST), the Panamerican Trauma Society (PTS), the Indian Society for Trauma and Acute Care (ISTAC), the Korean Society of Acute Care Surgery (KSACS), the World Society of Abdominal Compartment Syndrome (WSACS), the South African Society of Clinical Microbiology (SASCM), the Hellenic Society for Chemotherapy, the Italian Society of Anti-Infective Therapy (SITA), The Italian Society of Anesthesiology, Analgesia, Resuscitation and Intensive Therapy (SIAARTI), the Italian Society of Surgery (SIC), the Italian Association of Hospital Surgeons (ACOI), the Italian Society of Emergency Surgery and Trauma (SICUT), the Italian Society of Intensive Care (SITI) and the World Alliance Against Antibiotic Resistance (WAAAR). WAAAR is a non-profit non-governmental organization participating actively in the global fight against antibiotic resistance.

It is the intent of AGORA to actively raise awareness of healthcare providers and improve prescribing behaviors when treating patients with IAIs worldwide.

This position paper aims to review the consequences of antimicrobial use, the evidence behind the global phenomenon of antimicrobial resistance, and to summarize the general principles of antimicrobial therapy in the modern management of patients with intra-abdominal infections. A review of the scientific rationale of modern antimicrobial pharmacotherapy is presented.

Methods

An extensive review of the literature was conducted using the PubMed and MEDLINE databases, limited to the English language. The resulting information was shared by an international task force from 79 different countries combined in the AGORA (Antimicrobials: A Global Alliance for Optimizing their Rational Use in Intra-Abdominal Infections) project. The resulting document, detailing current knowledge and opinion, is presented in this position and consensus statement. The document is presented in light of the aim to facilitate clinical guidance in the rational use of antimicrobials for intra-abdominal infections.

Results

The development of antimicrobial resistance and the selection of pathogenic bacteria from use of antibiotics

Clinicians prescribing antibiotics have two potentially conflicting responsibilities. First, clinicians should offer optimal therapy for the individual patient under their care by offering antimicrobials. Second, they should preserve the efficacy of antimicrobials and minimize the development of resistance and the selection of resistant pathogens [1] by withholding antimicrobials.

Antimicrobials and resistance

The problem of antimicrobial resistance (AMR) is widespread worldwide. Clinicians should be aware of their role and responsibility for maintaining the effectiveness of current and future antimicrobials. Health workers can help tackle resistance by:

- *enhancing infection prevention and control;*
- *prescribing and dispensing antimicrobials when they are truly needed; and*
- *prescribing and dispensing the right antimicrobial(s) to treat the illness.*

Infections caused by antibiotic-resistant bacteria continue to be a challenge. Rice [2] in 2008 coined the acronym of "ESKAPE" pathogens including *Enterococcus faecium, Staphylococcus aureus, Klebsiella pneumoniae, Acinetobacter baumannii, Pseudomonas aeruginosa,* and *Enterobacter* species to emphasize that these bacteria currently cause the majority of hospital infections and effectively "escape" the effects of antibacterial drugs [3].

Although the phenomenon of AMR can be attributed to many factors, there is a well-established relationship between antimicrobial prescribing practices and the emergence of antimicrobial resistant pathogens [4–6]. After they have emerged, resistant pathogens may be transmitted from one individual to another [7]. While, the indigenous intestinal microbiota provides an important host-defense mechanism by preventing colonization of potentially pathogenic microorganisms, the intestinal tract is also an important reservoir for antibiotic-resistant bacteria [8, 9]. Antibiotics exert undue selective pressure on bacteria in the intestine through a two-step process. First, antibiotics kill susceptible bacteria from the commensal intestinal microbiota. This favors bacteria within the intestine that are already resistant, have become resistant through mutation or through the acquisition of exogenous DNA (e.g. plasmids) from cells colonized in, or passing through, the intestinal tract. Most feared by clinicians is the acquisition of multi-drug resistant organisms (MDRO) in the intestinal microbiota of patients [10]. Second, antibiotics promote the overgrowth of MDRO present in the intestinal microbiota [11, 12] thereby increasing the risks of cross-transmission between patients [13] and increasing the risk of untreatable or difficult-to-treat infectious outbreaks [14]. Selective pressure from antibiotics combined with ineffective infection control practices accelerates the spread of resistant bacteria [15]. Thus, with few new antibiotics being developed, particularly for Gram-negative organisms, prudent antibiotic use is vital for delaying the emergence of resistance [16].

Antibiotics and C. difficile infection

C. difficile infections have become more frequent, more severe and more difficult to treat.

The prolonged use of antibiotics induces a change in the intestinal flora and may result in a higher incidence of C. difficile infections.

C. difficile is an anaerobic, spore forming, Gram-positive bacillus, which may be part of the normal intestinal microbiota in healthy newborns but is rarely present in the gut of healthy adults [17]. A direct correlation between antibiotic use and *C. difficile* infection (CDI) has been well described [18]. Disruption of the normal gut flora as a consequence of antibiotic use provides an excellent setting for *C. difficile* to proliferate and produce toxins [19].

The risk of CDI is increased up to 6-fold during and in the subsequent month after antibiotic therapy [20]. Although nearly all antibiotics have been associated with CDI, clindamycin, amoxicillin-clavulanate, cephalosporins and fluoroquinolones have traditionally been considered to pose the greatest risk [21–38].

In 2014, a systematic review of observational epidemiological studies measuring associations between antibiotic classes and hospital acquired CDI was published [30]. Of 569 citations identified, 13 case–control and 1 cohort study (15,938 patients) were included. The strongest associations were found for third-generation cephalosporins, clindamycin, second-generation cephalosporins, fourth-generation cephalosporins, carbapenems, trimethoprim-sulphonamides, fluoroquinolones and penicillin combinations.

In the last two decades, the dramatic increase in incidence and severity of CDI in many countries worldwide [18], has made CDI a global public health challenge.

CDI represents the most common cause of diarrhea in hospitalized patients. *C. difficile* colitis can be treated by oral or intravenous metronidazole and/or oral or intracolonic vancomycin [29]. In severe colitis, surgery may be required [30].

In 2015, the WSES published guidelines for management of *C. difficile* infection in surgical patients [18].

Antibiotics and invasive candidiasis

Usually, Candida spp. are kept under control by the native bacteria and by the body's immune defenses.

Antibiotics disrupt normal bacterial colonization and may create an environment in which fungi can thrive.

The gastrointestinal tract is normally colonized by yeasts, mainly *Candida spp.* [31–33]. It is believed that invasive candidiasis predominantly originates from this reservoir [34]. The mechanisms that allow *Candida spp.* to cause invasive candidiasis and candidemia are quite complex. *Candida spp.* are commensal members of the gastrointestinal microflora and in homeostasis with the host. However, when this homeostasis is disrupted, the yeast can break through the intestinal mucosal barrier and cause dissemination [35, 36]. This process may involve many contributing factors and multiple mechanisms [35]. The immunocompetent human host, with his/her resident microbiota, is remarkably good at maintaining a healthy symbiotic equilibrium. However, chemotherapy and invasive surgical procedures, may result in a human host disequilibrium that facilitate fungal invasion.

The global burden of antimicrobial resistance

Antimicrobial Resistance (AMR) poses a global challenge. No single country, however effective it is at containing resistance within its boundaries, can protect itself from the importation of MDRO through travel and trade.

The global nature of AMR calls for a global response, both in the geographic sense and across the whole range of sectors involved. Nobody is exempt from the problem, nor from playing a role in the solution.

Despite an increasing prevalence of MDRO worldwide, the health and economic impact of these organisms is often underestimated.

The impact of AMR worldwide is significant, both in economic terms, and clinical morbidity and mortality because it may:

- *lead to some infections becoming untreatable;*
- *lead to inappropriate empirical treatment in critically ill patients where an appropriate and prompt treatment is mandatory;*
- *increase length of hospital stay, morbidity, mortality and cost; and*
- *make necessary alternative antimicrobials which are more toxic, less effective, or more expensive.*

Antimicrobial resistance is a natural phenomenon that occurs as microbes evolve. However, human activities have accelerated the pace at which microorganisms develop and disseminate resistance. Incorrect and injudicious use of antibiotics and other antimicrobials, as well as poor prevention and control of infections, are contributing to the development of such resistance.

The impact of AMR worldwide is significant, both in economic terms, and clinical morbidity and mortality [38–40].

Although the optimally effective and cost-effective strategy to reduce AMR is not known, a multifaceted approach is most likely to be successful [15].

Many calls to action on antimicrobial resistance have been made over the past years, but there has been very little progress. Countries with the strictest policies on antibiotic prescription including Scandinavian countries the Netherlands and Switzerland now report the lowest rates of bacterial resistance [41]. However in most high income countries, clinical use of antibiotics has not declined, despite frequent calls to curtail overuse.

The World Health Organization (WHO) is now leading a global effort to address antimicrobial resistance. At the 68th World Health Assembly in May 2015, the World Health Assembly endorsed a global action plan to tackle antimicrobial resistance [42]. It sets out five strategic objectives:

- to improve awareness and understanding of antimicrobial resistance;
- to strengthen knowledge through surveillance and research;
- to reduce the incidence of infection;
- to optimize the use of antimicrobial agents; and
- to develop the economic case for sustainable investment that takes account of the needs of all countries, and increase investment in new medicines, diagnostic tools, vaccines and other interventions.

An alarming pattern of resistance involving multi and pandrug-resistant Gram-negative bacteria is currently emerging; multi-resistant *Enterobacteriaceae* is an increasing major concern worldwide [43, 44]. Comparative antimicrobial resistance data worldwide are difficult to obtain and inevitably suffer from bias. In high income countries, MDRO have historically been confined to the hospital setting. Since the middle of the 2000s, however, MDRO such as the extended-spectrum (ESBL) producing beta-lactamase (ESBL) *Enterobacteriaceae* have been widespread in the community setting [45].

Throughout the 1980s and 1990s, prolonged hospital and intensive care unit stays were considered among the most important risk factors for harboring ESBL *Enterobacteriaceae* along with exposure to broad-spectrum antibiotics [46].

However, most ESBL producing infections are now also in the community and healthcare-associated settings as demonstrated in studies from Europe and the Southeastern USA [47, 48].

The burden of MDRO infections in low-middle income countries (LMIC) is difficult to quantify, because surveillance activities to guide interventions require resources [49].

In these countries, routine microbiologic culture and sensitivity testing, especially in rural hospitals, are not performed, due to lack of personnel, equipment and financial resources. As a result antimicrobial therapy is empirical and a small collection of antimicrobials may be overused. This approach, although relatively inexpensive, may further increase the emergence of AMR and hence sub-optimal clinical outcomes [49].

Therefore, although resistance containment interventions in healthcare structures have mostly been implemented in high-income countries, there is a pressing need to intervene in the resistance pandemic also in LMIC.

Mechanism of resistance

The treatment of infections is increasingly complicated by the ability of bacteria to develop resistance to antibiotics.

Bacteria may be intrinsically resistant to one or more classes of antibiotics, or may acquire resistance by de novo mutation or by the acquisition of resistance genes from other organisms.

Better understanding of mechanisms of antibiotic resistance would allow the development of control strategies to reduce the spread of resistant bacteria and their evolution.

Bacteria may be intrinsically resistant to a class of antibiotics or may acquire resistance.

Main mechanisms of resistance to antibiotics can be caused by [50]:

- the inactivation or modification of the antibiotic;
- an alteration or the protection of the target site of the antibiotic that reduces its binding capacity;
- the modification of metabolic pathways to circumvent the antibiotic effect; and
- the reduced intracellular antibiotic accumulation by decreasing permeability and/or increasing active efflux of the antibiotic.

Bacteria can develop resistance to antibiotics by mutating existing genes (vertical evolution) [51], or by acquiring new genes from other strains or species (horizontal gene transfer) [52].

Many of the antibiotic resistance genes are carried on genetic elements (plasmids, transposons or phages) that act as vectors that transfer these genes to other members of the same bacterial species, as well as to bacteria in another genus or species [52].

Evolution and dissemination of resistance

One of the main problems surrounding antibiotic resistance genes is their association with mobile genetic elements (MGEs) such as conjugative plasmids, transposons, and viruses or mobility genes from MGEs [53–55]. The MGEs allow resistance to spread horizontally and disseminate among different bacterial species. Although this association seems improbable, it appears to occur frequently and follows a series of evolutionary steps fueled by natural selection (antibiotic selection). The power of modern DNA sequence analysis allows us to better understand the process of emergence of these genetic structures.

Most families of antibiotics present in nature are compounds produced by fungi or bacteria; bacteria utilize these compounds to eliminate competitor microorganisms. As part of this arms race, many microorganisms code for genes whose products neutralize antibiotics; these genes may have been present in bacterial chromosomes for millions of years and they were probably not mobile, as evidenced by recent findings. The massive use of antibiotics probably favored selection of antibiotic resistant bacteria resulting in large numbers of bacteria coding for resistance genes. Additionally, genes with mutations conferring novel forms of antibiotic resistance may also rise in numbers under antibiotic pressure.

On the other hand, bacterial chromosomes are populated with transposable elements (insertion sequences known as *ISs*), which jump frequently and randomly, as demonstrated during in vitro experiments [56]. The existence of large numbers of bacteria containing resistance genes sets the stage for the next step which is the association of AR genes with *IS*, which may cause increased transcription of resistance genes (*IS* contain powerful promoters) [57]; antibiotic selection once again will then favor the survival of bacteria with higher expression of resistance genes. *IS*s are also known to promote the mobilization of contiguous pieces of DNA and once there is a large number of bacteria with resistance genes associated to *IS*s, the stage is set for the next step which is the mobilization of the resistance genes.

Antibiotic resistance genes could be mobilized to genetic structures, such as plasmids and phages, which can move horizontally between bacterial cells including different bacterial species. This is probably the path followed by many plasmid encoded genes such as CTX-M-type β-lactamase (found in plasmids in *Enterobacteriaceae*), which was probably mobilized by a transposon from its original location in the chromosome of the intestinal bacteria *Kluyvera* [58].

The association of resistance genes to these mobile structures could occur through *IS*s (as explained previously); this has been postulated as the origin of many MGE. Alternatively, plasmids or phages may also integrate in the bacterial chromosome in the vicinity of resistance genes and then mobilize the resistance genes as these structures excise from chromosomes [55].

Some of these gene associations are ancient and they have been dragging genes that confer bacteria with different abilities including protection from harmful compounds. Some of them have lost most of the genetic information retaining few MGE genes such as transposases, integrases or genes involved in conjugation (relaxosome) [55]. The examples of these ancient platforms are integrons which have integrases derived from phages [55] and conjugative integrative elements such as the staphylococcal SCC*mec* which contains genes allowing conjugation (similar to plasmids) [59]. Additionally, conjugal plasmid integration (formation of Hfr) and phages (generalized transduction) could promote the transfer of large sections of bacterial genome including resistance genes) [60, 61].

The antibiotic selection is responsible for large numbers of bacteria with antibiotic resistance genes; the combination of a large number of resistance genes and recombinant nature of bacterial chromosomes creates the ideal scenario for combination of genes. Antibiotic selection will influence every single genetic event (recombination, excision, conjugation, integration) allowing the survival of bacteria with ideal resistance gene expression; only changes that are meaningful (high benefits and low cost) will prevail, the rest of them will disappear or they will circulate at undetectable levels. The MGEs detected by the current gene detection analysis, including metagenomic analysis, correspond to the tip of the iceberg, as they represent the most successful gene associations. The more we use antibiotics, the more efficient MGEs will evolve.

Antibiotic resistance in Enterobacteriaceae

Resistance to beta-lactam antibiotics Resistance to beta-lactams in *Enterobacteriaceae* is mainly conferred by beta-lactamases. These enzymes inactivate beta-lactam antibiotics by hydrolysis. Beta-lactamases are commonly classified according to two systems: the Ambler molecular classification and the Bush–Jacoby–Medeiros functional classification [62].

The Ambler scheme classifies beta-lactamases into four classes according to the protein homology of enzymes. Beta-lactamases of class A, C, and D are serine beta-lactamase and class B enzymes are metallo-beta-lactamases [63]. The Bush–Jacoby–Medeiros functional scheme is based on functional properties of enzymes and on their ability to hydrolyze specific beta-lactam classes [64]. This classification was updated in 2010 [65]. The updated system includes group 1 (class C) cephalosporinases; group 2 (classes A and D) broad-spectrum, inhibitor-resistant, extended-spectrum beta-lactamases and serine carbapenemases; and group 3 (class B) metallo-beta-lactamases [65].

Group 1 enzymes are cephalosporinases belonging to molecular class C. They are more active on cephalosporins than benzylpenicillin. It includes AmpC beta-lactamases. AmpC beta-lactamases are clinically important cephalosporinases capable of inactivating cephalotin, cefazolin, cefoxitin, most penicillins, and beta-lactamase inhibitor-beta-lactam combinations. AmpC-hyperproducing mutants are resistant to penicillins, aztreonam, third generation cephalosporins including cefotaxime, ceftazidime, ceftriaxone and even ertapenem when the enzyme is massively expressed. Imipenem, meropenem and doripenem remain the most active beta-lactams against AmpC beta-lactamases [66].

Cefepime, a fourth-generation cephalosporin with broader spectrum activity compared to ceftriaxone, is a poor inducer of AmpC beta-lactamase. Many AmpC-producing organisms are susceptible to cefepime because cefepime is poorly hydrolyzed by the AmpC beta-lactamase enzyme [67]. However, the role of cefepime in treating infections caused by AmpC-producing organisms is controversial because of the inoculum effect. In vitro studies showed a high inoculum effect. If a 100-fold-higher inoculum is used, cefepime MIC increases dramatically for some AmpC producers [68]. Clinical studies demonstrated that cefepime may be a reasonable option for the treatment of invasive infections due to AmpC beta-lactamase-producing organisms when adequate source control is achieved [69].

Group 2 (classes A and D) represent the largest group of beta-lactamases, it includes ESBL producing *Enterobacteriaceae* and carbapenemases (class A) and OXA beta-lactamases (class D).

ESBL are enzymes capable of hydrolyzing and inactivating a wide variety of beta-lactams, including third-generation cephalosporins, penicillins, and aztreonam [70–72]. Most ESBLs of clinical interest are encoded by genes located on plasmids. These plasmids may also carry genes encoding resistance to other multiple drug classes including aminoglycosides and fluoroquinolones [73].

The main ESBL enzymes imparting antibiotic resistance are TEM-, SHV-, and CTX-M.

Although hyperproduction of beta-lactamases or additional resistance mechanisms may hamper the antibiotic effectiveness, most TEM, SHV and CTX-M variants remain susceptible in vitro to beta-lactam/beta-lactam inhibitor combinations (BLBLI) such as amoxicillin-clavulanate or piperacillin-tazobactam. However, the efficacy of BLBLI for treating serious ESBL infections is controversial [66]. For example, the increase in piperacillin/tazobactam MICs when bacterial inocula reach 10^7 colony forming units/mL is concerning, and may indicate the presence of other mechanisms of resistance [73]. Furthermore, in critically ill patients the pharmacokinetic properties of beta-lactams are modified and these patients may have adverse outcomes as a result of sub-optimal antibiotic exposure [74].

Rates of CTX-M infections have increased during the last decade compared with rates of TEM- and SHV-infections [75]. The diffusion of CTX-M-producing *Enterobacteriaceae* are common in Southeast Asia and Eastern Mediterranean countries (estimated rates of intestinal carriage, ~60 and ~30 %, respectively), therefore travel in these areas is a risk factor for acquisition [66, 76]. Carriage rates in the community are now above 5–10 % in many other geographic areas [76].

The OXA-type beta-lactamases are so named because of their oxacillin-hydrolyzing abilities. OXA beta-lactamases have resistance limited to the penicillins, but some became able to confer resistance to cephalosporins [77, 78]. OXA-1 and OXA-10 beta-lactamases have only a narrow hydrolytic spectrum. However, other OXA beta-lactamases including OXA-11, -14, -15, -16, -28, -31, -35 and -45 confer resistance to cefotaxime, ceftazidime and aztreonam [66]. OXA-23 and OXA-48 are classes of carbapenemases that belong to OXA-type beta-lactamases with carbapenem-hydrolyzing activities [79, 80]. While OXA-23 appears most frequently in *A. baumannii*, OXA-48 enzymes have now become widespread in the *Enterobacteriaceae*, especially in Mediterreanean countries [79].

K. pneumoniae carbapenemases (KPCs) are beta-lactamases produced by Gram-negative bacteria. They efficiently hydrolyse penicillins, all cephalosporins, monobactams, beta-lactamase inhibitors, and even carbapenems. KPCs are becoming an increasingly significant problem worldwide [81]. The first plasmid-encoded serine carbapenemase in the KPC enzyme family was discovered in the USA in 1996 and reported in 2001 [66]. KPC is the most common carbapenemase in the United States and in some European countries such as Italy. However, different groups of enzymes possessing carbapenemase properties have emerged, and are spreading worldwide. KPC-producing *K. pneumoniae* pose a serious threat in clinical situations where administration of effective empiric antibiotics is essential to prevent mortality following bacteraemia and infections in immunocompromised patients including organ transplant recipients and those with cancer [81–86]. A major concern is the emergence of colistin resistant KPC-positive *K pneumoniae* isolates. This is of particular clinical relevance, as colistin is currently a key component of treatment combinations. The selection of colistin resistant KPC producing strains probably results from the increasing use of colistin, in areas where KPC-positive *K pneumoniae* have spread [87]. In light of the emergence of a plasmid-borne colistin resistance gene, the prudent use of colistin is warranted [43].

Group 3 (Class B) metallo-beta-lactamases (MBLs) differ structurally from the other beta-lactamases by their requirement for a zinc ion at the active site. They are all capable of hydrolysing carbapenems. In contrast to the serine beta-lactamases, the MBLs have poor affinity or hydrolytic capability for monobactams and are not inhibited by clavulanic acid or tazobactam. The most common metallo-beta-lactamase families include the IMP, VIM and NDM. [88, 89]. A currently emerging MBL is the NDM (New Delhi metallo-beta-lactamase). NDM-1 was first detected in 2008 in a patient returning to Sweden from India [90, 91]. NDM-1 has been shown to be present at significant frequency within *Enterobacteriaceae* in India and has subsequently been shown to be present in bacterial isolates in a number of countries worldwide [91].

Resistance to fluoroquinolones All *Enterobacteriaceae* are naturally susceptible to fluoroquinolones. The process by which susceptible strains become highly fluoroquinolone resistant is thought to be a result of a series of sequential steps and several mutations are needed to produce a high level of fluoroquinolone resistance [92, 93]. High-level resistance emerges after successive chromosomal mutations in the DNA gyrase- encoding *gyrA* gene and topoisomerase IV-encoding *parC* gene [93]. The over-expression of efflux pumps may also play a role in the high level of resistance in certain strains. While there are many genes that are assumed to encode a drug transporter protein in *Enterobacteriaceae*, only AcrAB/TolC overexpression plays a major role in *E. coli* as a main efflux pump implicated in extruding fluoroquinolones [92]. Resistance to fluoroquinolones can also be mediated by the plasmid-encoded *qnr* genes, which confer protection of bacterial topoisomerases against fluoroquinolones, the plasmid-encoded efflux pump *qepA* and the aminoglycoside-modifying enzyme AAC(6′)-Ib-cr that partly inactivate ciprofloxacin [92].

Resistance to aminoglycosides Aminoglycosides resistance occurs through several mechanisms that can simultaneously coexist. Aminoglycosides resistance in *Enterobacteriaceae* relies mainly on the genes encoding aminoglycoside-modifying enzymes (AMEs). AMEs hamper antibiotic activity. AMEs are often located on plasmids that carry multiple resistance genes, including ESBL [66]. Current rates of co-resistance in hospital-acquired ESBL are 50–60 % for gentamicin and 10–20 % to amikacin [66]. Other described mechanisms of resistance include modification of the antibiotic target by mutation of the 16S rRNA or ribosomal proteins, methylation of 16S rRNA (by RNA methlysases which genes are often co-located with beta-lactamase encoding genes), reduced permeability and/or increasing active efflux of the antibiotic [94].

Antibiotic resistance in Non-fermenting gram-negative bacteria

Non-fermenting Gram-negative bacteria (*P. aeruginosa, S. maltophilia* and *A. baumannii*) are intrinsically resistant to many drugs and can acquire resistance to virtually any antimicrobial agent. A variety of resistance mechanisms have been identified in *P. aeruginosa* and other Gram-negative non-fermenting bacteria, including impermeable outer membranes, expression of efflux pumps, target alteration and production of antibiotic-hydrolyzing enzymes such as AmpC beta-lactamases that are either chromosomally encoded or acquired [95]. These mechanisms may be present simultaneously, conferring multiresistance to different classes of antibiotics. These mechanisms may also allow transmission to multiple strains of bacteria [66].

P. aeruginosa is intrinsically resistant to a number of beta-lactam antibiotics including amoxicillin, first and second generation cephalosporins, cefotaxime, ceftriaxone and ertapenem. Effective agents include ticarcillin, piperacillin, ceftazidime, cefepime, imipenem, meropenem and doripenem. Aztreonam activity is variable [66]. Unlike tazobactam, clavulanate is a strong inducer of AmpC in *P. aeruginosa* [96] *P. aeruginosa* also has the ability to acquire beta-lactamases, including ESBL and carbapenemases [66]. The *P. aeruginosa* genome contains several different multidrug resistance efflux pumps, which reside in the membrane and remove antimicrobials and toxins, thereby lowering their concentration inside the cell to sub-toxic levels. Overproduction of these pumps reduces susceptibility to a variety of antibiotics [97]. The most common system is MexAB-OprM. Its overexpression confers resistance to ticarcillin, aztreonam, and at a lesser extent, meropenem [98]. Reduced outer-membrane permeability caused by qualitative or quantitative alterations of the OprD porin, which manages the passage of imipenem through the outer membrane, confers *P. aeruginosa* a basal level of resistance to carbapenems, especially to imipenem [99].

The mechanisms of AMR in *A. baumannii* are various, and generally include production of beta-lactamases, impermeable outer membrane, expression of efflux pumps, and change of targets or cellular functions such as alterations in penicillin-binding proteins (PBPs). The PBPs play a crucial role in the synthesis of peptidoglycan, an essential component of the bacterial cell wall. *A. baumannii* naturally produces a non-inducible AmpC-type cephalosporinase (ACE-1 or ACE-2) and an OXA-51-like carbapenemase which confers, at basal levels of expression, intrinsic resistance to aminopenicillins, first and second generation cephalosporins and aztreonam. Ertapenem naturally lacks activity against non-fermenting Gram negative bacteria including *A. baumannii* [100]. Overproduction of the AmpC-type cephalosporinase confers acquired resistance to carboxypenicillins, ureidopenicillins and third generation cephalosporins. The emergence of carbapenem-resistant clones of *A baumannii* has been reported since the late 1980s. Carbapenem resistance can result from the over-expression of OXA-51-like oxacillinase, and from the acquisition of OXA-23-like, IMP, VIM, SIM or, more recently, NDM-type carbapenemases [101]. Acquired resistances to fluoroquinolones (mutations in *gyrA* and/or *parC*) and aminoglycosides (plasmid-borne AMEs) may be observed in ESBL as well as carbapenemase-producing *A. baumannii* strains [66]. Colistin resistant isolates are now increasing worldwide. Resistance to colistin is thought to be mediated by modifications of the lipopolysaccharides of the bacterial cell membrane that interfere with the agent's ability to bind bacterial targets [100].

Antibiotic resistance in Enterococci

Enterococci are intrinsically resistant to some penicillins, all cephalosporins, and, at a low level, to aminoglycosides. Additionally, they have acquired resistance to many other classes of antibiotics [102, 103].

Enterococci have intrinsic resistance to most beta-lactam antibiotics because of the low affinity penicillin binding proteins (PBPs). Attachment of beta-lactam agents to PBPs results in impaired cell wall synthesis and, in most cases, programmed cell death via creation of reactive oxygen species. Enterococci express low-affinity PBPs (PBP5 in *E. faecium*, PBP4 in *E. faecalis*) that bind weakly to beta-lactam antibiotics. Enterococci may develop increased resistance to penicillins through acquisition of beta-lactamases (very rare) or PBP4/5 mutations [104]. Higher level of resistance in *E. faecium* has been attributed to over production of low affinity PBP-5, a protein that can take over the function of all PBPs [104]. A variety of point mutations have been described in both *E. faecium* and *E. faecalis* [104]. In addition, enterococci are "tolerant" to the activity of beta-lactams, and may appear susceptible in vitro but develop tolerance after exposure to penicillin. This property is an acquired characteristic. Enterococci quickly develop tolerance after exposure to as few as five doses of penicillin [105, 106].

Enterococci exhibit intrinsic low-level resistance to all aminoglycosides, precluding their use as single agents. Intrinsic resistance is attributed to an inability of the aminoglycoside to enter the cell (where they act by inhibiting ribosomal protein synthesis) [104]. While intrinsic mechanisms result in low-level aminoglycoside resistance, acquisition of mobile genetic elements typically underlies high-level aminoglycoside resistance in both *E. faecium* and *E. faecalis*. High-level resistance most frequently occurs through acquisition of a bifunctional gene encoding aph(2'')-Ia-aac(6')-Ie, which inactivates aminoglycosides [106]. However, several other genes have been identified that confer gentamicin resistance, including aph(2′′)-Ic, aph(2′′)-Id and aph(2′′)-Ib [107]. These genes are minor contributors to resistance compared to aph(2′′)-Ia-aac(6′)-Ie. Their prevalence varies by geographical region [104].

The acquisition of glycopeptides resistance by enterococci has seriously affected the treatment and control of these organisms [108]. Glycopeptides act by binding to the pentapeptide precursors of enterococci, thereby inhibiting cell wall synthesis. Glycopeptide-resistant organisms modify these pentapeptide precursors, which bind glycopeptides with 1000-fold lower affinity than normal precursors [104]. Various phenotypes of vancomycin-resistant enterococci (VRE) have been characterized; VanA and VanB operons are by far the most prevalent in human glycopeptide-resistant enterococci (GRE) infections [104]. GRE have emerged as a major cause of nosocomial infections. The majority of GRE infections have been attributed to *E. faecium*, though glycopeptide resistance occurs in *E. faecalis* and other *Enterococcus* species as well [109].

Antibiotic resistance in Bacteroides fragilis

B. fragilis is the most frequently isolated anaerobic bacteria, perhaps because it is both one of the most prominent in the intestinal microbiota, and is one of the easiest to culture in routine laboratory conditions. Beta-lactam antibiotics and 5-nitroimidazoles have been extensively used against anaerobic bacteria. The classical mechanisms of resistance to beta-lactams include production of beta-lactamases, alteration of penicillin-binding proteins (PBPs), and changes in outer membrane permeability to beta-lactams [110]. The most common mechanism at this time is inactivation by one of the various groups of beta-lactamases encoded by the *cepA* gene. Many beta-lactamases from the *B. fragilis* group are cephalosporinases that may be inhibited by lactamase inhibitors (clavulanic acid, and tazobactam). This explains the susceptibilities of many *Bacteroides* strains to the beta-lactam/beta-lactamase inhibitor combinations [111, 112].

Bacterial resistance to carbapenems arises because of the production of metallo-beta-lactamase encoded by the *cfiA* gene [113]. *cfiA* is normally poorly expressed. However, increased expression of *cfiA*, caused by the acquisition of an insertion sequence (IS) upstream of the gene, can lead to high-level carbapenem resistance.

Metronidazole, the first 5-nitroimidazole to be used clinically, was introduced in 1960, but it was not until 1978 that Ingham et al. reported the first clinical isolate of *B. fragilis* that was metronidazole-resistant after long-term therapy [114]. A wide range of metronidazole resistance mechanisms have been described in *B. fragilis* including decreased activity or total inactivation of electron transport chain components [115], overexpression of multidrug efflux pumps [116] and overexpression of DNA repair protein (RecA protein). However, the most common mechanism of resistance consists in the expression of 5-nitroimidazole nitroreductases (encoded by the *nimA-G* genes) which are located on the chromosome or on a plasmid and transform 4- or 5-nitroimidazole genes to 4- or 5-aminoimidazoles [115]. Metronidazole-resistant strains of the *B. fragilis* group have been described in several countries, but in general, resistance is low [117]. As routine susceptibility testing of anaerobic bacteria in most laboratories is only performed in blood or other severe infections, it is difficult to estimate how frequent MDR *B. fragilis* group strain is.

Antibiotic resistance in intra-abdominal infections

Surveillance studies can help clinicians to identify trends in pathogens incidence and antimicrobial resistance, including identification of emerging pathogens at national and global levels.

Some epidemiological studies have monitored antimicrobial resistance in IAIs identifying changes in resistance patterns, mostly of Gram negative bacteria.

ESBL-producing Enterobacteriaceae

In the setting of intra-abdominal infections the main issue of resistance is due to ESBL producing *Enterobacteriaceae* [118]. Since 2002, the Study for Monitoring Antimicrobial Resistance Trends (SMART) has monitored the in vitro antibiotic susceptibility patterns of clinical Gram-negative collected worldwide from intra-abdominal cultures [119]. Limitations include the small number of contributing centers per country, and the characteristics of participating centers which are usually major teaching or tertiary-care centers.

From 2002 to 2011, the prevalence of MDR Gram negative bacilli, especially ESBL producers, has increased worldwide with regional variations in their distribution [119]. The prevalence of ESBLs producers in IAI isolates has steadily increased over time in Asia, Europe, Latin America, the Middle East, North America and the South Pacific. In contrast, the trend for ESBLs in intra-abdominal infection isolates from Africa has surprisingly, statistically significantly, decreased over time [119]. However only 7 African sites (3.9 %) (1 from Morocco, 2 from Tunisia and 4 from South Africa) were involved in the SMART Study.

Although ESBLs producing *Enterobacteriaceae* are common in hospital acquired IAIs, they are now being seen in community acquired IAIs as well as. In 2010, Hawser et al. [120] reported the incidence of ESBLs producers in community and hospital acquired IAI in Europe from 2002 to 2008. In order to differentiate community-acquired from hospital acquired IAIs, isolates were divided into those obtained from cultures collected <48 and ≥48 h after hospital admission, though this simple cut-off may result in mis-classification of some IAIs.

The SMART Study data showed a significant increase in ESBL-positive *E. coli* isolates (from 4.3 % in 2002 to 11.8 % in 2008 [$P < 0.001$]) with a smaller (and not statistically significant) increase in ESBL-positive *K. pneumoniae* isolates (increasing from 16.4 to 17.9 % [$p > 0.05$]) in Europe from 2002 to 2008. Hospital-acquired isolates were more common than community-acquired isolates, at 14.0 versus 6.5 %, respectively, for *E. coli* ($P < 0.001$) and 20.9 versus 5.3 %, respectively, for *K. pneumoniae* ($P < 0.01$) [120].

In the CIAOW Study [121] (Complicated intra-abdominal infections worldwide observational study), 68 medical institutions collaborated in a worldwide multi-center observational study, during a six-month study period (October 2012-March 2013). Among intra-operative isolates, ESBL producing *E. coli* isolates comprised 13.7 % (75/548) of all *E. coli* isolates, while ESBL producing *K. pneumoniae* isolates represented 18.6 % (26/140) of all *K. pneumoniae* isolates. ESBL producing *Enterobacteriaceae* were more prevalent in patients with healthcare-associated IAIs than they were in patients with community-acquired IAIs. Among healthcare associated infections, ESBL-positive *E. coli* isolates comprised 20.6 % (19/92) of all identified *E. coli* isolates, while ESBL-positive *K., pneumoniae* isolates made up 42.8 % (15/35) of all identified *K. pneumoniae* isolates.

Klebsiella pneumoniae Carbapenemases

K. pneumoniae carbapenemases (KPCs) are becoming an increasingly significant problem worldwide [122]. *E. coli* isolates from IAIs demonstrate consistently low resistance to carbapenems since the beginning of SMART. *K. pneumoniae* also continue to remain susceptible to carbapenems. Although carbapenem activity against *K. pneumoniae* from IAIs is also high, it is slightly lower than activity against *E. coli.* A total of 2841 clinical isolates of *K. pneumoniae* from intra-abdominal infections worldwide were collected in the SMART study during 2008 and 2009 [122]. Globally, 6.5 % of isolates were ertapenem resistant based on the June 2010 clinical breakpoints published by the Clinical and Laboratory Standards Institute, with MICs of ≥1 μg/ml [122].

Pseudomonas aeruginosa

P. aeruginosa was the third most common pathogen in IAIs at a rate of 5 % in the SMART Study [110]. In 2013, Babinchak et al. reported the trends in susceptibility of selected Gram-negative bacilli isolated from IAIs in North America from 2005 to 2010 [114]. The resistance of *P. aeruginosa* to fluoroquinolones significantly increased over time, from approximately 22 % in 2005, to 33 % in 2010. Imipenem activity remained unchanged with 20 % resistance. During this period, resistance to piperacillin-tazobactam, cefepime and ceftazidime remained unchanged at 23 to 26 %. [123]. However, the SMART Study demonstrated that the activity of select antimicrobials varied in different regions of the world. In South Africa during 2004–2009, *P. aeruginosa* resistance to piperacillin-tazobactam was 8 %, while it was approximately 25 % to cefepime, ceftazidime and imipenem, and 27 % to amikacin [119]. In China, during relatively the same time period (2002–2009), the resistance of *P. aeruginosa* to amikacin was 12 %, and to piperacillin-tazobactam was 8 % [119].

In the CIAOW study, among the microorganisms isolated from intraoperative samples, isolates of *P. aeruginosa* comprised 5.6 % of all aerobic identified bacteria. However, no significant differences between community acquired infections and healthcare associated infections (5.4 % in community acquired infections, versus 5.7 % healthcare associated infections) was demonstrated [121].

Enterococci

Among Gram-positive bacteria, enterococci play a significant role in IAI. Some studies have demonstrated poor outcomes among patients with documented enterococcal infections, particularly in those with post-operative IAI [124–127] where enterococci coverage should be always considered.

In 2012 the Dutch Peritonitis Study Group analyzing all patients from the RELAP trial found that the presence of only gram positive cocci, predominantly *Enterococcus* spp., was associated with worse outcome, although in secondary peritonitis microbial profiles did not predict ongoing abdominal infection after initial emergency laparotomy [128].

The Montravers EBIIA (Etude épidémiologique Bactério-clinique des Infections Intra-Abdominales) study [129] described the clinical, microbiological and resistance profiles of community-acquired and nosocomial IAI. This study reported an increase in the prevalence of nosocomial *E. faecalis* infections in patients (33 % in hospital-acquired infections, versus 19 % in community-acquired infections; $P < 0.05$). Although enterococci are found in community-acquired infections (11.8 %), they were far more prevalent in hospital-acquired infections (24.2 %).

In the CIAOW Study [121], among all the aerobic Gram-positive bacteria identified in the intraoperative samples, Enterococci (*E. faecalis and E. faecium*) were the most prevalent bacteria, representing 15.9 % of all aerobic isolates. Although Enterococci were also present in community-acquired infections, they were more prevalent in healthcare-associated infections (22.3 % in health-care IAIs versus 13.9 % in community-acquired infections).

Methicillin resistant Staphylococcus aureus (MRSA)

Methicillin resistant *Staphylococcus aureus* (MRSA) is not commonly isolated from patients with community-acquired intra-abdominal infection [121]. Although community-acquired MRSA has been reported in many settings, MRSA has less impact in community-acquired IAI. However, it should be always considered in the case of wound infections. MRSA should be suspected in patients with health care–associated IAI known colonized with the organism or who are at risk because of prior treatment failure and significant antibiotic exposure. The susceptibility pattern differs between community-acquired and hospital acquired MRSA.

Salmonella typhi

S. typhi infection may lead to diffuse peritonitis followed by ileal perforations in endemic countries [130].

The emergence of multidrug-resistant (MDR) typhoid fever is a major global health threat affecting many countries where the disease is endemic, such as countries in South-Central and Southeast Asia and many parts of Africa and Latin America [131]. In the past, *S. typhi* infections were routinely treated with chloramphenicol, ampicillin, or trimethoprim-sulfamethoxazole, but MDR to these antibiotics started to emerge in 1990 [132]. In response, a shift towards the prescription of fluoroquinolones or third-generation cephalosporins has occurred.

Singhal et al. [133] reported the trends in antimicrobial susceptibility of *S. typhi* from North India over a period of twelve years (2001–2012). In 852 isolates of *S. typhi*, a statistically significant decreased (p <0.001) resistance to chloramphenicol, ampicillin and and co-trimoxazole was observed. Resistance to nalidixic acid was found to be highest amongst all the antibiotics; it has been rising since 2005 and is presently 100 %. Ciprofloxacin resistance was relatively stable over the time period studied with a drastic increase from 5.8 % in 2008 to 10 % in 2009, since then it has increased in 2011–12 to 18.2 % [133].

Bacteroides fragilis

Anaerobes are the predominant components of the bacterial flora of normal human mucous membranes. *B. fragilis* strains are one of commonly isolated commensals in the setting of IAIs. Most clinical laboratories do not routinely perform the susceptibility testing of anaerobic isolates. In fact, their isolation requires appropriate methods of collection, transportation, and cultivation of specimens. Consequently, the treatment of anaerobic infections is often selected empirically [134].

B. fragilis strains are mostly sensitive to metronidazole, beta-lactam/beta-lactamase inhibitors and carbapenems. However, in the past years antibiotic resistance has increased among anaerobes and the susceptibility of anaerobic bacteria to antimicrobial agents has become less predictable [134].

Data of a national survey on antimicrobial resistance in *Bacteroides* strains, including 6574 isolates collected in 13 medical centers in United States from 1997 to 2007 were published in 2010 [135]. The study analyzed in vitro antimicrobial resistance to both frequently used and newly developed anti-anaerobic agents. Percent resistance was calculated using breakpoints recommended for the respective antibiotic by the CLSI or United States Food and Drug Administration. These data indicated that the carbapenems (imipenem, meropenem, ertapenem, and doripenem) and piperacillin-tazobactam were the most active agents against these pathogens, with resistance rates of 0.9–2.3 %. Metronidazole and tigecycline were the most active antibiotics among the non-beta-lactam agents. Metronidazole-resistant *Bacteroides* strains were also first reported during that period.

The susceptibilities of 824 *Bacteroides fragilis* group isolates against nine antibiotics were evaluated in a Europe-wide study involving 13 countries [136]. Piperacillin/Tazobactam was more active than amoxicillin/clavulanic acid (3.1 and 10.4 % resistance, respectively). Dramatic increases in resistance were observed for cefoxitin, clindamycin and moxifloxacin, with rates of 17.2, 32.4 and 13.6 %, respectively. The lowest resistances were found for imipenem, metronidazole and tigecycline (1.2, <1 and 1.7 %) [136].

Antimicrobial stewardship

Although most antimicrobial use occurs in the community, the intensity of use in hospitals is far higher; hospitals are therefore particularly important in the containment of antimicrobial resistance.

Hospital based Antibiotic Stewardship Programs (ASPs) can help clinicians both to optimize the treatment of infections and reduce adverse events associated with antibiotic use.

Given the urgent need to improve antimicrobial use in healthcare all acute care hospitals should implement Antibiotic Stewardship Programs.

Antimicrobial stewardship is an emerging strategy designed to optimize outcomes and reduce the emergence of resistant organisms through the pillars of surveillance, infection control and optimizing the use of antimicrobial therapy. Educating clinicians in the appropriate use of antimicrobials is an essential facet of antimicrobial stewardship [117].

Core principles of antimicrobial stewardship include the use of antibiotic prophylaxis only when there is proven efficacy, use of the narrowest spectrum of antimicrobial therapy with proven efficacy, use of the least number of agents and for the shortest length of therapy to achieve efficacy, and appropriate antimicrobial dosing to maximize efficacy and limit complications. However, the best strategies for an antimicrobial stewardship program (ASP) are not definitively established and are likely to vary based on local culture, policy and routine clinical practice [15]. Observational data support a significant association between stewardship practices and reduction of antibiotic resistance. In a retrospective before and after study design, analysis of two ICUs within a single institution (trauma and surgical) before and after the implementation of service specific antibiotic stewardship protocols, Dortch et al. demonstrated a significant reduction in the percentage of multidrug resistant gram negative pathogens isolated and a corresponding decrease in broad spectrum antibiotic use [137].

The Infectious Diseases Society of America/Society for Healthcare Epidemiology of America (IDSA/SHEA) guidelines identify two core proactive evidence-based strategies and several supplemental strategies for promoting antimicrobial stewardship [1]: first, a proactive strategy of either formulary restriction or a requirement for pre-approval for specific drugs or both, and second, a strategy of performing prospective audit with intervention and feedback to the prescriber. Restriction of antimicrobial use may be obtained either by limited access to available antimicrobials in the hospital through restriction of the hospital formulary, or implementation of a requirement for preapproval and a justification for prescribing drugs on the restricted list. Both methods have been shown to be effective in reducing the use and costs of restricted antimicrobials [138].

To estimate the effectiveness of antimicrobial stewardship programs and evaluate their impact on the incidence of antimicrobial-resistant pathogens or *C. difficile* infection and on clinical outcome a Cochrane meta-analysis was performed in 2013 [139]. Eighty-nine studies were included. The meta-analysis showed that interventions to decrease excessive antibiotic prescribing for hospital inpatients reduced antimicrobial resistance and hospital-acquired infections. Interventions to increase effective prescribing improved clinical outcomes. These data supported the use of restrictive interventions in urgent cases. However, persuasive and restrictive interventions were equally effective after six months.

Restrictive interventions do seem to have a greater immediate impact than persuasive interventions. However, with the passage of time, prescribers often find ways to circumvent restrictions [139].

Prescribing is a complex social process. Restriction is useful in urgent situations, but because of the reduced effects over time, programs and strategies should be balanced with positive actions. The ultimate goal of a stewardship should be to stimulate a behavioral change in prescribing practice.

In this context, education of prescribers is crucial to convince clinicians to use antibiotics judiciously.

The supplemental strategies employed in ASP include, implementation of guidelines and clinical pathways, antimicrobial order forms, streamlining or de-escalation, combination therapy, dose optimization, and IV-to-PO switch, therapeutic substitution, cycling, mixing and use of computer decision support. In general, several of these strategies are implemented in the daily practice simultaneously with one or both of the two core strategies.

Management of intra-abdominal infections

The treatment of patients with complicated IAI involves both timely source control and antimicrobial therapy.

Empiric antimicrobial therapy is important in the management of intra-abdominal infections and must be broad enough to cover all likely organisms. Adequate source control is mandatory in the management of complicated IAIs.

The treatment of patients with complicated IAI involves both source control and antimicrobial therapy. Source control encompasses all measures undertaken to eliminate the source of infection, reduce the bacterial inoculum and correct or control anatomic derangements to restore normal physiologic function [140]. Inadequate source control has been associated with increased mortality in patients with complicated IAI [141, 142]. Surgical source control entails resection or suture of a diseased or perforated viscus (e.g. diverticular perforation, gastroduodenal perforation), removal of the infected organ (e.g. appendix, gall bladder), debridement of necrotic tissue, resection of ischemic bowel and repair/resection of traumatic perforations, or drainage of infected fluid collections. The source control procedure will depend on the patient characteristics, organ affected, and specifically on the pathology that is encountered.

Ultrasound and CT guided percutaneous drainage of abdominal abscesses is safe and effective in selected patients [143–146], with 62–91 % cure rates and with morbidity and mortality rates equivalent to those of surgical drainage. Recent advances in interventional and more aggressive source control techniques, such as open abdomen strategy [147], could improve the outcome of patients with severe complicated IAI [148].

Although new surgical techniques, supported by innovative technology, have improved treatment for these patients, the markedly reduced development of new antibiotics has been unable to match the rapidly increasing phenomena of antimicrobial resistance making it a major ongoing challenge associated with the management of complicated IAI. Antimicrobial therapy plays an integral role in the management of complicated IAI. The main objectives of antimicrobial therapy in the treatment of IAI are to prevent local and haematogenous spread, and to reduce late complications.

Classifications

The term intra-abdominal infections (IAI), describes a wide heterogeneity of patient populations. A complete classification that includes all aspects of intra-abdominal infections does not exist. An ideal classification guiding clinicians in treatment should include:

- *the origin of source of infection;*
- *the anatomical extent of infection;*
- *the presumed pathogens involved and risk factors for major resistance patterns; and*
- *the patient's clinical condition.*

IAI encompass a variety of pathological conditions, ranging from uncomplicated appendicitis to faecal peritonitis. IAI are usually classified either as uncomplicated or complicated [149].

In uncomplicated IAI, the infection only involves a single organ and does not extend to the peritoneum. Such patients can be managed by either surgical resection or antibiotics [150]. In complicated IAI, the infectious process extends beyond the organ, causing either localized or diffuse peritonitis [150]. These situations require both source control and antimicrobial therapy.

A universally accepted classification divides infective peritonitis into primary peritonitis, secondary peritonitis and tertiary peritonitis [151]. Primary peritonitis is a diffuse bacterial infection (usually single organism) without loss of integrity of the gastrointestinal tract, typically seen in cirrhotic patients with ascites or patients with an indwelling peritoneal dialysis catheter. Secondary peritonitis, the most common form of peritonitis (>90 % cases), is an acute peritoneal infection resulting from loss of integrity of the gastrointestinal tract [152]. Examples include visceral perforations or necrosis of the gastrointestinal tract, blunt or penetrating trauma, and post-operative leakage of anastomoses or suture lines. Tertiary peritonitis is defined as a recurrent infection of the peritoneal cavity that occurs >48 h after apparently successful and adequate surgical source control of secondary peritonitis [153–155]. It is more common among critically ill or immunocompromised patients and may often be associated with highly resistant pathogens including *candida spp*. It is typically associated with high morbidity and mortality. Although tertiary peritonitis has been accepted as a distinct entity [153–155], it represents an evolution and complication of secondary peritonitis, therefore the term "ongoing peritonitis" may better indicate that it is not a different disease than secondary peritonitis, but rather represents secondary peritonitis lasting longer and harbouring other (selected) pathogen.

Traditionally, infections have been classified as, either community-acquired or hospital-acquired, dependent on the place of acquisition [155]. Hospital-acquired intra-abdominal infections (HA-IAI) are often associated with surgery or another invasive procedure (gastrointestinal endoscopy, invasive radiology). The most frequent type of HA-IAI is post-operative peritonitis (PP) [156–160], is the most common cause of which is anastomotic leakage [158]. In rare conditions, HA-IAI can occur in patients hospitalized for reasons unrelated to abdominal pathology and no prior abdominal surgery [161].

The term "healthcare-associated infection" (HCAI) is a new term for infections acquired during the course of receiving healthcare [162]. It includes hospital-acquired infections but also infections in patients living in skilled nursing facilities, having recent hospitalization within 90 days, using aggressive medical therapies (intravenous therapy, wound dressing) at home and invasive therapies (haemodialysis, chemotherapy, radiotherapy) in outpatient clinics within 30 days of the index infection [162].

However, in the years after the first proposal by Friedman et al. [162], a consensus definition of HCAI has not been reached. A systematic review of all definitions of HCAI used in clinical studies was published in 2014 [163]. The initial definition of HCAI seems to be increasingly accepted: "Attendance at a hospital or haemodialysis clinic in the previous 30 days and residence in a nursing home or long-term care facility" [163].

Differentiating community-acquired intra-abdominal infection (CA-IAIs) and healthcare-associated intra-abdominal infections (HCA-IAIs) is useful to define the presumed resistance patterns and specify patients with increased likelihood of infection caused by MDRO. Among patients with HCAI, those with hospital-acquired infections may be associated with increased mortality due to underlying patient health status and severity criteria at the time of diagnosis.

Grading of the clinical severity of patients with complicated IAI has been be well described by the sepsis definitions. Sepsis is a complex, multifactorial syndrome that may develop into conditions of varying and escalating severity [163–165].

Mortality rates increase in patients developing organ dysfunction and septic shock [166]. Mortality of septic patients from abdominal origin has decreased due to advances in management of the underlying infection and support of failing organs, but is still high [167]. The CIAOW study [121] described the epidemiological, clinical, and treatment profiles of complicated IAI worldwide. The overall mortality rate was 10.5 %, while it was significantly higher (36.5 %) for patients with organ dysfunction or septic shock at admission.

Recently, sepsis definitions were revised. Sepsis is defined as life-threatening organ dysfunction caused by a dysregulated host response to infection. Septic shock is defined as a subset of sepsis in which circulatory, cellular, and metabolic abnormalities are associated with a greater risk of mortality than with sepsis alone and should be clinically identified by a vasopressor requirement to maintain a mean arterial pressure of 65 mmHg or greater, and serum lactate level greater than 2 mmol/L (>18 mg/dL) in the absence of hypovolemia. Under this redefined terminology, "severe sepsis" has been abandoned [168].

Antimicrobial selection

Initial antimicrobial therapy for patients with IAIs is empiric in nature because critically-ill patients need immediate treatment and microbiological data (culture and susceptibility results) usually requires ≥24 h for the identification of pathogens and antibiotic susceptibility pattern.

Antimicrobials should be used after a treatable IAI has been recognized or when there is a high degree of suspicion for infection. Initial antimicrobial therapy in patients with IAIs is typically empirical in nature because they need immediate treatment (especially in critically-ill patients), and microbiological data (culture and susceptibility results) usually requires ≥24 h for the identification of pathogens and antibiotic susceptibility patterns. However, in non-critically ill patients survival benefit from adequate empiric antimicrobial therapy has not been consistently demonstrated, even in patients with Gram-negative bacteremia [169].

Knowledge of local rates of resistance and the risk factors that suggest an MDRO should be involved as essential components of the clinical decision-making process when deciding on which antimicrobial regimen to use for empiric treatment of infection [1]. Every clinician starting empiric therapy should know the local epidemiology. Surveillance initiatives are important, both in a local and in a global context. If local epidemiology suggests that a patient has been infected with a strain already known to be resistant to antibiotics, then inappropriate antimicrobial therapy, which fails to cover known resistance patterns risks further disruption of the natural flora and selecting for resistant variants without providing effective treatment.

Hospitals in the United States are required to publish an annual antibiogram that may be used as a source guideline for selecting appropriate antibiotics based on local resistance/susceptibility data.

Published guidelines

Different sets of guidelines for the management of patients with IAIs have been published.

Guidelines have a great impact on clinical care. They should incorporate stewardship principles.

Different sets of guidelines outlining the clinical management of IAIs have been published [170–178].

Historically, treatment guidelines have not taken into consideration antimicrobial stewardship principles when setting the priority order of antimicrobial options, and instead have focused primarily on safety and efficacy data.

Guidelines have major impact on delivery of clinical care, and on regulatory review of hospital performance. Hopefully, these guidelines will evolve to incorporate stewardship principles, in addition to safety and efficacy, when setting the priority order for recommended antimicrobial therapies.

Antimicrobial selection

Antimicrobial selection in community-acquired infections

For patients with CA-IAI, antimicrobial agents with a narrow spectrum of activity encompassing all likely organisms should be administered. However, a patient with risk factors for ESBL infection who is hemodynamically unstable may warrant empiric therapy to cover for ESBLs, with plans to de-escalate therapy once microbiology is known.

The major pathogens involved in community-acquired IAI (CA-IAI) are likely to be due to a patient's own flora. Therefore, they are predictable and include *Enterobacteriaceae* (predominantly *E. coli* and *Klebsiella* species), viridans group streptococci, and anaerobes (especially *B. fragilis*). For patients with CA-IAI, antimicrobial agents with a relatively narrower spectrum of activity encompassing wild-type strains from the above-mentioned species should be administered. However, if patients with CA-IAI have risk factors for infections due to ESBL producing *Enterobacteriaceae*, and in particular if the patient is hemodynamically unstable, antimicrobial agents that are effective against ESBLs may be warranted. Clinical stability and physiological well-being is an important factor, as compromised patients will suffer increased morbidity and mortality if initial therapy is ineffective [179]. In contrast, less severely ill patients may have more time for the clinician to know that initial therapy was not active. Specific risk factors for ESBL phenotype among infecting pathogens includes recent exposure to antibiotics (particularly beta-lactams or fluoroquinolones) within 90 days of IAI or known colonization with ESBL producing *Enterobacteriaceae*, [180, 181]. An additional risk may be represented by a recent trip to a region where MDR *Enterobacteriaceae* are widespread in the community [182].

Antimicrobial selection in health-care associated infections

For patients with HCA-IAI, empiric antimicrobial regimens with broader spectra of activity should be administered as these patients have a higher risk of infections due to MDRO.

By contrast, for patients with HCA-IAI, antimicrobial regimens with broader spectra of activity are preferable, as those patients have a higher risk of infections due to MDROs [183]. On receiving results of susceptibility testing, the clinician should opt for a narrow spectrum antimicrobial agent, which covers the likely causative organism. De-escalation of therapy must be weighed against the clinical significance of the culture results received as well as local epidemiology [184].

Antibiotic selection in critically Ill patients

An inadequate empiric antimicrobial regimen is associated with unfavorable outcomes in critical ill patients. In these patients the following strategies should be always implemented to obtain an optimal response to therapy:

- *early source control procedures when indicated;*
- *early initiation of therapy (ideally, within 1 h);*
- *correct dosing;*
- *considering risk factor for MDRO; and*
- *avoiding use of identical antibiotic and the same antibiotic class administered in the preceding 3 months.*

Infections are among the main factors contributing to mortality in intensive care units (ICU) [185]. Abdominal sepsis is a common indication for admission to the ICU. The abdomen is the second most common site of invasive infection among critically ill patients [186]. In 2014, the EPIC II study [187], including 13,796 adult patients from 1265 ICUs in 75 countries, revealed that mortality rate in patients who developed abdominal infections was significantly higher than in patients who had other infections (most of which were respiratory infections). Disease severity, need for organ support, and presence of co-morbidities were independently associated with mortality. In patients with organ dysfunction from septic shock, early appropriate empiric antimicrobial therapy has a significant impact on the outcome, independent of the site of infection [188]. The Surviving Sepsis Campaign guidelines recommend intravenous antimicrobials within the first hour of onset of sepsis and septic shock and the use of broad-spectrum agents with adequate penetration of the presumed site of infection [189]. An ineffective or otherwise inadequate antimicrobial regimen is one of the variables more strongly associated with unfavorable outcomes in critical ill patients [190]. Empiric antimicrobial therapy should be started as soon as possible in patients with organ dysfunction and septic shock [191–193].

De-escalation

The evidence on de-escalation strategies is largely restricted to patients with ventilator-associated pneumonia (VAP) [194–196] and patients with severe sepsis and septic shock, particularily in patients with IAIs [197, 198]. In 2013, a Cochrane review on de-escalation of antimicrobial treatment for adults with sepsis did not find adequate evidence to support this [199]. In 2014, a multicenter randomized trial investigating a strategy based on de-escalation of antibiotics resulted in prolonged duration of ICU stay and did not affect the mortality rate [198]. Several authors have associated antimicrobial de-escalation interventions in critically ill patients with reductions in length of hospitalization, inpatient antimicrobial use, adverse events, cost, and recovery of antimicrobial-resistant microorganisms [200, 201]. The safety and beneficial outcomes of carbapenem de-escalation as part of an antimicrobial stewardship program in an ESBL-endemic setting, was also recently confirmed [202].

Antibiotic armamentarium

The choice of empiric antibiotics in patients with IAI should be based on the severity of the infection, the individual risk for infection by resistant pathogens, and the local resistance epidemiology. Amoxicillin/clavulanate or cephalosporins in combination with metronidazole, are still good options for the treatment of non-severe IAIs, with piperacillin/tazobactam being a better choice if P. aeruginosa coverage is needed. The use of carbapenems should be limited so as to preserve activity of this class of antibiotics because of the concern of emerging carbapenem-resistance. Ciprofloxacin and levofloxacin are no longer appropriate first-line choices for empiric treatment in many regions because of the prevalence of fluoroquinolone resistance. Other options include aminoglycosides, particularly for suspected infections by Gram negative bacteria, and tigecycline especially when MDRO are suspected, though caution is advised for the latter, in the situation of a bacteremia.

Recent challenges in the management of multi-drug resistant Gram-negative infections, especially in critically ill patients, have reviewed the use of "old" antibiotics, such as polymyxins and fosfomycin.

Ceftolozone/tazobactam and ceftazidime/avibactam are new antibiotics that have been approved for treatment of cIAI infections (in combination with metronidazole) including infection by ESBLs and P. aeruginosa, though their role for the empirical therapy remains to be defined.

IAI may be managed by either single or multiple antimicrobial regimens. Table 1 presents the spectrum of activity of antimicrobial agents for common IAI pathogens, Table 2 presents recommended intravenous antimicrobial doses for patients with IAI and preserved renal function. These doses may not be adequate for patients with morbid obesity as there are currently no specific dosing recommendations for antibiotics in obese patients [203].

Beta-lactam/beta-lactamase inhibitor combinations

Beta-lactam/beta-lactamase inhibitor combinations (BLBLI), including ampicillin/sulbactam, amoxicillin/clavulanate, ticarcillin/clavulanate, piperacillin/tazobactam, have an in vitro activity against Gram-positive, Gram-negative and anaerobe organisms [204]. However, increasing antimicrobial resistance to ampicillin/sulbactam and amoxicillin/clavulanate among *E. coli* and other *Enterobacteriaceae* including community-acquired isolates, during the last decade, has compromised clinical utility of these agents for empirical therapy of serious Gram-negative infections [205, 206]. This is likely due to excessive use of amoxicillin and amoxicillin-clavulanate in both children and adults, particularly in the treatment of upper respiratory tract infection. The combination of over use of these oral antibiotics in the community and potential for household transmission of resistant *E. coli* strains among family members make ampicillin/sulbactam and amoxicillin/clavulanate resistance unpredictable [207]. Fortunately, most isolates remain susceptible to other beta-lactam/beta-lactamase inhibitors such as piperacillin/tazobactam. Broad-spectrum activity of piperacillin/tazobactam, including anti-pseudomonal and anaerobic coverage, still make it an attractive option in the management of severe IAIs [208].

A meta-analysis of PubMed and Scopus databases providing data for mortality among patients treated with carbapenems, BLBLI or non- BLBLI (mainly cephalosporins and fluoroquinolones), preferably as monotherapy was published in 2013 [209]. The study reported no statistically significant difference in mortality between carbapenems and BLBLI administered as either empiric or definitive therapy. The authors concluded that the role of BLBLI should be further evaluated for definitive treatment [209]. In a recent study of 331 unique patients with ESBL bacteremia, piperacillin/tazobactam appeared inferior to carbapenems in the treatment of ESBL bacteremia [210]; the use of piperacillin/tazobactam in ESBLs infections is still controversial [211].

Cephalosporins

Most isolates of *E. coli* and other *Enterobacteriaceae* remain susceptible to third-generation cephalosporins. Among this drug class, cefotaxime, ceftriaxone and ceftizoxime, in combination with metronidazole may be options for empirical therapy of CA-IAI, due to the relatively narrow spectrum of coverage bacause these agents lack activity against *P. aeruginosa*. On the other hand, ceftazidime and cefoperazone have activity against *P. aeruginosa*, but have relatively less activity against streptococci as compared to other third-generation cephalosporins. Cefepime, a fourth-generation cephalosporin, with broader spectrum activity compared to ceftriaxone is a poor inducer of AmpC beta-lactamase, and is poorly hydrolyzed by the enzyme, allowing it to be effective against AmpC-producing organisms [66]. For empiric therapy, cefepime must be combined with metronidazole [212] because it does not possess anti-anaerobic activity.

The newest "5th" generation cephalosporins such as ceftobiprole have very broad-spectrum activity, exhibiting potent in vitro activity against a number of Gram-positive pathogens including MRSA, penicillin-resistant *Streptococcus pneumoniae*, and Gram-negative pathogens including AmpC producing *E. coli* and *P. aeruginosa*. Their role towards *E. faecium* PBP 5 (PBP 5fm) is controversial [213]. Ceftobiprole medocaril is approved for the treatment of community-acquired pneumonia and hospital-acquired pneumonia (excluding ventilator-associated pneumonia), in the European Union [214, 215]. It has not been approved for the treatment of cIAI.

Fluoroquinolones

Fluoroquinolones (FQ) have been widely used in the treatment of intra-abdominal infections because of their excellent activity against aerobic Gram-negative bacteria and tissue penetration [216]. Ciprofloxacin has in vitro activity against *P. aeruginosa*. Ciprofloxacin has lowest MIC against *P. aeruginosa* among commonly used fluoroquinolones such as levofloxacin and moxifloxacin.

Except for moxifloxacin, the FQ have a moderate activity against anaerobes and have been used in combination with metronidazole in the empiric treatment of IAI.

FQ are rapidly, and almost completely, absorbed from the gastrointestinal tract, particularly levofloxacin and moxifloxacin. Peak serum concentrations obtained after oral administration are very near those achieved with intravenous administration [217]. Prior patient use of FQ has been demonstrated as an independent risk factor for FQ resistance [218]. Therefore, the empiric use of FQ for IAI is discouraged in patients with recent exposure to this class of antibiotics. In addition, the increasing use of FQ in aged care facilities, particularly for the treatment of urinary tract infections, has contributed to the emergence of *E. coli* virulent strains, such as O25b-ST131, with substantially high FQ resistance rates in patients living at those facilities [219]. In recent years, resistance of *E.coli* to FQ has risen over time [218]. The worldwide increase in FQ resistance among *E. coli* and other *Enterobacteriaceasaee* has limited the non-stratified use of FQ for empirical treatment of IAI, particularly in critically-ill patients and those with HCA-IAI [206].

Carbapenems

For decades, carbapenems have been the antibiotics of first choice for ESBLs. The best option for targeting ESBLs (though with no coverage of *P. aeruginosa)* is ertapenem, a once daily administered carbapenem that

Table 1 Antibiotics for treating patients with intra-abdominal infections based upon susceptibility. Use local antibiogram data for choosing optimal antibiotics in target population

Antibiotic	Enterococci	Ampicillin-resistant enterococci	Vancomycin-resistant enterococci	Enterobacteriaceae	ESBL-producing *Enterobactericeae*	*Pseudomonas aeruginosa*	Anaerobic Gram-negative bacilli
Penicillins/Beta-lactamase Inhibitors							
Amoxicillin/ clavulanate	+	–	–	+	–	–	+
Ampicillin/ Sulbactam	+	–	–	+	–	–	+/–
Piperacillin/ tazobactam	+	–	–	+	+/–	+	+
Carbapenems							
Ertapenem	–	–	–	+	+	–	+
Imipenem/ cilastatin	+/–[a]	–	–	+	+	+	+
Meropenem	–	–	–	+	+	+	+
Doripenem	–	–	–	+	+	+	+
Fluoroquinolones							
Ciprofloxacin	–	–	–	+	–	+[b]	–
Levofloxacin	+/–	–	–	+	–	+/–	–
Moxifloxacin	+/–	–	–	+	–	–	+/–
Cephalosporins							
Ceftriaxone	–	–	–	+	–	–	–
Ceftazidime	–	–	–	+	–	+	–
Cefepime	–	–	–	+	+/–	+	–
Ceftolozane/ tazobactam	–	–	–	+	+	+	–
Ceftazidime/ avibactam	–	–	–	+	+	+	–
Aminoglycosides							
Amikacin	c	c	c	+	+	+	
Gentamicin	c	c	c	+	+	+	–
Glycylcyclines							
Tigecycline	+	+	+	+[d]	+	–	+
5-nitroimidazole							
Metronidazole	–	–	–	–	–	–	+
Polymyxin							
Colistimethate (Colistin)	–	–	–	+[e]	+	+	–
Glycopeptides							
Teicoplanin	+	+	–	–	–	–	–
Vancomycin	+	+	–	–	–	–	–
Oxazolidines							
Linezolid	+	+	+	–	–	–	–

[a]"Imipenem/cilastatin" is more active against ampicillin-susceptible enterococci than ertapenem, meropenem and doripenem
[b]Ciprofloxacin is more active against *Pseudomonas aeruginosa* than levofloxacin
[c]Active in synergy with other agents
[d]Not active against *Proteus, Morganella* and *Providencia*
[e]Not active against *Morganella, Proteus, Providencia and Serratia*

Table 2 Recommended intravenous doses of the most commonly used antibiotics for patients with intra-abdominal infections and normal renal function (CrCl > 90 mL/min)

Intravenous Antibiotic	Intravenous dosing recommendation for patients with normal renal function *(CrCl > 90 mL/min)
Penicillins/ Beta-lactamase Inhibitors	
Amoxicillin/clavulanate	1.2 g 8-hourly
Ampicillin/Sulbactam	3 g 6-hourly
Piperacillin/tazobactam	4.5 g 6- 8-hourly or 3.375 g 6-hourly
Carbapenems	
Ertapenem	1 g 24-hourly
Imipenem/cilastatin	0.5 g 6-hourly (or1 g 8-hourly)
Meropenem	1 g 8-hourly
Fluoroquinolones	
Ciprofloxacin	400 mg 8–12 hourly
Levofloxacin	750 mg 24-hourly
Moxifloxacin	400 mg 24-hourly
Cephalosporins	
Ceftriaxone	1–2 g 24-hourly
Ceftazidime	2 g 8-hourly
Cefepime	1–2 g 8 hourly
Ceftolozane/tazobactam	1.5 g 8-hourly
Ceftazidime/avibactam	2.5 g 8-hourly
Glycylcyclines	
Tigecycline	100 mg initial dose, then 50 mg 12-hourly
Aminoglycosides	
Amikacin	15–20 mg/kg 24-hourly
Gentamicin	5–7 mg/kg 24-hourly
5-nitroimidazole	
Metronidazole	500 mg 6–8 hourly
Glycopeptides	
Teicoplanin	12 mg/kg 12-hourly times 3 loading dose then 12 mg/kg 24-hourly
Vancomycin	15–20 mg/kg/dose 8–12 hourly; in critically ill patients 25–30 mg/kg loading dose
Oxazolidinonees	
Linezolid	600 mg 12 hourly
Polymyxins	
Colistin	US: 2.5 to 5 mg/kg CBA 8–12 hourly Europe: 9 million IU 8–12 hourly as a slow intravenous; in critically ill patients 9 million IU loading dose as a slow intravenous infusion

Note–the above table provides general information, the susceptibility profile of individual organisms should be confirmed to guide antimicrobial therapy in all situations. Dosage should be adjusted according to the antibiotic's pharmacokinetic/pharmacodynamic profile in each patient
Higher dosages may be used in septic shock

otherwise shares the activity of imipenem, meropenem and doripenem against most species, including ESBL producing pathogens [220, 221]. Imipenem/cilastatin, meropenem and doripenem provide coverage for Gram-negative non-fermenting bacteria (e.g. *P. aeruginosa* and *A. baumannii*). However, inappropriate use of carbapenems should be avoided [222] because there is an association with the increase in carbapenem-resistant *Enterobacteriaceae*, e.g. the rapid spread of carbapenemases in *K. pneumoniae* or NDM-1 producing *Enterobacteriaceae* and *P. aeruginosa* [223].

Regarding *Enterococcus* coverage among carbapenems, impipenem/cilastatin is most active in vitro against ampicillin-susceptible *E. faecalis* while ertapenem, meropenem, and doripenem have limited activity against both *E. faecalis* and *E. faecium*. In addition, carbapenems are not generally recommended for use to treat bacteremia due to *Enterococcus* spp. In carbapenemase producing *K. pneumoniae* with an MIC ≤8 μg/ml, carbapenem-containing combinations, including meropenem or doripenem, is suggested [224].

Aminoglycosides

Aminoglycosides are particularly active against aerobic Gram-negative bacteria and act synergistically against certain Gram-positive organisms. They are effective against *P. aeruginosa,* but are ineffective against anaerobic bacteria. Because of their serious toxic side effects including nephrotoxicity and ototoxicity, some authors do not recommend aminoglycosides for the routine empiric treatment of community-acquired IAI. They may be reserved for patients with allergies to beta-lactam agents or when used in combination with beta-lactams for treatment of IAI secondary to MDRO [225]. However, other authors have questioned the clinical importance of the toxic side-effects [226], and their decreased activity in acidic environment such as pus. In any case, this class of antibiotics remains an important option in the antimicrobial armamentarium for combating Gram-negative bacteria and widening the spectrum of the empirical therapy when MDRO are suspected [178].

Tigecycline

Tigecycline, an antibiotic from the group of the tetracyclines, does not feature in vitro activity against *P. aeruginosa* or certain *Enterobacteriaceae* (*Proteus spp., Serratia spp., Morganella morganii, Providencia stuartii*). However, it remains a viable treatment option for complicated IAI due to its favorable in vitro activity against anaerobic organisms, enterococci, several ESBLs and some strains of carbapenemase-producing *Enterobacteriaceae* [227]. In several trials, excess mortality was seen in patients treated with tigecycline when compared with other drugs; in 12 of 13 phase 3 and 4 comparative clinical trials [228], all-cause mortality was found higher in the tigecycline group versus the comparison group. Study-level and patient-level analyses identified that patients in the hospital-acquired pneumonia trial, particularly those with ventilator-associated pneumonia with baseline bacteremia, were at a higher risk of clinical failure and mortality.

A mortality analysis was used to investigate the association of baseline factors in abdominal infections, including severity of illness at study entry and treatment assignment, with clinical failure and mortality. Mortality modelling identified multiple factors associated with death which did not include tigecycline and which were forced into the model.

Similarly, attributable mortality, among subjects who died of primary infection, in the cIAI studies, showed no difference among treatments. Combined with the four phase 3 and 4 cIAI trials that demonstrated the non-inferiority of tigecycline to the comparator regimens, these results suggest that deaths were less related to clinical failure and that other factors or patient co-morbidities were more likely to contribute to death [229].

Because of poor plasma concentration tigecycline performs poorly in bacteremic patients, with a much higher risk of failing clear bacteremia than the comparator. Tigecycline should not be considered first line for health care associated pneumonia, bacteremia or endocarditis. Nonetheless, tigecycline remains an important treatment option for patients with complicated IAI [230, 231]. Recently, tigecycline has been become an important option in managing infections due to MDR Gram negative bacteria [232] including NDMs, KPCs, and other carbapenemases, as some of these pathogens remain susceptible to tigecycline. However, high failure rates in cases of monotherapy with this antibiotic have occurred implying that combinations therapy should be recommended [233]. Higher-dose regimens have been associated with better outcomes than conventional administration due to Gram-negative MDR bacteria in a cohort of critically ill patients with severe infections [234].

Polymixins

Polymyxins, discovered in 1940s, are a group of polycationic peptide antibiotics that exhibit potent efficacy against most gram-negative bacteria. Among all the five chemical compounds (A–E) of polymyxins, only polymyxin B and E (colistin) are clinically used. Since the 1970s, these preparations were practically abandoned because of reports of severe adverse events. However, recent challenges in the management of multi-drug resistant (MDR) Gram-negative infections, especially in critically ill patients, have revived the clinical use of polymyxins [235–237]. The nephrotoxicity and neurotoxicity of polymyxins has been the major limiting factor in their clinical application. Challenging these earlier concerns, recent data, mainly from cases series, demonstrate that the use of polymyxins is relatively safe provided that recommended dosages are used and renal function is closely monitored [235, 238, 239].

Recently The US Food and Drug Administration (FDA) and European Medicines Agency (EMA) have approved updated dose recommendations for intravenous colistin in patients with various degrees of renal function [240].

The EMA recommendations were based on a review of the available clinical, pharmacological and pharmacokinetic data.

EMA recommended expression of colistin dose in IU of colistimethate sodium. Based on the limited available evidence the recommended dose in adults was 9 million IU (approximately 300 mg) daily in 2 or 3 divided doses as a slow intravenous infusion; in critically ill patients a loading dose of 9 million IU was suggested. EMA suggested to reduce dosage according to creatinine clearance in patients with renal impairment.

Also US Food and Drug Administration (FDA) approved changes to the dosage and administration section of the product label for colistimethate in the United States. The recommended dose was 2.5 to 5 mg/kg colistin base activity (CBA) per day in 2 to 4 divided doses for patients with normal renal function, depending on the severity of the infection. A loading dose was not recommended for critically ill patients. The FDA recommended dosing regimen accounts for renal function. The most significant difference regards loading dose suggested in the EU but not in the United States' recommendations.

Fosfomycin

Renewed interest in 'old' antibiotics has also focused interest in Fosfomycin. While traditionally fosfomycin disodium was administered parenterally, several countries have recently approved the oral administration of fosfomycin tromethamine for treating urinary tract infections (UTIs) caused by *Escherichia coli* and *E. faecalis*. Its use as a single agent is usually restricted in critically ill patients. However, intravenous fosfomycin has been administered in combination with other antibiotics for the treatment of MDR Gram-positive and Gram-negative bacteria including KPC [241].

The daily dose of intravenous fosfomycin disodium ranges from 12 to 16 g on average, administered in 2–4 infusions. Renal impairment significantly decreases the excretion of fosfomycin. For intravenous administration of fosfomycin, the doses should be reduced if the creatinine clearance is less than 50 ml/min [242].

The primary limitations of fosfomycin are the lack of established regimens for complicated infections and the lack of availability of the intravenous formulation in many countries [243].

New antibiotics

Ceftolozane/tazobactam [244, 245] and ceftazidime/avibactam [246, 247] have recently been approved in some national agencies for the treatment of intra-abdominal infections. By adding beta-lactamase inhibitor (tazobactam or avibactam), these new agents have strong activity against MDR Gram-negative pathogens. Unlike other beta-lactam and beta-lactamase inhibitor combination agents, these new agents should be combined with metronidazole for complicated IAI due to limited activity against some *Bacteroides* species.

These antibiotics will be valuable for treating infections caused by MDR Gram-negative bacteria in order to preserve carbapenems. Notably, ceftazidime/avibactam has demonstrated consistent activity against KPC-producing organisms [248].

In some instances that resistance can emerge to new antibiotics very rapidly after their first clinical trials, treatment with these new agents should be done in parallel with continued susceptibility testing [249]. Although many reviews have been written, their precise role as an empiric treatment for complicated IAI remains to be defined [250]. Cautious clinical use is advised, until their precise roles are further defined as empirical treatment.

The effect of fungal involvement in IAI

Empiric antifungal therapy should be considered in patients with clinical evidence of intra-abdominal infection and significant risk factors for candidiasis:

- *recent abdominal surgery;*
- *anastomotic leaks;*
- *necrotizing pancreatitis; and*
- *failure of treatment for bacterial infections.*

The epidemiological role of *Candida spp.* in IAI has not yet been conclusively defined [251]. However, recent data suggest that some specific subpopulations are at higher risk of fungal involvement, (i.e. complicated cases of bariatric surgery). In a recent study, Zappella et al. [252] reported 41 % of candida-positive patients with postoperative peritonitis following bariatric surgery. Isolation of *Candida* spp. in samples from IAI is associated with poor outcomes. In an observational study, Montravers et al. showed that isolation of *Candida* spp. was an independent risk factor of mortality in nosocomial peritonitis patients (odds ratio, 3; 95 % confidence interval, 1.3-6.7, $p < 0.001$). Antifungal treatment did not improve survival [253]. Recently, IDSA guidelines for the treatment of invasive candidiasis were developed and explicitly addressed candidal peritonitis [254]. Clinical evidence supporting the use of antifungal therapy for patients with suspected intra-abdominal invasive candidiasis is limited. Most studies are small and uncontrolled, single-center, or performed in specific patient cohorts. IDSA guidelines suggested considering empiric antifungal therapy for patients with clinical evidence of intra-abdominal infection and significant risk factors for candidiasis, including those with recent abdominal surgery, anastomotic leaks, or necrotizing pancreatitis, who are doing poorly despite treatment for bacterial infections.

Several meta-analyses of antifungal prophylaxis in high-risk surgical ICU patients have yielded conflicting results [255–258].

For the majority of ICU patients at high invasive candidiasis risk, a preemptive antifungal strategy, based on clinical risk factors and microbiologic evidence of substantial colonization, has been proposed [259].

A recent randomized, double-blind, placebo-controlled trial assessed a preemptive antifungal approach with an echinocandin in intensive care unit patients requiring surgery for intra-abdominal infection [260].

The study was unable to provide evidence that preemptive administration of an echinocandin was effective in preventing IC in high-risk surgical intensive care unit patients with intra-abdominal infections.

Preferred empiric therapy in critically ill patients or those previously exposed to an azole is an echinocandin (caspofungin: loading dose of 70 mg, then 50 mg daily; micafungin:100 mg daily; anidulafungin: loading dose of 200 mg, then 100 mg daily). However, fluconazole, 800-mg (12 mg/kg) loading dose, then 400 mg (6 mg/kg) daily, should be still considered first-line antifungal therapy, in hemodynamically stable patients who are colonized with azole susceptible Candida species or who have no prior exposure to azoles.

The duration of therapy should be determined by adequacy of source control and clinical response.

A role for echinocandin in the management of critically ill patients is confirmed by the increasing incidence of fluconazole-resistant and susceptible-dose dependent strains that should be taken into account when selecting empiric therapy in patients with severe sepsis or septic shock [261, 262].

Dosage

Knowledge of the pharmacokinetic and pharmacodynamic antimicrobial properties of each antimicrobial inform rational dosing.

Optimal use of the pharmacokinetic/pharmacodynamic characteristics of antimicrobial agents is important for obtaining good clinical outcomes and reduction of resistance.

The antimicrobial dosing regimen should be established depending on host factors and properties of antimicrobial agents. Antimicrobial pharmacodynamics integrates the complex relationship between organism susceptibility and patient pharmacokinetics. Pharmacokinetics describes the fundamental processes of absorption, distribution, metabolism, and elimination and the resulting concentration-versus-time profile of an agent administered in vivo. The achievement of appropriate target site concentrations of antimicrobials is essential to eradicate the relevant pathogen. Suboptimal target site concentrations may have important clinical implications, and may explain therapeutic failures, in particular, for bacteria for which in vitro MICs are high [263]. Antimicrobials typically need to reach a site of action outside the plasma. This requires the drug to pass through the capillary membranes. Disease and drug-related factors can contribute to differential tissue distribution [264]. Concentration gradient between the plasma and the peritoneal space has been studied for some antibiotics and have shown large variability [265–268]. Commonly encountered situations where pharmacokinetics change and dosing individualization may be necessary include renal and hepatic dysfunction. Dose reductions may be necessary to prevent accumulation and toxicity in patients with reduced renal or hepatic function.

Knowledge of the pharmacokinetic and pharmacodynamic antimicrobial properties of each drug including (inhibition of growth, rate and extent of bactericidal action, and post-antibiotic effect) may provide a more rational determination of optimal dosing regimens in terms of the dose and the dosing interval [269]. Optimal use of the pharmacokinetic/pharmacodynamic relationship of anti-infective agents is important for obtaining good clinical outcomes and reduction of resistance [270]. Dosing frequency is related to the concept of time-dependent versus concentration-dependent killing. Beta-lactams exhibit time-dependent activity and exert optimal bactericidal activity when drug concentrations are maintained above the MIC [271, 272]. Therefore, it is important that the serum concentration exceeds the MIC for appropriate duration of the dosing interval for the antimicrobial and the organism. Higher frequency dosing, prolonged infusions and continuous infusions have been utilized to achieve this effect [267]. For beta lactams, prolonged or continuous infusions have been advocated in order to maximize the time that the drug concentration exceeds the MIC, whereas high peak concentrations are not beneficial. However, large randomized controlled trials comparing continuous with intermittent infusion of piperacillin/tazobactam in patients with complicated IAI [273] as well as piperacillin/tazobactam, ticarcillin/clavulanate or meropenem in patients with severe sepsis [274], did not demonstrate different outcomes. These results may not be generalizable to patients with high severity of illness and infections caused by less susceptible pathogens with high MIC (e.g. *P. aeruginosa*), for which the greatest potential for a clinically relevant benefit is predicted by pharmacokinetic/pharmacodynamic theory, and has been supported by some retrospective studies [275, 276]. Prolonged or continuous infusions of beta lactams should therefore be considered for the treatment of critically ill patients with hospital-acquired IAI.

In contrast, antibiotics such as aminoglycosides exhibit concentration-dependent activity and should be administered in a once daily manner (or with the least possible number of daily administrations) in order to achieve high peak plasma concentrations.

With these agents, the peak serum concentration, and not the time the concentration remains above the MIC, is more closely associated with efficacy [271, 272]. In terms of toxicity, aminoglycosides nephrotoxicity is caused by a direct effect on the renal cortex and its uptake saturation. Thus, an extended interval dosing strategy reduces the renal cortex exposure to aminoglycosides and reduces the risk of nephrotoxicity [277].

In patients with septic shock, administering an optimal first dose is probably as equally important as to the timing of administration [271]. This optimal first dose could be described as a loading, or front-loaded dose and is calculated from the volume of distribution (Vd) of the drug and the desired plasma concentration. The Vd of hydrophilic agents (which disperse mainly in water such as beta-lactams, aminoglycosides and glycopeptides) in patients with septic shock may be altered by changes in the permeability of the microvascular endothelium and consequent alterations in extracellular body water. This may lead to lower than expected plasma concentrations during the first day of therapy resulting in sub-optimal achievement of antibiotic levels [271].

In the setting of alterations in the volume of distribution, loading doses and/or a higher overall total daily dose of beta-lactams, aminoglycosides, or glycopeptides are often required to maximize the pharmodynamics ensuring optimal drug exposure to the infection site in patients with severe sepsis or septic shock [271].

Tissue penetration is also an important aspect because high concentrations at the site of infection can potentially overcome "resistance". Albumin concentrations are crucial for highly protein-bound drugs [271].

When drains have been inserted, large drainage volume outputs may also affect antibiotic concentration, and may need to be accounted for when considering dosage and frequency of administration.

Once an appropriate initial loading dose is achieved, the antimicrobial regimen should be reassessed, at least daily, because pathophysiological changes may significantly affect drug availability in the critically ill patients. Lower than standard dosages of renally excreted drugs must be administered in the presence of impaired renal function, while higher than standard dosages of renally excreted drugs may be needed for optimal activity in patients with glomerular hyperfiltration [271]. It should be noted that in critically ill patients, plasma creatinine is an unreliable marker of renal function. The phenomenon of "augmented renal clearance" (creatinine clearance >130 ml/min/1.73 m^2) causes subtherapeutic concentrations. This phenomenon has high prevalence among critically ill patients [278].

The value of intra-operative specimens

Obtaining microbiological cultures from blood or fluid/ tissue allows:

- *to expand antimicrobial regimen if the initial choice is too narrow; and*
- *to perform a de-escalation is the empirical regimen is too broad.*

They should be always performed in patients with healthcare-associated infections or with community-acquired infections at risk for resistant pathogens.

When a microorganism is identified in clinical cultures, antimicrobial susceptibility testing (AST) should always be performed and reported to guide antibiotic therapy.

A lack of impact on patient outcomes by bacteriological cultures has been documented in patients with community-acquired IAI, especially in appendicitis [279, 280]. However, this observation may not address the issues surrounding the threats of antibiotic resistance. The results of microbiological testing may have great importance for the choice of therapeutic strategy of every patient, in particular in the adaptation of targeted antimicrobial treatment. While the yield of blood cultures may be relatively low in patients with IAI, clinicians should not miss an easy opportunity to establish the microbiologic etiology by obtaining two sets of blood cultures prior to starting antibiotics, particularly in patients admitted to the hospital in critically ill conditions. Fluid and/or tissue culture from the site of infection should be collected, particularly in the presence of an abscess. Sufficient fluid volume (usually at least 1 mL of fluid or tissue) must be collected, and then transported to the microbiology laboratory using a transport system that properly handles and preserves the samples to avoid damage or compromise their integrity.

Obtaining microbiological results from blood or fluid/ tissue culture from the site of infection has two advantages: a) it provides an opportunity to expand antimicrobial regimen if the initial choice was too narrow, and, b) it also allows de-escalation of antimicrobial therapy if the empirical regimen was too broad. When a microorganism is identified in clinical cultures, antimicrobial susceptibility testing (AST) should always be performed and reported to guide antibiotic therapy. AST measures the ability of a specific organism to grow in the presence of a particular drug using guidelines established by either the Clinical or Laboratory Standards Institute (CLSI) in United States or the European Committee for Antimicrobial Susceptibility Testing (EUCAST) in Europe. By the end of 2012, in several European Countries, CLSI guidelines had been replaced by EUCAST [281]. In vitro susceptibility results are correlated with the clinical success or failure of an antibiotic against a particular organism. Data are reported in the form of MIC, which is the lowest concentration of an antibiotic that inhibits visible growth of a microorganism. The numerical MIC number, expressed as micrograms/ml, is usually reported by microbiology laboratories as a categorical guide for clinicians, ie as "susceptible", "resistant", or "intermediate", according to CLSI and EUCAST criteria. In general, EUCAST supports lower, more stringent, resistance MIC breakpoints than CLSI, in particular for Gram-negative bacteria [282]. However, in only a few cases have these differences been translated into major interpretive category discrepancies [283]. Both CLSI and EUCAST periodically update their recommendations concerning the interpretation of in vitro AST [284]. Recently, both CLSI and EUCAST published new AST guidelines, but some differences in terms of the categorization of ESBLs still remain in the EUCAST guidelines [285]. In general, it may be a wise practice to communicate directly with the microbiology laboratory when antimicrobial susceptibility patterns appear unusual.

Antimicrobial duration

In patients with uncomplicated IAI, and where the source of infection is treated definitively, post-operative antimicrobial therapy is not necessary.

In patients with complicated IAI undergoing an adequate source-control procedure, post-operative therapy should be shortened as much as possible after the resolution of physiological abnormalities.

In the event of uncomplicated IAIs, the infection involves a single organ and does not extend to the peritoneum. When the source of infection is treated effectively by surgical excision, post-operative antimicrobial therapy is not necessary, as demonstrated in managing uncomplicated acute appendicitis or cholecystitis [177, 286–288]. In complicated IAI, the infectious process extends beyond the organ, causing either localized or diffuse peritonitis (examples include: perforated appendicitis, perforated peptic ulcer, perforated diverticulitis, and post-operative anastomotic leaks) [289, 290]. Treatment of patients with complicated IAI generally involves both source control and antimicrobial therapy. Antibiotics to treat IAI with antimicrobials can prevent local and hematogenous spread and may reduce late complications.

The optimal duration of antibiotic therapy for cIAIs is debated. Guidelines by Surgical Infection Society (SIS) and Infectious Diseases Society of America (IDSA), published in 2010 [171], recommended a treatment course of 4 to 7 days, depending on the clinical response. French guidelines also recommended 5 to 7 days of treatment [178]. The World Society of Emergency Surgery (WSES) [174] recommended shortened antibiotic therapy in those patients demonstrating a positive response to treatment, without signs of persistent leukocytosis or fever. The recent prospective trial by Sawyer et al. demonstrated that in patients with complicated IAI undergoing an adequate source-control procedure, the outcomes after approximately 4 days fixed-duration antibiotic therapy were similar to those after a longer course of antibiotics that extended until after the resolution of physiological abnormalities [291]. Finally, protracted antibiotic administration may not be safe; for IAI in which a duration of therapy >7 days was prescribed, an association with increased risk of subsequent extra-abdominal infections and increased mortality, was recently observed [292].

Duration of therapy should be shortened as much as possible unless there are special circumstances that require prolonging antimicrobial therapy such as immunosuppression, or ongoing infections. Oral antimicrobials, can substitute IV agents as soon as the patient is tolerating an oral diet so as to minimize the adverse effects which are associated with intravenous access devices. Where possible, conversion to oral antimicrobial agents having high oral bioavailability (e.g. fluoroquinolones) should be considered. Patients who have signs of sepsis beyond 5 to 7 days of treatment warrant aggressive diagnostic investigation to determine if an ongoing uncontrolled source of infection or antimicrobial treatment failure is present. In the management of critically ill patients with sepsis and septic shock clinical signs and symptoms as well as inflammatory response markers such as procalcitonin, although debatable, may assist in guiding antibiotic treatment [293].

Recently, a systematic review of preclinical and clinical studies of mediators in intra-abdominal sepsis/injury was published [294].

Persistently high PCT in plasma was associated with infection or with a significant increase in mortality in patients with sepsis [295, 296].

Therefore, PCT has been used as a guide for interventions or antibiotic therapy for patients with abdominal sepsis [297]. However, other studies have not consistently confirmed PCT as an accurate marker for sepsis or to predict patient's response to the initial treatment [298].

Conclusions

An optimal antimicrobial approach to treating IAI involves a delicate balance between the optimization of empiric therapy, which improves clinical outcomes, and the reduction of excessive antimicrobial use, which increases the rate of emergence of antimicrobial-resistant strains. Increasing resistance rates among Gram-negative pathogens that are responsible for serious nosocomial infections, including ESBL *Enterobacteriaceae,* MDR *P. aeruginosa* and carbapenem-resistant *Enterobacteriaceae* is a consequence of increasing acquisition of carbapenemase genes worldwide [299]. These organisms represent an emerging threat due to the limited availability of viable therapeutic options. This complicates the choice of the most appropriate empiric treatment for patients with IAI. The clinical challenge remains to find the balance between ensuring that each individual patient is appropriately covered for the most likely pathogens of their IAI, while avoiding the use of overtly broad-spectrum antimicrobials in order to preserve them for future use. The appropriateness and need for antimicrobial treatment should be reassessed daily. Treatment duration as short as 4 days may be sufficient for a vast majority of patients suffering from complicated IAIs, when coupled with effective source control.

Although most clinicians are aware of the problem of antimicrobial resistance, most underestimate its importance; judicious antimicrobial management decisions is an integral part of responsible medication prescribing behavior.

In Appendix recommendations for appropriate therapy in patients with intra-abdominal infections are reported.

Appendix

Recommendations for appropriate therapy in patients with intra-abdominal infections

- Antimicrobials should be used after a treatable IAI has been recognized or if there is a high degree of suspicion of an infection.
- Patient factors, the nature of the infection and disease, and the environment all affect appropriate planning of antimicrobial therapy.
- Empiric antimicrobial therapy should be started in patients with IAI.
- Knowledge of local rates of resistance is an essential component in the determination of the empiric antimicrobial regimen for IAI.
- For patients with community-acquired IAI, empiric agents with a narrower spectrum of activity are sufficient.
- For patients with hospital-acquired IAI, antimicrobial regimens with broader spectrum of activity are preferred.
- Targeted antimicrobial therapy regimens are appropriate when culture and antimicrobial susceptibility test results are available.
- In uncomplicated IAI, post-operative therapy is not usually necessary following source control.

- In complicated IAIs, antimicrobial therapy is usually continued after source control.
- The antimicrobial therapy should be shortened in patients demonstrating a positive response to treatment.
- Patients having signs of sepsis beyond 5 to 7 days of antibiotic treatment should undergo aggressive diagnostic investigation to determine ongoing uncontrolled sources of infection, or antimicrobial treatment failure.
- Where possible, conversion to oral antimicrobial agents with high oral bioavailability should be considered to minimize the adverse effects associated with intravenous access devices.
- Sufficient knowledge of the general principles of antimicrobial therapy is necessary for clinicians treating intra-abdominal infections; this may minimize treatment failures, and minimize the development of antimicrobial resistance.

Abbreviations

AMR, antimicrobial resistance; IAIs, intra-abdominal infections; CDI, *C. difficile* infection; ESBL, extended-spectrum beta-lactamases; KPC, *K. pneumoniae* carbapenemase; MDRO, multidrug resistant organism; CA-IAIs, community-acquired intra-abdominal infections; HCA-IAIs, healthcare-associated intra-abdominal infections

Acknowledgements

Not applicable.

Funding

No fundings to declare.

Authors' contributions

MS designed the manuscript and wrote the first draft of the manuscript. All authors reviewed and approved the final manuscript. The views expressed in this article are those of the authors and do not necessarily reflect the official policy or position of the Department of the Navy, Department of Defense, nor the U.S. Government. Copyright Statement.

Competing interests

The authors declare that they have no competing interest.

Author details

[1]Department of Surgery, Macerata Hospital, Via Santa Lucia 2, 62100 Macerata, Italy. [2]Department of Trauma Surgery, Royal Perth Hospital, Perth, Australia. [3]Genomic Research Laboratory, Geneva University Hospitals, Geneva, Switzerland. [4]Infectious Diseases Division, Santa Maria Misericordia University Hospital, Udine, Italy. [5]Department of Emergency Medicine and Surgery, Stony Brook University School of Medicine, Stony Brook, NY, USA. [6]General Surgery Department, Papa Giovanni XXIII Hospital, Bergamo, Italy. [7]Department of General, Maggiore Hospital, Parma, Italy. [8]Department of Surgery, "Infermi" Hospital, Rimini, Italy. [9]Department of Surgery, College of Medicine and Health Sciences, UAE University, Al-Ain, United Arab Emirates. [10]Department of Surgery, UC San Diego Medical Center, San Diego, USA. [11]Department of Surgery, University of Colorado, Denver Health Medical Center, Denver, CO, USA. [12]Department of Surgery, Division of Acute Care Surgery, and Center for Sepsis and Critical Illness Research, University of Florida College of Medicine, Gainesville, FL, USA. [13]Department of Surgery, University of Washington, Seattle, WA, USA. [14]Department of Critical Care Medicine, Ghent University Hospital, Ghent, Belgium. [15]General, Acute Care, and Trauma Surgery, Foothills Medical Centre, Calgary, AB, Canada. [16]General and Upper GI Surgery, Queen Elizabeth Hospital, Birmingham, UK. [17]Department of General, Visceral, and Thoracic Surgery, Klinikum Peine, Academic Hospital of Medical University Hannover, Peine, Germany. [18]Department of Clinical microbiology, Ampath National Laboratory Services, Milpark Hospital, Johannesburg, South Africa. [19]Department of Surgery, School of Medicine, Washington University in Saint Louis, Missouri, USA. [20]Departments of Surgery and Anesthesiology, Division of Trauma and Surgical Critical Care, Vanderbilt University Medical Center, Nashville, TN, USA. [21]Department of Surgery, University of Virginia Health System, Charlottesville, VA, USA. [22]Departments of Medicine, Clinical Epidemiology and Biostatistics, and Pathology and Molecular Medicine, McMaster University, Hamilton, ON, Canada. [23]Département d'Anesthésie-Réanimation, CHU Bichat Claude-Bernard-HUPNVS, Assistance Publique-Hôpitaux de Paris, University Denis Diderot, Paris, France. [24]Section of Critical Care Medicine and Section of Infectious Diseases, Department of Medicine, Medical Microbiology and Pharmacology/Therapeutics, University of Manitoba, Winnipeg, MB, Canada. [25]Australia Pharmacy Department, Royal Brisbane and Womens' Hospital; Burns, Trauma, and Critical Care Research Centre, Australia School of Pharmacy, The University of Queensland, Brisbane, QLD, Australia. [26]Department of Intensive Care, Erasme Hospital, Université libre de Bruxelles, Brussels, Belgium. [27]Department of Internal Medicine, Division of Infectious Diseases, Akron General Medical Center, Northeast Ohio Medical University, Akron, OH, USA. [28]Clinical Microbiology and Infectious Diseases, School of Pathology, Faculty of Health Sciences, University of the Witwatersrand, Johannesburg, South Africa. [29]Division of Infectious Diseases, Los Angeles County-University of Southern California (USC) Medical Center, Keck School of Medicine at USC, Los Angeles, CA, USA. [30]Department of Infectious Diseases, Alfred Hospital, Melbourne, VIC, Australia. [31]Department of Surgery, College of Health Sciences, Obafemi Awolowo University, Ile-Ife, Nigeria. [32]Division of Clinical and Administrative Sciences, College of Pharmacy, Xavier University of Louisiana, New Orleans, LA, USA. [33]Department of Medicine, Division of Infectious Diseases, University of South Carolina School of Medicine, Columbia, SC, USA. [34]General Surgery, ULSS19 del Veneto, Adria Hospital, RO, Italy. [35]Biomedical Research Center, Qatar University, Doha, Qatar. [36]Departments of Microbiology, Chitwan Medical College, Bharatpur, Chitwan, Nepal and Depertments of Environmental and Preventative Medicine, Oita University, Oita, Japan. [37]Centre for Neglected Tropical Diseases, Liverpool School of Tropical Medicine, University of Liverpool, and Mercy Hospital Research Laboratory, Njala University, Bo, Sierra Leone. [38]Department of Surgery, University Hospital Center, Zagreb, Croatia. [39]Trauma and Acute Care Surgery Unit, Hadassah Hebrew University Medical Center, Jerusalem, Israel. [40]Department of Traumatology, John Hunter Hospital and University of Newcastle, Newcastle, NSW, Australia. [41]Department of Surgery, Bizerte Hospital, Bizerte, Tunisia. [42]Academic Department of Surgery, Queen Elizabeth Hospital, Birmingham, UK. [43]Department of General Surgery, Hospital San Juan de Dios de La Serena, La Serena, Chile. [44]Emergency Department, University of Leipzig, Leipzig, Germany. [45]Department of Surgery, University of Colorado, Denver, CO, USA. [46]Department of Surgery, Academic Medical Centre, Amsterdam, The Netherlands. [47]Department of Pathology and Laboratory Medicine, VA Boston HealthCare System, and Department of Pathology and Laboratory Medicine, Boston University School of Medicine, Boston, MA, USA. [48]Division of Acute Care Surgery, Department of Surgery, University of Michigan, Ann Arbor, MI, USA. [49]Department of Surgery, Radboud University Nijmegen Medical Center, Nijmegen, The Netherlands. [50]Department of Surgery, Hospital Clínico Universitario, Santiago de Compostela, Spain. [51]Pharmacy Department, Alfred Health, Melbourne, VIC, Australia. [52]Hospital Epidemiology and Infectious Diseases, Hospital Universitario Dr Jose Eleuterio Gonzalez, Monterrey, Mexico. [53]Department of Pharmacology, Pushpagiri Institute of Medical Sciences and Research Centre, Thiruvalla, Kerala, India. [54]Department of General Surgery, Kuala Krai Hospital, Kuala Krai, Kelantan, Malaysia. [55]Department of Surgery and Obstetrics/Gynaecology, Regional Hospital, Limbe, Cameroon. [56]Department of Mathematics, Imperial College London, London, UK. [57]Department of Laparoscopic and Robotic Surgery, Colli-Monaldi Hospital, Naples, Italy. [58]Department of Surgery, Tianjin Nankai

Hospital, Nankai Clinical School of Medicine, Tianjin Medical University, Tianjin, China. [59]Infectología Institucional SRL, Hospital Municipal Chivilcoy, Buenos Aires, Argentina. [60]Department of Surgery, University Clinical Center of Tuzla, Tuzla, Bosnia and Herzegovina. [61]Department General Surgery, Kipshidze Central University Hospital, Tbilisi, Georgia. [62]Department of Surgery, Quatre Villes Hospital, St Cloud, France. [63]School of Pharmacy, Faculty of Medical Sciences, The University of the West Indies, St. Augustine, Eric Williams Medical Sciences Complex, Uriah Butler Highway, Champ Fleurs, Trinidad and Tobago. [64]Division of Acute Care Surgery, Program in Trauma, R Adams Cowley Shock Trauma Center, University of Maryland, Baltimore, MD, USA. [65]Department of Surgical Sciences, Cannizzaro Hospital, University of Catania, Catania, Italy. [66]Ifakara Health Institute, Dar es Salaam, Tanzania. [67]Department of Surgery, Maggiore Hospital, Bologna, Italy. [68]Center for Food Safety, Department of Food Science and Technology, University of Georgia, Griffin, GA, USA. [69]School of Pharmacy and Biomedicine, Mongolian National University of Medical Sciences, Ulaanbaatar, Mongolia. [70]Department of Surgery, University Hospital of Trauma, Tirana, Albania. [71]Département d'Anesthésie-Réanimation, CHU Amiens-Picardie, and INSERM U1088, Université de Picardie Jules Verne, Amiens, France. [72]Department of Surgery, Division of Burn, Critical Care, and Trauma Surgery (K.P.S., S.R.E.), Weill Cornell Medical College/New York-Presbyterian Hospital, New York, USA. [73]Department of Medicine, Infectious Disease Division, King Fahad Medical City, Riyadh, Saudi Arabia. [74]Department of Surgery, Pirogov Russian National Research Medical University, Moscow, Russian Federation. [75]Sudan National Public Health Laboratory, Federal Ministry of Health, Khartoum, Sudan. [76]Department of Surgery, Virginia Commonwealth University, Richmond, VA, USA. [77]Department of Global Health and Population, Harvard T.H. Chan School of Public Health, Boston, MA, USA. [78]Division of Trauma Surgery, Department of Surgery, School of Medical Sciences, University of Campinas (Unicamp), Campinas, SP, Brazil. [79]Institut Pasteur, Abidjan, Ivory Coast. [80]6th Department of Internal Medicine, Hygeia General Hospital, Athens, Greece. [81]Department of General Surgery, Mansoura Faculty of Medicine, Mansoura University, Mansoura, Egypt. [82]2nd Department of Surgery, Aretaieion University Hospital, National and Kapodistrian University of Athens, Athens, Greece. [83]Department of Surgery, Hospital Universitário Terezinha de Jesus, Faculdade de Ciências Médicas e da Saúde de Juiz de Fora, Juiz de Fora, Brazil. [84]Center for Global Health, Mito Kyodo General Hospital, University of Tsukuba, Mito, Ibaraki, Japan. [85]Hospital Privado Centro Médico de Caracas and Hospital Vargas de Caracas, Caracas, Venezuela. [86]Unit of Pharmacology, Faculty of Medicine and Defense Health, National Defence University of Malaysia, Kuala Lumpur, Malaysia. [87]Institute of Hygiene, Charité-Universitätsmedizin Berlin, Hindenburgdamm 27, 12203 Berlin, Germany. [88]Department of General and Thoracic Surgery, University Hospital Giessen, Giessen, Germany. [89]Orgamed Consulting, Bad Griesbach, Germany. [90]Department of Surgery, St. Josef Hospital, Ruhr University Bochum, Bochum, Germany. [91]Department of Surgery, Faculté de médecine, Université de Parakou, BP 123 Parakou, Bénin. [92]Division of Trauma and Surgical Critical Care, Department of Surgery, Asan Medical Center, University of Ulsan College of Medicine, Seoul, Republic of Korea. [93]Department of Visceral, Transplant and Thoracic Surgery, Innsbruck Medical University, Innsbruck, Austria. [94]Department of Surgery Philadelphia VA Medical Center, Perelman School of Medicine, University of Pennsylvania, Philadelphia, PA, USA. [95]Department of Microbiology, Gandhi Medical College, Bhopal, India. [96]Clinic for Emergency Surgery, Medical Faculty University of Belgrade, Belgrade, Serbia. [97]Department of Anesthesiology and Intensive Care, Charité Universitätsmedizin Berlin, Campus Benjamin Franklin, Berlin, Germany. [98]3rd Department of General Surgery, Jagiellonian University Medical College, Krakow, Poland. [99]Department of Pharmacology and Therapeutics, College of Health Sciences, Makerere University, Kampala, Uganda. [100]Department of Surgery, Albert Einstein College of Medicine and Jacobi Medical Center, Bronx, NY, USA. [101]Department of General Surgery, Division of Surgery, Rambam Health Care Campus, Haifa, Israel. [102]Department of Emergency Surgery, City Hospital, Mozyr, Belarus. [103]Department of Primary Care and Emergency Medicine, Kyoto University Graduate School of Medicine, Kyoto, Japan. [104]Department of Surgery, The Brunei Cancer Centre, Jerudong Park, Brunei. [105]Department of Surgery, Edendale Hospital, Pietermaritzburg, South Africa. [106]School of Medicine, Western Sydney University, Campbelltown, NSW, Australia. [107]Division of Acute Care Surgery and Surgical Critical Care, Department of Surgery, Los Angeles County and University of Southern California Medical Center, University of Southern California, Los Angeles, CA, USA. [108]Department of General Surgery, Erzincan University, Faculty of Medicine, Erzincan, Turkey. [109]Department of Pharmacy, Lebanese International University, Beirut, Lebanon. [110]School of Life Science and The ithree Institute, University of Technology, Sydney, NSW, Australia. [111]Department of Biomedical Sciences and Public Health, Unit of Hygiene, Preventive Medicine and Public Health, UNIVMP, Ancona, Italy. [112]Department of Critical Care Medicine, Cliniques Universitaires Saint Luc, Université Catholique de Louvain (UCL), Brussels, Belgium. [113]Department of Surgery, Division of Trauma, University of Arizona, Tucson, AZ, USA. [114]Department of Surgery, Yonsei University College of Medicine, Seoul, South Korea. [115]Texas Tech University Health Sciences Center School of Pharmacy, Abilene, TX, USA. [116]Department of Anaesthesiology and Critical Care, Hôpital Nord, Assistance Publique-Hôpitaux de Marseille, Aix Marseille Université, Marseille, France. [117]Abdominal Center, University Hospital Meilahti, Helsinki, Finland. [118]Department of Surgery, Inling Hospital, Nanjing University School of Medicine, Nanjing, China. [119]Division of Infectious Diseases, Division of Emergency Medicine, Washington University School of Medicine, St. Louis, MO, USA. [120]Division of Infectious Diseases, Department of Clinical Pathology, Faculty of Medicine, University of Indonesia, Cipto Mangunkusumo General Hospital, Jakarta, Indonesia. [121]Department for Traumatology and Orthopedic Surgery, Cologne Merheim Medical Center (CMMC), University of Witten/Herdecke (UW/H), Cologne, Germany. [122]Health Research Program, Institute of Economic and Social Research, University of Zambia, Lusaka, Zambia. [123]Multidisciplinary Intensive Care Research Organization (MICRO), Wellcome Trust-HRB Clinical Research, Department of Clinical Medicine, Trinity Centre for Health Sciences, St James' University Hospital, Dublin, Ireland. [124]Department of Surgery, Post-Graduate Institute of Medical Sciences, Rohtak, India. [125]Department of Clinical Pharmacology, School of Medicine, University of Botswana, Gaborone, Botswana. [126]Department of Surgery, Radiology, University Hospital of the West Indies, Kingston, Jamaica. [127]General Surgery Department, Centro Hospitalar de São João, Porto, Portugal. [128]Department of Surgery, Emergency Hospital of Bucharest, Bucharest, Romania. [129]Center of Anti-Infective Research and Development, Hartford, CT, USA. [130]Department of Laboratory Medicine, Division of Clinical Microbiology, Karolinska University Hospital Huddinge, Stockholm, Sweden. [131]Research Unit, Health Policy Consult, Weija-Accra, Ghana. [132]Department of Surgery, King Abdullah University Hospital, Irbid, Jordan. [133]Department of Surgery and Critical Care, Universidad del Valle, Fundación Valle del Lili, Cali, Colombia. [134]Department of Surgery, Hassan II University Hospital, Medical School of Fez, Sidi Mohamed Benabdellah University, Fez, Morocco. [135]Division of Emergency and Trauma Surgery, Ribeirão Preto Medical School, Ribeirão Preto, Brazil. [136]Division of Surgery, Vittorio Emanuele Hospital, Catania, Italy. [137]Department of General and Emergency Surgery, Riga East University Hospital 'Gailezers', Riga, Latvia. [138]National Institute for Health Research, Health Protection Research Unit in Healthcare Associated Infections and Antimicrobial Resistance, Imperial College London, Hammersmith Campus, London, UK. [139]Department of General Surgery, Jesenice General Hospital, Jesenice, Slovenia. [140]Trauma and Acute Care Service, St Michael's Hospital, University of Toronto, Toronto, Canada. [141]U.S. Naval Medical Research Unit N° 6, Callao, Peru. [142]General Surgery Department, Medical University, University Hospital St George, Plovdiv, Bulgaria. [143]Intensive Care Department, Hospital Clínico San Carlos, Madrid, Spain. [144]II Cátedra de Clínica Quirúrgica, Hospital de Clínicas, Universidad Nacional de Asunción, San Lorenzo, Paraguay. [145]Department of Surgery, Catholic University of Sacred Heart, Policlinico A Gemelli, Rome, Italy. [146]Department of Surgery, Faculty of Medicine, Thammasat University Hospital, Thammasat University, Pathum Thani, Thailand. [147]Department of General Surgery, Tan Tock Seng Hospital, Tan Tock Seng, Singapore. [148]Department of Gastrointestinal Surgery, Stavanger University Hospital, Stavanger, Department of Clinical Medicine, University of Bergen, Bergen, Norway. [149]Department of Emergency Surgery and Critical Care, Centro Medico Imbanaco, Cali, Colombia. [150]Department of Surgery, North Estonia Medical Center, Tallinn, Estonia. [151]Surgery Health Care Group, Hull and East Yorkshire Hospitals NHS Trust, Hull, UK. [152]APHP medical and infectious diseases ICU, Bichat Hospital, Paris, France. [153]Institute of Microbiology, Biological and Environmental Sciences College, University San Francisco de Quito, Quito, Ecuador. [154]Department of Molecular Biology, Tran Hung Dao Hospital, No 1, Tran Hung Dao Street, Hai Ba Trung Dist, Hanoi, Vietnam. [155]1st Department of Surgery - Department of Abdominal, Thoracic Surgery and Traumatology, General University Hospital, Prague, Czech Republic. [156]Department of Surgery, Medical School University of Pécs, Pécs, Hungary. [157]Nottingham Oesophago-Gastric Unit, Nottingham University Hospitals,

Nottingham, UK. [158]Department of Surgery, Sheri-Kashmir Institute of Medical Sciences, Srinagar, India. [159]State Key Laboratory for Diagnosis and Treatment of Infectious Diseases, The First Affilliated Hospital, Zhejiang University, Zhejiang, China. [160]Trauma and Emergency Surgery Department, Chang Gung Memorial Hospital, Taoyuan City, Taiwan. [161]Department of Surgery, MOSC Medical College Kolenchery, Cochin, India. [162]Infection Control Unit, Angers University, CHU d'Angers, Angers, France. [163]Division of Trauma and Surgical Critical Care, DeWitt Daughtry Family Department of Surgry, University of Miami, Miami, FL, USA. [164]Anesthesia and Intensive Care Unit, AORN dei Colli Vincenzo Monaldi Hospital, Naples, Italy. [165]Anesthesiology and Intensive Care Unit, Sant'Orsola University Hospital, Bologna, Italy. [166]Infectious Diseases Unit, University of Genoa (DISSAL) and IRCCS San Martino-IST, Genoa, Italy. [167]Infectious Diseases Unit, Department of Medical and Surgical Sciences, Sant' Orsola Hospital, University of Bologna, Bologna, Italy.

References

1. Dellit TH, Owens RC, McGowan Jr JE, Gerding DN, Weinstein RA, Burke JP, et al. Infectious Diseases Society of America. Society for Healthcare Epidemiology of America Infectious Diseases Society of America and the Society for Healthcare Epidemiology of America guidelines for developing an institutional program to enhance antimicrobial stewardship. Clin Infect Dis. 2007;44:159–77.
2. Rice LB. Federal funding for the study of antimicrobial resistance in nosocomial pathogens: no ESKAPE. J Infect Dis. 2008;197:1079–81.
3. Boucher HW, Talbot GH, Bradley JS, Edwards JE, Gilbert D, Rice LB, et al. Bad bugs, no drugs: no ESKAPE! An update from the Infectious Diseases Society of America. Clin Infect Dis. 2009;48:1–12.
4. Rao GG. Risk factors for the spread of antibiotic-resistant bacteria. Drugs. 1998;55:323–30.
5. Deege MP, Paterson DL. Reducing the development of antibiotic resistance in critical care units. Curr Pharm Biotechnol. 2011;12:2062–9.
6. Septimus EJ, Owens Jr RC. Need and potential of antimicrobial stewardship in community hospitals. Clin Infect Dis. 2011;53 Suppl 1:S8–S14.
7. Recommendations for preventing the spread of vancomycin resistance: recommendations of the Hospital Infection Control Practices Advisory Committee (HICPAC). Am J Infect Control. 1995;23:87–94.
8. Donskey CJ. Antibiotic regimens and intestinal colonization with antibiotic-resistant gram-negative bacilli. Clin Infect Dis. 2006;43 Suppl 2:S62–9.
9. Salyers AA, Gupta A, Wang Y. Human intestinal bacteria as reservoirs for antibiotic resistance genes. Trends Microbiol. 2004;12:412–6.
10. Vollaard EJ, Clasener HA. Colonization resistance. Antimicrob Agents Chemother. 1994;38:409–14.
11. Bhalla A, Pultz NJ, Ray AJ, Hoyen CK, Eckstein EC, Donskey CJ. Antianaerobic antibiotic therapy promotes overgrowth of antibiotic-resistant, gram-negative bacilli and vancomycin-resistant enterococci in the stool of colonized patients. Infect Control Hosp Epidemiol. 2003;24:644–9.
12. Donskey CJ, Chowdhry TK, Hecker MT, Hoyen CK, Hanrahan JA, Hujer AM, et al. Effect of antibiotic therapy on the density of vancomycin-resistant enterococci in the stool of colonized patients. N Engl J Med. 2000;343:1925–32.
13. Taur Y, Xavier JB, Lipuma L, Ubeda C, Goldberg J, Gobourne A, et al. Intestinal domination and the risk of bacteremia in patients undergoing allogeneic hematopoietic stem cell transplantation. Clin Infect Dis. 2012;55:905–14.
14. Ruppé E, Lixandru B, Cojocaru R, Büke C, Paramythiotou E, Angebault C, et al. Relative fecal abundance of extended-spectrum-beta-lactamase-producing Escherichia coli strains and their occurrence in urinary tract infections in women. Antimicrob Agents Chemother. 2013;57:4512–7.
15. Paphitou NI. Antimicrobial resistance: action to combat the rising microbial challenges. Int J Antimicrob Agents. 2013;42(Suppl):S25–8.
16. Pulcini C, Gyssens IC. How to educate prescribers in antimicrobial stewardship practices. Virulence. 2013;4:192–202.
17. Viscidi R, Willey S, Bartlett JG. Isolation rates and toxigenic potential of Clostridium difficile isolates from various patient populations. Gastroenterology. 1981;81:5–9.
18. Sartelli M, Malangoni MA, Abu-Zidan FM, Griffiths EA, Di Bella S, McFarland LV, et al. WSES guidelines for management of Clostridium difficile infection in surgical patients. World J Emerg Surg. 2015;10:38.
19. Farrell RJ, LaMont JT. Pathogenesis and clinical manifestations of Clostridium difficile diarrhea and colitis. Curr Top Microbiol Immunol. 2000;250:109–25.
20. Hensgens MP, Goorhuis A, Dekkers OM, Kuijper EJ. Time interval of increased risk for Clostridium difficile infection after exposure to antibiotics. J Antimicrob Chemother. 2012;67:742–8.
21. Muto CA, Pokrywka M, Shutt K, Mendelshon AB, Nouri K, Posey K, et al. A large outbreak of Clostridium difficile–associated disease with an unexpected proportion of deaths and colectomies at a teaching hospital following increased fluoroquinolone use. Infect Control Hosp Epidemiol. 2005;26:273–80.
22. Loo VG, Poirier L, Miller MA, Oughton M, Libman MB, Michaud S, et al. A predominately clonal multi-institutional outbreak of Clostridium difficile-associated diarrhea with high morbidity and mortality. N Engl J Med. 2005;353:2442–9.
23. Pépin J, Saheb N, Coulombe MA, Alary ME, Corriveau MP, Authier S, et al. Emergence of fluoroquinolones as the predominant risk factor for Clostridium difficile-associated diarrhea: a cohort study during an epidemic in Quebec. Clin Infect Dis. 2005;41:1254–60.
24. Dubberke ER, Reske KA, Yan Y, Olsen MA, McDonald LC, Fraser VJ. Clostridium difficile-associated disease in a setting of endemicity: identification of novel risk factors. Clin Infect Dis. 2007;45:1543–9.
25. Owens RC, Donskey CJ, Gaynes RP, Loo VG, Muto CA. Antimicrobial-associated risk factors for Clostridium difficile infection. Clin Infect Dis. 2008;46:19–31.
26. McCusker ME, Harris AD, Perencevich E, Roghmann M. Fluoroquinolone use and Clostridium difficile-associated diarrhea. Emerg Infect Dis. 2003;9:730–3.
27. Leffler DA, Lamont JT. Clostridium difficile infection. N Engl J Med. 2015;16(372):1539–48.
28. Slimings C, Riley TV. Antibiotics and hospital-acquired Clostridium difficile infection: update of systematic review and meta-analysis. J Antimicrob Chemother. 2014;69:881–91.
29. Kim PK, Huh HC, Cohen HW, Feinberg EJ, Ahmad S, Coyle C, et al. Intracolonic vancomycin for severe Clostridium difficile colitis. Surg Infect (Larchmt). 2013;14:532–9.
30. Neal MD, Alverdy JC, Hall DE, Simmons RL, Zuckerbraun BS. Diverting loop ileostomy and colonic lavage: an alternative to total abdominal colectomy for the treatment of severe, complicated Clostrodium difficile associated disease. Ann Surg. 2011;254:423–7.
31. Bougnoux ME, Diogo D, François N, Sendid B, Veirmeire S, Colombel JF, et al. Multilocus sequence typing reveals intrafamilial transmission and microevolutions of Candida albicans isolates from the human digestive tract. J Clin Microbiol. 2006;44:1810–20.
32. Kam AP, Xu J. Diversity of commensal yeasts within and among healthy hosts. Diagn Microbiol Infect Dis. 2002;43:19–28.
33. Xu J, Boyd CM, Livingston E, Meyer W, Madden JF, Mitchell TG. Species and genotypic diversities and similarities of pathogenic yeasts colonizing women. J Clin Microbiol. 1999;37:3835–43.
34. Miranda LN, Van Der Heijden IM, Costa SF, Sousa AP, Sienra RA, Gobara S, et al. Candida colonisation as a source for candidaemia. J Hosp Infect. 2009;72:9–16.
35. Yan L, Yang C, Tang J. Disruption of the intestinal mucosal barrier in Candida albicans infections. Microbiol Res. 2013;168:389–95.
36. Schulte DM, Sethi A, Gangnon R, Duster M, Maki DG, Safdar N. Risk factors for Candida colonization and Co-colonization with multi-drug resistant organisms at admission. Antimicrob Resist Infect Control. 2015;4:46.
37. Aly M, Balkhy HH. The prevalence of antimicrobial resistance in clinical isolates from gulf corporation council countries. Antimicrob Resist Infect Control. 2012;1:26.
38. Laxminarayan R, Duse A, Wattal C, Zaidi AK, Wertheim HF, Sumpradit N, et al. Antibiotic resistance-the need for global solutions. Lancet Infect Dis. 2013;13:1057–98.
39. Ashiru-Oredope D, Cookson B, Fry C, Advisory Committee on Antimicrobial Resistance and Healthcare Associated Infection Professional Education Subgroup. Developing the first national antimicrobial prescribing and stewardship competences. J Antimicrob Chemother. 2014;69:2886–8.
40. Allegranzi B, Pittet D. Preventing infections acquired during health-care delivery. Lancet. 2008;372:1719–20.
41. ECDC. Annual epidemiological report. Antimicrobial resistance and healthcare-associated infections. http://ecdc.europa.eu/en/publications/Publications/antimicrobial-resistance-annual-epidemiological-report.pdf. Accessed 03 Apr 2016.

42. World Health Organization (WHO). Global action plan on antimicrobial resistance. http://apps.who.int/iris/bitstream/10665/193736/1/9789241509763_eng.pdf?ua=1. Accessed 03 Apr 2016.
43. Huttner A, Harbarth S, Carlet J, Cosgrove S, Goossens H, Holmes A, et al. Antimicrobial resistance: a global view from the 2013 World Healthcare-Associated Infections Forum. Antimicrob Resist Infect Control. 2013;2:31.
44. Liu YY, Wang Y, Walsh TR, Yi LX, Zhang R, Spencer J, et al. Emergence of plasmid-mediated colistin resistance mechanism MCR-1 in animals and human beings in China: a microbiological and molecular biological study. Lancet Infect Dis. 2016;16:161–8.
45. Pitout JD, Laupland KB. Extended-spectrum beta-lactamase-producing Enterobacteriaceae: an emerging public-health concern. Lancet Infect Dis. 2008;8:159–66.
46. Jacoby GA. Extended-spectrum beta-lactamases and other enzymes providing resistance to oxyimino-beta-lactams. Infect Dis Clin North Am. 1997;11:875–87.
47. Courpon-Claudinon A, Lefort A, Panhard X, Clermont O, Dornic Q, Fantin B, et al. Bacteraemia caused by third-generation cephalosporin-resistant Escherichia coli in France: prevalence, molecular epidemiology and clinical features. Clin Microbiol Infect. 2011;17:557–65.
48. Thaden JT, Fowler VG, Sexton DJ, Anderson DJ. Increasing Incidence of Extended-Spectrum beta-lactamase-Producing Escherichia coli in Community Hospitals throughout the Southeastern United States. Infect Control Hosp Epidemiol. 2016;37:49–54.
49. Makoka MH, Miller WC, Hoffman IF, Cholera R, Gilligan PH, Kamwendo D, et al. Bacterial infections in Lilongwe, Malawi: aetiology and antibiotic resistance. BMC Infect Dis. 2012;12:67.
50. McManus MC. Mechanisms of bacterial resistance to antimicrobial agents. Am J Health Syst Pharm. 1997;54:1420–33.
51. Martinez JL, Baquero F. Mutation frequencies and antibiotic resistance. Antimicrob Agents Chemother. 2000;44:1771–7.
52. Palmer KL, Kos VN, Gilmore MS. Horizontal gene transfer and the genomics of enterococcal antibiotic resistance. Curr Opin Microbiol. 2010;13:632–9.
53. Billard-Pomares T, Fouteau S, Jacquet ME, Roche D, Barbe V, Castellanos M, et al. Characterization of a P1-like bacteriophage carrying an SHV-2 extended-spectrum β-lactamase from an *Escherichia coli* strain. Antimicrob Agents Chemother. 2014;58(11):6550–7.
54. Brown-Jaque M, Calero-Cáceres W, Muniesa M. Transfer of antibiotic-resistance genes via phage-related mobile elements. Plasmid. 2015;79:1–7.
55. Trueba G. Chapter Ten: The forces behind the dissemination of bacterial virulence and antibiotic resistance. In: Why does Evolution Matter? The Importance of Understanding Evolution. UK: Cambridge Scholars Publishing; 2014.
56. Iida S, Meyer J, Arber W. Genesis and natural history of IS-mediated transposons. Cold Spring Harb Symp Quant Biol. 1981;45(Pt 1):27–43.
57. Poirel L, Marqué S, Héritier C, Segonds C, Chabanon G, Nordmann P. OXA-58, a novel class D β-lactamase involved in resistance to carbapenems in *Acinetobacter baumannii*. Antimicrob Agents Chemother. 2005;49(1):202–8.
58. Humeniuk C, Arlet G, Gautier V, Grimont P, Labia R, Philippon A. Beta-lactamases of *Kluyvera ascorbata*, probable progenitors of some plasmid-encoded CTX-M types. Antimicrob Agents Chemother. 2002;46(9):3045–9.
59. Ray MD, Boundy S, Archer GL. Transfer of the methicillin resistance genomic island among staphylococci by conjugation. Mol Microbiol. 2016;100:675–85.
60. Chen L, Mathema B, Pitout JD, DeLeo FR, Kreiswirth BN. Epidemic *Klebsiella pneumoniae* ST258 is a hybrid strain. MBio. 2014;5(3):e01355–14.
61. Smyth DS, McDougal LK, Gran FW, Manoharan A, Enright MC, Song JH, et al. Population structure of a hybrid clonal group of methicillin-resistant *Staphylococcus aureus*, ST239-MRSA-III. PLoS One. 2010;5(1), e8582.
62. Bush K, Fisher JF. Epidemiological expansion, structural studies, and clinical challenges of new beta-lactamases from Gram-negative bacteria. Annu Rev Microbiol. 2011;65:455–78.
63. Ambler RP. The structure of beta-lactamases. Philos Trans R Soc Lond B Biol Sci. 1980;289:321–31.
64. Bush K, Jacoby GA, Medeiros AA. A functional classification scheme for beta-lactamases and its correlation with molecular structure. Antimicrob Agents Chemother. 1995;39:1211–33.
65. Bush K, Jacoby GA. Updated Functional Classification of beta-Lactamases. Antimicrob Agents Chemother. 2010;54:969–76.
66. Ruppé É, Woerther PL, Barbier F. Mechanisms of antimicrobial resistance in Gram-negative bacilli. Ann Intensive Care. 2015;5:61.
67. Jacoby GA. AmpC beta-lactamases. Clin Microbiol Rev. 2009;22:161–82.
68. Kang CI, Pai H, Kim SH, Kim HB, Kim EC, Oh MD, et al. Cefepime and the inoculum effect in tests with Klebsiella pneumoniae producing plasmid-mediatedAmpC-type beta-lactamase. J Antimicrob Chemother. 2004;54:1130–3.
69. Tamma PD, Girdwood SC, Gopaul R, Tekle T, Roberts AA, Harris AD, et al. The use of cefepime for treating AmpC beta-lactamase-producing Enterobacteriaceae. Clin Infect Dis. 2013;57:781–8.
70. Schultsz C, Geerlings S. Plasmid-mediated resistance in Enterobacteriaceae: changing landscape and implications for therapy. Drugs. 2012;72:1–16.
71. Dalhoff A. Global fluoroquinolone resistance epidemiology and implictions for clinical use. Interdiscip Perspect Infect Dis. 2012;2012:976273.
72. Brolund A. Overview of ESBL-producing Enterobacteriaceae from a Nordic perspective. Infect Ecol Epidemiol. 2014;1:4.
73. Perez F, Bonomo RA. Can we really use beta-lactam/beta-lactam inhibitor combinations for the treatment of infections caused by extended-spectrum beta-lactamase-producing bacteria? Clin Infect Dis. 2012;54:175–7.
74. Roberts JA, Paul SK, Akova M, Bassetti M, De Waele JJ, Dimopoulos G, et al. DALI: defining antibiotic levels in intensive care unit patients: are current beta-lactam antibiotic doses sufficient for critically ill patients? Clin Infect Dis. 2014;58:1072–83.
75. Paterson D, Bonomo R. Extended spectrum beta-lactmases. Clin Microbiol Rev. 2005;18:657–86.
76. Woerther PL, Burdet C, Chachaty E, Andremont A. Trends in human fecal carriage of extended-spectrum beta-lactamases in the community: toward the globalization of CTX-M. Clin Microbiol Rev. 2013;26:744–58.
77. Weldhagen GF, Poirel L, Nordmann P. Ambler class A extended-spectrum beta-lactamases in Pseudomonas aeruginosa: novel developments and clinical impact. Antimicrob Agents Chemother. 2003;47:2385–92.
78. Livermore DM. Beta-lactamases in laboratory and clinical resistance. Clin Microbiol Rev. 1995;8:557–84.
79. Hammoudi D, Ayoub Moubareck C, Aires J, Adaime A, Barakat A, Fayad N, et al. Countrywide spread of OXA-48 carbapenemase in Lebanon: surveillance and genetic characterization of carbapenem-non-susceptible Enterobacteriaceae in 10 hospitals over a one-year period. Int J Infect Dis. 2014;29:139–44.
80. Poirel L, Héritier C, Tolün V, Nordmann P. Emergence of oxacillinase-mediated resistance to imipenem in Klebsiella pneumoniae. Antimicrob Agents Chemother. 2004;48:15–22.
81. Lee J, Patel G, Huprikar S, Calfee DP, Jenkins SG. Decreased susceptibility to polymyxin B during treatment of carbapenem-resistant Klebsiella pneumoniae infection. J Clin Microbiol. 2009;47:1611–2.
82. Yigit H, Queenan AM, Anderson GJ, Domenech-Sanchez A, Biddle JW, Steward CD, et al. Novel carbapenem-hydrolyzing beta-lactamase, KPC-1, from a carbapenem-resistant strain of Klebsiella pneumoniae. Antimicrob Agents Chemother. 2001;45:1151–61.
83. Ducomble T, Faucheux S, Helbig U, Kaisers UX, König B, Knaust A, et al. Large hospital outbreak of KPC-2-producing Klebsiella pneumoniae: investigating mortality and the impact of screening for KPC-2 with polymerase chain reaction. J Hosp Infect. 2015;89:179–85.
84. Lübbert C, Lippmann N, Busch T, Kaisers UX, Ducomble T, Eckmanns T, et al. Long-term carriage of Klebsiella pneumoniae carbapenemase-2-producing K pneumoniae after a large single-center outbreak in Germany. Am J Infect Control. 2014;42:376–80.
85. Lübbert C, Rodloff AC, Laudi S, Simon P, Busch T, Mössner J, et al. Lessons learned from excess mortality associated with Klebsiella pneumoniae carbapenemase 2-producing K. pneumoniae in liver transplant recipients. Liver Transpl. 2014;20:736–8.
86. Tzouvelekis LS, Markogiannakis A, Piperaki E, Souli M, Daikos GL. Treating infections caused by carbapenemase-producing Enterobacteriaceae. Clin Microbiol Infect. 2014;20:862–72.
87. Munoz-Price LS, Poirel L, Bonomo RA, Schwaber MJ, Daikos GL, Cormican M, et al. Clinical epidemiology of the global expansion of Klebsiella pneumoniae carbapenemases. Lancet Infect Dis. 2013;13:785–96.
88. Palzkill T. Metallo-beta-lactamase structure and function. Ann N Y Acad Sci. 2013;1277:91–104.
89. Cornaglia G, Giamarellou H, Rossolini GM. Metallo-beta-lactamases a last frontier for beta-lactams? Lancet Inf Dis. 2011;11:381–93.
90. Yong D, Toleman MA, Giske CG, Cho HS, Sundman K, Lee K, et al. Characterization of a new metallo-beta-lactamase gene, bla(NDM-1), and a novel erythromycin esterase gene carried on a unique genetic structure in

Klebsiella pneumoniae sequence type 14 from India. Antimicrob Agents Chemother. 2009;53:5046–54.

91. Brink AJ, Coetzee J, Clay CG, Sithole S, Richards GA, Poirel L, et al. Emergence of New Delhi Metallo-Beta-Lactamase (NDM-1) and Klebsiella pneumoniae Carbapenemase (KPC-2) in South Africa. J Clin Microbiol. 2012;50:525–7.
92. Fàbrega A, Madurga S, Giralt E, Vila J. Mechanism of action of and resistance to quinolones. Microb Biotechnol. 2009;2:40–61.
93. Jacoby GA. Mechanisms of resistance to quinolones. Clin Infect Dis. 2005;41 Suppl 2:S120–6.
94. Ramirez MS, Tolmasky ME. Aminoglycoside Modifying Enzymes. Drug Resist Updat. 2010;13:151–71.
95. Kumari H, Balasubramanian D, Zincke D, Mathee K. Role of Pseudomonas aeruginosa AmpR on beta-lactam and non-beta-lactam transient cross-resistance upon pre-exposure to subinhibitory concentrations of antibiotics. J Med Microbiol. 2014;63:544–55.
96. Lister PD, Gardner VM, Sanders CC. Clavulanate induces expression of the Pseudomonas aeruginosa AmpC cephalosporinase at physiologically relevant concentrations and antagonizes the antibacterial activity of ticarcillin. Antimicrob Agents Chemother. 1999;43:882–9.
97. Poole K. Efflux-mediated multiresistance in Gram-negative bacteria. Clin Microbiol Infect. 2004;10:12–26.
98. Venter H, Mowla R, Ohene-Agyei T, Ma S. RND-type drug efflux pumps from Gram-negative bacteria: molecular mechanism and inhibition. Front Microbiol. 2015;6:377.
99. Li H, Luo YF, Williams BJ, Blackwell TS, Xie CM. Structure and function of OprD protein in Pseudomonas aeruginosa: from antibiotic resistance to novel therapies. Int J Med Microbiol. 2012;302:63–8.
100. Manchanda V, Sanchaita S, Singh N. Multidrug resistant acinetobacter. J Glob Infect Dis. 2010;2:291–304.
101. Potron A, Poirel L, Nordmann P. Emerging broad-spectrum resistance in Pseudomonas aeruginosa and Acinetobacter baumannii: mechanisms and epidemiology. Int J Antimicrob Agents. 2015;45:568–85.
102. Linden PK. Optimizing therapy for vancomycin-resistant Enterococci (VRE). Semin Respir Crit Care Med. 2007;28:632–45.
103. Chou YY, Lin TY, Lin JC, Wang NC, Peng MY, Chang FY. Vancomycin-resistant enterococcal bacteremia: Comparison of clinical features and outcome between Enterococcus faecium and Enterococcus faecalis. J Microbiol Immunol Infect. 2008;41:124–9.
104. Hollenbeck BL, Rice LB. Intrinsic and acquired resistance mechanisms in enterococcus. Virulence. 2012;3:421–569.
105. Hodges TL, Zighelboim-Daum S, Eliopoulos GM, Wennersten C, Moellering Jr RC. Antimicrobial susceptibility changes in Enterococcus faecalis following various penicillin exposure regimens. Antimicrob Agents Chemother. 1992;36:121–5.
106. Marothi YA, Agnihotri H, Dubey D. Enterococcal resistance-an overview. Indian J Med Microbiol. 2005;23:214–9.
107. Mahbub Alam M, Kobayashi N, Ishino M, Sumi A, Kobayashi K, Uehara N, et al. Detection of a novel aph(2″) allele (aph[2″]-Ie) conferring high-level gentamicin resistance and a spectinomycin resistance gene ant(9)-Ia (aad 9) in clinical isolates of enterococci. Microb Drug Resist. 2005;11:239–47.
108. Depardieu F, Podglajen I, Leclercq R, Collatz E, Courvalin P. Modes and modulations of antibiotic resistance gene expression. Clin Microbiol Rev. 2007;20:79–114.
109. Noskin GA. Vancomycin-resistant Enterococci: Clinical, microbiologic, and epidemiologic features. J Lab Clin Med. 1997;130:14–20.
110. Fang H, Edlund C, Hedberg M, Nord CE. New findings in beta-lactam and metronidazole resistant Bacteroides fragilis group. Int J Antimicrob Agents. 2002;19:361–70.
111. Rasmussen BA, Bush K, Tally FP. Antimicrobial resistance in anaerobes. Clin Infect Dis. 1997;24 Suppl 1:S110–20.
112. Gutacker M, Valsangiacomo C, Piffaretti JC. Identification of two genetic groups in Bacteroides fragilis by multilocus enzyme electrophoresis: distribution of antibiotic resistance (cfiA, cepA) and enterotoxin (bft) encoding genes. Microbiology. 2000;146:1241–54.
113. Ang L, Brenwald NP, Walker RM, Andrews J, Fraise A. Carbapenem resistance in Bacteroides fragilis. J Antimicrob Chemother. 2007;59:1042–4.
114. Ingham HR, Eaton S, Venables CW, Adams PC. Bacteroides fragilis resistant to metronidazole after long-term therapy. Lancet. 1978;1:214.
115. Diniz CG, Farias LM, Carvalho MA, Rocha ER, Smith CJ. Differential gene expression in a Bacteroides fragilis metronidazole-resistant mutant. J Antimicrob Chemother. 2004;54:100–8.
116. Pumbwe L, Chang A, Smith RL, Wexler HM. BmeRABC5 is a multidrug efflux system that can confer metronidazole resistance in Bacteroides fragilis. Microb Drug Resist. 2007;13:96–101.
117. Nagy E, Urbán E, Nord CE, ESCMID Study Group on Antimicrobial Resistance in Anaerobic Bacteria. Antimicrobial susceptibility of Bacteroides fragilis group isolates in Europe: 20 years of experience. Clin Microbiol Infect. 2011;17:371–9.
118. Sartelli M, Catena F, Di Saverio S, Ansaloni L, Coccolini F, Tranà C, et al. The Challenge of antimicrobial resistance in managing intra-abdominal infections. Surg Infect (Larchmt). 2015;16:213–20.
119. Morrissey I, Hackel M, Badal R, Bouchillon S, Hawser S, Biedenbach D. A review of ten years of the study for monitoring antimicrobial resistance trends (SMART) from 2002 to 2011. Pharmaceuticals (Basel). 2013;6:1335–46.
120. Hawser SP, Bouchillon SK, Hoban DJ, Badal RE, Cantón R, Baquero F. Incidence and antimicrobial susceptibility of Escherichia coli and Klebsiella pneumoniae with extended-spectrum beta-lactamases in community- and hospital-associated intra-abdominal infections in Europe: results of the 2008 Study for Monitoring Antimicrobial Resistance Trends (SMART). Antimicrob Agents Chemother. 2010;54:3043–6.
121. Sartelli M, Catena F, Ansaloni L, Coccolini F, Corbella D, Moore EE, et al. Complicated intra-abdominal infections worldwide: the definitive data of the CIAOW Study. World J Emerg Surg. 2014;9:37.
122. Hawser SP, Bouchillon SK, Lascols C, Hackel M, Hoban DJ, Badal RE, et al. Susceptibility of Klebsiella pneumoniae isolates from intra-abdominal infections and molecular characterization of ertapenem-resistant isolates. Antimicrob Agents Chemother. 2011;55:3917–21.
123. Babinchak T, Badal R, Hoban D, Hackel M, Hawser S, Lob S, et al. Trends in susceptibility of selected gram-negative bacilli isolated from intra-abdominal infections in North America: SMART 2005–2010. Diagn Microbiol Infect Dis. 2013;76:379–81.
124. Sitges-Serra A, Lopez MJ, Girvent M, Almirall S, Sancho JJ. Postoperative enterococcal infection after treatment of complicated intra-abdominal sepsis. Br J Surg. 2002;89:361–7.
125. Burnett RJ, Haverstock DC, Dellinger EP, Reinhart HH, Bohnen JM, Rotstein OD, et al. Definition of the role of enterococcus in intraabdominal infection: analysis of a prospective randomized trial. Surgery. 1995;118:716–21.
126. Dupont H, Friggeri A, Touzeau J, Airapetian N, Tinturier F, Lobjoie E, et al. Enterococci increase the morbidity and mortality associated with severe intra-abdominal infections in elderly patients hospitalized in the intensive care unit. J Antimicrob Chemother. 2011;66:2379–85.
127. Kaffarnik MF, Urban M, Hopt UT, Utzolino S. Impact of enterococcus on immunocompetent and immunosuppressed patients with perforation of the small or large bowel. Technol Health Care. 2012;20:37–48.
128. Van Ruler O, Kiewiet JJ, Van Ketel RJ, Boermeester MA, Dutch Peritonitis Study Group. Initial microbial spectrum in severe secondary peritonitis and relevance for treatment. Eur J Clin Microbiol Infect Dis. 2012;31:671–82.
129. Montravers P, Lepape A, Dubreuil L, Gauzit R, Pean Y, Benchimol D, et al. Clinical and microbiological profiles of community-acquired and nosocomial intra-abdominal infections: results of the French prospective, observational EBIIA study. J Antimicrob Chemother. 2009;63:785–94.
130. Verma H, Pandey S, Sheoran KD, Marwah S. Surgical audit of patients with ileal perforations requiring ileostomy in a Tertiary Care Hospital in India. Surg Res Pract. 2015;2015:351548.
131. Mirza SH, Beeching NJ, Hart CA. Multi-drug resistant typhoid: a global problem. J Med Microbiol. 1996;44:317–9.
132. Hammad OM, Abdel Wahab MF, Zaky S, Abdel Baki AM, Afify A, El Tantawi MA. Multidrug resistant typhoid fever in Egypt. J Med Lab Sci. 2007;16:57–63.
133. Singhal L, Gupta PK, Kale P, Gautam V, Ray P. Trends in antimicrobial susceptibility of Salmonella typhi from North India (2001–2012). Indian J Med Microbiol. 2014;32:149–52.
134. Brook I, Wexler HM, Goldstein EJ. Antianaerobic antimicrobials: spectrum and susceptibility testing. Clin Microbiol Rev. 2013;26:526–46.
135. Snydman DR, Jacobus NV, McDermott LA, Golan Y, Hecht DW, Goldstein EJ, et al. Lessons learned from the anaerobe survey: historical perspective and review of the most recent data (2005–2007). Clin Infect Dis. 2010;50 Suppl 1:S26–33.
136. Ramsay C, Brown E, Hartman G, Davey P. Room for improvement: a systematic review of the quality of evaluations of interventions to improve hospital antibiotic prescribing. J Antimicrob Chemother. 2003;52:764–71.
137. Dortch MJ, Fleming SB, Kauffmann RM, Dossett LA, Talbot TR, May AK. Infection reduction strategies including antibiotic stewardship protocols in surgical and trauma intensive care units are associated with reduced

resistant gram-negative healthcare-associated infections. Surg Infect (Larchmt). 2011;12:15–25.

138. White Jr AC, Atmar RL, Wilson J, Cate TR, Stager CE, Greenberg SB. Effects of requiring prior authorization for selected antimicrobials: expenditures, susceptibilities, and clinical outcomes. Clin Infect Dis. 1997;25:230–9.
139. Davey P, Brown E, Charani E, Fenelon L, Gould IM, Holmes A, et al. Interventions to improve antibiotic prescribing practices for hospital inpatients. Cochrane Database Syst Rev. 2013;4, CD003543.
140. Marshall JC. Principles of source control in the early management of sepsis. Curr Infect Dis Rep. 2010;12:345–53.
141. Wacha H, Hau T, Dittmer R, Ohmann C. Risk factors associated with intraabdominal infections: a prospective multicenter study. Peritonitis Study Group. Langenbecks Arch Surg. 1999;384:24–32.
142. Sartelli M, Abu-Zidan FM, Catena F, Griffiths EA, Di Saverio S, Coimbra R, et al. Global validation of the WSES Sepsis Severity Score for patients with complicated intra-abdominal infections: a prospective multicentre study (WISS Study). World J Emerg Surg. 2015;10:61.
143. VanSonnenberg E, Ferrucci JT, Mueller PR, Wittenberg J, Simeone JF. Percutaneous drainage of abscesses and fluid collections: Technique, results, and applications. Radiology. 1982;142:1–10.
144. Bouali K, Magotteaux P, Jadot A, Saive C, Lombard R, Weerts J, et al. Percutaneous catheter drainage of abdominal abscess after abdominal surgery: Results in 121 cases. J Belg Radiol. 1993;76:11–4.
145. VanSonnenberg E, Wing VW, Casola G, Coons HG, Nakamoto SK, Mueller PR, et al. Temporizing effect of percutaneous drainage of complicated abscesses in critically ill patients. Am J Roentgenol. 1984;142:821–6.
146. Jaffe TA, Nelson RC, DeLong D, Paulson EK. Practice Patterns in Percutaneous Image-guided Intra-abdominal Abscess Drainage: Survey of Academic and Private Practice Centres. Radiology. 2004;233:750–6.
147. Kirkpatrick AW, Roberts DJ, De Waele J, Jaeschke R, Malbrain ML, De Keulenaer B, et al. Intra-abdominal hypertension and the abdominal compartment syndrome: updated consensus definitions and clinical practice guidelines from the World Society of the Abdominal Compartment Syndrome. Intensive Care Med. 2013;39:1190–206.
148. Kirkpatrick AW, Roberts DJ, Faris PD, Ball CG, Kubes P, Tiruta C, et al. Active Negative Pressure Peritoneal Therapy After Abbreviated Laparotomy: The Intraperitoneal Vacuum Randomized Controlled Trial. Ann Surg. 2015;262:38–46.
149. Menichetti F, Sganga G. Definition and classification of intra-abdominal infections. J Chemother. 2009;21 Suppl 1:3–4.
150. Sartelli M. A focus on intra-abdominal infections. World J Emerg Surg. 2010;5:9.
151. Gupta S, Kaushik R. Peritonitis–the Eastern experience. World J Emerg Surg. 2006;1:13.
152. Mishra SP, Tiwary SK, Mishra M, Gupta SK. An introduction of Tertiary Peritonitis. J Emerg Trauma Shock. 2014;7:121–3.
153. Reemst PH, Van Goor H, Goris RJ. SIRS, MODS and tertiary peritonitis. Eur J Surg Suppl. 1996;576:47–8. discussion 49.
154. Chromik AM, Meiser A, Hölling J, Sülberg D, Daigeler A, Meurer K, et al. Identification of patients at risk for development of tertiary peritonitis on a surgical intensive care unit. J Gastrointest Surg. 2009;13:1358–67.
155. Herzog T, Chromik AM, Uhl W. Treatment of complicated intra-abdominal infections in the era of multi-drug resistant bacteria. Eur J Med Res. 2010;15:525–32.
156. Roehrborn A, Thomas L, Potreck O, Ebener C, Ohmann C, Goretzki PE, et al. The microbiology of postoperative peritonitis. Clin Infect Dis. 2001;33:1513–9.
157. Mulier S, Penninckx F, Verwaest C, Filez L, Aerts R, Fieuws S, et al. Factors affecting mortality in generalized postoperative peritonitis: multivariate analysis in 96 patients. World J Surg. 2003;27:379–84.
158. Ordoñez CA, Puyana JC. Management of peritonitis in the critically ill patient. Surg Clin North Am. 2006;86:1323–49.
159. Seguin P, Fédun Y, Laviolle B, Nesseler N, Donnio PY, Mallédant Y. Risk factors for multidrug-resistant bacteria in patients with post-operative peritonitis requiring intensive care. J Antimicrob Chemother. 2010;65:342–6.
160. Augustin P, Kermarrec N, Muller-Serieys C, Lasocki S, Chosidow D, Marmuse JP, et al. Risk factors for multi drug resistant bacteria and optimization of empirical antibiotic therapy in postoperative peritonitis. Crit Care. 2010;14(1):R20.
161. Montravers P, Chalfine A, Gauzit R, Lepape A, Pierre Marmuse J, Vouillot C, et al. Clinical and therapeutic features of nonpostoperative nosocomial intra-abdominal infections. Ann Surg. 2004;239:409–16.
162. Friedman ND, Kaye KS, Stout JE, McGarry SA, Trivette SL, Briggs JP, et al. Health care-associated bloodstream infections in adults: a reason to change the accepted definition of community-acquired infections. Ann Intern Med. 2002;137:791–7.
163. Cardoso T, Almeida M, Friedman ND, Aragão I, Costa-Pereira A, Sarmento E, et al. Classification of healthcare-associated infection: a systematic review 10 years after the first proposal. BMC Med. 2014;12:40.
164. Bone RC, Balk RA, Cerra FB, Dellinger RP, Fein AM, Knaus WA, et al. American College of Chest Physicians/Society of Critical Care Medicine Consensus Conference: Definitions for sepsis and organ failure and guidlines for the use of innovative therapies in sepsis. Chest. 1992;101:1644–55.
165. Levy MM, Fink MP, Marshall JC, Abraham E, Angus D, Cook D, et al. 2001 SCCM/ ESICM/ACCP/ATS/SIS International Sepsis Definitions Conference. Crit Care Med. 2003;31:1250–6.
166. Esteban A, Frutos-Vivar F, Ferguson ND, Peñuelas O, Lorente JA, Gordo F, et al. Sepsis incidence and outcome: contrasting the intensive care unit with the hospital ward. Crit Care Med. 2007;35:1284–9.
167. Sartelli M, Catena F, Di Saverio S, Ansaloni L, Malangoni M, Moore EE, et al. Current concept of abdominal sepsis: WSES position paper. World J Emerg Surg. 2014;9:22.
168. Singer M, Deutschman CS, Seymour CW, Shankar-Hari M, Annane D, Bauer M, et al. The Third International Consensus Definitions for Sepsis and Septic Shock (Sepsis-3). JAMA. 2016;315:801–10.
169. Cain SE, Kohn J, Bookstaver PB, Albrecht H, Al-Hasan MN. Stratification of the impact of inappropriate empirical antimicrobial therapy for Gram-negative bloodstream infections by predicted prognosis. Antimicrob Agents Chemother. 2015;59:245–50.
170. Guirao X, Arias J, Badía JM, García-Rodríguez JA, Mensa J, Alvarez-Lerma F, et al. Recommendations in the empiric anti-infective agents of intra-abdominal infection. Rev Esp Quimioter. 2009;22:151–72.
171. Solomkin JS, Mazuski JE, Bradley JS, Rodvold KA, Goldstein EJ, Baron EJ, et al. Diagnosis and management of complicated intra-abdominal infection in adults and children: guidelines by the Surgical Infection Society and the Infectious Diseases Society of America. Surg Infect (Larchmt). 2010;11:79–109.
172. Solomkin JS, Mazuski JE, Baron EJ, Sawyer RG, Nathens AB, DiPiro JT, et al. Guidelines for the selection of anti-infective agents for complicated intra-abdominal infections. Clin Infect Dis. 2003;37:997–1005.
173. Mazuski JE, Sawyer RG, Nathens AB, DiPiro JT, Schein M, Kudsk KA, et al. The Surgical Infection Society guidelines on antimicrobial therapy for intra-abdominal infections: an executive summary. Surg Infect (Larchmt). 2002;3:161–73.
174. Sartelli M, Viale P, Catena F, Ansaloni L, Moore E, Malangoni M, et al. 2013 WSES guidelines for management of intra-abdominal infections. World J Emerg Surg. 2013;8:3.
175. Sartelli M, Viale P, Koike K, Pea F, Tumietto F, Van Goor H, et al. WSES consensus conference: Guidelines for first-line management of intra-abdominal infections. World J Emerg Surg. 2011;6:2.
176. Chow AW, Evans GA, Nathens AB, Ball CG, Hansen G, Harding GK, et al. Canadian practice guidelines for surgical intra-abdominal infections. Can J Infect Dis Med Microbiol. 2010;21:11–37.
177. Gomi H, Solomkin JS, Takada T, Strasberg SM, Pitt HA, Yoshida M, et al. TG13 antimicrobial therapy for acute cholangitis and cholecystitis. J Hepatobiliary Pancreat Sci. 2013;20:60–70.
178. Montravers P, Dupont H, Leone M, Constantin JM, Mertes PM, Société française d'anesthésie et de réanimation (Sfar), et al. Guidelines for management of intra-abdominal infections. Anaesth Crit Care Pain Med. 2015;34:117–30.
179. Kumar A, Ellis P, Arabi Y, Roberts D, Light B, Parrillo JE, et al. Initiation of inappropriate antimicrobial therapy results in a five-fold reduction of survival in human septic shock. Chest. 2009;136:1237–48.
180. Tumbarello M, Trecarichi EM, Bassetti M, De Rosa FG, Spanu T, Di Meco E, et al. Identifying patients harboring extended-spectrum-beta-lactamase-producing Enterobacteriaceae on hospital admission: derivation and validation of a scoring system. Antimicrob Agents Chemother. 2011;55:3485–90.
181. Al-Hasan MN, Eckel-Passow JE, Baddour LM. Impact of healthcare-associated acquisition on community-onset Gram-negative bloodstream infection: a population-based study. Eur J Clin Microbiol Infect Dis. 2012;31:1163–71.
182. Ruppé E, Armand-Lefèvre L, Estellat C, Consigny PH, El Mniai A, Boussadia Y, et al. High Rate of Acquisition but Short Duration of Carriage of Multidrug-Resistant Enterobacteriaceae After ravel to the Tropics. Clin Infect Dis. 2015;61:593–600.

183. McDonald LC. Trends in antimicrobial resistance in health care-associated pathogens and effect on treatment. Clin Infect Dis. 2006;42 Suppl 2:S65–71.
184. Montravers P, Augustin P, Grall N, Desmard M, Allou N, Marmuse JP, Guglielminotti J. Characteristics and outcomes of anti-infective de-escalation during health care-associated intra-abdominal infections. Crit Care. 2016;20(1):83.
185. Angus DC, Linde-Zwirble WT, Lidicker J, Clermont G, Carcillo J, Pinsky MR. Epidemiology of severe sepsis in the United States: analysis of incidence, outcome, and associated costs of care. Crit Care Med. 2001;29:1303–10.
186. Vincent JL, Rello J, Marshall J, Silva E, Anzueto A, Martin CD, et al. International study of the prevalence and outcomes of infection in intensive care units. JAMA. 2009;302:2323–9.
187. De Waele J, Lipman J, Sakr Y, Marshall JC, Vanhems P, Barrera Groba C, et al. Abdominal infections in the intensive care unit: characteristics, treatment and determinants of outcome. BMC Infect Dis. 2014;14:420.
188. Kumar A, Roberts D, Wood KE, Light B, Parrillo JE, Sharma S, et al. Duration of hypotension before initiation of effective antimicrobial therapy is the critical determinant of survival in human septic shock. Crit Care Med. 2006;34:1589–96.
189. Dellinger RP, Levy MM, Rhodes A, Annane D, Gerlach H, Opal SM, et al. Surviving Sepsis Campaign: international guidelines for management of severe sepsis and septic shock, 2012. Intensive Care Med. 2013;39:165–228.
190. Shani V, Muchtar E, Kariv G, Robenshtok E, Leibovici L. Systematic review and meta-analysis of the efficacy of appropriate empiric antibiotic therapy for sepsis. Antimicrob Agents Chemother. 2010;54:4851–63.
191. Ferrer R, Artigas A, Suarez D, Palencia E, Levy MM, Arenzana A, et al. Edusepsis Study Group: Effectiveness of treatments for severe sepsis: A prospective, multicenter, observational study. Am J Respir Crit Care Med. 2009;180:861–6.
192. Castellanos-Ortega A, Suberviola B, García-Astudillo LA, Holanda MS, Ortiz F, Llorca J, et al. Impact of the Surviving Sepsis Campaign protocols on hospital length of stay and mortality in septic shock patients: Results of a three-year follow-up quasi-experimental study. Crit Care Med. 2010;38:1036–43.
193. Puskarich MA, Trzeciak S, Shapiro NI, Arnold RC, Horton JM, Studnek JR, et al. Association between timing of antibiotic administration and mortality from septic shock in patients treated with a quantitative resuscitation protocol. Crit Care Med. 2011;39:2066–71.
194. Rello J, Vidaur L, Sandiumenge A, Rodriguez A, Gualis B, Boque C, et al. De-escalation therapy in ventilator-associated pneumonia. Crit Care Med. 2004;32:2183–90.
195. Alvarez-Lerma F, Alvarez B, Luque P, Ruiz F, Dominguez-Roldan JM, Quintana E, et al. Empiric broad-spectrum antibiotic therapy of nosocomial pneumonia in the intensive care unit: a prospective observational study. Crit Care. 2006;10:R78.
196. Eachempati SR, Hydo LJ, Shou J, Barie PS. Does de-escalation of antibiotic therapy for ventilator-associated pneumonia affect the likelihood of recurrent pneumonia or mortality in critically ill surgical patients? J Trauma. 2009;66:1343–8.
197. Garnacho-Montero J, Gutiérrez-Pizarraya A, Escoresca-Ortega A, Corcia-Palomo Y, Fernández-Delgado E, Herrera-Melero I, et al. De-escalation of empirical therapy is associated with lower mortality in patients with severe sepsis and septic shock. Intensive Care Med. 2014;40:32–40.
198. Leone M, Bechis C, Baumstarck K, Lefrant JY, Albanèse J, Jaber S, et al. De-escalation versus continuation of empirical antimicrobial treatment in severe sepsis: a multicenter non-blinded randomized noninferiority trial. Intensive Care Med. 2014;40:1399–408.
199. Silva BN, Andriolo RB, Atallah AN, Salomão R. De-escalation of antimicrobial treatment for adults with sepsis, severe sepsis or septic shock. Cochrane Database Syst Rev. 2013;3, CD007934.
200. Madaras-Kelly K, Jones M, Remington R, Caplinger C, Huttner B, Samore M. Description and validation of a spectrum score method to measure antimicrobial de-escalation in healthcare associated pneumonia from electronic medical records data. BMC Infect Dis. 2015;15:197.
201. Cisneros JM, Neth O, Gil-Navarro MV, Lepe JA, Jiménez-Parrilla F, Cordero E, et al. Global impact of an educational antimicrobial stewardship programme on prescribing practice in a tertiary hospital centre. Clin Microbiol Infect. 2014;20:82–8.
202. Lew KY, Ng TM, Tan M, Tan SH, Lew EL, Ling LM, et al. Safety and clinical outcomes of carbapenem de-escalation as part of anantimicrobial stewardship programme in an ESBL-endemic setting. J Antimicrob Chemother. 2015;70:1219–25.
203. Tucker CE, Lockwood AM, Nguyen NH. Antibiotic dosing in obesity: the search for optimum dosing strategies. Clin Obes. 2014;4:287–95.
204. Hackel MA, Badal RE, Bouchillon SK, Biedenbach DJ, Hoban DJ. Resistance rates of intra-abdominal isolates from intensive care units and non-intensive care units in the United States: the study for monitoring antimicrobial resistance trends 2010–2012. Surg Infect (Larchmt). 2015;16:298–304.
205. Powell LL, Wilson SE. The role of beta-lactam antimicrobials as single agents in treatment of intra-abdominal infection. Surg Infect (Larchmt). 2000;1:57–63.
206. Al-Hasan MN, Lahr BD, Eckel-Passow JE, Baddour LM. Antimicrobial resistance trends of Escherichia coli bloodstream isolates: a population-based study, 1998–2007. J Antimicrob Chemother. 2009;64:169–74.
207. Johnson JR, Owens K, Gajewski A, Clabots C. Escherichia coli colonization patterns among human household members and pets, with attention to acute urinary tract infection. J Infect Dis. 2008;197:218–24.
208. Gin A, Dilay L, Karlowsky JA, Walkty A, Rubinstein E, Zhanel GG. Piperacillin-tazobactam: a beta-lactam/beta-lactamase inhibitor combination. Expert Rev Anti Infect Ther. 2007;5:365–83.
209. Vardakas KZ, Tansarli GS, Rafailidis PI, Falagas ME. Carbapenems versus alternative antibiotics for the treatment of bacteraemia due to Enterobacteriaceae producing extended-spectrum beta-lactamases: a systematic review and meta-analysis. J Antimicrob Chemother. 2012;67:2793–803.
210. Tamma PD, Han JH, Rock C, Harris AD, Lautenbach E, Hsu AJ, et al. Carbapenem therapy is associated with improved survival compared with piperacillin-tazobactam for patients with extended-spectrum beta-lactamase bacteremia. Clin Infect Dis. 2015;60:1319–25.
211. Harris PN, Tambyah PA, Paterson DL. Beta-lactam and beta-lactamase inhibitor combinations in the treatment of extended-spectrum beta-lactamase producing Enterobacteriaceae: time for a reappraisal in the era of few antibiotic options? Lancet Infect Dis. 2015;15:475–85.
212. Garbino J, Villiger P, Caviezel A, Matulionyte R, Uckay I, Morel P, et al. A randomized prospective study of cefepime plus metronidazole with imipenem-cilastatin in the treatment of intra-abdominal infections. Infection. 2007;35:161–6.
213. Henry X, Amoroso A, Coyette J, Joris B. Interaction of ceftobiprole with the low-affinity PBP 5 of Enterococcus faecium. Antimicrob Agents Chemother. 2010;54:953–5.
214. Liapikou A, Cillóniz C, Torres A. Ceftobiprole for the treatment of pneumonia: a European perspective. Drug Design, Development and Therapy. 2015;9:4565–72.
215. Queenan AM, Shang W, Kania M, Page MG, Bush K. Interactions of ceftobiprole with beta-lactamases from molecular classes A to D. Antimicrob Agents Chemother. 2007;51:3089–95.
216. Falagas ME, Matthaiou DK, Bliziotis IA. Systematic review: Fluoroquinolones for the treatment of intra-abdominal surgical infections. Aliment Pharmacol Ther. 2007;25:123–31.
217. Borcherding SM, Stevens R, Nicholas RA, Corley CR, Self T. Quinolones: A practical review of clinical uses, dosing considerations, and drug interactions. J Fam Pract. 1996;42:69–78.
218. Ortega M, Marco F, Soriano A, Almela M, Martínez JA, Muñoz A, et al. Analysis of 4758 Escherichia coli bacteraemia episodes: predictive factors for isolation of an antibiotic-resistant strain and their impact on the outcome. J Antimicrob Chemother. 2009;63:568–74.
219. Banerjee R, Johnston B, Lohse C, Porter SB, Clabots C, Johnson JR. Escherichia coli sequence type 131 is a dominant, antimicrobial-resistant clonal group associated with healthcare and elderly hosts. Infect Control Hosp Epidemiol. 2013;34:361–9.
220. Patterson JE. Antibiotic utilization: is there an effect on antimicrobial resistance? Chest. 2001;119(2 Suppl):426S–30S.
221. Sartelli M, Catena F, Coccolini F, Pinna AD. Antimicrobial management of intra-abdominal infections: literature's guidelines. World J Gastroenterol. 2012;18:865–71.
222. Falagas ME, Peppas G, Makris GC, Karageorgopoulos DE, Matthaiou DK. Meta-analysis: Ertapenem for complicated intra-abdominal infections. Aliment Pharmacol Ther. 2008;27:919–31.
223. Lepper PM, Grusa E, Reichl H, Högel J, Trautmann M. Consumption of imipenem correlates with beta-lactam resistance in Pseudomonas aeruginosa. Antimicrob Agents Chemother. 2002;46:2920–5.
224. Daikos GL, Tsaousi S, Tzouvelekis LS, Anyfantis I, Psichogiou M, Argyropoulou A, et al. Carbapenemase-producing Klebsiella pneumoniae bloodstream infections: lowering mortality by antibiotic combination

schemes and the role of carbapenems. Antimicrob Agents Chemother. 2014;58:2322–8.

225. Trivedi M, Patel V, Soman R, Rodriguez C, Singhal T. The outcome of treating ESBL infections with carbapenems vs. non carbapenem antimicrobials. J Assoc Physicians India. 2012;60:28–30.
226. Dupont H, Carbon C, Carlet J. Monotherapy with a broad-spectrum beta-lactam is as effective as its combination with an aminoglycoside in treatment of severe generalized peritonitis: a multicenter randomized controlled trial. The Severe Generalized Peritonitis Study Group. Antimicrob Agents Chemother. 2000;44:2028–33.
227. Heizmann WR, Löschmann PA, Eckmann C, Von Eiff C, Bodmann KF, Petrik C. Clinical efficacy of tigecycline used as monotherapy or in combination regimens for complicated infections with documented involvement of multiresistant bacteria. Infection. 2015;43:37–43.
228. McGovern PC, Wible M, El-Tahtawy A, Biswas P, Meyer RD. All-cause mortality imbalance in the tigecycline phase 3 and 4 clinical trials. Int J Antimicrob Agents. 2013;41:463–7.
229. Bassetti M, McGovern PC, Wenisch C, Meyer RD, Yan JL, Wible M, et al. Clinical response and mortality in tigecycline complicated intra-abdominal infection and complicated skin and soft-tissue infection trials. Int J Antimicrob Agents. 2015;46:346–50.
230. Montravers P, Dupont H, Bedos JP, Bret P. Tigecycline Group. Tigecycline use in critically ill patients: a multicentre prospective observational study in the intensive care setting. Intensive Care Med. 2014;40:988–97.
231. Eckmann C, Montravers P, Bassetti M, Bodmann KF, Heizmann WR, Sánchez García M, et al. Efficacy of tigecycline for the treatment of complicated intra-abdominal infections in real-life clinical practice from five European observational studies. J Antimicrob Chemother. 2013;68 Suppl 2:ii25–35.
232. Chen YH, Hsueh PR. Changing bacteriology of abdominal and surgical sepsis. Curr Opin Infect Dis. 2012;25:590–5.
233. Tzouvelekis LS, Markogiannakis A, Psichogiou M, Tassios PT, Daikos GL. Carbapenemases in Klebsiella pneumoniae and other Enterobacteriaceae: an evolving crisis of global dimensions. Clin Microbiol Rev. 2012;25:682–707.
234. De Pascale G, Montini L, Pennisi M, Bernini V, Maviglia R, Bello G, et al. High dose tigecycline in critically ill patients with severe infections due to multidrug-resistant bacteria. Crit Care. 2014;18:R90.
235. Falagas ME, Rafailidis PI. Re-emergence of colistin in today's world of multidrug-resistant organisms: personal perspectives. Expert Opin Investig Drugs. 2008;17:973–81.
236. Falagas ME, Kasiakou SK, Kofteridis DP, Roditakis G, Samonis G. Effectiveness and nephrotoxicity of intravenous colistin for treatment of patients with infections due to polymyxin-only-susceptible (POS) gram-negative bacteria. Eur J Clin Microbiol Infect Dis. 2006;25:596–9.
237. Ruiz J, Núñez ML, Pérez J, Simarro E, Martínez-Campos L, Gómez J. Evolution of resistance among clinical isolates of Acinetobacter over a 6-year period. Eur J Clin Microbiol Infect Dis. 1999;18:292–5.
238. Garnacho-Montero J, Ortiz-Leyba C, Jimenez-Jimenez FJ, Barrero-Almodovar AE, Garcia-Garmendia JL, Bernabeu-Wittell M, et al. Treatment of multidrug-resistant Acinetobacter baumannii ventilator-associated pneumonia (VAP) with intravenous colistin: a comparison with imipenem-susceptible VAP. Clin Infect Dis. 2003;36:1111–8.
239. Plachouras D, Karvanen M, Friberg LE, Papadomichelakis E, Antoniadou A, Tsangaris I, et al. Population pharmacokinetic analysis of colistin methanesulfonate and colistin after intravenous administration in critically ill patients with infections caused by gram-negative bacteria. Antimicrob Agents Chemother. 2009;53(8):3430–6.
240. Nation RL, Garonzik SM, Li J, Thamlikitkul V, Giamarellos-Bourboulis EJ, Paterson DL, et al. Updated US and European Dose Recommendations for Intravenous Colistin: How Do They Perform? Clin Infect Dis. 2016;62:552–8.
241. Pontikis K, Karaiskos I, Bastani S, Dimopoulos G, Kalogirou M, Katsiari M, et al. Outcomes of critically ill intensive care unit patients treated with fosfomycin for infections due to pandrug-resistant and extensively drug-resistant carbapenemase-producing Gram-negative bacteria. Int J Antimicrob Agents. 2014;43(1):52–9.
242. Michalopoulos AS, Livaditis IG, Gougoutas V. The revival of fosfomycin. Int J Infect Dis. 2011;15:e732–9.
243. Reffert JL, Smith WJ. Fosfomycin for the treatment of resistant gram-negative bacterial infections. Insights from the Society of Infectious Diseases Pharmacists. Pharmacotherapy. 2014;34:845–57.
244. Eckmann C, Solomkin J. Ceftolozane/tazobactam for the treatment of complicated intra-abdominal infections. Expert Opin Pharmacother. 2015;16:271–80.
245. Solomkin J, Hershberger E, Miller B, Popejoy M, Friedland I, Steenbergen J, et al. Ceftolozane/Tazobactam Plus Metronidazole for Complicated Intra-abdominal Infections in an Era of Multidrug Resistance: Results From a Randomized, Double-Blind, Phase 3 Trial (ASPECT-cIAI). Clin Infect Dis. 2015;60:1462–71.
246. Mawal Y, Critchley IA, Riccobene TA, Talley AK. Ceftazidime-avibactam for the treatment of complicated urinary tract infections and complicated intra-bdominal infections. Expert Rev Clin Pharmacol. 2015;8:691–707.
247. Mazuski JE, Gasink LB, Armstrong J, Broadhurst H, Stone GG, Rank D, et al. Efficacy and safety of ceftazidime-avibactam plus metronidazole versus meropenem in the treatment of complicated intra-abdominal infection–results from a randomized, controlled, double-blind, phase 3 program. Clin Infect Dis. 2016 [Epub ahead of print]
248. Liscio JL, Mahoney MV, Hirsch EB. Ceftolozane/tazobactam and Ceftazidime/avibactam: two novel beta-lactam/beta-lactamase inhibitor combination agents for the treatment of resistant Gram-negative bacterial infections. Int J Antimicrob Agents. 2015;46:266–71.
249. Holden MT, Hsu LY, Kurt K, Weinert LA, Mather AE, Harris SR, et al. A genomic portrait of the emergence, evolution, and global spread of a methicillin-resistant Staphylococcus aureus pandemic. Genome Res. 2013;23:653–64.
250. Skalweit MJ. Profile of ceftolozane/tazobactam and its potential in the treatment of complicated intra-abdominal infections. Drug Des Devel Ther. 2015;9:2919–25.
251. Montravers P, Dupont H, Gauzit R, Veber B, Auboyer C, Blin P, et al. Candida as a risk factor for mortality in peritonitis. Crit Care Med. 2006;34:646–52.
252. Zappella N, Desmard M, Chochillon C, Ribeiro-Parenti L, Houze S, Marmuse JP, et al. Positive peritoneal fluid fungal cultures in postoperative peritonitis after bariatric surgery. Clin Microbiol Infect. 2015;21:853.e1-3.
253. Montravers P, Mira JP, Gangneux JP, Leroy O, Lortholary O. AmarCand study group. A multicentre study of antifungal strategies and outcome of Candida spp. peritonitis in intensive-care units. Clin Microbiol Infect. 2011;17:1061–7.
254. Pappas PG, Kauffman CA, Andes D, Benjamin DK, Calandra TF, Edwards JE, et al. Clinical practice guidelines for the management of candidiasis: 2009 update by the Infectious Diseases Society of America. Clin Infect Dis. 2009;48:503–35.
255. Playford EG, Webster AC, Sorrell TC, Craig JC. Antifungal agents for preventing fungal infections in non-neutropenic critically ill and surgical patients: systematic review and meta-analysis of randomized clinical trials. J Antimicrob Chemother. 2006;57:628–38.
256. Shorr AF, Chung K, Jackson WL, Waterman PE, Kollef MH. Fluconazole prophylaxis in critically ill surgical patients: a meta-analysis. Crit Care Med. 2005;33:1928–35.
257. Vardakas KZ, Samonis G, Michalopoulos A, Soteriades ES, Falagas ME. Antifungal prophylaxis with azoles in high-risk, surgical intensive care unit patients: a meta-analysis of randomized, placebo-controlled trials. Crit Care Med. 2006;34:1216–24.
258. Cruciani M, De Lalla F, Mengoli C. Prophylaxis of Candida infections in adult trauma and surgical intensive care patients: a systematic review and meta-analysis. Intensive Care Med. 2005;31:1479–87.
259. Cornely OA, Bassetti M, Calandra T, Garbino J, Kullberg BJ, Lortholary O, et al. ESCMID Fungal Infection Study Group. ESCMID* guideline for the diagnosis and management of Candida diseases 2012: non-neutropenic adult patients. Clin Microbiol Infect. 2012;18 Suppl 7:19–37.
260. Knitsch W, Vincent JL, Utzolino S, François B, Dinya T, Dimopoulos G, et al. A randomized, placebo-controlled trial of preemptive antifungal therapy for the prevention of invasive candidiasis following gastrointestinal surgery for intra-abdominal infections. Clin Infect Dis. 2015;61(11):1671–8.
261. Allou N, Allyn J, Montravers P. When and how to cover for fungal infections in patients with severe sepsis and septic shock. Curr Infect Dis Rep. 2011;13:426–32.
262. Shields RK, Nguyen MH, Press EG, Clancy CJ. Abdominal candidiasis is a hidden reservoir of echinocandin resistance. Antimicrob Agents Chemother. 2014;58:7601–5.
263. Müller M, Dela Peña A, Derendorf H. Issues in pharmacokinetics and pharmacodynamics of anti-infective agents: distribution in tissue. Antimicrob Agents Chemother. 2004;48:1441–53.

264. Gonzalez D, Schmidt S, Derendorf H. Importance of relating efficacy measures to unbound drug concentrations for anti-infective agents. Clin Microbiol Rev. 2013;26:274–88.
265. Seguin P, Verdier MC, Chanavaz C, Engrand C, Laviolle B, Donnio PY, et al. Plasma and peritoneal concentration following continuous infusion of cefotaxime in patients with secondary peritonitis. J Antimicrob Chemother. 2009;63:564–7.
266. Buijk SL, Gyssens IC, Mouton JW, Van Vliet A, Verbrugh HA, Bruining HA. Pharmacokinetics of ceftazidime in serum and peritoneal exudate during continuous versus intermittent administration to patients with severe intra-abdominal infections. J Antimicrob Chemother. 2002;49:121–8.
267. Dahyot-Fizelier C, Lefeuvre S, Laksiri L, Marchand S, Sawchuk RJ, Couet W, et al. Kinetics of imipenem distribution into the peritoneal fluid of patients with severe peritonitis studied by microdialysis. Clin Pharmacokinet. 2010;49:323–34.
268. Karjagin J, Lefeuvre S, Oselin K, Kipper K, Marchand S, Tikkerberi A, et al. Pharmacokinetics of meropenem determined by icrodialysis in the peritoneal fluid of patients with severe peritonitis associated with septic shock. Clin Pharmacol Ther. 2008;83:452–9.
269. Levison ME. Pharmacodynamics of antimicrobial drugs. Infect Dis Clin North Am. 2004;18:451–65.
270. Roberts JA, Abdul-Aziz MH, Lipman J, Mouton JW, Vinks AA, Felton TW, et al. Individualised antibiotic dosing for patients who are critically ill: challenges and potential solutions. Lancet Infect Dis. 2014;14:498–509.
271. Leekha S, Terrell CL, Edson RS. General principles of antimicrobial therapy. Mayo Clin Proc. 2011;86:156–67.
272. Pea F, Viale P. Bench-to-bedside review: appropriate antibiotic therapy in severe sepsis and septic shock-does the dose matter? Crit Care. 2009;13:214.
273. Lau WK, Mercer D, Itani KM, Nicolau DP, Kuti JL, Mansfield D, et al. Randomized, open-label, comparative study of piperacillin-tazobactam administered by continuous infusion versus intermittent infusion for treatment of hospitalized patients with complicated intra-abdominal infection. Antimicrob Agents Chemother. 2006;50:3556–61.
274. Dulhunty JM, Roberts JA, Davis JS, Webb SA, Bellomo R, Gomersall C, et al. A Multicenter Randomized Trial of Continuous versus Intermittent beta-lactam Infusion in Severe Sepsis. Am J Respir Crit Care Med. 2015;192:1298–305.
275. Lodise Jr TP, Lomaestro B, Drusano GL. Piperacillin-tazobactam for Pseudomonas aeruginosa infection: clinical implications of an extended-infusion dosing strategy. Clin Infect Dis. 2007;44:357–63.
276. Lorente L, Jiménez A, Martín MM, Iribarren JL, Jiménez JJ, Mora ML. Clinical cure of ventilator-associated pneumonia treated with piperacillin/tazobactam administered by continuous or intermittent infusion. Int J Antimicrob Agents. 2009;33:464–8.
277. Hatala R, Dinh T, Cook DJ. Once-daily aminoglycoside dosing in immunocompetent adults: a meta-analysis. Ann Intern Med. 1996;124:717–25.
278. Udy AA, Baptista JP, Lim NL, Joynt GM, Jarrett P, Wockner L, et al. Augmented renal clearance in the ICU: results of a multicenter observational study of renal function in critically ill patients with normal plasma creatinine concentrations. Crit Care Med. 2014;42:520–7.
279. Gladman MA, Knowles CH, Gladman LJ, Payne JG. Intra-operative culture in appendicitis: traditional practice challenged. Ann R Coll Surg Engl. 2004;86:196–201.
280. Davies HO, Alkhamesi NA, Dawson PM. Peritoneal fluid culture in appendicitis: review in changing times. Int J Surg. 2010;8:426–9.
281. Marchese A, Esposito S, Barbieri R, Bassetti M, Debbia E. Does the adoption of EUCAST susceptibility breakpoints affect the selection of antimicrobials to treat acute community-acquired respiratory tract infections? BMC Infect Dis. 2012;12:181.
282. Wolfensberger A, Sax H, Weber R, Zbinden R, Kuster SP, Hombach M. Change of antibiotic susceptibility testing guidelines from CLSI to EUCAST: influence on cumulative hospital antibiograms. PLoS One. 2013;8, e79130.
283. Van der Bij AK, Van Dijk K, Muilwijk J, Thijsen SF, Notermans DW, De Greeff S, et al. Clinical breakpoint changes and their impact on surveillance of antimicrobial resistance in Escherichia coli causing bacteraemia. Clin Microbiol Infect. 2012;18:E466–72.
284. Polsfuss S, Bloemberg GV, Giger J, Meyer V, Hombach M. Comparison of European Committee on Antimicrobial Susceptibility Testing (EUCAST) and CLSI screening parameters for the detection of extended-spectrum beta-lactamase production in clinical Enterobacteriaceae isolates. J Antimicrob Chemother. 2012;67:159–66.
285. Hombach M, Mouttet B, Bloemberg GV. Consequences of revised CLSI and EUCAST guidelines for antibiotic susceptibility patterns of ESBL- and AmpC beta-lactamase-producing clinical Enterobacteriaceae isolates. J Antimicrob Chemother. 2013;68:2092–8.
286. Andersen BR, Kallehave FL, Andersen HK. Antibiotics versus placebo for prevention of postoperative infection after appendicectomy. Cochrane Database Syst Rev. 2005;3, CD001439.
287. Mazeh H, Mizrahi I, Dior U, Simanovsky N, Shapiro M, Freund HR, et al. Role of antibiotic therapy in mild acute calculus cholecystitis: a prospective andomized controlled trial. World J Surg. 2012;36:1750–9.
288. Regimbeau JM, Fuks D, Pautrat K, Mauvais F, Haccart V, Msika S, et al. Effect of postoperative antibiotic administration on postoperative infection following cholecystectomy for acute calculous cholecystitis: a randomized clinical trial. JAMA. 2014;312:145–54.
289. Bhangu A, Søreide K, Di Saverio S, Assarsson JH, Drake FT. Acute appendicitis: modern understanding of pathogenesis, diagnosis, and management. Lancet. 2015;386:1278–87.
290. Søreide K, Thorsen K, Harrison EM, Bingener J, Møller MH, Ohene-Yeboah M, et al. Perforated peptic ulcer. Lancet. 2015;386:1288–98.
291. Sawyer RG, Claridge JA, Nathens AB, Rotstein OD, Duane TM, Evans HL, et al. Trial of short-course antimicrobial therapy for intraabdominal infection. N Engl J Med. 2015;372:1996–2005.
292. Riccio LM, Popovsky KA, Hranjec T, Politano AD, Rosenberger LH, Tura KC, et al. Association of excessive duration of antibiotic therapy for intra-abdominal infection with subsequent extra-abdominal infection and death: a study of 2,552 consecutive infections. Surg Infect (Larchmt). 2014;15:417–24.
293. Hochreiter M, Köhler T, Schweiger AM, Keck FS, Bein B, von Spiegel T, et al. Procalcitonin to guide duration of antibiotic therapy in intensive care patients: a randomized prospective controlled trial. Crit Care. 2009;13:R83.
294. Xiao Z, Wilson C, Robertson HL, Roberts DJ, Ball CG, Jenne CN, et al. Inflammatory mediators in intra-abdominal sepsis or injury–a scoping review. Crit Care. 2015;19:373.
295. Tschaikowsky K, Hedwig-Geissing M, Braun GG, Radespiel-Troeger M. Predictive value of procalcitonin, interleukin-6, and C-reactive protein for survival in postoperative patients with severe sepsis. J Crit Care. 2011;26:54–64.
296. Azevedo JR, Torres OJ, Czeczko NG, Tuon FF, Nassif PA, Souza GD. Procalcitonin as a prognostic biomarker of severe sepsis and septic shock. Rev Col Bras Cir. 2012;39:456–61.
297. Schroeder S, Hochreiter M, Koehler T, Schweiger AM, Bein B, Keck FS, et al. Procalcitonin (PCT)-guided algorithm reduces length of antibiotic treatment in surgical intensive care patients with severe sepsis: results of a prospective randomized study. Langenbecks Arch Surg. 2009;394:221–6.
298. Jung B, Molinari N, Nasri M, Hajjej Z, Chanques G, Jean-Pierre H, et al. Procalcitonin biomarker kinetics fails to predict treatment response in perioperative abdominal infection with septic shock. Crit Care. 2013;17:R255.
299. Centers for Disease Control and Prevention (CDC). Guidance for control of infections with carbapenem-resistant or carbapenemase-producing Enterobacteriaceae in acute care facilities. Morb Mortal Wkly Rep. 2009;58:256–60.

10

2013 WSES guidelines for management of intra-abdominal infections

Massimo Sartelli[1*], Pierluigi Viale[2], Fausto Catena[3], Luca Ansaloni[4], Ernest Moore[5], Mark Malangoni[6], Frederick A Moore[7], George Velmahos[8], Raul Coimbra[9], Rao Ivatury[10], Andrew Peitzman[11], Kaoru Koike[12], Ari Leppaniemi[13], Walter Biffl[5], Clay Cothren Burlew[5], Zsolt J Balogh[14], Ken Boffard[15], Cino Bendinelli[14], Sanjay Gupta[16], Yoram Kluger[17], Ferdinando Agresta[18], Salomone Di Saverio[19], Imtiaz Wani[20], Alex Escalona[21], Carlos Ordonez[22], Gustavo P Fraga[23], Gerson Alves Pereira Junior[24], Miklosh Bala[25], Yunfeng Cui[26], Sanjay Marwah[27], Boris Sakakushev[28], Victor Kong[29], Noel Naidoo[30], Adamu Ahmed[31], Ashraf Abbas[32], Gianluca Guercioni[33], Nereo Vettoretto[34], Rafael Díaz-Nieto[35], Ihor Gerych[36], Cristian Tranà[37], Mario Paulo Faro[38], Kuo-Ching Yuan[39], Kenneth Yuh Yen Kok[40], Alain Chichom Mefire[41], Jae Gil Lee[42], Suk-Kyung Hong[43], Wagih Ghnnam[44], Boonying Siribumrungwong[45], Norio Sato[11], Kiyoshi Murata[46], Takayuki Irahara[47], Federico Coccolini[4], Helmut A Segovia Lohse[48], Alfredo Verni[49] and Tomohisa Shoko[50]

Abstract

Despite advances in diagnosis, surgery, and antimicrobial therapy, mortality rates associated with complicated intra-abdominal infections remain exceedingly high.

The 2013 update of the World Society of Emergency Surgery (WSES) guidelines for the management of intra-abdominal infections contains evidence-based recommendations for management of patients with intra-abdominal infections.

Introduction

The clinical recommendations discussed in these guidelines are based on research conducted by members of the WSES Expert Panel. These updated guidelines replace those previously published in 2010 [1]. The guidelines outline clinical recommendations based on the Grading of Recommendations Assessment, Development, and Evaluation (GRADE) hierarchy criteria summarized in Table 1 [2,3].

Principles of surgical management

Intra-abdominal infections (IAIs) encompass a variety of pathological conditions, ranging from uncomplicated appendicitis to fecal peritonitis [4].

As a general principle, every verified source of infection should be controlled as soon as possible. The level of urgency of treatment is determined by the affected organ(s), the relative speed at which clinical symptoms progress and worsen, and the underlying physiological stability of the patient.

The procedure used to treat the infection depends on the anatomical site of infection, the degree of peritoneal inflammation, the generalized septic response, the patient's underlying condition, and the available resources of the treatment center. IAIs are subcategorized in 2 groups: uncomplicated and complicated IAIs [5].

In the event of an uncomplicated case of IAI, the infection involves a single organ and does not spread to the peritoneum. Patients with such infections can be treated with either surgical intervention or antibiotics. When the infection is effectively resolved by means of surgery, a 24-hour regimen of perioperative antibiotics is typically sufficient. Patients with uncomplicated intra-abdominal infections, such as acute diverticulitis, acute cholecystitis, and acute appendicitis, may be treated non-operatively by means of antimicrobial therapy.

In the event of complicated IAI, the infectious process proceeds beyond a single organ, causing either localized or diffuse peritonitis. The treatment of patients with

* Correspondence: m.sartelli@virgilio.it
[1]Department of Surgery, Macerata Hospital, Macerata, Italy
Full list of author information is available at the end of the article

Table 1 Grading of recommendations from Guyatt and colleagues [1,2]

Grade of recommendation	Clarity of risk/benefit	Quality of supporting evidence	Implications
1A			
Strong recommendation, high-quality evidence	Benefits clearly outweigh risk and burdens, or vice versa	RCTs without important limitations or overwhelming evidence from observational studies	Strong recommendation, applies to most patients in most circumstances without reservation
1B			
Strong recommendation, moderate-quality evidence	Benefits clearly outweigh risk and burdens, or vice versa	RCTs with important limitations (inconsistent results, methodological flaws, indirect or imprecise) or exceptionally strong evidence from observational studies	Strong recommendation, applies to most patients in most circumstances without reservation
1C			
Strong recommendation, low-quality or very low-quality evidence	Benefits clearly outweigh risk and burdens, or vice versa	Observational studies or case series	Strong recommendation based on limited evidence; recommendations may change when higher quality or more extensive evidence becomes available
2A			
Weak recommendation, high-quality evidence	Benefits closely balanced with risks and burdens	RCTs without important limitations or overwhelming evidence from observational studies	Weak recommendation, best action may differ depending on circumstances, expertise of clinician, the patient in question, or other social issues
2B			
Weak recommendation, moderate-quality evidence	Benefits closely balanced with risks and burdens	RCTs with important limitations (inconsistent results, methodological flaws, indirect or imprecise) or exceptionally strong evidence from observational studies	Weak recommendation, best action may differ depending on circumstances, expertise of clinician, the patient in question, or other social issues
2C			
Weak recommendation, Low-quality or very low-quality evidence	Uncertainty in the estimates of benefits, risks, and burdens; benefits, risks, and burdens may be closely balanced	Observational studies or case series	Very weak recommendation; other alternatives may be equally reasonable

complicated intra-abdominal infections involves both surgical and antibiotic therapy [5].

The safety and efficacy of ultrasound- and CT-guided percutaneous drainage of abdominal abscesses has been documented in patients with appendiceal and diverticular abscesses. Percutaneous image-guided drainage may also be used to address cases of advanced acute cholecystitis.

Sepsis management

Patients with severe sepsis or septic shock of abdominal origin require early hemodynamic support, source control, and antimicrobial therapy (Recommendation 1A).

Abdominal sepsis occurs as result of intra-abdominal or retroperitoneal infection. Early detection of the site of infection and timely therapeutic intervention are crucial steps for improving the treatment outcome of sepsis patients.

Sepsis is a complex, multifactorial, evolutive syndrome that can progress to conditions of varying severity. If improperly treated, it may cause the functional impairment of one or more vital organs or systems, which could lead to multiple organ failure [6]. Previous studies have demonstrated that there is an increased risk of death as patients transition from sepsis to severe sepsis and septic shock [7]. In the context of intra-abdominal infections, severe sepsis represents the diagnostic threshold separating stable and critical clinical conditions.

Thus, early detection of severe sepsis and prompt, aggressive treatment of the underlying organ dysfunction is an essential component of improving patient outcome. If untreated, sepsis dysfunction can lead to global tissue hypoxia, direct tissue damage, and ultimately to multiple organ failure [8-10].

Sepsis in the surgical patient continues to be a common and potentially lethal problem. Early identification of patients and timely implementation of evidence-based therapies continue to represent significant clinical challenges for care providers. The implementation of a sepsis screening program in conjunction with protocol for the delivery of evidence-based care and rapid source control can improve patient outcomes [11].

Early, correctly administered resuscitation can improve the outcome of patients with severe sepsis and septic shock (Recommendation 1A).

Rivers et al. demonstrated that a strategy of early goal-directed therapy (EGDT) decreases the in-hospital mortality of patients admitted to the emergency department in septic shock [9].

In surgical patients early intervention and implementation of evidence-based guidelines for the management of severe sepsis and septic shock improve outcomes in patients with sepsis [12].

Patients with severe sepsis and septic shock may present with inadequate perfusion. Poor tissue perfusion can lead to global tissue hypoxia and, in turn, to elevated levels of serum lactate. Fluid resuscitation should be initiated as early as possible in patients with severe sepsis.

The Surviving Sepsis Campaign guidelines [10] recommend that fluid challenge in patients with suspected hypovolemia begin with >1000 mL of crystalloids or 300–500 mL of colloids administered over a period of 30 minutes. Quicker administration and greater volumes of fluid may be required for patients with sepsis-induced tissue hypoperfusion. Given that the volume of distribution is smaller for colloids than it is for crystalloids, colloid-mediated resuscitation requires less fluid to achieve the same results. A colloid equivalent is an acceptable alternative to crystalloid, though it should be noted that crystalloids are typically less expensive.

When fluid challenge fails to restore adequate arterial pressure and organ perfusion, clinicians should resort to vasopressor agents. Vasopressor drugs maintain adequate blood pressure and preserve perfusion pressure, thereby optimizing blood flow in various organs.

Both norepinephrine and dopamine are the first-line vasopressor agents to correct hypotension in septic shock. Both norepinephrine and dopamine can increase blood pressure in shock states, although norepinephrine seems to be more powerful. Dopamine may be useful in patients with compromised cardiac function and cardiac reserve [13], but norepinephrine is more effective than dopamine in reversing hypotension in patients with septic shock. Dopamine has also potentially detrimental effects on the release of pituitary hormones and especially prolactin, although the clinical relevance of these effects is still unclear and can have unintended effects such as tachyarrhythmias. Dopamine has different effects based on the doses [14].

A dose of less than 5 μg/kg/min results in vasodilation of renal, mesenteric, and coronary districts. At a dose of 5–10 μg/kg/min, beta-1-adrenergic effects increase cardiac contractility and heart rate. At doses about 10 μg/kg/min, alpha-adrenergic effects lead to arterial vasoconstriction and increase blood pressure. Its major side effects are tachycardia and arrhythmogenesis.

The use of renal-dose dopamine in sepsis is a controversial issue. In the past, low-dose dopamine was routinely used because of the possible renal protective effects. Dopamine at a dose of 2–3 μg/kg/min was known to stimulate diuresis by increasing renal blood flow.

A meta-analysis of literature from 1966 to 2000 for studies addressing the use of dopamine in the prevention and/or treatment of renal dysfunction [15] concluded that the use of low-dose dopamine for the treatment or prevention of acute renal failure was not justified on the basis of available evidence.

Norepinephrine is a potent alpha-adrenergic agonist with minimal beta-adrenergic agonist effects. Norepinephrine can successfully increase blood pressure in patients who are septic and remain hypotensive following fluid resuscitation. Norepinephrine is effective to treat hypotension in septic shock patients. In many studies norepinephrine administration at doses 0.01 to 0.3 μg/kg/min has been shown may be effective [16,17].

Martin and coll. [18] published a randomized trial comparing norepinephrine vs dopamine. 32 volume-resuscitated septic patients were given either dopamine or norepinephrine to achieve and maintain normal hemodynamic and oxygen transport parameters for at least 6 h. Dopamine administration was successful in only 31% of patients, whereas norepinephrine administration was successful in 93%. Of the 11 patients who did not respond to dopamine, 10 responded when norepinephrine was added to therapy. Serum lactate levels were decreased as well, suggesting that norepinephrine therapy improved tissue oxygenation.

Recently a prospective trial by Patel and coll. compared dopamine to norepinephrine as the initial vasopressor in fluid resuscitated 252 adult patients with septic shock [19]. If the maximum dose of the initial vasopressor was unable to maintain the hemodynamic goal, then fixed dose vasopressin was added to each regimen. If additional vasopressor support was needed to achieve the hemodynamic goal, then phenylephrine was added. In this study dopamine and norepinephrine were equally effective as initial agents as judged by 28-day mortality rates. However, there were significantly more cardiac arrhythmias with dopamine treatment.

The Surviving Sepsis Campaign guidelines [10] state that there is no sufficient evidence to suggest which agent is better as initial vasopressor in the management of patients with septic shock.

Phenylephrine is a selective alpha-1 adrenergic receptor agonist primarily used in anesthesia to increase blood pressure. Although studies are limited [20], its rapid onset, short duration, and primary vascular effects make it an important agent in the management of sepsis-associated hypotension; however, it should be noted that there are concerns regarding its potential to reduce cardiac output in certain patients.

Epinephrine is a potent α-adrenergic and β-adrenergic agent that increases mean arterial pressure by increasing both cardiac index and peripheral vascular tone. The primary concern regarding the use of epinephrine in septic patients is its potential to decrease regional blood flow, particularly in the splanchnic circulation [21].

Vasopressin infusion of 0.01 to 0.04 U/min in patients with septic shock increases plasma vasopressin levels to those observed in patients with hypotension attributable to other etiologies, such as cardiogenic shock. Increased vasopressin levels are associated with a reduced demand for other vasopressors. Urinary output may increase, and pulmonary vascular resistance may decrease. Infusions >0.04 U/min may lead to adverse, vasoconstriction-mediated events [22]. Low doses of vasopressin (0.03 U/min) may be effective in raising blood pressure in patients refractory to other vasopressors and may convey other therapeutic benefits.

Dobutamine is frequently used to treat septic shock patients as an inotropic agent that increases cardiac output, stroke index, and oxygen delivery (Do_2). However, the tendency of dobutamine to increase Do_2 to supranormal values in critically ill patients has raised serious questions regarding its saftey in the treatment of septic shock. The Surviving Sepsis Campaign Guidelines [10] recommend that a dobutamine infusion be administered in the event of myocardial dysfunction as indicated by elevated cardiac filling pressures and low cardiac output

The clinical benefits of corticosteroids in the treatment of severe sepsis and septic shock remain controversial.

A systematic review of corticosteroids in the treatment of severe sepsis and septic shock in adult patients was recently published in which the authors discussed 17 randomized trials (2138 patients) and 3 quasi-randomized trials (n = 246) of acceptable methodological quality and pooled the results in a subsequent meta-analysis [23]. The authors concluded that corticosteroid therapy has been used in varied doses for treating sepsis and related syndromes for more than 50 years, but its ability to reduce mortality rates has never been conclusively proven. Since 1998, studies have consistently used prolonged low-dose corticosteroid therapy, and follow-up analyses of this subgroup have found that such regimens tend to reduce short-term mortality.

According to the findings of the meta-analysis, corticosteroids should be considered at daily doses of 200–300 mg of hydrocortisone (or equivalent), administered as either an intravenous bolus or continuous infusion. Although the evidence supporting this claim was not particularly robust, the authors nevertheless suggested that treatment be administered at full dosage for at least 100 hours in adult patients presenting with vasopressor-dependent septic shock.

Diagnosis

Early diagnosis and prompt treatment of intra-abdominal infections can minimize complications (Recommendation 1C).

Detection of complicated intra-abdominal infections is primarily a clinical diagnosis. However, critically ill patients may be difficult to evaluate due to distracting injuries, respiratory failure, obtundation, or other comorbidities.

Initially, the pain may be dull and poorly localized (visceral peritoneum) before progressing to steady, severe, and more localized pain (parietal peritoneum).

Signs of hypotension and hypoperfusion such as lactic acidosis, oliguria, and acute alteration of mental status are indicative of a patient's transition to severe sepsis.

Diffuse abdominal rigidity suggests peritonitis and should be addressed promptly by means of aggressive resuscitation and surgical intervention.

Plain films of the abdomen are often the first imaging analyses obtained for patients presenting with intra-abdominal infections.

Upright films are useful for identifying free air beneath the diaphragm (most often on the right side) as an indication of perforated viscera.

The diagnostic approach to confirming the source of abdominal infection in septic patients depends largely on the hemodynamic stability of the patient [24].

For unstable patients who do not undergo an immediate laparotomy and whose critical condition prevents them from leaving the ICU for further imaging analysis, ultrasound is the best available imaging modality (Recommendation 1B).

For stable, adult patients who do not undergo an immediate laparotomy, computerized tomography (CT) is the imaging modality of choice for diagnosing intra-abdominal infections. In children and young adults, exposure to CT radiation is of particular concern and must be taken into consideration (Recommendation 1B).

When patients are stable, computerized tomography (CT) is the optimal imaging modality for assessing most intra-abdominal conditions [24,25].

When possible, computed tomography (CT) of the abdomen and pelvis is the most effective means of diagnosing intra-abdominal infections.

The value of both CT imaging and ultrasound in the diagnostic work-up of intra-abdominal infections has been comprehensively studied in the context of acute appendicitis.

In 2006, a meta-analysis by Doria et al. demonstrated that CT imaging featured significantly higher sensitivity and resolution than ultrasound in studies of both children and adults with acute appendicitis [26].

However, when examining children and young adults, clinicians must always take into account the risk of radiation exposure associated with CT.

Although CT scans are very useful in a clinical setting, children are more radiosensitive than adults and their exposure to ionizing radiation should be minimized [27].

Recently, a single-blind, noninferiority trial, evaluated the rate of negative (unnecessary) appendectomies following low-dose and standard-dose abdominal CTs in young adults with suspected appendicitis. Low-dose CTs were noninferior to standard-dose CTs with respect to negative appendectomy rates in young adults with suspected appendicitis [18]. However low-dose CTs could not detect perforated viscera as effectively as their standard-dose counterparts.

When CT and abdominal ultrasound are not available diagnostic options, diagnostic peritoneal lavage may be useful for the diagnosis of complicated IAIs [24].

Acute appendicitis

The appendectomy remains the treatment of choice for acute appendicitis. Antibiotic therapy is a safe means of primary treatment for patients with uncomplicated acute appendicitis, but this conservative approach is less effective in the long-term due to significant recurrence rates. (Recommendation 1A).

Although the standard treatment for acute appendicitis has historically been the appendectomy, the medical community has recently seen a notable increase in the use of antibiotic therapy as a primary means of treatment.

Several meta-analyses have been published overviewing a series of randomized trials comparing antibiotic therapy to appendectomies for acute uncomplicated appendicitis (cases without abscesses or phlegmon) [28-31].

Although non-operative, antibioitic-mediated treatments of uncomplicated appendicitis are associated with significantly fewer complications, more manageable pain control, and shorter patient sick leave, this conservative approach features high rates of recurrence and is therefore inferior to the traditional appendectomy.

Considering that only a small number of RCTs of poor methodological quality are currently available, well-designed RCTs are required to better assess the effects of an antibiotic-based approach in conservative treatments of uncomplicated acute appendicitis.

Given this controversy, the appendectomy remains the treatment of choice for acute appendicitis. Non-operative antibiotic treatment may be used as an alternative treatment for specific patients for whom surgery is contraindicated.

Both open and laparoscopic appendectomies are viable approaches to surgical treatment of acute appendicitis (Recommendation 1A).

Several randomized trials have compared the diagnostic and therapeutic advantages of laparoscopic and conventional open appendectomies in the treatment of acute appendicitis.

While the trials demonstrated a reduction in wound infections for the laparoscopic appendectomy group, they also exhibited a threefold increase in intra-abdominal abscesses.

In 2010, Sauerland et al. updated a previously published meta-analysis comparing the diagnostic and therapeutic results of laparoscopic and conventional open surgery [32]. 56 studies comparing laparoscopic appendectomies (with or without diagnostic laparoscopy) to open appendectomies for adult patients were included in the meta-analysis. Wound infections were less likely following a laparoscopic appendectomy (LA) than they were following an open appendectomy (OA), but the laparoscopic procedure showed an increased prevalence of intra-abdominal abscesses. The duration of surgery was on average 10 minutes longer for LAs that it was for open procedures. Compared to OAs, LAs typically resulted in less post-operative pain; on day 1 after surgery, patients who underwent a laparoscopic procedure reported reduced pain by 8 mm on a 100 mm visual analogue scale compared to patients who had undergone the open procedure. Further, the overall hospital stay was reduced for patients who underwent LAs compared to those who underwent OAs. While the operational costs of LAs were significantly higher, the costs associated with recovery were substantially reduced. 7 studies of children were included in the review, but the results did not differ significantly from those of similar adult-focused studies. Diagnostic laparoscopy reduced the risk of unnecessary appendectomies, though this trend was most common in fertile women as compared to unselected adults [33].

However, in many cases the strong predictive power of CT and ultrasound analysis renders the diagnostic laparoscopy clinically superfluous.

In 2011, Masoomi et al. used the Nationwide Inpatient Sample Database to evaluate the clinical data of adult patients in the United States who had undergone either LAs or OAs for suspected acute appendicitis from 2006 to 2008 [34].

A total of 573,244 adults underwent emergency appendectomies during this 3-year period. Overall, 65.2% of all appendectomies were performed laparoscopically. Use of the laparoscopic approach increased 23.7% from 58.2% in 2006 to 72% in 2008. In the context of acute non-perforated appendicitis, LAs featured lower overall complication rates, lower in-hospital mortality rates, and a shorter mean length of hospitalization compared to the open procedure.

Routine use of intraoperative irrigation for appendectomies does not prevent intra-abdominal abscess formation, adds extra costs, and may be avoided (Recommendation 2B).

Recently a retrospective review of 176 consecutive appendectomies, open (39%) and laparoscopic (61%), at a university affiliated tertiary care facility from July 2007 to November 2008 investigated routine use of intraoperative irrigation for appendectomies. The results did not show decrease in postoperative intra-abdominal abscess with use of intraoperative irrigation. Thirteen patients developed postoperative abscess: 11 with irrigation, two without irrigation. Ten of 13 patients who developed abscess were perforated; nine with irrigation and one without [35].

Patients with periappendiceal abscesses should be treated with percutaneous image-guided drainage. (Recommendation 1B).

Current evidence demonstrates that an interval appendectomy is not routinely necessary following initial non-operative treatment of complicated appendicitis. However, interval appendicectomies should always be performed for patients with recurrent symptoms (Recommendation 2B).

For patients with acute appendicitis presenting with abscesses, the optimal management strategy is somewhat controversial.

Percutaneous drainage to address periappendiceal abscesses results in fewer complications and shorter overall hospitalization [36-38].

In 2010, a meta-analysis was published comparing conservative treatment (i.e., antibiotic therapy +/– percutanteous abscess drainage) to appendectomies in the treatment of complicated appendicitis (cases exhibiting abscesses or phlegmon) [39].

17 studies (16 non-randomized/retrospective and 1 non-randomized/prospective) reported clinical data for 1572 patients: 847 patients received conservative treatment and 725 underwent acute appendectomies. Conservative treatment was associated with significantly fewer complications, wound infections, abdominal/pelvic abscesses, ileal/bowel obstructions, and additional follow-up surgeries. No significant differences were found in the overall length of hospitalization or in the duration of intravenous antibiotic infusion. Overall, several clinical studies demonstrated that there were significantly fewer complications in the conservative treatment group than there were in the appendectomy group.

The authors concluded that conservative treatment of complicated appendicitis was associated with decreased complication rates and fewer repeat surgeries ("re-operations") compared to traditional appendectomies, while both treatments featured comparable lengths of hospitalization.

Traditional management is initially conservative followed by interval appendectomies performed after resolution of the mass.

Recently, the efficacy of interval appendicectomies has been called into question, and there is disagreement in the medical community regarding whether or not the procedure is appropriate for adults with appendiceal abscesses. The main dispute involves the recurrence and complication rates following interval appendectomies as well as the procedure's ability to address underlying malignancy. The literature provides little evidence that an interval appendicectomy is routinely necessary; findings instead demonstrate that the procedure is unnecessary in 75%-90% of cases [40-42]. The results of a review by Andersonn and Petzold [41] based primarily on retrospective studies supported the practice of nonsurgical treatment without interval appendectomies in patients with appendiceal abscesses or phlegmon. Appendiceal abscesses or phlegmon were found in 3.8% of patients with appendicitis. Nonsurgical treatment failed in 7.2% of these cases, and abscess drainage was required in 19.7%. Immediate surgery was associated with higher morbidity rates compared to nonsurgical treatment. After successful nonsurgical treatments, malignancy and serious benign diseases were detected in 1.2% and 0.7% of cases, respectively, during follow-up analyses.

Following successful conservative treatment, interval appendicectomies were only performed for patients with recurrent symptoms. In patients over 40 years of age, other pathological causes of right iliac masses could be excluded by means of further investigation (colonoscopy and computerized tomography scans).

Studies investigating interval appendectomies after conservative treatment of appendiceal masses are typically retrospective in nature. The risk of recurrence of symptoms is only 7.2%, which suggests that appendectomies may not be routinely necessary [29]. Due to significant variability between studies and their retrospective natures, additional studies are needed to confirm these findings.

Diverticulitis

Patients with uncomplicated acute diverticulitis should be treated with antibiotic therapy to address gram-negative and anaerobic pathogens (Recommendation 2C).

The routine use of antibiotics for patients with uncomplicated acute diverticulitis is a point of controversy in the medical community.

In 2011, a systematic review was published overviewing antibiotic use in cases of uncomplicated diverticulitis [43]. Relevant data regarding the use of antibiotics in mild or uncomplicated cases of diverticulitis were sparse and of poor methodological quality. There was no concrete evidence to support the routine use of antibiotics in the treatment of uncomplicated diverticulitis.

Recently a prospective, multicenter, randomized trial involving 10 surgical departments in Sweden and 1 in Iceland investigated the use of antibiotic treatment in cases of acute uncomplicated diverticulitis. Antibiotic treatment for acute uncomplicated diverticulitis neither accelerated recovery nor prevented complications or recurrence [44].

However, even in the absence of evidence supporting the routine use of antibiotics for patients with uncomplicated acute diverticulitis, we recommend adequate antimicrobial coverage for gram-negative and anaerobic microorganisms.

Mild cases of uncomplicated acute diverticulitis should be treated in an outpatient setting. Outpatient treatment of uncomplicated acute diverticulitis depends on the condition and compliance of the patient as well as his or her availability for follow-up analysis. The treatment involves orally administered antibiotics to combat gram-negative and anaerobic bacteria. If symptoms persist or worsen, the patient should be admitted for more aggressive inpatient treatment.

Hospitalized patients with uncomplicated acute diverticulitis should be treated with intravenous fluids and antibiotic infusion.

The clinical value of antibiotics in the treatment of acute uncomplicated left-sided diverticulitis is poorly understood by the medical community and therefore merits further study.

The grade and stage of diverticulitis are determined by clinical severity and Hinchey classification of disease, and used to identify patents likely to fail medical management or require surgery. Hinchey's classification provides a means of consistent classification of severity of disease for clinical description and decision making. Perforation with operative findings of purulent peritonitis corresponds to Hinchey stage III, and feculent peritonitis to Hinchey stage IV. Stage I and Stage II refer to inflammatory phlegmon and paracolic abscesses [45].

Systemic antibiotic treatment alone is usually the most appropriate treatment for patients with small (< 4 cm in diameter) diverticular abscesses; image-guided (ultrasound- or CT-guided) percutaneous drainage is suggested for patients with large diverticular abscesses (> 4 cm in diameter) (Recommendation 2B).

For patients with diverticulitis complicated by peridiverticular abscesses, the size of an abscess is an important factor in determining the proper course of action and in deciding whether or not percutaneous drainage is the optimal approach [46].

Patients with small pericolic abscesses (< 4 cm in diameter) without generalized peritonitis (Hinchey Stage 1) can be treated conservatively with bowel rest and broad-spectrum antibiotics [47].

For patients with peridiverticular abscesses larger than 4 cm in diameter, observational studies indicate that CT-guided percutaneous drainage is the treatment of choice [48-51].

Recommendations for elective sigmoid colectomy following recovery from acute diverticulitis should be made on a case-by-case basis (Recommendation 1C).

The role of prophylactic surgery following conservatively managed diverticulitis remains unclear and controversial.

Although elective resection is often recommended after single episodes of complicated acute diverticulits that were resolved with conservative treatment, such an invasive procedure following a favorable response to noninvasive methods has serious implications and should be made on an individual basis [52-55].

Acute diverticulitis has a low rate of recurrence and rarely progresses to more serious complications, and as such, elective surgery to prevent recurrence and development of further complications should be used sparingly.

To investigate recurrence rates and post-operative complications following conservatively managed diverticulitis, Eglinton et al. retrospectively analyzed clinical data from all patients with diverticulitis admitted to their department from 1997 to 2002 [56]. After an initial episode of uncomplicated diverticulitis, only 5% of patients went on to develop the complicated form of the disease. Complicated diverticulitis recurred in 24% of patients, compared to a recurrence rate of 23.4% in those with uncomplicated diverticulitis. Recurrence typically occurred within 12 months of the initial episode.

Recently, Makela et al. published a review of 977 patients admitted for acute diverticulitis during a 20-year period [57]. The authors found that even with 2 or more previous admissions for acute diverticulitis, sigmoid resection remained unjustifiably excessive.

Elective surgery is recommended for patients with pelvic abscesses treated by means of percutaneous drainage due to the poor long-term outcomes of conservative treatment. However, minor mesocolic abscesses that typically resolve when treated conservatively are not always grounds for surgical intervention (Recommendation 1B).

Given the poor outcomes of pelvic abscesses associated with acute left-sided colonic diverticulitis, percutaneous drainage followed by secondary colectomy is recommended [58].

In the event of a colectomy performed to address diverticular disease, a laparoscopic approach is appropriate for select patients (Recommendation 1B).

Laparoscopic colectomies may have some advantages over open colectomies, including less post-operative pain, fewer cosmetic considerations, and a shorter average length of hospitalization. However, there appears to be no significant difference in early or late complication rates between the laparoscopic and open procedures [59,60].

The cost and outcome of the laparoscopic approach are both comparable to those of the open resection [61].

Laparoscopic surgery is recommended for elderly patients [62] and appears to be safe for select patients with complicated diverticulitis [63].

Emergency surgery is required for patients with acute diverticulitis associated with diffuse peritonitis as well as for patients with acute diverticulitis whose initial non-operative management has failed (Recommendation 1B).

Hartmann's resection is recommended in the event of severe acute diverticulitis with generalized, purulent, or fecal peritonitis as well as for patients with poor prognostic criteria. In the event of diffuse peritonitis, resection with primary anastomosis and peritoneal lavage is a suitable approach for patients with promising prognostic criteria or for those whose non-operative management of acute diverticulitis has failed.

Hartmann's procedure has historically been the standard treatment for complicated acute diverticulitis [64].

However, bowel reconstruction following Hartmann's procedure requires additional surgeries, which many patients cannot undergo due to complicated medical conditions; therefore, many of these patients remain with permanent stoma [65].

The optimal approach for treating left colonic perforation is a one-stage procedure involving primary anastomosis.

In an emergency setting, intraoperative lavage of the colon and primary anastomosis are safe procedures for addressing complicated diverticulitis, though Hartmann's procedure is still recommended for cases of diffuse or fecal peritonitis, immunocompromised patients, or patients experiencing septic shock and multiorgan failure [66].

Many studies have demonstrated that, for select patients, primary anastamosis can be safely performed in the presence of localized or diffuse peritonitis [67].

Primary anastomosis is not recommended for patients in high-risk categories [67-73].

In 2010, Tabbara et al. reviewed the medical records of 194 patients with complicated acute diverticulitis from 1996 to 2006 who required a colectomy within 48 hours of hospital admission [74].

The independent criteria predictive of eventual resection with primary anastomosis included the following: age less than 55 years, period between hospital admission and surgery lasting longer than 4 hours, and a Hinchey score of I or II.

There were patients featuring many of these indicators of primary anastomosis who instead underwent fecal diversion. The conditions and characteristics of these patients were comparable to those of the primary anastomosis patients, yet the former group experienced poorer clinical outcomes than the latter.

In the event of either intraoperative difficulty or extraperitoneal anastomosis, a diverting loop ileostomy following resection and primary anastomosis ,may suggested for high-risk patients who are hemodynamically stable; in this case, high risk is defined by immunosuppression, fecal peritonitis, and/or ASA grade IV [71].

Masoomi et al. [75] using the National Inpatient Sample database, examined the clinical data of patients who underwent an urgent open colorectal resection (sigmoidectomy or anterior resection) for acute diverticulitis from 2002 to 2007 in the United States. A total of 99,259 patients underwent urgent surgery for acute diverticulitis during these years [Primary anastomosis without diversion: 39.3%; Hartman's procedure (HP): 57.3% and primary anastomosis with proximal diversion (PAD): 3.4%]. The overall complication rate was lower in the PAD group compared with the HP group (PAD: 39.06% vs. HP: 40.84%; $p = 0.04$). Patients in the HP group had a shorter mean length of stay (12.5 vs.14.4 days, $p < 0.001$) and lower mean hospital costs (USD 65,037 vs. USD 73,440, $p < 0.01$) compared with the PAD group. Mortality was higher in the HP group (4.82 vs. 3.99%, $p = 0.03$).

PAD improved outcomes compared with HP, and should be considered in patients who are deemed candidates for two-stage operations for acute diverticulitis.

Laparoscopic peritoneal lavage with placement of drainage tubes is a safe approach for cases of perforated diverticulitis (Recommendation 2B).

Several case series and prospective studies have demonstrated that laparoscopic peritoneal lavage is a safe alternative to conventional management in the treatment of perforated diverticulitis with diffuse purulent peritonitis [76-79].

Recently a retrospective population study used an Irish national database to identify patients acutely admitted with diverticulitis, was published. Demographics, procedures, comorbidities, and outcomes were obtained for the years 1995 to 2008 [80].

Two thousand four hundred fifty-five patients underwent surgery for diverticulitis, of whom 427 underwent laparoscopic lavage. Patients selected for laparoscopic lavage had lower mortality (4.0% vs 10.4%, $p < 0.001$), complications (14.1% vs 25.0%, $p < 0.001$), and length of stay (10 days vs 20 days, $p < 0.001$) than those requiring laparotomy/resection. Patients older than 65 years were more likely to die (OR 4.1, $p < 0.001$), as were those with connective tissue disease (OR 7.3, $p < 0.05$) or chronic kidney disease (OR 8.0, $p < 0.001$).

Colonic carcinoma perforation

Patients with perforated colonic carcinoma represent the highest risk cases of colonic perforation [81].

Treatments for perforated colonic carcinoma should both stabilize the emergency condition of the peritonitis and fulfil the technical objectives of oncological intervention (Recommendation 1B).

Treating perforated colorectal cancer is a complicated procedure and the prognosis is rarely straightforward. Colorectal cancer-induced perforation is considered an advanced stage disease due to the potential for peritoneal dissemination of tumor cells throughout the site of perforation [82].

The stage of illness, proximity of the perforation to the tumor, and the number of metastatic lymph nodes are positively correlated with reduced procedural and cancer-free survival rates [83].

Hartmann's procedure has been widely accepted as an effective means of treating carcinoma of the left colon (with adequate R0 resection) in certain emergency scenarios [84].

A diverting ileostomy is recommended when anastomosis is performed for high-risk patients.

Colonic perforation following colonoscopy

Early detection and prompt treatment are essential in optimizing the treatment of colonic post-colonoscopy perforations. Patients presenting with such perforations should undergo immediate surgical intervention, which typically involves primary repair or resection (Recommendation 1B).

Recently, the frequency of colonic perforation has increased due to routinely performed advanced therapeutic endoscopy.

Over the last decade, many advancements have been streamlined to better address these perforations, yet there are no definitive guidelines for their optimal management [85].

Choosing a conservative or surgical approach depends on a variety of clinical factors [86].

Conservative management is typically used to treat patients in stable clinical condition without any signs of peritonitis. In published literature, fewer than 20% of patients with colonoscopy-related perforations were successfully treated with a non-surgical approach [87-89].

Although select patients may be responsive to non-operative therapy, most cases warrant prompt surgical intervention to minimize the extent of intraperitoneal contamination, thereby facilitating a single-step procedure that will likely reduce post-operative complications [88].

Further, timely intervention (shortened timeframe between perforation and treatment) results in improved patient outcome [90-92].

An early laparoscopic approach is a safe and effective treatment for colonoscopy-related colonic perforation (Recommendation 1C).

Laparoscopic surgery is a prudent compromise that minimizes the risks of invasive surgery as well as those of insufficiently aggressive non-operative therapy [93,94].

If the area of perforation cannot be localized laparoscopically, the surgeon should begin with a laparotomy before proceeding further [95].

Post-traumatic bowel injuries

The time between incidence and surgery is a significant determinant of morbidity in patients with injuries to visceral lumens (Hollow Viscus Injuries, HVIs). An expeditious diagnosis and prompt surgical intervention are recommended to improve the prognosis of patients presenting with HVIs (Recommendation 1C).

Hollow Viscus Injuries (HVIs) are associated with significant rates of morbidity and mortality. HVIs can occur by means of penetrating injury or blunt trauma, but they are less common in patients who have experienced blunt trauma than they are in those who have suffered a penetrating injury. In patients who have experienced blunt trauma, an accurate and timely diagnosis is often a difficult undertaking.

Several mechanisms of bowel injury have been documented in the wake of blunt abdominal trauma. The most common injury is the posterior crushing of the bowel segment between the seat belt and vertebra or pelvis. It results in local lacerations of the bowel wall, mural and mesenteric hematomas, transection of the bowel, localized devascularization, and full-thickness contusions. Devitalization of the areas of contusion may subsequently result in late perforation.

An important determinant of morbidity in patients with HVIs appears to be the interim time between injury and surgery. Only expeditious evaluation and prompt surgical action can improve the prognosis of these patients [96].

Older age, elevated Abdominal Abbreviated Injury Scores, significant extra-abdominal injuries, and delays exceeding 5 hours between admission and laparotomy were identified as significant risk factors predictive of patient mortality [97].

Colonic non-destructive injuries should be primarily repaired. Although Delayed Anastomosis (DA) is suggested for patients with Destructive Colon Injuries (DCI) who must undergo a Damage Control Laparotomy (CDL), this strategy is not suggested for high risk patients (Recommendation 2C).

Management pathway of colonic injury has been evolving over last three decades. There has been general agreement that injury location does not affect the outcome.

Sharp and Coll. stratified 469 consecutive patients with full thickness penetrating colon injuries for 13 years by age, injury location and mechanism, and severity of shock.

314 (67%) patients underwent primary repair and 155 (33%) underwent resection. Most injuries involved the transverse colon (39%), followed by the ascending colon (26%), the descending colon (21%), and the sigmoid colon (14%). Overall, there were 13 suture line failures (3%) and 72 abscesses (15%). Most suture line failures involved injuries to the descending colon ($p = 0.06$), whereas most abscesses followed injuries to the ascending colon ($p = 0.37$). Injury location did not affect morbidity or mortality after penetrating colon injuries. For destructive injuries, operative decisions based on a defined algorithm

rather than injury location achieved an acceptably low morbidity and mortality rate and simplifies management [98].

Colon injuries in the context of a Damage Control Laparotomy (DCL) are associated with high complication rates and an increased incidence of leakage [99]. Performing a Delayed Anastomosis (DA) during DCL for patients with Destructive Colon Injuries (DCI) who require surgical resection is an effective approach with complication rates comparable to those of conventional laparotomy and primary anastomosis and/or standard colostomy. However, in the event of extensive damage with vascular and visceral involvement, the surgical outcome depends largely on the damage control strategy. Hollow-organ injury following penetrating trauma should be transiently managed with suture ligation, staples, or simple suturing of the proximal and distal ends of the affected organ, while more definitive repairs (such as anastomosis, reconstruction, and colostomy) are typically deferred to later procedures [100-102]. Small bowel or colonic perforations are repaired with sutured closure. If the bowel requires resection and anastomosis, these steps are implemented at a later time and are not performed during initial management; this stepwise approach allows for better control of intestinal leakage without prolonging surgical time or increasing physiological stress. While the colostomy is a relatively quick procedure, it is not always recommended given that, during reanimation, the already edematous abdominal wall often swells to an even greater size, and the intestinal loop that is used to create the stoma may become necrotic due to hindered blood supply. Further, these circumstances can substantially prolong surgical time [100-102].

In 2011, Ordonez et al. performed a retrospective review of patients with penetrating DCI. The authors concluded that DAs should be performed for all patients presenting with DCI who undergo DCL; however, DAs are not recommended for patients with recurrent intra-abdominal abscesses, severe bowel wall edema and inflammation, or persistent metabolic acidosis. In these patients, a colostomy is a more appropriate alternative [103].

In 2011 Burlew et al. [104] reviewed patients requiring an open abdomen after trauma from January 1, 2002 to December 31, 2007. Type of bowel repair was stratified as immediate repair, immediate anastomosis, delayed anastomosis, stoma and a combination.

During the 6-year study period, 204 patients suffered enteric injuries and were managed with an open abdomen.

Enteric injuries were managed with immediate repair (58), immediate anastomosis (15), delayed anastomosis (96), stoma (10), and a combination (22); three patients died before definitive repair. Sixty-one patients suffered intra-abdominal complications: 35 (17%) abscesses, 15 (7%) leaks, and 11 (5%) enterocutaneous fistulas. The majority of patients with leaks had a delayed anastomosis. Leak rate increased as one progresses toward the left colon (small bowel anastomoses, 3% leak rate; right colon, 3%; transverse colon, 20%; left colon, 45%). There was a significant trend toward higher incidence of leak with closure day, with closure after day 5 having a four times higher likelihood of developing leak (3% vs. 12%, $p = 0.02$).

Gastroduodenal perforation

Surgery is the treatment of choice for perforated peptic ulcers. In selected cases (patients younger than 70 years of age without septic shock or peritonitis and showing no spillage of water-soluble contrast medium in a gastroduodenogram), non-operative management may be appropriate. However, if there is no improvement of clinical condition within 24 hours of initial non-operative treatment, the patient should undergo surgery (Recommendation 1A).

Research has shown that surgery is the most effective means of source control in patients with peptic ulcer perforations [105-107].

Patients with perforated peptic ulcers may respond to conservative treatment without surgery. Such conservative treatment consists of nasogastric aspiration, antibiotics, and antisecretory therapy. However, patients older than 70 years of age with significant comorbidities, septic shock upon admission, and longstanding perforation (> 24 hours) are associated with higher mortality rates when non-operative treatment is attempted [107-109].

Delaying the time of surgery beyond 12 hours after the onset of clinical symptoms reduces the efficacy of the procedure, resulting in poorer patient outcome [110].

Simple closure with or without an omental patch is a safe and effective procedure to address small perforated ulcers (< 2 cm) (Recommendation 1A).

In the event of large perforated ulcers, concomitant bleeding or stricture, resectional gastroduodenal surgery may be required. Intraoperative assessment enables the surgeon to determine whether or not resection is the proper course of action (Recommendation 1B).

Different techniques for simple closure of perforations have been described and documented in detail.

In 2010, Lo et al. conducted a study to determine if an omental patch offers any clinical benefit that is not offered by simple closure alone [111].

The study demonstrated that, in terms of leakage rates and overall surgical outcome, covering the repaired perforated peptic ulcer with an omental patch did not convey additional advantages compared to simple closure alone. The authors of the investigation concluded that further prospective, randomized studies were needed to clarify the safety and feasibility of simple closure without the support of an omental patch.

In the event of a small perforated gastroduodenal peptic ulcer, no significant differences in immediate post-operative conditions were reported when comparing simple closure and surgery [106,111-115]

The role of resectional surgery in the treatment of perforated peptic gastroduodenal disease is poorly understood; many reports recommend gastrectomy only in select patients with large gastric perforations and concomitant bleeding or stricture [116-120].

Laparoscopic repair of perforated peptic ulcers can be a safe and effective procedure for experienced surgeons (Recommendation 1A).

Aside from reduced post-operative analgesic demands, the post-operative outcome of the laparoscopic approach does not differ significantly from that of open surgery. In all reported studies, patients presented with small ulcers and received simple sutures, and many also received an omental patch. There were no studies reporting emergency laparoscopic resection or laparoscopic repair of large ulcers [121-126].

When a pathologist is available, frozen sections should be prepared from biopsied tissue to better assess the nature of gastric perforations (Recommendation 2C).

If a patient has a curable tumor and is of a stable clinical condition (no septic shock, localized peritonitis, or other comorbidities) the ideal treatment is a gastrectomy (total or sub-total) with D2 lymph-node dissection. For patients with a curable tumor complicated by poor underlying conditions, a two-stage radical gastrectomy is recommended (first step: simple repair, second step: elective gastrectomy). By contrast, simple repair is recommended for patients in poor clinical condition with non-curable tumors (Recommendation 2C).

Surgery is the treatment of choice for cases of perforated gastric cancer. In most instances, gastric carcinoma is not suspected as the cause of perforation prior to an emergency laparotomy, and the diagnosis of malignancy is often made following intra- and post-operative examination. The treatment is intended to both manage the emergency condition of peritonitis and fulfil the technical demands of oncological intervention. Perforation alone does not significantly affect long-term survival rates following gastrectomies [127]; similarly, differed resections (i.e. two-stage radical gastrectomy) do not typically affect long-term recovery [128,129].

The presence of pre-operative shock appears to be the most significant prognostic factor adversely affecting post-operative survival rates following surgery for perforated gastric cancer [130].

Even in the presence of concurrent peritonitis, patients with perforated gastric cancer should undergo gastric resection; the only exception to this recommendation occurs when a patient is hemodynamically unstable or has unresectable cancer [131-133].

Early detection and prompt treatment are essential in optimizing the management of patients with post-Endoscopic Retrograde Cholangiopancreatography (ERCP) duodenal perforation.

Stable patients may be managed non-operatively. The timing of surgery following failed conservative treatment greatly influences the outcome of patients with post-ERCP duodenal perforation (Recommendation 2C).

The use of ERCP has transitioned from a diagnostic tool to a primarily therapeutic intervention in the treatment of pancreaticobiliary disorders. Several studies [134-137] have reported an elevated rate of ERCP-related perforation, increasing from 0.3% to 1.0%. Duodenal perforations may be retroperitoneal (typically in the periampullary region following sphincterotomy) or intraperitoneal (typically in the lateral wall following adjacent endoscope passage). Intraperitoneal perforations are often large, and affected patients may require immediate surgery [138].

Diagnoses of nosocomial, procedure-related perforations are made by evaluating clinical findings, particularly radiographic imaging with contrast examinations (preferably CT). The presence of retroperitoneal air upon CT analysis does not linearly correlate with the severity of the condition or the need for surgery [139,140].

If there is any suspicion of perforation, the surgeon must promptly diagnose the patient and immediately initiate systemic support, including broad-spectrum antibiotics and intravenous resuscitation. Following clinical and radiographic examination, the mechanism, site, and extent of injury should be taken into account when selecting a conservative or surgical approach [141].

Despite extensive retroperitoneal air observed in CT analysis, successful non-operative management of sphincterotomy-related retroperitoneal perforations is possible, provided that the patient remains stable [142,143]. In contrast, if a patient develops abdominal pain, becomes febrile, or appears critically ill, surgical exploration should be considered for repair or drainage, especially in the case of elderly or chronically ill patients who are less able to withstand physiological stress.

Early surgical intervention often facilitates ensuing primary repair strategies, similar in principle to closure of duodenal perforations secondary to duodenal ulcers. Delayed repair following failed non-operative treatment can be devastating and may require duodenal diversion and drainage without repair of the actual perforation.

Several novel methods of managing ERCP-induced perforation have been reported in recent literature [143,144]. Some patients have been managed successfully with an endoclipping device; however, this procedure is somewhat precarious given that adequate closure requires inclusion of the submucosal layer of the bowel wall, which clips cannot reliably ensure. Patients must be carefully selected for this procedure; the clipping method is only appropriate for patients who meet the criteria for conservative management (such as the absence of peritoneal signs) and who present with small, well-defined perforations detected without delay. The majority of pancreaticobiliary and duodenal perforations (70%) secondary to periampullary endoscopic interventions can be treated non-operatively [144] by means of nasogastric drainage, antibiotic coverage and nutritional support.

Small bowel perforations

Jejunoileal perforations are a relatively uncommon source of peritonitis in Western countries compared to less developed regions where such intestinal perforations are a frequent contributor to high morbidity and mortality rates [145,146].

Although prompt surgery correlates with better clinical outcomes, there is widespread disagreement among the medical community regarding the proper surgical course of action; surgeons advocate a wide array of procedures, including simple closure, wedge excision or segmental resection and anastomosis, ileostomy, and side-to-side ileo-transverse anastomosis following primary perforation repair.

Surgery is the treatment of choice for patients with small bowel perforations (Recommendation 1A).

In the event of small perforations, primary repair is recommended. However, when resection is required, subsequent anastomosis has not been shown to reduce post-operative morbidity and mortality rates. (Recommendation 2B).

Further, only treatment centers with surgeons who are experienced in laparoscopic procedures should utilize the laparoscopic approach (Recommendation 2C).

Primary repair of perforated bowels is preferable to resection and anastomosis due to lower complication rates, although it should be noted that the optimal outcome in these cases may be attributable to the limited tissue injury of minor perforations [145,146].

Patients with malignant lesions, necrotic bowels, perforations associated with mesenteric vascular injuries, or multiple contiguous perforations should not undergo primary repair [147].

During resection, the entire diseased segment is excised, leaving healthy, well perfused ends for anastomosis. The technique used for the enteroenterostomy (stapled or hand-sewn) seems to have little impact on the anastomotic complication rate.

Primary bowel anastomosis must be approached cautiously in the presence of gross purulent or feculent peritonitis due to high rates of serious complications [146].

While laparoscopic management of small bowel perforations was extensively reported in published literature, there were no studies comparing laparoscopy to open surgery [147].

Among small bowel perforations, typhoid ileal perforation remains a serious complication of typhoid enteritis in many tropical countries, with mortality rates as high as 20-40% [148]. Furthermore, the increased incidence of *S. typhi* infections in patients with Acquired Immunodeficiency Syndrome (AIDS) raises the possibility of resurgent typhoid fever in the developed world [149].

No meta-analyses have been published on the subject of typhoid ileal perforation. In a recent prospective study, 53 consecutive patients with typhoid perforation were surgically treated; the morbidity rate for this series of procedures was 49.1%, and the most common post-operative complications included wound infection, wound dehiscence, burst abdomen, residual intra-abdominal abscesses, and enterocutaneous fistulae. The mortality rate was 15.1% and was significantly affected by the presence of multiple perforations, severe peritoneal contamination, and burst abdomen (p value < 0.05, odds ratio > 1) [150].

The morbidity and mortality rates do not depend on the surgical technique, but rather on the general status of the patient, the virulence of the pathogens, and the duration and character of disease evolution preceding surgical treatment. It is therefore important to provide attentive pre-operative management, including aggressive resuscitation by means of intravenous hydration and adequate antibiotic coverage. During surgery, thorough abdominal lavage is important in cases of serious abdominal suppuration [151]. Surgical treatment includes simple closure of the perforation, ileal resection, and side-to-side ileo-transverse colostomy or diverting ileostomy [148,152,153].

Primary repair should be performed for patients with minor symptoms and with perioperative findings of minimal fecal contamination of the peritoneal cavity. In the event of enteric perforation, early repair is typically more effective than a temporary ileostomy given that repair is more cost effective and is free of ileostomy-related complications. However, in delayed cases, there can be severe inflammation and edema of the bowel, resulting in friable tissue that complicates handling and suturing of the bowel. Primary closure of the perforation is therefore likely to leak, which is the etiological basis of the high incidence of fecal peritonitis and fecal fistulae associated with the procedure. Surgeons should perform a protective ileostomy to address fecal peritonitis and reduce mortality rates in the immediate term. The ileostomy serves to divert, decompress, and exteriorize, and in doing so, appears to have lower overall morbidity and mortality rates than other surgical procedures. The ileostomy is particularly useful for patients in critical condition presenting late in the course of illness when it often proves to be a life saving procedure.

Acute cholecystitis

A laparoscopic cholecystectomy is a safe and effective treatment for acute cholecystitis. (Recommendation 1A).

The laparoscopic versus open cholecystectomy debate has been extensively investigated. Beginning in the early 1990s, techniques for laparoscopic treatment of the acutely inflamed gallbladder were streamlined and today the laparoscopic cholecystectomy is employed worldwide to treat acute cholecystitis.

Many prospective trials have demonstrated that the laparoscopic cholecystectomy is a safe and effective treatment for acute cholecystitis [154-158].

An early laparoscopic cholecystectomy is a safe treatment for acute cholecystitis and generally results in shorter recovery time and hospitalization compared to delayed laparoscopic cholecystectomies. (Recommendation 1A).

Timing is perhaps the most important factor in the surgical treatment of acute gallstone cholecystitis (AGC).

Evidence from published literature [159-162] demonstrates that, compared to delayed laparoscopic cholecystectomies, early laparoscopic cholecystectomies performed to treat acute cholecystitis reduce both recurrence rates and the overall length of hospital stay. A promptly performed laparoscopic cholecystectomy is therefore the most cost-effective means of treating acute cholecystitis.

In recent years, the medical community has debated the possible risk factors predictive of perioperative conversion to an open cholecystectomy from a laparoscopic approach in cases of acute cholecystitis [163,164].

Systematic evaluation of risk factors for laparoscopic to open conversion during cholecystectomies in patients with acute cholecystitis may help predict procedural difficulties and optimize surgical strategies of high-risk cases.

A delayed laparoscopic cholecystectomy is perhaps the most significant risk factor predictive of eventual laparoscopic to open conversion during a cholecystectomy in cases of acute cholecystitis [165].

In 2011, researchers published an analysis of patients undergoing urgent laparoscopic cholecystectomies (LCs) for acute cholecystitis based on the prospective database of the Swiss Association of Laparoscopic and Thoracoscopic Surgery [166]. The patients were grouped according to the time lapsed between hospital admission and laparoscopic cholecystectomy (admission day: d0, subsequent days of hospitalization: d1, d2, d3, d4/5, $d \geq 6$). Delaying LC resulted in the following shifts in patient outcome: significantly higher conversion rates (increasing from 11.9% at d0 to 27.9% at $d \geq 6$, $P < 0.001$), increased postoperative complications (increasing from 5.7% to 13%, $P < 0.001$), elevated repeat operation rates (increasing from 0.9% to 3%, $P = 0.007$), and significantly longer postoperative hospitalization ($P < 0.001$).

Percutaneous cholecystostomy can be used to safely and effectively treat acute cholecystitis patients who are ineligible for open surgery. Whenever possible, percutaneous cholecystostomies should be followed by laparoscopic cholecystectomies (Recommendation 2C).

No randomized studies have been published that compare the clinical outcomes of percutaneous and traditional cholecystostomies. It is not currently possible to make definitive recommendations regarding percutaneous cholecystostomies (PC) or traditional cholecystectomies in elderly or critically ill patients with acute cholecystitis.

Whenever possible, percutaneous cholecystostomies should be followed by laparoscopic cholecystectomies.

A literature database search was performed on the subject of percutaneous cholecystostomies in the elderly population [167].

Successful intervention was observed in 85.6% of patients with acute cholecystitis. A total of 40% of the patients treated with PC were later cholecystectomized, resulting in a mortality rate of 1.96%. The overall mortality rate of the procedure was 0.36%, but 30-day mortality rates were 15.4% in patients treated with PC and 4.5% in those treated with a traditional cholecystectomy ($P < 0.001$).

Recently, several studies have confirmed the effects of cholecystostomies in critically ill patients [168], elderly patients [169], and surgically high-risk patients [170-174].

Early diagnosis of gallbladder perforation and immediate surgical intervention may substantially decrease morbidity and mortality rates (Recommendation 1C).

Gallbladder perforation is an unusual form of gallbladder disease. Early diagnosis of gallbladder perforation and immediate surgical intervention are of utmost importance in decreasing morbidity and mortality rates associated with this condition.

Perforation is rarely diagnosed pre-operatively. Delayed surgical intervention is associated with elevated morbidity and mortality rates, increased likelihood of ICU admission, and prolonged post-operative hospitalization [175-179].

Ascending cholangitis

Ascending cholangitis is a life-threatening condition that must be treated in a timely manner.

Early treatment, which includes appropriate antibiotic coverage, hydratation, and biliary decompression, is of utmost importance in the management of acute cholangitis (Recommendation 1A).

The appropriatness of biliary drainage in patients with acute cholangitis depends on specific clinical findings, and this procedure may be secondary to a previous failed treatment.

Cholangitis varies greatly in severity, ranging from a mild form requiring parenteral antibiotics to severe or suppurative cholangitis, which requires early drainage of the biliary tree to prevent further complications [180].

Retrospective studies have shown that, 20–30 years ago, when biliary drainage was not available, the mortality rate of conservatively treated acute cholangitis was extremely high [181].

Given that emergency biliary drainage in patients with acute cholangitis is not always necessary or feasible, it is very important that surgeons promptly and effectively triage patients, distinguishing those who require this urgent procedure from those who do not.

In 2001, Hui et al. [182] published a prospective study investigating predictive criteria for emergency biliary decompression for 142 patients with acute cholangitis. Emergency ERCP was associated with fever, a maximum heart rate exceeding 100 beats per minute, albumin less than 30 g/L, bilirubin greater than 50 µmol/L, and prothrombin time exceeding 14 seconds.

There are 3 common methods used to perform biliary drainage: endoscopic drainage, percutaneous transhepatic drainage, and open drainage.

Endoscopic drainage of the biliary tree is safer and more effective than open drainage (Recommendation A).

Endoscopic biliary drainage is a well-established means of biliary decompression for patients with acute cholangitis caused by malignant or benign biliary disease and associated biliary obstruction [183,184].

Many retrospective case-series studies have also demonstrated the efficacy of percutaneous transhepatic drainage.

Endoscopic modalities of biliary drainage are currently favored over percutaneous procedures due to reduced complication rates. There are currently no RCTs comparing endoscopic and percutaneous drainage. (Recommendation 2C).

Currently, only retrospective studies have been published comparing the safety and effectiveness of endoscopic and percutaneous transhepatic biliary drainage in the treatment of acute obstructive suppurative cholangitis. These reports confirmed the clinical efficacy of endoscopic drainage as well as its ability to facilitate subsequent endoscopic or surgical intervention [185].

Open drainage should only be performed for patients for whom endoscopic or percutaneous transhepatic drainage has failed or is otherwise contraindicated (Recommendation 2C).

Given the shortened length of hospitalization and the rarity of serious complications such as intraperitoneal hemorrhage and biliary peritonitis, endoscopic drainage is preferred to open drainage [186-189].

Post-operative intra-abdominal infections

Post-operative peritonitis can be a life-threatening complication of abdominal surgery associated with high rates of organ failure and mortality. Treating patients with post-operative peritonitis requires supportive therapy of organ dysfunction, source control of infection via surgery and/or drainage, and intensive antimicrobial therapy [190].

Treatment recommendations are of little value given that randomized clinical trials are extremely difficult to perform for this particular pathology, and consequently, little relevant literature is available on the subject.

Percutaneous drainage is the optimal means of treating post-operative localized intra-abdominal abscesses when there are no signs of generalized peritonitis (Recommendation 2C).

Several retrospective studies in the fields of surgery and radiology have documented the effectiveness of percutaneous drainage in the treatment of post-operative localized intra-abdominal abscesses [191-193].

Source control should be initiated as promptly as possible following detection and diagnosis of post-operative intra-abdominal peritonitis. Ineffective control of the septic source is associated with significantly elevated mortality rates (Recommendation 1C).

Inability to control the septic source is associated with significant increases in patient mortality.

Organ failure and/or subsequent re-laparotomies that have been delayed for more than 24 hours both result in higher rates of mortality for patients affected by post-operative intra-abdominal infections [194].

Physical and laboratory tests are of limited value in diagnosing abdominal sepsis. CT scans typically offer the greatest diagnostic accuracy. Early re-laparotomies appear to be the most effective means of treating post-operative peritonitis [195].

Re-laparotomy strategy

In certain instances infection can lead to an excessive immune response and sepsis may progress to severe sepsis, septic shock, or multiple organ dysfunction syndrome (MODS).

In these cases, patients are severely destabilized by the septic shock and will likely experience increased complication and mortality rates [196].

These patients benefit from aggressive surgical treatment, prompt intervention, and successive follow-up surgeries ("re-operations") to better control MODS triggered by the ongoing intra-abdominal infection [197].

Deciding if and when to perform a re-laparotomy in cases of secondary peritonitis is largely subjective and based on professional experience. Factors indicative of progressive or persistent organ failure during early post-operative follow-up analysis are the best indicators of ongoing infection [198].

Three methods are currently employed for local mechanical management of abdominal sepsis following an initial laparotomy:

(1) Open abdomen
(2) Planned re-laparotomy
(3) On-demand re-laparotomy

Given the procedure's ability to streamline healthcare resources, reduce overall medical costs, and prevent the need for further re-laparotomies, the on-demand re-laparotomy is recommended for patients with severe peritonitis. (Recommendation 1A).

In 2007, van Ruler et al. [199] published a randomized, clinical study comparing planned and on-demand re-laparotomy strategies for patients with severe peritonitis.

In this trial, a total of 232 patients with severe intra-abdominal infections were randomized (116 planned and 116 on-demand).

In the planned re-laparotomy group, procedures were performed every 36 to 48 hours following the index laparotomy to inspect, drain, lavage, and perform other necessary abdominal interventions to address residual peritonitis or new infectious focuses.

In the on-demand re-laparotomy group, procedures were only performed for patients who demonstrated clinical deterioration or lack of improvement that was likely attributable to persistent intra-abdominal pathology.

Patients in the on-demand re-laparotomy group did not exhibit a significantly lower rate of adverse outcomes compared to patients in the planned re-laparotomy group, but they did show a substantial reduction in subsequent re-laparotomies and overall healthcare costs.

The on-demand group featured a shorter median ICU stay (7 days for on-demand group < 11 days for planned group; P = 0.001) and a shorter median length of hospitalization (27 days for on-demand group < 35 days for planned group; P = 0.008). Direct per-patient medical costs were reduced by 23% using the on-demand approach.

Members of our Expert Panel emphasize, however, that an on-demand strategy is not a forgone conclusion for all patients presenting with severe secondary peritonitis; that is, secondary peritonitis alone isn't necessary and sufficient to automatically preclude other alternatives. The decision to implement an on-demand strategy is based on contextual criteria and should be determined on a case-by-case basis.

For "wait-and-see" management of on-demand patients requiring follow-up surgery, early re-laparotomies appear to be the most effective means of treating post-operative peritonitis and controlling the septic source [200-202].

Organ failure and/or subsequent re-laparotomies delayed for more than 24 hours both correlate with higher mortality rates for patients affected by post-operative intra-abdominal infections [203].

Deciding whether or not to perform additional surgeries is context sensitive and depends on the surgeon and on his or her professional experience; no telltale clinical parameters are available [204,205].

The findings of a single RTC are hardly concrete, and further studies are therefore required to better define the optimal re-laparotomy strategy.

The open abdomen remains a viable option for treating intra-abdominal sepsis. The benefits of maintaining an open abdomen include ease of subsequent exploration, control of abdominal contents, reduced risk of intra-abdominal hypertension and abdominal compartment syndrome, and fascial preservation to ensure proper closure of the abdominal wall. However, prolonged exposure of abdominal viscera can result in additional complications, including infection, sepsis, and fistula formation (Recommendation 1C).

The open abdomen is the most technically straightforward means of conducting a planned follow-up procedure.

Open treatment was first used to manage severe intra-abdominal infections and pancreatic necrosis [200].

However, severe complications such as evisceration, fistula formation, and the development of giant incisional hernias were frequently observed in this procedure.

Temporary closure of the abdomen may be achieved by using gauze and large, impermeable, self-adhesive membrane dressings, both absorbable and non-absorbable meshes, and negative pressure therapy devices.

At present, negative pressure techniques (NPT) have become the most extensively employed means of temporary closure of the abdominal wall.

In recent years, open abdomen procedures have increased dramatically due to streamlined "damage control" techniques in life-threatening conditions, recognition and treatment of intra-abdominal hypertension and abdominal compartment syndrome, and important clinical findings regarding the management of severe intra-abdominal sepsis.

A more comprehensive understanding of the pathophysiology of open abdomen conditions as well as the development of new technologies for temporary abdominal wall closure have improved the management and outcome of patients undergoing this procedure [203].

Severe intra-abdominal infection is a progressive condition; affected patients progress from sepsis to severe sepsis with organ dysfunction and ultimately to septic shock.

This stepwise progression is characterized by excessive proinflammation, which causes vasodilation, hypotension, and myocardial depression. These effects combined with endothelial activation and Diffused Intravascular Coagulopathy (DIC), cause ongoing endothelial leakage, cellular shock, and microvascular thrombosis. Outwardly, clinical manifestations are characterized by septic shock and progressive MOF. In this situation, a surgeon must decide whether or not to perform a "damage control" laparotomy, thereby providing prompt and aggressive source control to curb the momentum of crescendoing sepsis.

Advantages of the open abdomen include prevention of abdominal compartment syndrome (ACS). In the event of septic shock, massive fluid resuscitation, bowel edema and forced closure of a non-compliant abdominal wall all contribute to intra-abdominal hypertension (IAH). Elevated intra-abdominal pressure (IAP) adversely affects the physiological processes of pulmonary, cardiovascular, renal, splanchnic, and central nervous systems. The combination of IAH and other physiological stressors contributes to significantly elevated morbidity and mortality rates.

Several studies have investigated open abdomen in the context of intra-abdominal infections, generating great interest and optimism in the medical community [206-209].

However, in 2007 a randomized study compared open and closed "on-demand" management of severe peritonitis. The study was terminated following the inclusion of only 40 patients after acknowledging the clearly discernable clinical disadvantages of the open abdomen group (55% and 30% mortality rates for open and closed procedures, respectively). It should be noted that, in this study, the open abdomen was managed exclusively with non-absorbable polypropylene mesh and without negative pressure therapy [210].

Following stabilization of the patient, surgeons should attempt early, definitive closure of the abdomen. Primary fascial closure may be possible when there is minimal risk of excessive tension or recurrence of IAH (Recommendation 1C).

When early, definitive fascial closure is not possible, progressive closure should be attempted each time the patient returns for subsequent procedures.

For patients with persistent large fascial defects, it is suggested that surgeons implement bridging with biological materials (Recommendation 1C).

Following stabilization of the patient, the primary objective is early and definitive closure of the abdomen to minimize complications associated with OA [206].

For many patients, primary fascial closure may be possible within a few days of the initial operation [206].

In other patients, early definitive fascial closure may not be possible. In these cases, surgeons should attempt progressive closure, in which the abdomen is incrimentally closed each time the patient undergoes a subsequent surgery.

Many methods of fascial closure have been described in medical literature [211-216]. In many cases abdominal closure is only partially achieved, resulting in large, debilitating hernias of the abdominal wall that will eventually require complex surgical repair. In these cases, bridging with biological mesh is recommended [217].

Antimicrobial therapy

Initial antibiotic therapy for IAIs is typically empirical in nature because the patient needs immediate attention, and microbiological data (culture and susceptibility results) can require up to 48 hours before they are available for a more detailed analysis.

IAIs can be treated with either single or multiple antimicrobial regimens depending on the range requirements of antimicrobial coverage.

Beta-lactam/beta-lactamase inhibitor combinations exhibit in vitro activity against gram-positive, gram-negative, and anaerobic organisms [218,219] and are viable options for empirical treatment of IAIs [218]. However, the increasing prevalence of drug-resistant Enterobacteriaceae observed in community-acquired infections restricts this regimen's empirical use to patients who are not at risk for these drug-resistant microorganisms [220].

In the past, Cephalosporins have often been used in the treatment of intra-abdominal infections. Among third generation cephalosporins, subgroups with both limited and strong activity against *Pseudomonas aeruginosa* (cefepime and ceftazidime) have been used in conjunction with metronidazole to treat IAIs. Enterobacteriaceae can have acquired resistance to both cephalosporins, while such resistance is intrinsic in Enterococci [221-223].

In light of the increasing prevalence of ESBL-producing enterobacteriaceae due to selection pressures related to overuse of cephalosporins, routine use of these antibiotics is strongly discouraged.

Aztreonam is a parenteral synthetic beta-lactam antibiotic and the first monobactam marketed for clinical use. The drug exhibits potent in vitro activity against a wide spectrum of gram-negative aerobic pathogens (including *Pseudomonas aeruginosa*), but its routine use is discouraged due to selection pressures favoring resistant strains, and it therefore shares the same constraints associated with cephalosporin use.

Carbapenems offer a wide spectrum of antimicrobial activity against gram-positive and gram-negative aerobic and anaerobic pathogens (with the exception of MDR resistant gram-positive cocci). For more than 2 decades, carbapenems have been considered the agents of "last resort" for multidrug-resistant infections caused by Enterobacteriaceae. In the last decade, increased carbapenem consumption has been associated with an increased emergence of carbapenem resistance among Enterobacteriacea, particularly in *Klebsiella pneumoniae.*

The recent and rapid spread of serine carbapenemases in *Klebsiella pneumoniae* (known as Klebsiella pneumoniae carbapenemases or KPCs) has become an issue of crucial importantance in hospitals worldwide [224].

Group 1 carbapenems include ertapenem, a once-a-day carbapenem that shares the activity of imipenem and meropenem against most species, including extended-spectrum beta-lactamase (ESBL)-producing pathogens, but is not active against Pseudomonas and Enterococcus species [225,226].

Group 2 includes imipenem/cilastatin, meropenem, and doripenem, which share activity against non-fermentative gram-negative bacilli. Researchers have reported doripenem's slightly elevated in vitro activity against certain Pseudomonas strains in registrative trials [227].

Further, given their excellent tissue penetration and strong activity against aerobic gram-negative bacteria, fluoroquinolones have been widely used in recent years for treatment of IAIs. It should also be noted that all fluoroquinolones are rapidly and almost completely absorbed from the gastrointestinal tract.

A combination of ciprofloxacin/metronidazole has been perhaps the most commonly used regimen for complicated IAIs in recent years. The latest quinolone, Moxifloxacin, has demonstrated to be active against a wide range of aerobic gram-positive and gram-negative species [228]. Compared to ciprofloxacin, moxifloxacin has enhanced activity against gram-positive bacteria and decreased activity against gram-negative bacteria [229]. Among quinolones, moxifloxacin appears to also be effective against *Bacterioides fragilis,* suggesting that the drug may be equally effective without co-administered antianaerobic agents [230-232]. However, in recent years, the ever-increasing incidence of drug resistance among Enterobacteriaceae and non-fermentative gram-negative bacilli has discouraged the drug's use in empirical regimens.

Aminoglycosides are particularly active against aerobic gram-negative bacteria and act synergistically against certain gram-positive organisms. They are effective against *Pseudomonas aeruginosa* but are ineffective against anaerobic bacteria. Aminoglycosides may be suboptimal for treatment of abscesses or intra-abdominal infections due to their low penetration in acidic environments [233].

Tigecycline is a parenteral glycylcycline antibiotic derived from minocycline. It is the first representative of the glycylcycline class of antibacterial agents to be marketed for clinical use [234,235].

While tigecycline does not feature in vitro activity against *P. aeruginosa* or *P. mirabilis,* it remains a viable treatment option for complicated IAIs due to its favorable in vitro activity against anaerobic organisms, Enterococci, several ESBL- and carbapenemase-producing Enterobacteriaceae, Acinetobacter species, and *Stenotrophomonas maltophilia* [236-238].

The use of tigecycline to treat IAIs is particularly useful in light of its unique pharmacokinetic properties; the drug is eliminated by active biliary secretion and is therefore able to establish high biliary and fecal concentrations [239].

Cultures from the site of infection are always recommended for patients with healthcare-associated infections or with community-acquired infections at risk for resistant pathogens. In these patients, the causative pathogens and the related resistance patterns are not readily predictable and therefore require further analysis (Recommendation 1C).

The results of microbiological analysis are helpful in designing therapeutic strategies for individual patients to customize antibiotic treatments and ensure adequate antimicrobial coverage.

Although it has been documented that bacteriological cultures have little impact on the course of treatment of common conditions like appendicitis [240], in this era of prevalent drug-resistant microorganisms involved in both nosocomial and community-acquired infections, the threat of resistance is a source of major concern that cannot be ignored.

In 2010, a review was published investigating the value of peritoneal fluid cultures in cases of appendicitis [241]. All included studies focusing on the use of intra-peritoneal swabs were open, non-randomized, and retrospective; further, they featured incompletely matched control groups and non-standardized swab collection techniques, and therefore offered limited statistical power with which to suggest modifications of surgical practice. Until controlled trial data of more reliable methodological quality become available, clinicians should continue the use of peritoneal swabs, especially for high-risk patients.

Cultures should be taken from intra-abdominal samples during surgical or interventional drainage procedures. Surgeons must ensure sufficient volume (a minimum of 1 mL of fluid or tissue) before sending the samples to a clinical laboratory by means of a transport system that properly handles the samples so as not to damage them or compromise their integrity.

The empirically designed antimicrobial regimen depends on the underlying severity of infection, the pathogens presumed to be involved, and the risk factors indicative of major resistance patterns (Recommendation 1B).

Predicting the pathogens and potential resistance patterns of a given infection begins by establishing whether the infection is community-acquired or healthcare-associated (nosocomial).

The major pathogens involved in community-acquired intra-abdominal infections are Enterobacteriaceae, Streptococcus species, and anaerobes (especially *B. fragilis*).

Contrastingly, the spectrum of microorganisms involved in nosocomial infections is significantly broader. In the past 20 years, the incidence of healthcare-associated infections caused by drug-resistant microorganisms has risen dramatically, probably in correlation with escalating levels of antibiotic exposure and increasing frequency of patients with one or more predisposing conditions, including elevated severity of illness, advanced age, degree of organ dysfunction, low albumin levels, poor nutritional status, immunodepression, presence of malignancy, and other comorbidities.

Although the transmission of multidrug-resistant organisms is most frequently observed in acute care facilities, all healthcare settings are affected by the emergence of drug-resistant pathogens.

In past decades, an increased prevalence of infections caused by antibiotic-resistant pathogens, including methicillin-resistant *Staphylococcus aureus*, vancomycin-resistant Enterococcus species, carbapenem-resistant *Pseudomonas aeruginosa*, extended-spectrum beta-lactamase (ESBL)-producing *Escherichia coli* and Klebsiella species, multidrug-resistant Acinetobacter species, and Candida species has been observed, particularly in cases of intra-abdominal infection [242-244].

For patients with severe sepsis or septic shock, early and properly administered empirical antimicrobial therapy can have a significant impact on the outcome, independent of the anatomical site of infection [245].

These data confirm the results of Riché et al. whose prospective observational study involving 180 consecutive patients with secondary generalized peritonitis demonstrated a significantly higher mortality rate for patients in septic shock (35% and 8% for patients with and without shock, respectively) [246].

International guidelines for the management of severe sepsis and septic shock (the Surviving Sepsis Campaign) recommend intravenously administered antibiotics within the first hour of onset of severe sepsis and septic shock and the use of broad-spectrum agents with adequate penetration of the presumed site of infection. Additionally, the employed antimicrobial regimen should be reassessed daily in order to optimize efficacy, prevent toxicity, minimize cost, and reduce selection pressures favoring resistant strains [10].

To ensure timely and effective administration of antimicrobial therapy for critically ill patients, clinicians must consider the pathophysiological and immunological status of the patient as well as the pharmacokinetic properties of the employed antibiotics (Recommendation 1C).

In the event of abdominal sepsis, clinicians must be aware that drug pharmacokinetics may be altered significantly in critically ill patients due to the pathophysiology of sepsis. The "dilution effect," also known as the "third spacing phenomenon," is very important for hydrophilic agents. Higher than standard loading doses of hydrophilic agents such as beta-lactams, aminoglycosides, and glycopeptides should be administered to ensure optimal exposure at the infection site, maintaining a therapeutic threshold that withstands the effects of renal function [247].

For lipophilic antibiotics such as fluoroquinolones and tetracyclines, the "dilution effect" in extracellular fluids may be mitigated during severe sepsis by the rapid redistribution of drugs to the interstitium from the intracellular compartment. Unlike observations of subtherapeutic administration of standard-dose hydrophilic antimicrobials, standard dosages of lipophilic antimicrobials are often sufficient to ensure adequate loading, even in patients with severe sepsis or septic shock [248].

Once initial loading is achieved, it is recommended that clinicians reassess the antimicrobial regimen daily, given that pathophysiological changes may occur that significantly alter drug disposition in critically ill patients.

Lower-than-standard dosages of renally excreted drugs must be administered in the presence of impaired renal function, while higher-than-standard dosages of renally excreted drugs may be required for optimal exposure in patients with glomerular hyperfiltration [249].

Table 2 overviews recommended dosing regimens of the most commonly used renally excreted antimicrobials.

The therapeutic approach undertaken by clinicians must take into account the activity of employed antimicrobials.

Antibiotics such as quinolones, daptomycin, tigecycline, aminoglycosides, polienes, and echinocandins exhibit concentration-dependent activity; as such, the dose should be administered in a once-a-day manner (or with the lowest possible daily administrations) in order to achieve zenithal plasma levels [249].

Beta-lactams, glycopeptides, oxazolidinones, and azoles exhibit time-dependent activity and exert optimal bactericidal activity when drug concentrations are maintained above the Minimum Inhibitory Concentration (MIC).

Table 2 Recommended dosing regimens (according to renal function) of the most commonly used renally excreted antimicrobials [248]

	Renal function			
Antibiotic	**Increased**	**Normal**	**Moderately impaired**	**Severely impaired**
Piperacillin/tazobatam	16/2 g q24 h CI or 3.375 q6 h EI over 4 hours	4/0.5 g q6 h	3/0.375 g q6 h	2/0.25 g q6 h
Imipenem	500 mg q4 h or 250 mg q3 h over 3 hours CI	500 mg q6 h	250 mg q6 h	250 mg q12 h
Meropenem	1 g q6 h over 6 hours CI	500 mg q6 h	250 mg q6 h	250 mg q12 h
Ertapenem	ND	1 g q24 h	1 g q24 h	500 mg q24 h
Gentamycin	9 to 10 mg/kg q24 h[b]	7 mg/kg q24 h	7 mg/kg q36–48 h	7 mg/kg q48–96 h
Amikacin	20 mg/kg q24 h	15 mg/kg q24 h	15 mg/kg q36–48 h[b]	15 mg/kg q48–96 h
Ciprofloxacin	600 mg q12 h or 400 mg q8 h	400 mg q12 h	400 mg q12 h	400 mg q24 h
Levofloxacin	500 mg q12 h	750 mg q24 h	500 mg q24 h	500 mg q48 h
Vancomycin	30 mg/kg q24 h CI	500 mg q6 h	500 mg q12 h	500 mg q24–72 h
Teicoplanin	LD 12 mg/kg q12 h for 3 to 4 doses; MD 6 mg/kg q12 h	LD 12 mg/kg q12 h for 3 to 4 doses; MD 4 to 6 mg/kg q12 h	LD 12 mg/kg q12 h for 3 to 4 doses; MD 2 to 4 mg/kg q12 h	LD 12 mg/kg q12 h for 3 to 4 doses; MD 2 to 4 mg/kg q24 h
Tigecycline	LD 100 mg; MD 50 mg q12 h	LD 100 mg; MD 50 mg q12 h	LD 100 mg; MD 50 mg q12 h	LD 100 mg; MD 50 mg q12 h

The efficacy of time-dependent antibacterial agents in severely ill patients is related primarily to the maintenance of supra-inhibitory concentrations, and therefore multiple daily dosing may be appropriate.

For these drugs, continuous intravenous infusion ensures the highest steady-state concentration under the same dosage constraints and may therefore be the most effective means of maximizing pharmacodynamic exposure [250,251].

For patients with community-acquired intra-abdominal infections (CA-IAIs), agents with a narrower spectrum of activity are preferred. However, if CA-IAI patients have prior exposure to antibiotics or serious comorbidities requiring concurrent antibioitic therapy, anti-ESBL-producer converage may be warranted. By contrast, for patients with healthcare-associated infections, antimicrobial regimens with broader spectra of activity are preferred (Recommendation 1B).

In the context of intra-abdominal infections, the main resistance problem is posed by ESBL-producing Enterobacteriaceae, which are alarmingly prevalent in nosocomial infections and frequently observed in community-acquired infections, albeit to a lesser extent.

The Study for Monitoring Antimicrobial Resistance Trends (SMART) program monitors the activity of antibiotics against aerobic gram-negative intra-abdominal infections. Hawser et al. reported susceptibility levels of key intra-abdominal pathogens in Europe in 2008 and noted that the number of viable treatment options available for empirical treatment of intra-abdominal infections had fallen dramatically [252].

Although a variety of factors can increase the risk of selection for ESBL producers, the most significant risk factors include prior exposure to antibiotics (especially third generation cephalosporins) and comorbidities requiring concurrent antibiotic therapy.

In a study published by Ben-Ami et al., researchers evaluated risk factors for non-hospitalized patients that increased susceptibility to ESBL-producing infections; the study compiled data from 6 treatment centers in Europe, Asia, and North America [253].

A total of 983 patient-specific isolates were analyzed; 890 [90.5%] were *Escherichia coli*; 68 [6.9%] were Klebsiella species; and 25 [2.5%] were *Proteus mirabilis*. Overall, 339 [34.5%] of the observed isolates produced ESBLs. Significant risk factors identified by multivariate analysis included recent antibiotic exposure, residence in long-term care facilities, recent hospitalization, and advanced age greater than 65 years. Additionally, men appeared to be more prone to these infections than women.

However, 34% of the analyzed ESBL isolates were derived from patients with no recent healthcare exposure.

Bacteria producing Klebsiella pneumoniae carbapenemases (KPCs) are rapidly emerging as a major source of multidrug-resistant infections worldwide. The recent emergence of carbapenem resistance among Enterobacteriaceae poses a considerable threat to hospitalized patients.

In addition to hydrolyzing carbapenems, KPC-producing strains are often resistant to a variety of other antibiotics, and effective treatment of these versatile and resilient pathogens has therefore become an important challenge for clinicians in acute care settings [254].

KPC-producing bacteria have become commonplace in nosocomial infections, especially in patients with previous exposure to antibiotics [255].

Further, *Pseudomonas aeruginosa* and *Acinetobacter baumannii* have exhibited alarming rates of increased resistance to a variety of antibiotics in hospitals and healthcare facilities worldwide. Both species are intrinsically resistant to several drugs and could acquire additional resistances to other important antimicrobial agents [256].

Although no supportive data are currently available, *P. aeruginosa* coverage is only generally recommended for patients with nosocomial intra-abdominal infections, despite the fact that, in certain subpopulations, an inexplicably high prevalence of *Pseudomonas aeruginosa* has been documented in association with community-acquired appendicitis, which may complicate empirical antibiotic therapy [257].

Among multidrug-resistant gram-positive bacteria, Enterococci remain a considerable challenge.

Empirical coverage of Enterococci is not generally recommended for patients with community-acquired IAIs. Studies have demonstrated that coverage against Enterococci offers little therapeutic benefit for patients with community-acquired infections [258,259].

In the context of community-acquired IAIs, antimicrobial therapy for Enterococci should be considered for immunocompromised patients, patients with valvular heart disease or prosthetic materials, and critically ill patients for whom empirical antimicrobial therapy has a significant impact on clinical outcome.

Methicillin-resistant *Staphylococcus aureus* (MRSA) is another multidrug-resistant gram-positive nosocomial pathogen known to cause severe morbidity and mortality worldwide [260].

Although community-acquired MRSA has been reported in other settings, there are no studies that have systematically documented MRSA in community-acquired intra-abdominal infections.

Patients with nosocomial intra-abdominal infections should not be treated empirically for MRSA unless the patient has a history of infections by this organism or there is reason to believe that the infection is associated with MRSA.

Appendices 1, 2, 3, 4, 5, 6, 7, 8, 9, 10 list recommended antimicrobial regimens.

Empirical antifungal therapy for Candida species is recommended for patients with nosocomial infections and for critically ill patients with community-acquired infections. An echinocandin regimen is recommended for critically ill patients with nosocomial infections (Recommendation 1B).

Although the epidemiological profile of Candida species has not yet been defined in the context of nosocomial peritonitis, its presence is clinically significant and is usually associated with poor prognoses.

Empirical antifungal therapy for Candida species is typically not recommended for patients with community-acquired intra-abdominal infections, with the notable exceptions of patients recently exposed to broad-spectrum antimicrobials and immunocompromised patients (due to neutropenia or concurrent administration of immunosuppressive agents, such as glucocorticosteroids, chemotherapeutic agents, and immunomodulators) [261].

However, considering the high mortality rate of Candida-related peritonitis, and given the poor outcome that could result from inadequate antimicrobial therapy for critically ill patients, antifungal coverage is recommended for these patients

In 2006, Montravers et al. published a retrospective, case–control study involving critically ill patients admitted to 17 French intensive care units (ICUs) [262].

The study demonstrated an increased mortality rate in cases of nosocomial peritonitis in which fungal isolates had been identified (48% and 28% mortality rates for fungal peritonitis and control groups, respectively $p < 0.01$). Upper gastrointestinal tract sites and positive identification of Candida species were found to be independent variables predictive of mortality for patients with nosocomial peritonitis.

More recently, Montravers et al. published the results of a prospective, non-interventional study involving 271 adult ICU patients with invasive Candida infections who received systemic antifungal therapy; the authors reported a mortality rate of 38% in a prospective cohort of 93 patients admitted to the ICU with candidal peritonitis [261].

Given the results of these studies, the inclusion of an anticandidal drug in empirical regimens for nosocomial IAIs seems appropriate.

The recently published Pappas IDSA guidelines for the treatment of invasive candidiasis do not dedicate a specific section to candidal peritonitis [263]. However, the use of echinocandins is generally recommended as a first-line empirical treatment for critically ill patients, while fluconazole is typically recommended for less severe conditions.

Applying these trends to IAIs, the use of echinocandins is recommended as a first-line treatment in cases of severe nosocomial IAI.

Knowledge of mechanisms of secretion of antibiotics into bile is helpful in designing the optimal therapeutic regimen for patients with biliary-related intra-abdominal infections (Recommendation 1C).

The bacteria most often isolated in biliary infections are *Escherichia coli* and *Klebsiella pneumonia*, gram-negative aerobes,, as well as certain anaerobes, particularly *Bacteroides fragilis*. Given that the pathogenicity of Enterococci in biliary tract infections remains unclear, specific coverage against these microorganisms is not routinely advised [264-266].

The efficacy of antibiotics in the treatment of biliary infections depends largely on the therapeutic level of drug concentrations [267-271].

The medical community has debated the use of antimicrobials with effective biliary penetration to address biliary infections. However, no clinical or experimental evidence is available to support the recommendation of biliary-penetrative antimicrobials for these patients. Other important factors include the antimicrobial potency of individual compounds and the effect of bile on antibacterial activity [270].

If there are no signs of persistent leukocytosis or fever, antimicrobial therapy for intra-abdominal infections should be shortened for patients demonstrating a positive response to treatment (Recommendation 1C).

An antimicrobial-based approach involves both optimizing empirical therapy and curbing excessive antimicrobial use to minimize selective pressures favoring drug resistance [271].

Shortening the duration of antimicrobial therapy in the treatment of intra-abdominal infections is an important strategy for optimizing patient care and reducing the spread of antimicrobial resistance.

The optimal duration of antibiotic therapy for intra-abdominal infections has been extensively debated.

Shorter durations of therapy have proven to be as effective as longer durations for many common infections. A prospective, randomized, double-blind trial comparing 3- and ≥ 5-day ertapenem regimens in 111 patients with community-acquired intra-abdominal infections reported similar cure and eradication rates (93% vs. 90% and 95% vs. 94% for 3- and > 5-day regimens, respectively) [272].

Studies have demonstrated a low likelihood of infection recurrence or treatment failure when antimicrobial therapy is discontinued in patients with complicated intra-abdominal infection who no longer show signs of infection.

Lennard et al. [273] compared post-operative outcomes in 65 intra-abdominal sepsis patients with and without leukocytosis and fever at the conclusion of antimicrobial therapy. Intra-abdominal sepsis patients at risk for post-operative infection were those who were afebrile with persistent leukocytosis or those who remained febrile after the antibiotics were discontinued.

Hedrick et al. [274] retrospectively analyzed the relationship between the duration of antibiotic therapy and infectious complications (i.e., recurrent infection by the same organism or renewed infectious focus at the same anatomical site). In the study, 929 patients with intra-abdominal infections associated with fever or leukocytosis were categorized into quartiles on the basis of either the total duration of antibiotic therapy or the duration of treatment following resolution of fever and leukocytosis. Shorter courses of antibiotics were associated with comparable or fewer complications than prolonged therapy.

These results suggest that antimicrobial therapy to address intra-abdominal infections should be shortened for patients who demonstrate a positive response to treatment, show no signs of persistent leukocytosis or fever, and are able to resume an oral diet.

Conclusions

Despite advances in diagnosis, surgery, and antimicrobial therapy, mortality rates associated with complicated intra-abdominal infections remain exceedingly high.

WSES guidelines represent a contribution on this debated topic by specialists worldwide.

Appendix 1. Antimicrobial therapy for community-acquired extra-biliary IAIs in stable, non-critical patients presenting with no ESBL-associated risk factors (WSES recommendations)

Community-acquired extra-biliary IAIs
Stable, non-critical patients
No risk factors for ESBL
AMOXICILLIN/CLAVULANATE
Daily schedule: 2.2 g every 6 hours (2-hour infusion time)
OR (in the event of patients allergic to beta-lactams):
CIPROFLOXACIN
Daily schedule: 400 mg every 8 hours (30-minute infusion time)
\+
METRONIDAZOLE
Daily schedule: 500 mg every 6 hours (1-hour infusion time)

Appendix 2. Antimicrobial therapy for community-acquired extra-biliary IAIs in stable, non-critical patients presenting with ESBL-associated risk factors (WSES recommendations)

Community-acquired extra-biliary IAIs
Stable, non-critical patients
ESBL-associated risk factors
ERTAPENEM
Daily schedule: 1 g every 24 hours (2-hour infusion time)
OR
TIGECYCLINE
Daily schedule: 100 mg LD then 50 mg every 12 hours

Appendix 3. Antimicrobial therapy for community-acquired extra-biliary IAIs in critically ill patients presenting with no ESBL-associated risk factors (WSES recommendations)

Community-acquired extra-biliary IAIs
Critically ill patients (≥ SEVERE SEPSIS)
No risk factors for ESBL

PIPERACILLIN/TAZOBACTAM
Daily schedule: 8/2 g LD then 16/4 g/day via continuous infusion or 4.5 g every 6 hours (4-hour infusion time)

Appendix 4. Antimicrobial therapy for community-acquired extra-biliary IAIs in critically ill patients presenting with ESBL-associated risk factors (WSES recommendations)

Community-acquired IAIs
Critically ill patients (≥ SEVERE SEPSIS)
ESBL-associated risk factors
MEROPENEM
Daily schedule: 500 mg every 6 hours (6-hour infusion time)
OR
IMIPENEM
Daily schedule: 500 mg every 4 hours (3-hour infusion time)
+/−
FLUCONAZOLE
Daily schedule: 600 mg LD then 400 mg every 24 hours (2-hour infusion time)

Appendix 5. Antimicrobial therapy for biliary IAI in stable, non-critical patients presenting with no ESBL-associated risk factors (WSES recommendations)

Community-acquired biliary IAIs
Stable, non-critical patients
No risk factors for ESBL
AMOXICILLIN/CLAVULANATE
Daily schedule: 2.2 g every 6 hours (2-hour infusion time)
OR (in the event of patients allergic to beta-lactams)
CIPROFLOXACIN
Daily schedule: 400 mg every 8 hours (30-minute infusion time)
+
METRONIDAZOLE
Daily schedule: 500 mg every 6 hours (1-hour infusion time)

Appendix 6. Antimicrobial therapy for biliary IAIs in stable, non-critical patients presenting with ESBL-associated risk factors (WSES recommendations)

Community-acquired biliary IAIs
Stable, non-critical patients.
Risk factors for ESBL
TIGECYCLINE
Daily schedule: 100 mg LD then 50 mg every 12 hours (2-hour infusion time)

Appendix 7. Antimicrobial therapy for biliary IAIs in critically ill patients presenting with no ESBL-associated risk factors (WSES recommendations)

Community-acquired biliary IAIs
Critically ill patients (≥ SEVERE SEPSIS)
No risk factors for ESBL
PIPERACILLIN/TAZOBACTAM
Daily schedule: 8/2 g LD then 16/4 g/day via continuous infusion or 4.5 g every 6 hours (4-hour infusion time)

Appendix 8. Antimicrobial therapy for biliary IAIs in critically ill patients presenting with ESBL-associated risk factors (WSES recommendations)

Community-acquired biliary IAIs
Critically ill patients (SEVERE SEPSIS)
Risk factors for ESBL
PIPERACILLIN
Daily schedule: 8 g by LD then 16 g via continuous infusion or 4 g every 6 hours (4-hour infusion time)
+
TIGECYCLINE
Daily schedule: 100 mg LD then 50 mg every 12 hours (2-hour infusion time)
+/−
FLUCONAZOLE
Daily schedule: 600 mg LD then 400 mg every 24 hours (2-hour infusion time)

Appendix 9. Antimicrobial therapy for nosocomial IAIs in stable, non-critical patients (WSES recommendations)

Hospital-acquired IAIs
Stable, non-critical patients (< SEVERE SEPSIS)
Risk factors for MDR pathogens
PIPERACILLIN
Daily schedule: 8 g by LD then 16 g via continuous infusion or 4 g every 6 hours (4-hour infusion time)
+
TIGECYCLINE
Daily schedule: 100 mg LD then 50 mg every 12 hours (2-hour infusion time)
+
FLUCONAZOLE
Daily Schedule: 600 mg LD then 400 mg every 24 hours (2-hour infusion time)

Appendix 10. Antimicrobial therapy for nosocomial IAI in critically ill patients. (WSES recommendations)

Hospital-acquired extra-biliary IAIs
Critically ill patients (≥SEVERE SEPSIS)
Risk factors for MDR pathogens
PIPERACILLIN
Daily schedule: 8 g by LD then 16 g via continuous infusion or 4 g every 6 hours (4-hour infusion time)
+
TIGECYCLINE
Daily schedule: 100 mg LD then 50 mg every 12 hours (2-hour infusion time)
+
ECHINOCANDIN
caspofungin (70 mg LD, then 50 mg daily),
anidulafungin (200 mg LD, then 100 mg daily),
micafungin (100 mg daily)
OR
MEROPENEM
Daily Schedule: 500 mg every 6 hours (6-hour infusion time)
IMIPENEM
Daily Schedule: 500 mg every 4 hours (3-hour infusion time)
DORIPENEM
Daily Schedule: 500 mg every 8 hours (4-hour infusion time)
+
TEICOPLANIN
Daily Schedule: LD 12 mg/kg/12 h for 3 doses then 6 mg/kg every 12 hours (with TDM corrections/ adjustments – PD target 20–30 mg/L)
+
ECHINOCANDIN
caspofungin (70 mg LD, then 50 mg daily),
anidulafungin (200 mg LD, then 100 mg daily),
micafungin (100 mg daily)

Competing interests
The authors declare that they have no competing interests.

Authors' contributions
MS wrote the manuscript. All authors read and approved the final manuscript.

Author details
[1]Department of Surgery, Macerata Hospital, Macerata, Italy. [2]Clinic of Infectious Diseases, Department of Internal Medicine Geriatrics and Nephrologic Diseases, St Orsola-Malpighi University Hospital, Bologna, Italy. [3]Emergency Surgery, Maggiore Parma Hospital, Parma, Italy. [4]Department of General Surgery, Ospedali Riuniti, Bergamo, Italy. [5]Department of Surgery, Denver Health Medical Center, Denver, CO, USA. [6]American Board of Surgery, Philadelphia, PA, USA. [7]University of Texas Health Science Center, Houston, TX, USA. [8]Harvard Medical School, Division of Trauma, Emergency Surgery and Surgical Critical Care Massachusetts General Hospital, Boston, MA, USA. [9]Department of Surgery, UC San Diego Health System, San Diego, CA, USA. [10]Department of Surgery, Virginia Commonwealth University Medical Center, Richmond, VA, USA. [11]Division of General Surgery, University of Pittsburgh Medical Center, Pittsburgh, PA, USA. [12]Department of Primary Care & Emergency Medicine, Kyoto University Graduate School of Medicine, Kyoto, Japan. [13]Department of Abdominal Surgery, University Hospital Meilahti, Helsinki, Finland. [14]Department of Surgery, University of Newcastle, Newcastle, NSW, Australia. [15]Department of Surgery, Charlotte Maxeke Johannesburg Hospital University of the Witwatersrand, Johannesburg, South Africa. [16]Department of Surgery, Govt Medical College and Hospital, Chandigarh, India. [17]Department of General Surgery, Rambam Health Care Campus, Haifa, Israel. [18]Department of Surgery, Adria Hospital, Adria, Italy. [19]Department of Surgery, Maggiore Hospital, Bologna, Italy. [20]Department of Digestive Surgery Faculty of Medicine Pontificia Universidad Católica de Chile, Santiago, Chile. [21]Department of Surgery, Sheri-Kashmir Institute of Medical Sciences, Srinagar, India. [22]Department of Surgery, Universidad del Valle, Fundacion Valle del Lili, Cali, Colombia. [23]Division of Trauma Surgery, Hospital de Clinicas - University of Campinas, Campinas, Brazil. [24]Emergency Unit, Department of Surgery, Ribeirão Preto, Brazil. [25]Department of General Surgery, Hadassah Medical Center, Jerusalem, Israel. [26]Department of Surgery, Tianjin Nankai Hospital, Nankai Clinical School of Medicine, Tianjin Medical University, Tianjin, China. [27]Department of Surgery, Pt BDS Post-graduate Institute of Medical Sciences, Rohtak, India. [28]First Clinic of General Surgery, University Hospital /UMBAL/ St George Plovdiv, Plovdiv, Bulgaria. [29]Department of Surgery, Edendale Hospital, Pietermaritzburg, Republic of South Africa. [30]Department of Surgery, Port Shepstone Hospital, Kwazulu Natal, South Africa. [31]Department of Surgery, Ahmadu Bello University Teaching Hospital Zaria, Kaduna, Nigeria. [32]Department of Surgery, Mansoura University Hospital, Mansoura, Egypt. [33]Department of Surgery, Mazzoni Hospital, Ascoli Piceno, Italy. [34]Department of Surgery, Mellini Hospital, Chiari (BS), Italy. [35]Department of General and Digestive Surgery, University Hospital, Malaga, Spain. [36]Department of General Surgery, Lviv Emergency Hospital, Lviv, Ukraine. [37]Department of Surgery, Ancona University, Ancona, Italy. [38]Division of General and Emergency Surgery, Faculdade de Medicina da Fundação do ABC, São Paulo, Santo André, Brazil. [39]Department of Surgery, Chang Gung Memorial Hospital, Taoyuan, Taiwan. [40]Department of Surgery, Ripas Hospital, Bandar Seri Begawan, Brunei. [41]Clinical Sciences, Regional Hospitals Limbe and Buea, Limbe, Cameroon. [42]Department of Surgery, Severance Hospital, Yonsei University College of Medicine, Seoul, Republic of Korea. [43]Division of Trauma and Surgical Critical Care, Department of Surgery, University of Ulsan, Seoul, Republic of Korea. [44]Wagih Ghnnam, Department of Surgery, Khamis Mushayt General Hospital, Khamis Mushayt, Saudi Arabia. [45]Boonying Siribumrungwong, Department of Surgery, Thammasat University Hospital, Pathumthani, Thailand. [46]Department of Acute and Critical Care Medicine, Tokyo Medical and Dental University, Tokyo, Japan. [47]Department of Emergency and Critical Care Medicine, Nippon Medical School, Emergency and Critical Care Center of Nippon Medical School, Tama-Nagayama Hospital, Tokyo, Japan. [48]II Catedra de Clinica Quirúrgica, Hospital de Clínicas, San Lorenzo, Paraguay. [49]Department of Surgery, Cutral Co Clinic, Neuquen, Argentina. [50]The Shock Trauma and Emergency Medical Center, Matsudo City Hospital, Chiba, Japan.

References
1. Sartelli M, Viale P, Koike K, Pea F, Tumietto F, van Goor H, Guercioni G, Nespoli A, Tranà C, Catena F, Ansaloni L, Leppaniemi A, Biffl W, Moore FA, Poggetti R, Pinna AD, Moore EE: **WSES consensus conference: Guidelines for first-line management of intra-abdominal infections.** *World J Emerg Surg* 2011, **6**:2.
2. Guyatt G, Gutterman D, Baumann MH, Addrizzo-Harris D, Hylek EM, Phillips B, Raskob G, Lewis SZ, Schunemann H: **Grading strength of recommendations and quality of evidence in clinical guidelines: report from an American college of chest physicians task force.** *Chest* 2006, **129**:174–181.
3. Brozek JL, Akl EA, Jaeschke R, Lang DM, Bossuyt P, Glasziou P, Helfand M, Ueffing E, Alonso-Coello P, Meerpohl J, Phillips B, Horvath AR, Bousquet J, Guyatt GH, Schunemann HJ: **Grading quality of evidence and strength of recommendations in clinical practice guidelines: part 2 of 3. The GRADE approach to grading quality of evidence about diagnostic tests and strategies.** *Allergy* 2009, **64**:1109–1116.

4. Menichetti F, Sganga G: **Definition and classification of intra-abdominal infections.** *J Chemother* 2009, **21**:3–4.
5. Pieracci FM, Barie PS: **Management of severe sepsis of abdominal origin.** *Scand J Surg* 2007, **96**(3):184–196.
6. Bone RC, Balk RA, Cerra FB, Dellinger RP, Fein AM, Knaus WA, Schein RM, Sibbald WJ, American College of Chest Physicians/Society of Critical Care Medicine Consensus Conference: **Definitions for sepsis and organ failure and guidlines for the use of innovative therapies in sepsis.** *Chest* 1992, **101**:1644–1655.
7. Levy MM, Fink MP, Marshall JC, Abraham E, Angus D, Cook D, Cohen J, Opal SM, Vincent JL, Ramsay G: **2001 SCCM/ ESICM/ACCP/ATS/ SIS international sepsis definitions conference.** *Crit Care Med* 2003, **31**:1250–1256.
8. Esteban A, Frutos-Vivar F, Ferguson ND, Peñuelas O, Lorente JA, Gordo F, Honrubia T, Algora A, Bustos A, García G, Diaz-Regañón IR, de Luna RR: **Sepsis incidence and outcome: contrasting the intensive care unit with the hospital ward.** *Crit Care Med* 2007, **35**(5):1284–1289.
9. Rivers E, Nguyen B, Havstad S, Ressler J, Muzzin A, Knoblich B, Peterson E, Tomlanovich M, Early Goal-Directed Therapy Collaborative Group: **Early goal-directed therapy in the treatment of severe sepsis and septic shock.** *N Eng J Med* 2001, **345**:1368–1377.
10. Emergency Physicians, Canadian Critical Care Society, European Society of Clinical Microbiology and Infectious Diseases, European Society of Intensive Care Medicine, European Respiratory Society, International Sepsis Forum, Japanese Association for Acute Medicine, Japanese Society of Intensive Care Medicine, Society of Critical Care Medicine, Society of Hospital Medicine, Surgical Infection Society, World Federation of Societies of Intensive and Critical Care Medicine, Dellinger RP, Levy MM, Carlet JM, Bion J, Parker MM, Jaeschke R, Reinhart K, Angus DC, Brun-Buisson C, Beale R, Calandra T, Dhainaut JF, Gerlach H, Harvey M, Marini JJ, Marshall J, Ranieri M, Ramsay G, Sevransky J, Thompson BT, Townsend S, Vender JS, Zimmerman JL, Vincent JL: **Surviving sepsis campaign: international guidelines for management of severe sepsis and septic shock: 2008.** *Crit Care Med* 2008, **36**(1):296–327.
11. Moore LJ, Moore FA: **Epidemiology of sepsis in surgical patients.** *Surg Clin North Am* 2012, **92**(6):1425–1443.
12. Moore LJ, Moore FA, Jones SL, Xu J, Bass BL: **Sepsis in general surgery: a deadly complication.** *Am J Surg* 2009, **198**(6):868–874.
13. Vincent JL, Biston P, Devriendt J, Brasseur A, De Backer D: **Dopamine versus norepinephrine: is one better?** *Minerva Anestesiol* 2009, **75**(5):333–337.
14. Hollenberg SM: **Vasopressor support in septic shock.** *Chest* 2007, **132**(5):1678–1687.
15. Kellum J, Decker J: **Use of dopamine in acute renal failure: a meta-analysis.** *Crit Care Med* 2001, **29**:1526–1531.
16. Hesselvik JF, Brodin B: **Low dose norepinephrine in patients with septic shock and oliguria: effects on afterload, urine flow, and oxygen transport.** *Crit Care Med* 1989, **17**:179–180.
17. Meadows D, Edwards JD, Wilkins RG, Nightingale P: **Reversal of intractable septic shock with norepinephrine therapy.** *Crit Care Med* 1988, **16**:663–667.
18. Martin C, Papazian L, Perrin G, Saux P, Gouin F: **Norepinephrine or dopamine for the treatment of hyperdynamic septic shock.** *Chest* 1993, **103**:1826–1831.
19. Patel GP, Grahe JS, Sperry M, Singla S, Elpern E, Lateef O, Balk RA: **Efficacy and safety of dopamine versus norepinephrine in the management of septic shock.** *Shock* 2010, **33**(4):375–380.
20. Flancbaum L, Dick M, Dasta J, Sinha R, Choban P: **A dose–response study of Phenylephrine in critically ill, septic surgical patients.** *Eur J Clin Pharmacol* 1997, **51**:461–465.
21. De Backer D, Creteur J, Silva E, Vincent JL: **Effects of dopamine, norepinephrine, and epinephrine on the splanchnic circulation in septic shock: which is best?** *Crit Care Med* 2003, **31**(6):1659–1667.
22. Holmes CL, Patel BM, Russell JA, Walley KR: **Physiology of vasopressin relevant to management of septic shock.** *Chest* 2001, **120**(3):989–1002.
23. Annane D, Bellissant E, Bollaert PE, Briegel J, Confalonieri M, De Gaudio R, Keh D, Kupfer Y, Oppert M, Meduri GU: **Corticosteroids in the treatment of severe sepsis and septic shock in adults: a systematic review.** *JAMA* 2009, **301**(22):2362–2375.
24. Emmi V, Sganga G: **Diagnosis of intra-abdominal infections: clinical findings and imaging.** *Infez Med* 2008, **16**(Suppl 1):19–30.
25. Foinant M, Lipiecka E, Buc E, Boire JY, Schmidt J, Garcier JM, Pezet D, Boyer L: **Impact of computed tomography on patient's care in non-traumatic acute abdomen: 90 patients.** *J Radiol* 2007, **88**(4):559–566.
26. Doria AS, Moineddin R, Kellenberger CJ, Epelman M, Beyene J, Schuh S, Babyn PS, Dick PT: **US or CT for diagnosis of appendicitis in children and adults? a meta-analysis.** *Radiology* 2006, **241**:83–94.
27. Pearce MS, Salotti JA, Little MP, McHugh K, Lee C, Kim KP, Howe NL, Ronckers CM, Rajaraman P, Sir Craft AW, Parker L, de González AB: **Radiation exposure from CT scans in childhood and subsequent risk of leukaemia and brain tumours: a retrospective cohort study.** *Lancet* 2012, **380**(9840):499–505.
28. Varadhan KK, Neal KR, Lobo DN: **Safety and efficacy of antibiotics compared with appendicectomy for treatment of uncomplicated acute appendicitis: meta-analysis of randomised controlled trials.** *BMJ* 2012, **344**:e2156.
29. Mason RJ, Moazzez A, Sohn H, Katkhouda N: **Meta-analysis of randomized trials comparing antibiotic therapy with appendectomy for acute uncomplicated (no abscess or phlegmon) appendicitis.** *Surg Infect (Larchmt)* 2012, **13**(2):74–84.
30. Ansaloni L, Catena F, Coccolini F, Ercolani G, Gazzotti F, Pasqualini E, Pinna AD: **Surgery versus conservative antibiotic treatment in acute appendicitis: a systematic review and meta-analysis of randomized controlled trials.** *Dig Surg* 2011, **28**(3):210–221.
31. Liu K, Fogg L: **Use of antibiotics alone for treatment of uncomplicated acute appendicitis: a systematic review and meta-analysis.** *Surgery* 2011, **150**(4):673–683.
32. Sauerland S, Jaschinski T, Neugebauer EA: **Laparoscopic versus open surgery for suspected appendicitis.** *Cochrane Database Syst Rev* 2010, **6**(10):CD001546. Review.
33. Agresta F, Ansaloni L, Baiocchi GL, Bergamini C, Campanile FC, Carlucci M, Cocorullo G, Corradi A, Franzato B, Lupo M, Mandalà V, Mirabella A, Pernazza G, Piccoli M, Staudacher C, Vettoretto N, Zago M, Lettieri E, Levati A, Pietrini D, Scaglione M, De Masi S, De Placido G, Francucci M, Rasi M, Fingerhut A, Uranüs S, Garattini S: **Laparoscopic approach to acute abdomen from the consensus development conference of the società italiana di chirurgia endoscopica e nuove tecnologie (SICE), associazione chirurghi ospedalieri italiani (ACOI), società italiana di chirurgia (SIC), società italiana di chirurgia d'Urgenza e del trauma (SICUT), società italiana di chirurgia nell'Ospedalità privata (SICOP), and the european association for endoscopic surgery (EAES).** *Surg Endosc* 2012, **26**(8):2134–2164.
34. Masoomi H, Mills S, Dolich MO, Ketana N, Carmichael JC, Nguyen NT, Stamos MJ: **Comparison of outcomes of laparoscopic versus open appendectomy in adults: data from the nationwide inpatient sample (NIS), 2006–2008.** *J Gastrointest Surg* 2011, **15**(12):2226–2231.
35. Moore CB, Smith RS, Herbertson R, Toevs C: **Does use of intraoperative irrigation with open or laparoscopic appendectomy reduce post-operative intra-abdominal abscess?** *Am Surg* 2011, **77**(1):78–80.
36. Oliak D, Yamini D, Udani VM, Lewis RJ, Arnell T, Vargas H, Stamos MJ: **Initial nonoperative management for periappendiceal abscess.** *Dis Colon Rectum* 2001, **44**:936–941.
37. Brown CV, Abrishami M, Muller M, Velmahos GC: **Appendiceal abscess: immediate operation or percutaneous drainage?** *Am Surg* 2003, **69**:829–832.
38. Kim JK, Ryoo S, Oh HK, Kim JS, Shin R, Choe EK, Jeong SY, Park KJ: **Management of appendicitis presenting with abscess or mass.** *J Korean Soc Coloproctol* 2010, **26**:413–419.
39. Simillis C, Symeonides P, Shorthouse AJ, Tekkis PP: **A meta-analysis comparing conservative treatment versus acute appendectomy for complicated appendicitis (abscess or phlegmon).** *Surgery* 2010, **147**(6):818–829.
40. Corfield L: **Interval appendicectomy after appendiceal mass or abscess in adults: what is "best practice"?** *Surg Today* 2007, **37**(1):1–4.
41. Andersson RE, Petzold MG: **Nonsurgical treatment of appendiceal abscess or phlegmon: a systematic review and meta-analysis.** *Ann Surg* 2007, **246**(5):741–748.
42. Meshikhes AW: **Appendiceal mass: is interval appendicectomy "something of the past"?** *World J Gastroenterol* 2011, **17**(25):2977–2980.
43. de Korte N, Unlü C, Boermeester MA, Cuesta MA, Vrouenreats BC, Stockmann HB: **Use of antibiotics in uncomplicated diverticulitis.** *Br J Surg* 2011, **98**(6):761–767.
44. Chabok A, Pahlman L, Hjern F, Haapaniemi S, Smedh K, AVOD Study Group: **Randomized clinical trial of antibiotics in acute uncomplicated diverticulitis.** *Br J Surg* 2012, **99**(4):532–539.

45. Bauer VP: **Emergency management of diverticulitis.** *Clin Colon Rectal Surg* 2009, **22**(3):161–168.
46. Jacobs DO: **Clinical practice.** *Diverticulitis. N Engl J Med* 2007, **357:**2057–2066.
47. Ambrosetti P, Robert J, Witzig JA, Mirescu D, de Gautard R, Borst F, Rohner A: **Incidence, outcome, and proposed management of isolated abscesses complicating acute left-sided colonic diverticulitis: a prospective study of 140 patients.** *Dis Colon Rectum* 1992, **35:**1072–1076.
48. Siewert B, Tye G, Kruskal J, Sosna J, Opelka F, Raptopoulos V, Goldberg SN: **Impact of CT-guided drainage in the treatment of diverticular abscesses: size matters.** *AJR Am J Roentgenol* 2006, **186:**680–686 [Erratum, *AJR Am J Roentgenol* 2007; **189:**512].
49. Kumar RR, Kim JT, Haukoos JS, Macias LH, Dixon MR, Stamos MJ, Konyalian VR: **Factors affecting the successful management of intraabdominal abscesses with antibiotics and the need for percutaneous drainage.** *Dis Colon Rectum* 2006, **49:**183–189.
50. Stabile BE, Puccio E, van Sonnenberg E, Neff CC: **Preoperative percutaneous drainage of diverticular abscesses.** *Am J Surg* 1990, **159:**99–104.
51. Kaiser AM, Jiang JK, Lake JP, Ault G, Artinyan A, Gonzalez-Ruiz C, Essani R, Beart RW Jr: **The management of complicated diverticulitis and the role of computed tomography.** *Am J Gastroenterol* 2005, **100:**910–917.
52. Salem L, Veenestra DL, Sullivan SD, Flum DR: **The timing of elective colectomy in diverticulitis: a decision análisis.** *J Am Coll Surg* 2004, **199:**904–912.
53. Janes S, Meagher A, Frizelle FA: **Elective surgery after acute diverticulitis.** *Br J Surg* 2005, **92:**133–142.
54. Rafferty J, Sellito P, Hyman NH, Buie WD: **Practice parameters for sigmoid diverticulitis.** *Dis Colon Rectum* 2006, **49:**939–944.
55. Holmer C, Lehmann KS, Gröne J, Buhr HJ, Ritz JP: **Perforation risk and patient age. [Risk analysis in acute sigmoid diverticulitis].** *Chirurg* 2011, **82**(4):359–366.
56. Eglinton T, Nguyen T, Raniga S, Dixon L, Dobbs B, Frizelle FA: **Patterns of recurrence in patients with acute diverticulitis.** *Br J Surg* 2010, **97:**952–957.
57. Makela JT, Kiviniemi HO, Laitinen ST: **Spectrum of disease and outcome among patients with acute diverticulitis.** *Dig Surg* 2010, **27:**190–196.
58. Ambrosetti P, Chautems R, Soravia C, Peiris-Waser N, Terrier F: **Long-term outcome of mesocolic and pelvic diverticular abscesses of the left colon. A prospective study of 73 cases.** *Dis Colon Rectum* 2005, **48:**787–791.
59. Schwandner O, Farke S, Fischer F, Eckmann C, Schiedeck TH, Bruch HP: **Laparoscopic colectomy for recurrent and complicated diverticulitis: a prospective study of 396 patients.** *Langenbecks Arch Surg* 2004, **389:**97–103.
60. Guller U, Jain N, Hervey S, Purves H, Pictoobon R: **Laparoscopic vs. Open colectomy: outcomes comparison based on large nationwide databases.** *Arch Surg* 2003, **138:**1179–1186.
61. Dwivedi A, Chahin F, Agrawal S, Chau WY, Tootla A, Tootla F, Silva YJ: **Laparoscopic colectomy vs. Open colectomy for sigmoid diverticular disease.** *Dis Colon Rectum* 2002, **45:**1309–1314.
62. Tuech JJ, Pessaux P, Rouge C, Regenet N, Bergamaschi R, Arnaud JP: **Laparoscopic vs. Open colectomy for sigmoid diverticulitis: a prospective comparative study in the elderly.** *Surg Endosc* 2000, **14:**1031–1033.
63. Bartus CM, Lipof T, Sarwar CM, Vignati PV, Johnson KH, Sardella WV, Cohen JL: **Colovesicle fistula: not a contraindication to elective laparoscopic colectomy.** *Dis Colon Rectum* 2005, **48:**233–236.
64. Fleming FJ, Gillen P: **Reversal of Hartmann's procedure following acute diverticulitis: is timing everything?** *Int J Colorectal Dis* 2009, **24:**1219–1225.
65. Roig JV, Cantos M, Balciscueta Z, Uribe N, Espinosa J, Roselló V, García-Calvo R, Hernandis J, Landete F: **Sociedad valenciana de cirugía cooperative group. Hartmann's Operation: how often is it reversed and at what cost? a multicentre study.** *Colorectal Dis* 2011, **13**(12):396–402.
66. Lee EC, Murray JJ, Coller JA, Roberts PL, Schoetz DL Jr: **Intraoperative colonic lavage in nonelective surgery for diverticular disease.** *Dis Colon Rectum* 1997, **40:**669–674.
67. Herzog T, Janot M, Belyaev O, Sülberg D, Chromik AM, Bergmann U, Mueller CA, Uhl W: **Complicated sigmoid diverticulitis–Hartmann's procedure or primary anastomosis?** *Acta Chir Belg* 2011, **111**(6):378–383.
68. Myers E, Winter DC: **Adieu to Henri Hartmann?** *Colorectal Dis* 2010, **12:**849–850.
69. Trenti L, Biondo S, Golda T, Monica M, Kreisler E, Fraccalvieri D, Frago R, Jaurrieta E: **Generalized peritonitis due to perforated diverticulitis: Hartmann's procedure or primary anastomosis?** *Int J Colorectal Dis* 2011, **26**(3):377–384.
70. Biondo S, Jaurrieta E, Martí Ragué J, Ramos E, Deiros M, Moreno P, Farran L: **Role of resection and primary anastomosis of the left colon in the presence of peritonitis.** *Br J Surg* 2000, **87**(11):1580–1584.
71. Salem L, Flum DR: **Primary anastomosis or Hartmann's procedure for patients with diverticular peritonitis? A systematic review.** *Dis Colon Rectum* 2004, **47:**1953–1964.
72. Zorcolo L, Covotta L, Carlomagno N, Bartolo DCC: **Safety of primary anastomosis in emergency Colo-rectal surgery.** *Colorectal Dis* 2003, **5:**262–269.
73. Kreis ME, Mueller MH, Thasler WH: **Hartmann's Procedure or primary anastomosis?** *Dig Dis* 2012, **30**(1):83–85.
74. Tabbara M, Velmahos GC, Butt MU, Chang Y, Spaniolas K, Demoya M, King DR, Alam HB: **Missed opportunities for primary repair in complicated acute diverticulitis.** *Surgery* 2010, **148**(5):919–924.
75. Masoomi H, Stamos MJ, Carmichael JC, Nguyen B, Buchberg B, Mills S: **Does primary anastomosis with diversion have Any advantages over Hartmann's procedure in acute diverticulitis?** *Dig Surg* 2012, **29**(4):315–320.
76. Taylor CJ, Layani L, Ghusn MA, White SI: **Perforated diverticulitis managed by laparoscopic lavage.** *ANZ J Surg* 2006, **76:**962–965.
77. Myers E, Hurley M, O'Sullivan GC, Kavanagh D, Wilson I, Winter DC: **Laparoscopic peritoneal lavage for generalized peritonitis due to perforated diverticulitis.** *Br J Surg* 2008, **95:**97–101.
78. Favuzza J, Frield JC, Kelly JJ, Perugini R, Counihan TC: **Benefits of laparoscopic peritoneal lavage for complicated sigmoid diverticulitis.** *Int J Colorectal Dis* 2009, **24:**799–801.
79. Karoui M, Champault A, Pautrat K, Valleur P, Cherqui D, Champault G: **Laparoscopic peritoneal lavage or primary anastomosis with defuctioning stoma for Hinchey 3 complicated diverticulitis: results of a comparative study.** *Dis Colon Rectum* 2009, **52:**609–615.
80. Rogers AC, Collins D, O'Sullivan GC, Winter DC: **Laparoscopic lavage for perforated diverticulitis: a population analysis.** *Dis Colon Rectum* 2012, **55**(9):932–938.
81. Kriwanek S, Armbruster C, Dittrich K, Beckerhinn P: **Perforated colorectal cancer.** *Dis Colon Rectum* 1996, **39**(12):1409–1414.
82. Khan S, Pawlak SE, Eggenberger JC, Lee CS, Szilagy EJ, Margolin DA: **Acute colonic perforation associated with colorectal cancer.** *Am Surg* 2001, **67**(3):261–264.
83. Lee IK, Sung NY, Lee YS, Lee SC, Kang WK, Cho HM, Ahn CH, Lee do S, Oh ST, Kim JG, Jeon HM, Chang SK: **The survival rate and prognostic factors in 26 perforated colorectal cancer patients.** *Int J Colorectal Dis* 2007, **22**(5):467–473.
84. Meyer F, Marusch F, Koch A, Meyer L, Führer S, Köckerling F, Lippert H, Gastinger I: **German study group "colorectal carcinoma (primary tumor)". emergency operation in carcinomas of the left colon: value of Hartmann's procedure.** *Tech Coloproctol* 2004, **8**(Suppl 1):s226–s229.
85. Won DY, Lee IK, Lee YS, Cheung DY, Choi SB, Jung H, Oh ST: **The indications for nonsurgical management in patients with colorectal perforation after colonoscopy.** *Am Surg* 2012, **78**(5):550–554.
86. Donckier V, André R: **Treatment of colon endoscopic perforations.** *Acta Chir Belg* 1993, **93**(2):60–62.
87. Cobb WS, Heniford BT, Sigmon LB, Hasan R, Simms C, Kercher KW, Matthews BD: **Colonoscopic perforations: incidence, management, and outcomes.** *Am Surg* 2004, **70**(9):750–757. discussion 757–8.
88. Iqbal CW, Cullinane DC, Schiller HJ, Sawyer MD, Zietlow SP, Farley DR: **Surgical management and outcomes of 165 colonoscopic perforations from a single institution.** *Arch Surg* 2008, **143**(7):701–706. discussion 706–7.
89. Lohsiriwat V, Sujarittanakarn S, Akaraviputh T, Lertakyamanee N, Lohsiriwat D, Kachinthorn U: **Colonoscopic perforation: a report from world gastroenterology organization endoscopy training center in Thailand.** *World J Gastroenterol* 2008, **14**(43):6722–6725.
90. Araujo SE, Seid VE, Caravatto PP, Dumarco R: **Incidence and management of colonoscopic colon perforations: 10 years' experience.** *Hepatogastroenterology* 2009, **56**(96):1633–1636.
91. Lüning TH, Keemers-Gels ME, Barendregt WB, Tan AC, Rosman C: **Colonoscopic perforations: a review of 30,366 patients.** *Surg Endosc* 2007, **21**(6):994–997. Epub 2007 Apr 24. Review.
92. Rumstadt B, Schilling D: **Optimizing time management after perforation by colonoscopy results in better outcome for the patients.** *Hepatogastroenterology* 2008, **55**(85):1308–1310.

93. Coimbra C, Bouffioux L, Kohnen L, Deroover A, Dresse D, Denoël A, Honoré P, Detry O: **Laparoscopic repair of colonoscopic perforation: a new standard?** *Surg Endosc* 2011, **25**(5):1514–1517.
94. Rumstadt B, Schilling D, Sturm J: **The role of laparoscopy in the treatment of complications after colonoscopy.** *Surg Laparosc Endosc Percutan Tech* 2008, **18**(6):561–564.
95. Hansen AJ, Tessier DJ, Anderson ML, Schlinkert RT: **Laparoscopic repair of colonoscopic perforations: indications and guidelines.** *J Gastrointest Surg* 2007, **11**(5):655–659.
96. Faria GR, Almeida AB, Moreira H, Barbosa E, Correia-da-Silva P, Costa-Maia J: **Prognostic factors for traumatic bowel injuries: killing time.** *World J Surg* 2012, **36**(4):807–812.
97. Malinoski DJ, Patel MS, Yakar DO, Green D, Qureshi F, Inaba K, Brown CV, Salim A: **A diagnostic delay of 5 hours increases the risk of death after blunt hollow viscus injury.** *J Trauma* 2010, **69**(1):84–87.
98. Sharpe JP, Magnotti LJ, Weinberg JA, Zarzaur BL, Shahan CP, Parks NA, Fabian TC, Croce MA: **Impact of location on outcome after penetrating colon injuries.** *J Trauma Acute Care Surg* 2012, **73**(6):1426–1431.
99. Weinberg JA, Griffin RL, Vandromme MJ, Melton SM, George RL, Reiff DA, *et al*: **Management of colon wounds in the setting of damage control laparotomy: a cautionary tale.** *J Trauma* 2009, **67**(5):929–935.
100. Johnson JW, Gracias VH, Schwab CW, Reilly PM, Kauder DR, Shapiro MB, *et al*: **Evolution in damage control for exsanguinating penetrating abdominal injury.** *J Trauma* 2001, **51**(2):261–269. discussion 269–71.
101. Sasaki LS, Allaben RD, Golwala R, Mittal VK: **Primary repair of colon injuries: a prospective randomized study.** *J Trauma* 1995, **39**(5):895–901.
102. Miller PR, Chang MC, Hoth JJ, Holmes JH, Meredith JW: **Colonic resection in the setting of damage control laparotomy: is delayed anastomosis safe?** *Am Surg* 2007, **73**(6):606–609. discussion 609–10.
103. Ordoñez CA, Pino LF, Badiel M, Sánchez AI, Loaiza J, Ballestas L, *et al*: **Safety of performing a delayed anastomosis during damage control laparotomy in patients with destructive colon injuries.** *J Trauma* 2011, **71**(6):1512–1517. discussion 1517–8.
104. Burlew CC, Moore EE, Cuschieri J, Jurkovich GJ, Codner P, Crowell K, Nirula R, Haan J, Rowell SE, Kato CM, MacNew H, Ochsner MG, Harrison PB, Fusco C, Sauaia A, Kaups KL, WTA Study Group: **Sew it up! a western trauma association multi-institutional study of enteric injury management in the postinjury open abdomen.** *J Trauma* 2011, **70**(2):273–277.
105. Crofts TJ, Park KG, Steele RJ, Chung SS, Li AK: **A randomized trial of nonoperative treatment for perforated peptic ulcer.** *N Engl J Med* 1989, **320**:970–973.
106. Boey J, Lee NW, Koo J, Lam PH, Wong J, Ong GB: **Immediate definitive surgery for perforated duodenal ulcers: a prospective controlled trial.** *Ann Surg* 1982, **196**:338–344.
107. Millat B, Fingerhut A, Borie F: **Surgical treatment of complicated duodenal ulcers: controlled trials.** *World J Surg* 2000, **24**:299–306.
108. Bucher P, Oulhaci W, Morel P, Ris F, Huber O: **Results of conservative treatment for perforated gastroduodenal ulcers in patients not eligible for surgical repair.** *Swiss Med Wkly* 2007, **137**:337–340.
109. Sogne B, Jean F, Foulatier O, Khalil H, Scotté M: **Non operative treatment for perforated peptic ulcer: results of a prospective study.** *Ann Chir* 2004, **129**:578–582.
110. Svanes C, Lie RT, Svanes K, Lie SA, Soreide O: **Adverse effects of delayed treatment for perforated peptic ulcer.** *Ann Surg* 1994, **220**(2):168–175.
111. Lo HC, Wu SC, Huang HC, Yeh CC, Huang JC, Hsieh CH: **Laparoscopic simple closure alone is adequate for low risk patients with perforated peptic ulcer.** *World J Surg* 2011, **35**(8):1873–1878.
112. Tanphiphat C, Tanprayoon T, Nathalong A: **Surgical treatment of perforated duodenal ulcer: a prospective trial between simple closure and definitive surgery.** *Br J Surg* 1985, **72**:370.
113. Christiansen J, Andersen OB, Bonnesen T, Baekgaard N: **Perforated duodenal ulcer managed by simple closure versus closure and proximal gastric vagotomy.** *Br J Surg* 1987, **74**(4):286–287.
114. Hay JM, Lacaine F, Kohlmann G, Fingerhut A: **Immediate definitive surgery for perforated duodenal ulcer does not increase operative mortality: a prospective controlled trial.** *World J Surg* 1988, **12**(5):705–709.
115. Kuwabara K, Matsuda S, Fushimi K, Ishikawa KB, Horiguchi H, Fujimori K: **Reappraising the surgical approach on the perforated gastroduodenal ulcer: should gastric resection be abandoned?** *J Clin Med Res* 2011, **3**(5):213–222.
116. Sarath Chandra SS, Kumar SS: **Definitive or conservative surgery for perforated gastric ulcer? an unresolved problem.** *Int J Surg* 2009, **7**:136–139.
117. Turner WW Jr, Thompson WM Jr, Thal ER: **Perforated gastric ulcers. A plea for management by simple closures.** *Arch Surg* 1988, **123**(8):960–964.
118. Wysocki A, Biesiada Z, Beben P, Budzynski A: **Perforated gastric ulcer.** *Dig Surg* 2000, **17**:132–137.
119. Tsugawa K, Koyanagi N, Hashizume M, Tomikawa M, Akahoshi K, Ayukawa K, *et al*: **The therapeutic strategies in performing emergency surgery for gastroduodenal ulcer perforation in 130 patients over 70 years of age.** *Hepatogastroenterology* 2001, **48**(37):156–162.
120. Cheng M, Li WH, Cheung MT: **Early outcome after emergency gastrectomy for complicated peptic ulcer disease.** *Hong Kong Med J* 2012, **18**(4):291–298.
121. Sanabria AE, Morales CH, Villegas MI: **Laparoscopic repair for perforated peptic ulcer disease.** *Cochrane Database Syst Rev* 2005, **19**(4):CD004778.
122. Lau H: **Laparoscopic repair of perforated peptic ulcer: a meta-analysis.** *Surg Endosc* 2004, **18**(7):1013–1021.
123. Lau WY, Leung KL, Kwong KH, Davey IC, Robertson C, Dawson JJ, Chung SC, Li AK: **A randomized study comparing laparoscopic versus open repair of perforated peptic ulcer using suture or sutureless technique.** *Ann Surg* 1996, **224**:131–138.
124. Siu WT, Leong HT, Law BK, Chau CH, Li AC, Fung KH, Tai YP, Li MK: **Laparoscopic repair for perforated peptic ulcer: a randomized controlled trial.** *Ann Surg* 2002, **235**:313–319.
125. Bertleff MJ, Halm JA, Bemelman WA, van der Ham AC, van der Harst E, Oei HI, Smulders JF, Steyerberg EW, Lange JF: **Randomized clinical trial of laparoscopic versus open repair of the perforated peptic ulcer: the LAMA trial.** *World J Surg* 2009, **33**:1368–1373.
126. Bertleff MJ, Lange JF: **Laparoscopic correction of perforated peptic ulcer: first choice? a review of literature.** *Surg Endosc* 2010, **24**(6):1231–1239. Epub 2009 Dec 24. Review.
127. Gertsch P, Choe LWC, Yuen ST, Chau KY, Lauder IJ: **Long term survival after gastrectomy for advanced bleeding or perforated gastric carcinoma.** *Eur J Surg* 1996, **162**:723–727.
128. Lehnert T, Buhl K, Dueck M, Hinz U, Herfarth C: **Two-stage radical gastrectomy for perforated gastric cancer.** *Eur J Surg Oncol* 2000, **26**:780–784.
129. Ozmen MM, Zulfikaroglu B, Kece C, Aslar AK, Ozalp N, Koc M: **Factors influencing mortality in spontaneous gastric tumour perforations.** *J Int Med Res* 2002, **30**:180–184.
130. So JBY, Yam A, Cheah WK, Kum CK, Goh PM: **Risk factors related to operative mortality and morbidity in patients undergoing emergency gastrectomy.** *Br J Surg* 2000, **87**:1702–1707.
131. Roviello F, Simone R, Marrelli D, *et al*: **Perforated gastric carcinoma: a report of 10 cases and review of the literature.** *World J Surg Oncol* 2006, **4**:19–24.
132. Jwo S, Chien R, Chao T, *et al*: **Clinicopathological features, surgical management, and disease outcome of perforated gastric cancer.** *J Surg Oncol* 2005, **91**:219–225.
133. Adachi Y, Mori M, Maehara Y, *et al*: **Surgical results of perforated gastric carcinoma: an analysis of 155 Japanese patients.** *Am J Gastroenterol* 1997, **92**:516–518.
134. Christensen M, Matzen P, Schulze S, Rosenberg J: **Complications of ERCP: a prospective study.** *Gastrointest Endosc* 2004, **60**:721–731.
135. Stapfer M, Selby RR, Stain SC, *et al*: **Management of duodenal perforation after endoscopic retrograde cholangiopancreatography and sphincterotomy.** *Ann Surg* 2000, **232**:191–198.
136. Enns R, Eloubeidi MA, Mergener K, *et al*: **ERCP-related perforations: risk factors and management.** *Endoscopy* 2002, **34**:293–298.
137. Pungpapong S, Kongkam P, Rerknimitr R, Kullavanijaya P: **Experience on endoscopic retrograde cholangiopancreatography at tertiary referral center in Thailand: risks and complications.** *J Med Assoc Thai* 2005, **88**:238–246.
138. Cohen SA, Siegel JH, Kasmin FE: **Complications of diagnostic and therapeutic ERCP.** *Abdom Imaging* 1996, **21**:385–394.
139. Jacob KM, Helzberg JH: **Significance of retroperitoneal air after endoscopic retrograde cholangiopancreatography with sphincterotomy.** *Am J Gastroenterol* 1999, **94**:1267–1270.
140. Machado NO: **Management of duodenal perforation post-endoscopic retrograde cholangiopancreatography. When and whom to operate and**

what factors determine the outcome? a review article. *JOP* 2012, **13**(1):18–25.
141. Nam JS, Yi SY: **Massive pneumoperitoneum and pneumomediastinum with subcutaneous emphysema after endoscopic sphincterotomy.** *Clin Gastroenterol Hepatol* 2004, **2:**xxii.
142. Baron TH, Gostout CJ, Herman L: **Hemoclip repair of a sphincterotomy-induced duodenal perforation.** *Gastrointest Endosc* 2000, **52:**566–568.
143. Mutignani M, Iacopini F, Dokas S, Larghi A, Familiari P, Tringoli A, *et al*: **Successful endoscopic closure of a lateral duodenal wall perforation at ERCP with fibrin glue.** *Gastrointest Endosc* 2006, **63**(4):725–727.
144. Fatima J, Baron TH, Topazian MD, Houghton SG, Iqbal CW, Ott BJ, Farley DR, Farnell MB, Sarr MG: **Pancreaticobiliary and duodenal perforations after periampullary endoscopic procedures: diagnosis and management.** *Arch Surg* 2007, **142**(5):448–454. discussion 454–5.
145. Ayite A, Dosseh DE, Tekou HA, James K: **Surgical treatment of single non traumatic perforation of small bowel: excision-suture or resection anastomosis.** *Ann Chir* 2005, **131**(2):91–95.
146. Kirkpatrick AW, Baxter KA, Simons RK, Germann E, Lucas CE, Ledgerwood AM: **Intra-abdominal complications after surgical repair of small bowel injuries: an international rreiew.** *J Trauma* 2003, **55**(3):399–406.
147. Sinha R, Sharma N, Joshi M: **Laparoscopic repair of small bowel perforation.** *JSLS* 2005, **9:**399–402.
148. Mock CN, Amaral J, Visser LE: **Improvement in survival from typhoid ileal perforation. Results of 221 operative cases.** *Ann Surg* 1992, **215**(3):244–249.
149. Gotuzzo E, Frisancho O, Sanchez J, Liendo G, Carrillo C, Black RE, Morris JG Jr: **Association between the acquired immunodeficiency syndrome and infection with salmonella typhi or salmonella paratyphi in an endemic typhoid area.** *Arch Intern Med* 1991, **151**(2):381–382.
150. Edino ST, Yakubu AA, Mohammed AZ, Abubakar IS: **Prognostic factors in typhoid ileal perforation: a prospective study of 53 cases.** *J National Med Assoc* 2007, **99:**1042–1045.
151. Kouame J, Adio LK, Turquin HT: **Typhoid ileal perforation: surgical experience of 64 cases.** *Acta Chir Belg* 2004, **104:**445–447.
152. Eggleston FC, Santoshi B, Singh CM: **Typhoid perforation of the bowel.** *Ann Surg* 1979, **190:**31–35.
153. Malik AM, Laghari AA, Mallah Q, Qureshi GA, Talpur AH, Effendi S, *et al*: **Different surgical options and ileostomy in typhoid perforation.** *World J Med Sci* 2006, **1:**112–116.
154. Kiviluoto T, Sirén J, Luukkonen P, Kivilaakso E: **Randomised trial of laparoscopic versus open cholecystectomy for acute and gangrenous cholecystitis.** *Lancet* 1998, **351**(9099):321–325.
155. Johansson M, Thune A, Nelvin L, Stiernstam M, Westman B, Lundell L: **Randomized clinical trial of open versus laparoscopic cholecystectomy in the treatment of acute cholecystitis.** *Br J Surg* 2005, **92**(1):44–49.
156. Kum CK, Goh PMY, Isaac JR, Tekant Y, Ngoi SS: **Laparoscopic cholecystectomy for acute cholecystitis.** *Br J Surg* 1994, **81:**1651–1654.
157. Pessaux P, Regenet N, Tuech JJ, Rouge C, Bergamaschi R, Arnaud JP: **Laparoscopic versus open cholecystectomy: a prospective comparative study in the elderly with acute cholecystitis.** *Surg Laparosc Endosc Percutan Tech* 2001, **11:**252–255.
158. Lujan JA, Parrilla P, Robles R, Marin P, Torralba JA, Garcia-Ayllon J: **Laparoscopic cholecystectomy vs open cholecystectomy in the treatment of acute cholecystitis: a prospective study.** *Arch Surg* 1998, **133:**173–175.
159. Gurusamy K, Samraj K, Gluud C, Wilson E, Davidson BR: **Meta-analysis of randomized controlled trials on the safety and effectiveness of early versus delayed laparoscopic cholecystectomy for acute cholecystitis.** *Br J Surg* 2010, **97**(2):141–150.
160. Siddiqui T, MacDonald A, Chong PS, Jenkins JT: **Early versus delayed laparoscopic cholecystectomy for acute cholecystitis: a meta-analysis of randomized clinical trials.** *Am J Surg* 2008, **195**(1):40–47.
161. Lau H, Lo CY, Patil NG, Yuen WK: **Early versus delayed-interval laparoscopic cholecystectomy for acute cholecystitis: a meta-analysis.** *Surg Endosc* 2006, **20**(1):82–87.
162. Papi C, Catarci M, D'Ambrosio L, Gili L, Koch M, Grassi GB, Capurso L: **Timing of cholecystectomy for acute calculous cholecystitis: a meta-analysis.** *Am J Gastroenterol* 2004, **99**(1):147–155.
163. Lee NW, Collins J, Britt R, Britt LD: **Evaluation of preoperative risk factors for converting laparoscopic to open cholecystectomy.** *Am Surg* 2012, **78**(8):831–833.
164. Domínguez LC, Rivera A, Bermúdez C: **Herrera W: [Analysis of factors for conversion of laparoscopic to open cholecystectomy: a prospective study of 703 patients with acute cholecystitis].** *Cir Esp* 2011, **89**(5):300–306.
165. Hadad SM, Vaidya JS, Baker L, Koh HC, Heron TP, Hussain K, Thompson AM: **Delay from symptom onset increases the conversion rate in laparoscopic cholecystectomy for acute cholecystitis.** *World J Surg* 2007, **31**(6):1298–1301.
166. Banz V, Gsponer T, Candinas D, Güller U: **Population-based analysis of 4113 patients with acute cholecystitis: defining the optimal time-point for laparoscopic cholecystectomy.** *Ann Surg* 2011, **254**(6):964–970.
167. Winbladh A, Gullstrand P, Svanvik J, Sandström P: **Systematic review of cholecystostomy as a treatment option in acute cholecystitis.** *HPB (Oxford)* 2009, **11**(3):183–193.
168. Morse BC, Smith JB, Lawdahl RB, Roettger RH: **Management of acute cholecystitis in critically ill patients: contemporary role for cholecystostomy and subsequent cholecystectomy.** *Am Surg* 2010, **76**(7):708–712.
169. McGillicuddy EA, Schuster KM, Barre K, Suarez L, Hall MR, Kaml GJ, Davis KA, Longo WE: **Non-operative management of acute cholecystitis in the elderly.** *Br J Surg* 2012, **99**(9):1254–1261.
170. Abi-Haidar Y, Sanchez V, Williams SA, Itani KM: **Revisiting percutaneous cholecystostomy for acute cholecystitis based on a 10-year experience.** *Arch Surg* 2012, **147**(5):416–422.
171. McKay A, Abulfaraj M, Lipschitz J: **Short- and long-term outcomes following percutaneous cholecystostomy for acute cholecystitis in high-risk patients.** *Surg Endosc* 2012, **26**(5):1343–1351.
172. Rodríguez-Sanjuán JC, Arruabarrena A, Sánchez-Moreno L, González-Sánchez F, Herrera LA, Gómez-Fleitas M: **Acute cholecystitis in high surgical risk patients: percutaneous cholecystostomy or emergency cholecystectomy?** *Am J Surg* 2012, **204**(1):54–59.
173. Nasim S, Khan S, Alvi R, Chaudhary M: **Emerging indications for percutaneous cholecystostomy for the management of acute cholecystitis–a retrospective review.** *Int J Surg* 2011, **9**(6):456–459.
174. Kortram K, de Vries Reilingh TS, Wiezer MJ, van Ramshorst B, Boerma D: **Percutaneous drainage for acute calculous cholecystitis.** *Surg Endosc* 2011, **25**(11):3642–3646.
175. Derici H, Kara C, Bozdag AD, Nazli O, Tansug T, Akca E: **Diagnosis and treatment of gallbladder perforation.** *World J Gastroenterol* 2006, **12**(48):7832–7836.
176. Menakuru SR, Kaman L, Behera A, Singh R, Katariya RN: **Current management of gall bladder perforations.** *ANZ J Surg* 2004, **74:**843–846.
177. Roslyn JJ, Thompson JE Jr, Darvin H, DenBesten L: **Risk factors for gallbladder perforation.** *Am J Gastroenterol* 1987, **82:**636–640.
178. Ong CL, Wong TH, Rauff A: **Acute gall bladder perforation-a dilemma in early diagnosis.** *Gut* 1991, **32:**956–958.
179. Stefanidis D, Sirinek KR, Bingener J: **Gallbladder perforation: risk factors and outcome.** *J Surg Res* 2006, **131**(2):204–208. Epub 2006 Jan 18.
180. van Lent AU, Bartelsman JF, Tytgat GN, Speelman P, Prins JM: **Duration of antibiotic therapy for cholangitis after successful endoscopic drainage of the biliary tract.** *Gastrointest Endosc* 2002, **55:**518–522.
181. Leung JWC, Chung SCS, Sung JJY, Banez VP, Li AKC: **Urgent endoscopic drainage for acute suppurative cholangitis.** *Lancet* 1989, **1:**1307–1309.
182. Hui CK, Lai KC, Yuen MF, Ng M, Lai CL, Lam SK: **Acute cholangitis—predictive factors for emergency ERCP.** *Aliment Pharmacol Ther* 2001, **15**(10):1633–1637.
183. Lai EC, Mok FP, Tan ES, Lo CM, Fan ST, You KT, Wong J: **Endoscopic biliary drainage for severe acute cholangitis.** *N Engl J Med* 1992, **24:**1582–1586.
184. Kumar R, Sharma BC, Singh J, Sarin SK: **Endoscopic biliary drainage for severe acute cholangitis in biliary obstruction as a result of malignant and benign diseases.** *J Gastroenterol Hepatol* 2004, **19**(9):994–997.
185. Ou-Yang B, Zeng KW, Hua HW, Zhang XQ, Chen FL: **Endoscopic nasobiliary drainage and percutaneous transhepatic biliary drainage for the treatment of acute obstructive suppurative cholangitis: a retrospective study of 37 cases.** *Hepatogastroenterology* 2012, **17:**59(120).
186. Lee DWH, Chung SCS: **Biliary infection.** *Baillieres Clin Gastroenterol* 1997, **11:**707–724.
187. Lipsett PA, Pitt HA: **Acute cholangitis.** *Surg Clin North Am* 1990, **70:**1297–1312.
188. Hanau LH, Steigbigel NH: **Acute cholangitis.** *Infect Dis Clin North Am* 2000, **14:**521–546.
189. Lee JG: **Diagnosis and management of acute cholangitis.** *Nat Rev Gastroenterol Hepatol* 2009, **6**(9):533–541.

190. Augustin P, Kermarrec N, Muller-Serieys C, Lasocki S, Chosidow D, Marmuse JP, Valin N, Desmonts JM, Montravers P: **Risk factors for multidrug resistant bacteria and optimization of empirical antibiotic therapy in postoperative peritonitis.** *Crit Care* 2010, **14**(1):R20.
191. Theisen J, Bartels H, Weiss W, Berger H, Stein HJ, Siewert JR: **Current concepts of percutaneous abscess drainage in postoperative retention.** *J Gastrointest Surg* 2005, **9**(2):280–283.
192. Khurrum Baig M, Hua Zhao R, Batista O, Uriburu JP, Singh JJ, Weiss EG, Nogueras JJ, Wexner SD: **Percutaneous postoperative intra-abdominal abscess drainage after elective colorectal surgery.** *Tech Coloproctol* 2002, **6**(3):159–164.
193. Benoist S, Panis Y, Pannegeon V, Soyer P, Watrin T, Boudiaf M, Valleur P: **Can failure of percutaneous drainage of postoperative abdominal abscesses be predicted?** *Am J Surg* 2002, **184**(2):148–153.
194. Torer N, Yorganci K, Elker D, Sayek I: **Prognostic factors of the mortality of postoperative intraabdominal infections.** *Infection* 2010, **38**(4):255–260.
195. Koperna T, Schulz F: **Prognosis and treatment of peritonitis. Do we need new scoring systems?** *Arch Surg* 1996, **131**(2):180–186.
196. van Ruler O, Lamme B, Gouma DJ, Reitsma JB, Boermeester MA: **Variables associated with positive findings at relaparotomy in patients with secondary peritonitis.** *Crit Care Med* 2007, **35**(2):468–476.
197. Hutchins RR, Gunning MP, Lucas DN, Allen-Mersh TG, Soni NC: **Relaparotomy for suspected Intraperitoneal sepsis after abdominal surgery.** *World J Surg* 2004, **28**(2):137–141.
198. Lamme B, Mahler CW, van Ruler O, Gouma DJ, Reitsma JB, Boermeester MA: **Clinical predictors of ongoing infection in secondary peritonitis: systematic review.** *World J Surg* 2006, **30**(12):2170–2181.
199. Van Ruler O, Mahler CW, Boer KR, Reuland EA, Gooszen HG, Opmeer BC, de Graaf PW, Lamme B, Gerhards MF, Steller EP, van Till JW, de Borgie CJ, Gouma DJ, Reitsma JB, Boermeester MA: **Comparison of on-demand vs planned relaparotomy strategy in patients with severe peritonitis: a randomized trial.** *JAMA* 2007, **298:**865–872.
200. Schein M: **Planned reoperations and open management in critical intra-abdominal infections: prospective experience in 52 cases.** *World J Surg* 1991, **15**(4):537–545.
201. Mulier S, Penninckx F, Verwaest C, Filez L, Aerts R, Fieuws S, *et al*: **Factors affecting mortality in generalized postoperative peritonitis: multivariate analysis in 96 patients.** *World J Surg* 2003, **27**(4):379–384.
202. Bader FG, Schröder M, Kujath P, Muhl E, Bruch H-P, Eckmann C: **Diffuse postoperative peritonitis – value of diagnostic parameters and impact of early indication for relaparotomy.** *Eur J Med Res* 2009, **14**(11):491–496.
203. Demetriades D: **Total management of the open abdomen.** *Int Wound J* 2012, **9**(Suppl 1):17–24.
204. Uggeri FR, Perego E, Franciosi C, Uggeri FA: **Surgical approach to the intraabdominal infections.** *Minerva Anestesiol* 2004, **70**(4):175–179.
205. van Ruler O, Kiewiet JJS, van Ketel RJ, Boermeester MA: **Initial microbial spectrum in severe secondary peritonitis and relevance for treatment.** *Eur J Clin Microbiol Infect Dis* 2012, **31**(5):671–682.
206. Duff JH, Moffat J: **Abdominal sepsis managed by leaving abdomen open.** *Surgery* 1981, **90:**774–778.
207. Adkins AL, Robbins J, Villalba M, Bendick P, Shanley CJ: **Open abdomen management of intra-abdominal sepsis.** *Am Surg* 2004, **70:**137–140.
208. Jansen JO, Loudon MA: **Damage control surgery in a non-trauma setting.** *Br J Surg* 2007, **94**(7):789–790.
209. Wild T, Stortecky S, Stremitzer S, Lechner P, Humpel G, Glaser K, Fortelny R, Karner J, Sautner T: **[Abdominal dressing – a new standard in therapy of the open abdomen following secondary peritonitis?].** *Zentralbl Chir* 2006, **131**(Suppl 1):S111–S114.
210. Robledo FA, Luque-de-León E, Suárez R, Sánchez P, de-la-Fuente M, Vargas A, Mier J: **Open versus closed management of the abdomen in the surgical treatment of severe secondary peritonitis: a randomized clinical trial.** *Surg Infect (Larchmt)* 2007, **8:**63–72.
211. Boele van Hensbroek P, Wind J, Dijkgraaf MG, *et al*: **Temporary closure of the open abdomen: a systematic review on delayed primary fascial closure in patients with an open abdomen.** *World J Surg* 2009, **33:**199–207.
212. Tsuei BJ, Skinner JC, Bernard AC, *et al*: **The open peritoneal cavity: etiology correlates with the likelihood of fascial closure.** *Am Surg* 2004, **70:**652–656.
213. Reimer MW, Yelle JD, Reitsma B, *et al*: **Management of open abdominal wounds with a dynamic fascial closure system.** *Can J Surg* 2008, **51:**209–214.
214. Urbaniak RM, Khuthaila DK, Khalil AJ, *et al*: **Closure of massive abdominal wall defects: a case report using the abdominal reapproximation anchor (ABRA) system.** *Ann Plast Surg* 2006, **57:**573–577.
215. Rasilainen SK, Mentula PJ, Leppäniemi AK: **Vacuum and mesh-mediated fascial traction for primary closure of the open abdomen in critically ill surgical patients.** *Br J Surg* 2012, **99**(12):1725–1732.
216. Leppäniemi A, Tukiainen E: **Planned hernia repair and late abdominal wall reconstruction.** *World J Surg* 2012, **36**(3):511–515.
217. Kissane NA, Itani KM: **A decade of ventral incisional hernia repairs with biologic acellular dermal matrix: what have we learned?** *Plast Reconstr Surg* 2012, **130**(5 Suppl 2):194S–202S.
218. Powell LL, Wilson SE: **The role of beta-lactam antimicrobials as single agents in treatment of intra-abdominal infection.** *Surg Infect (Larchmt)* 2000, **1**(1):57–63.
219. Lode HM: **Rational antibiotic therapy and the position of ampicillin/sulbactam.** *Int J Antimicrob Agents* 2008, **32**(1):10–28.
220. Al-Hasan MN, Lahr BD, Eckel-Passow JE, Baddour LM: **Antimicrobial resistance trends of Escherichia coli bloodstream isolates: a population-based study, 1998–2007.** *J Antimicrob Chemother* 2009, **64**(1):169–174.
221. Paterson DL: **Resistance in gram-negative bacteria: Enterobacteriaceae.** *Am J Infect Control* 2006, **34**(5 Suppl 1):S20–S28.
222. Murray BE: **The life and times of the Enterococcus.** *Clin Microbiol Rev* 1990, **3:**45–65.
223. Garbino J, Villiger P, Caviezel A, Matulionyte R, Uckay I, Morel P, Lew D: **A randomized prospective study of cefepime plus metronidazole with imipenem-cilastatin in the treatment of intra-abdominal infections.** *Infection* 2007, **35**(3):161–166.
224. Souli M, Galani I, Antoniadou A, Papadomichelakis E, Poulakou G, Panagea T, Vourli S, Zerva L, Armaganidis A, Kanellakopoulou K, Giamarellou H: **An outbreak of infection due to beta-Lactamase Klebsiella pneumoniae Carbapenemase 2-producing K. pneumoniae in a Greek University Hospital: molecular characterization, epidemiology, and outcomes.** *Clin Infect Dis* 2010, **50**(3):364–373.
225. Hammond ML: **Ertapenem: a group 1 carbapenem with distinct antibacterial and pharmacological properties.** *J Antimicrob Chemother* 2004, **53**(Suppl 2):ii7–ii9.
226. Falagas ME, Peppas G, Makris GC, Karageorgopoulos DE, Matthaiou DK: **Meta-analysis: ertapenem for complicated intra-abdominal infections.** *Aliment Pharmacol Ther* 2008, **27**(10):919–931.
227. Chahine EB, Ferrill MJ, Poulakos MN: **Doripenem: a new carbapenem antibiotic.** *Am J Health Syst Pharm* 2010, **67**(23):2015–2024.
228. Weiss G, Reimnitz P, Hampel B, Muehlhofer E, Lippert H, AIDA Study Group: **Moxifloxacin for the treatment of patients with complicated intra-abdominal infections (the AIDA study).** *J Chemother* 2009, **21**(2):170–180.
229. Stein GE: **Pharmacokinetics and pharmacodynamics of newer fluoroquinolones.** *Clin Infect Dis* 1996, **23**(suppl 1):S19–S24.
230. Edmiston CE, Krepel CJ, Seabrook GR, Somberg LR, Nakeeb A, Cambria RA, Towne JB: **In vitro activities of moxifloxacin against 900 aerobic and anaerobic surgical isolates from patients with intra-abdominal and diabetic foot infections.** *Antimicrob Agents Chemother* 2004, **48**(3):1012–1016.
231. Goldstein EJ, Citron DM, Warren YA, Tyrrell KL, Merriam CV, Fernandez H: **In vitro activity of moxifloxacin against 923 anaerobes isolated from human intra-abdominal infections.** *Antimicrob Agents Chemother* 2006, **50**(1):148–155.
232. Solomkin J, Zhao YP, Ma EL, Chen MJ, Hampel B: **DRAGON study team.** *Int J Antimicrob Agents* 2009, **34**(5):439–445.
233. Wagner C, Sauermann R, Joukhadar C: **Principles of antibiotic penetration into abscess fluid.** *Pharmacology* 2006, **78**(1):1–10.
234. Bradford PA: **Tigecycline: a first in class glycylcycline.** *Clin Microbiol Newsl* 2004, **26:**163–168.
235. Townsend ML, Pound MW, Drew RH: **Tigecycline in the treatment of complicated intra-abdominal and complicated skin and skin structure infections.** *Ther Clin Risk Manag* 2007, **3**(6):1059–1070.
236. Boucher HW, Wennersten CB, Eliopoulos GM: **In vitro activities of the glycylcycline GAR-936 against gram-positive bacteria.** *Antimicrob Agents Chemother* 2000, **44:**2225–2229.
237. Papaparaskevas J, Tzouvelekis LS, Tsakris A, Pittaras TE, Legakis NJ, Hellenic Tigecycline Study Group: **In vitro activity of tigecycline against 2423 clinical isolates and comparison of the available interpretation breakpoints.** *Diagn Microbiol Infect Dis* 2010, **66**(2):187–194.

238. Giamarellou H, Poulakou G: **Multidrug-resistant gram-negative infections: what are the treatment options?** *Drugs* 2009, **69**(14):1879–1901.
239. Hoffmann M, DeMaio W, Jordan RA, Talaat R, Harper D, Speth J, Scatina J: **Metabolism, excretion, and pharmacokinetics of [14C] tigecycline, a first-in-class glycylcycline antibiotic, after intravenous infusion to healthy male subjects.** *Drug Metab Dispos* 2007, **35**(9):1543–1553.
240. Gladman MA, Knowles CH, Gladman LJ, Payne JG: **Intra-operative culture in appendicitis: traditional practice challenged.** *Ann R Coll Surg Engl* 2004, **86**(3):196–201.
241. Davies HO, Alkhamesi NA, Dawson PM: **Peritoneal fluid culture in appendicitis: review in changing times.** *Int J Surg* 2010, **8**(6):426–429.
242. Sartelli M, Catena F, Ansaloni L, Leppäniemi A, Taviloglu K, van Goor H, Viale P, Lazzareschi DV, de Werra C, Marrelli D, Colizza S, Scibé R, Alis H, Torer N, Navarro S, Catani M, Kauhanen S, Augustin G, Sakakushev B, Massalou D, Pletinckx P, Kenig J, Di Saverio S, Guercioni G, Rausei S, Laine S, Major P, Skrovina M, Angst E, Pittet O, Gerych I, Tepp J, Weiss G, Vasquez G, Vladov N, Tranà C, Vettoretto N, Delibegovic S, Dziki A, Giraudo G, Pereira J, Poiasina E, Tzerbinis H, Hutan M, Vereczkei A, Krasniqi A, Seretis C, Diaz-Nieto R, Mesina C, Rems M, Campanile FC, Agresta F, Coletta P, Uotila-Nieminen M, Dente M, Bouliaris K, Lasithiotakis K, Khokha V, *et al*: **Complicated intra-abdominal infections in Europe: preliminary data from the first three months of the CIAO study.** *World J Emerg Surg* 2012, **7**(1):15.
243. Montravers P, Lepape A, Dubreuil L, Gauzit R, Pean Y, Benchimol D, Dupont H: **Clinical and microbiological profiles of community-acquired and nosocomial intra-abdominal infections: results of the French prospective, observational EBIIA study.** *J Antimicrob Chemother* 2009, **63**(4):785–794.
244. Seguin P, Laviolle B, Chanavaz C, Donnio PY, Gautier-Lerestif AL, Campion JP, Mallédant Y: **Factors associated with multidrug-resistant bacteria in secondary peritonitis: impact on antibiotic therapy.** *Clin Microbiol Infect* 2006, **12**(10):980–985.
245. Gaieski DF, Mikkelsen ME, Band RA, Pines JM, Massone R, Furia FF, Shofer FS, Goyal M: **Impact of time to antibiotics on survival in patients with severe sepsis or septic shock in whom early goal-directed therapy was initiated in the emergency department.** *Crit Care Med* 2010, **38**(4):1045–1053.
246. Riché FC, Dray X, Laisné MJ, Matéo J, Raskine L, Sanson-Le Pors MJ, Payen D, Valleur P, Cholley BP: **Factors associated with septic shock and mortality in generalized peritonitis: comparison between community-acquired and postoperative peritonitis.** *Crit Care* 2009, **13**(3):R99.
247. Taccone FS, Laterre PF, Dugernier T, Spapen H, Delattre I, Wittebole X, De Backer D, Layeux B, Wallemacq P, Vincent JL, Jacobs F: **Insufficient β-lactam concentrations in the early phase of severe sepsis and septic shock.** *Crit Care* 2010, **14**(4):R126. Epub 2010 Jul 1.
248. Pea F, Viale P: **Bench-to-bedside review: appropriate antibiotic therapy in severe sepsis and septic shock–does the dose matter?** *Crit Care* 2009, **13**(3):214.
249. Mueller EW, Boucher BA: **The use of extended-interval aminoglycoside dosing strategies for the treatment of moderate-to-severe infections encountered in critically ill surgical patients.** *Surg Infect* 2009, **10**(6):563–570.
250. Lorente L, Jiménez A, Martín MM, Iribarren JL, Jiménez JJ, Mora ML: **Clinicalcure of ventilator-associated pneumonia treated with piperacillin/tazobactam administered by continuous or intermittent infusion.** *Int J Antimicrob Agents* 2009, **33**(5):464–468.
251. Roberts JA, Lipman J, Blot S, Rello J: **Better outcomes through continuous infusion of time-dependent antibiotics to critically ill patients?** *Curr Opin Crit Care* 2008, **14**(4):390–396.
252. Hawser SP, Bouchillon SK, Hoban DJ, Badal RE, Cantón R, Baquero F: **Incidence and antimicrobial susceptibility of Escherichia coli and Klebsiella pneumoniae with extended-spectrum beta-lactamases in community- and hospital-associated intra-abdominal infections in Europe: results of the 2008 study for monitoring antimicrobial resistance trends (SMART).** *Antimicrob Agents Chemother* 2010, **54**(7):3043–3046.
253. Ben-Ami R, Rodriguez-Bano J, Arsian H, Pitout JD, Quentin C, Calbo ES, Azap OK, Arpin C, Pascual A, Livermore DM, Garau J, Carmeli Y: **A multinational survey of risk factors for infection with extended-spectrum β-lactamase-producing Enterobacteriaceae in nonhospitalized patients.** *Clin Infect Dis* 2009, **49**:682–690.
254. Nordmann P, Cuzon G, Naas T: **The real threat of Klebsiella pneumoniae carbapenemase-producing bacteria.** *Lancet Infect Dis* 2009, **9**(4):228–236.
255. Patel N, Harrington S, Dihmess A, Woo B, Masoud R, Martis P, Fiorenza M, Graffunder E, Evans A, McNutt LA, Lodise TP: **Clinical epidemiology of carbapenem-intermediate or -resistant Enterobacteriaceae.** *J Antimicrob Chemother* 2011, **66**(7):1600–1608.
256. Ho J, Tambyah PA, Paterson DL: **Multiresistant gram-negative infections: a global perspective.** *Curr Opin Infect Dis* 2010, **23**(6):546–553.
257. Lin WJ, Lo WT, Chu CC, Chu ML, Wang CC: **Bacteriology and antibiotic susceptibility of community-acquired intra-abdominal infection in children.** *J Microbiol Immunol Infect* 2006, **39**:249–254.
258. Solomkin JS, Yellin AE, Rotstein OD, Christou NV, Dellinger EP, Tellado JM, Malafaia O, Fernandez A, Choe KA, Carides A, Satishchandran V, Teppler H, Protocol 017 study group: **Ertapenem versus piperacillin/tazobactam in the treatment of complicated intraabdominal infections: results of a double-blind, randomized comparative phase III trial.** *Ann Surg* 2003, **237**(2):235–245.
259. Malangoni MA, Song J, Herrington J, Choudhri S, Pertel P: **Randomized controlled trial of moxifloxacin compared with piperacillin-tazobactam and amoxicillin-clavulanate for the treatment of complicated intra-abdominal infections.** *Ann Surg* 2006, **244**(2):204–211.
260. Levi J, Martinez O, Malinin T, Zeppa R, Livingstone A, Hutson D, *et al*: **Decreased biliary excretion of cefamandole after percutaneous biliary decompression in patients with total common bile duct obstruction.** *Antimicrob Agents Chemother* 1984, **26**:944–946.
261. Montravers P, Mira JP, Gangneux JP, Leroy O, Lortholary O, for the AmarCand study group: **A multicentre study of antifungal strategies and outcome of Candida spp. peritonitis in intensive-care units.** *Clin Microbiol Infect* 2011, **17**(7):1061–1067.
262. Montravers P, Dupont H, Gauzit R, Veber B, Auboyer C, Blin P, Hennequin C, Martin C: **Candida as a risk factor for mortality in peritonitis.** *Crit Care Med* 2006, **34**(3):646–652.
263. Pappas PG, Kauffman CA, Andes D, Benjamin DK Jr, Calandra TF, Edwards JE Jr, Filler SG, Fisher JF, Kullberg BJ, Ostrosky-Zeichner L, Reboli AC, Rex JH, Walsh TJ, Sobel JD: **Infectious diseases society of America: clinical practice guidelines for the management of candidiasis: 2009 update by the infectious diseases society of America.** *Clin Infect Dis* 2009, **48**(5):503–535.
264. Westphal JF, Brogard JM: **Biliary tract infections: a guide to drug treatment.** *Drugs* 1999, **57**(1):81–91.
265. Jarvinen H: **Biliary bacteremia at various stages of acute cholecystitis.** *Acta Chir Scand* 1980, **146**:427–430.
266. Hanau L, Steigbigel N: **Acute (ascending) cholangitis.** *Infect Dis Clin North Am* 2000, **14**:521–546.
267. Sinanan M: **Acute cholangitis.** *Infect Dis Clin North Am* 1992, **6**:571–599.
268. Blenkharn J, Habib N, Mok D, John L, McPherson G, Gibson R, *et al*: **Decreased biliary excretion of piperacillin after percutaneous relief of extrahepatic obstructive jaundice.** *Antimicrob Agents Chemother* 1985, **28**:778–780.
269. van den Hazel S, De Vries X, Speelman P, Dankert J, Tytgat G, Huibregtse K, *et al*: **Biliary excretion of ciprofloxacin and piperacillin in the obstructed biliary tract.** *Antimicrob Agents Chemother* 1996, **40**:2658–2660.
270. Tanaka A, Takada T, Kawarada Y, Nimura Y, Yoshida M, Miura F, Hirota M, Wada K, Mayumi T, Gomi H, Solomkin JS, Strasberg SM, Pitt HA, Belghiti J, de Santibanes E, Padbury R, Chen MF, Belli G, Ker CG, Hilvano SC, Fan ST, Liau KH: **Antimicrobial therapy for acute cholangitis: Tokyo guidelines.** *J Hepatobiliary Pancreat Surg* 2007, **14**(1):59–67. Epub 2007 Jan 30.
271. Sartelli M, Catena F, Coccolini F, Pinna AD: **Antimicrobial management of intra-abdominal infections: literature's guidelines.** *World J Gastroenterol* 2012, **18**(9):865–871.
272. Basoli A, Chirletti P, Cirino E, D'Ovidio NG, Doglietto GB, Giglio D, Giulini SM, Malizia A, Taffurelli M, Petrovic J, Ecari M, Italian Study Group: **A prospective, double-blind, multicenter, randomized trial comparing ertapenem 3 vs > or = 5 days in community-acquired intraabdominal infection.** *J Gastrointest Surg* 2008, **12**(3):592–600.
273. Lennard ES, Dellinger EP, Wertz MJ, Minshew BH: **Implications of leukocytosis and fever at conclusion of antibiotic therapy for intra-abdominal sepsis.** *Ann Surg* 1982, **195**(1):19–24.
274. Hedrick TL, Evans HL, Smith RL, McElearney ST, Schulman AS, Chong TW, Pruett TL, Sawyer RG: **Can we define the ideal duration of antibiotic therapy?** *Surg Infect (Larchmt)* 2006, **7**(5):419–432.

11

Clinical profile and outcome of surgical treatment of perforated peptic ulcers in Northwestern Tanzania: A tertiary hospital experience

Phillipo L Chalya[1*], Joseph B Mabula[1†], Mheta Koy[2†], Mabula D Mchembe[3†], Hyasinta M Jaka[2†], Rodrick Kabangila[2†], Alphonce B Chandika[1†] and Japhet M Gilyoma[1†]

Abstract

Background: Perforated peptic ulcer is a serious complication of peptic ulcers with potential risk of grave complications. There is paucity of published reports on perforated peptic ulcer disease in our local environment. This study was conducted to evaluate the clinical presentation, management and outcome of patients with peptic ulcer perforation in our setting and to identify predictors of outcome of these patients.

Methods: This was a combined retrospective and prospective study of patients who were operated for perforated peptic ulcers at Bugando Medical Centre between April 2006 and March 2011. Data were collected using a pre-tested and coded questionnaire and analyzed using SPSS computer software version 15.0. Ethical approval to conduct the study was obtained from relevant authority before the commencement of the study.

Results: A total of 84 patients were studied. Males outnumbered females by a ratio of 1.3: 1. Their median age was 28 years and the modal age group was 21-30 years. The median duration of illness was 5.8 days. The majority of patients (69.0%) had no previous history of treatment for peptic ulcer disease. The use of non-steroidal anti-inflammatory drugs, alcohol and smoking was reported in 10.7%, 85.7% and 64.3% respectively. Eight (9.5%) patients were HIV positive with a median CD4 count of 220 cells/μl. Most perforations were located on the duodenum {90.4%) with the duodenal to gastric ulcers ratio of 12.7: 1. Graham's omental patch (Graham's omentopexy) of the perforations was performed in 83.3% of cases. Complication and mortality rates were 29.8% and 10.7% respectively. The factors significantly related to complications were premorbid illness, HIV status, CD 4 count < 200 cells/μl, treatment delay and acute perforation (P < 0.001). Mortality rate was high in patients who had age ≥ 40 years, delayed presentation (>24 hrs), shock at admission (systolic BP < 90 mmHg), HIV positivity, low CD4 count (<200 cells/μl), gastric ulcers, concomitant diseases and presence of complications (P < 0.001). The median overall length of hospital stay was 14 days. Excellent results using Visick's grading system were obtained in 82.6% of surviving patients.

Conclusion: Perforation of peptic ulcer remains a frequent clinical problem in our environment predominantly affecting young males not known to suffer from PUD. Simple closure with omental patch followed by *Helicobacter pylori* eradication was effective with excellent results in majority of survivors despite patients' late presentation in our center.

Keywords: Perforated peptic ulcers, clinical profile, surgical management, outcome, Tanzania

* Correspondence: drphillipoleo@yahoo.com
† Contributed equally
[1]Department of Surgery, Weill-Bugando University College of Health Sciences, Mwanza, Tanzania
Full list of author information is available at the end of the article

Background

Peptic ulcer disease (PUD) represents a worldwide health problem because of its high morbidity, mortality and economic loss [1]. In the United States, approximately 5 million adults suffer annually from peptic ulcer disease and 500.000 new cases with 4 million recurrences are reported each year [1,2].

Globally, the incidence of peptic ulcer disease has fallen in recent years [3-5]. Despite this and recent advances in both diagnosis and management of peptic ulcer disease, namely the improvement in endoscopic facilities, eradication of H. pylori and the introduction of the proton pump inhibitors, complications such as peptic ulcer perforation remain a substantial healthcare problem. This may be due to an increase in the risk factors for peptic ulcer complications [3,6].

Peptic ulcer perforation is a serious complication which affects almost 2-10% of peptic ulcer patients on the average [7,8]. Peptic ulcer perforation presents with an overall mortality of 10% [9] although some authors report ranges between 1.3% and 20% [10,11]. Being a life threatening complication of peptic ulcer disease, it needs special attention with prompt resuscitation and appropriate surgical management if morbidity and mortality are to be avoided [3,11].

The pattern of perforated PUD has been reported to vary from one geographical area to another depending on the prevailing socio-demographic and environmental factors [12]. In the developing world, the patient population is young with male predominance, patients present late, and there is a strong association with smoking [13]. In the west the patients tend to be elderly and there is a high incidence of ulcerogenic drug ingestion [14].

The diagnosis of perforated PUD poses a diagnostic challenge in most of cases. The spillage of duodenal or gastric contents into peritoneal cavity causing abdominal pain, shock, peritonitis, marked tenderness and decreased liver dullness offers little difficulty in diagnosis of perforations [15].The presence of gas under the diaphragm on plain abdominal erect X-ray is diagnostic in 75% of the cases [16].

Since the first description of surgery for acute perforated peptic ulcer disease, many techniques have been recommended. The recent advances in antiulcer therapy have shown that simple closure of perforation with omental patch followed by eradication of *H. Pylori* is a simple and safe option in many centers and have changed the old trend of truncal vagotomy and drainage procedures [17]. The definitive operation for perforated PUD is performed by few surgeons.

Delay in diagnosis and initiation of surgical treatment of perforated PUD has been reported to be associated with high morbidity and mortality after surgery for perforated PUD [4,17]. Early recognition and prompt surgical treatment of perforated PUD is of paramount importance if morbidity and mortality associated with perforated PUD are to be avoided [4,11]. A successful outcome is obtained by prompt recognition of the diagnosis, aggressive resuscitation and early institution of surgical management.

Little work has been done on the surgical management of perforated peptic ulcer disease in our local environment despite increase in the number of admissions of this condition. The aim of this study was to describe our experience on the surgical management of perforated peptic ulcer disease in our local environment outlining the incidence, clinical presentation, management and outcome of patients with peptic ulcer perforation in our setting and to identify predictors of outcome of these patients.

Methods

Study design and setting

This was a combined retrospective and prospective study of patients operated for peptic ulcer perforations at Bugando Medical Centre (BMC) in Northwestern Tanzania from April 2006 to March 2011. BMC is a tertiary care hospital in Mwanza City that also receives patients from its six neighboring regions around Lake Victoria. It is a 1000 bed, consultant and teaching hospital for the Weill-Bugando University Collage of Health Sciences (WBUCHS) and other paramedics.

Study subject

The subjects of this study included all patients who were operated for perforated peptic ulcers at Bugando Medical Centre during the period under study. Patients with incomplete data were excluded from the study. Patients treated conservatively and those who failed to consent for HIV infection were also excluded from the study. The details of patients who presented from April 2006 to March 2008 were retrieved retrospectively from patient registers kept in the Medical record departments, the surgical wards, and operating theatre. Patients who presented to the A & E department between April 2008 and March 2011 were prospectively enrolled in the study after signing an informed written consent for the study. A detailed history and thorough physical examination were followed by investigations like full blood count, blood grouping, serum urea, serum creatinine and random blood sugar. Patients were also screened for HIV infection using rapid test/ELISA test. A determination of CD 4 count was also performed in all HIV positive patients. Radiological investigations like X-ray abdomen erect and chest X-ray were done in all patients on the suspicion of diagnosis of perforated PUD. Other investigations included hematological profile, serum urea and electrolytes and urinalysis. The diagnosis of perforated PUD was made from history, plain abdominal and chest radiographs, and confirmed at laparotomy. Patients were put on intra-venous fluids, nasogastric suction, intravenous antibiotics and intravenous anti-ulcer drugs; adequate hydration was indicated by an hourly urine output of 30 ml/hour. After adequate resuscitation, laparotomy was done through midline incision and identified the perforation site. Simple closure of the perforation and reinforcement with pedicled omental patch (Graham's omentopexy) was done. Thorough peritoneal lavage with 3 to 4 liters of normal saline was followed by placement of intraperitoneal drain. The operations were performed either by a consultant surgeon or a senior resident under the direct supervision of a consultant surgeon. The Boey score [11] as a tool for outcome prediction was calculated based on data recorded at the time of admission to hospital. The Boey risk stratification in perforated peptic ulcer consists of associated medical illness, preoperative shock and long-standing perforation (more than 24 hours). Preoperative shock was defined as a preoperative systolic blood pressure of less than 90 mmHg. All the patients were put on triple regime consisting of Amoxicillin (500 mg TID), Metranidazole(400 mg TID) and Omeprazole (20 mg BID), all given orally for 14 days to eradicate *H. Pylori.* Patients were followed up on an out patient basis for up to 12 months after surgery. Depending upon their symptoms at each visit, patients were graded using a modified Visick classification [18] as follows:-

Grade I: No symptoms, excellent results.
II: Mild symptoms, good results.
III: Moderate symptoms, easily controlled by medications.
IV: Severe symptoms, requiring constant medication or re-operation

Data collection

Data were collected using a preformed questionnaire. variables included in the questionnaire were; patient's demographic data (age, sex), associated medical premorbid illness, duration of illness, previous history of PUD, NSAID use, alcohol use and cigarette smoking, HIV status, CD 4 count, timing of surgical treatment, site of perforation, size of perforation, type of surgical procedure, postoperative complication, length of hospital stay, mortality. The duration of symptoms was defined as the time span between the initial pain perception due to perforation and the operation.

Statistical analysis

The statistical analysis was performed using statistical package for social sciences (SPSS) version 15.0 for Windows (SPSS, Chicago IL, U.S.A).The mean ± standard deviation (SD), median and ranges were calculated for continuous variables whereas proportions and frequency tables were used to summarize categorical variables. Continuous variables were categorized. Chi-square ($\chi 2$) test were used to test for the significance of association between the independent (predictor) and dependent (outcome) variables in the categorical variables. The level of significance was considered as $P < 0.05$. Multivariate logistic regression analysis was used to determine predictor variables that predict the outcome.

Ethical consideration

Ethical approval to conduct the study was obtained from the WBUCHS/BMC joint institutional ethic review committee before the commencement of the study. Patients recruited prospectively were required to sign a written informed consent for the study and for HIV testing.

Results

Out of 1124 patients who presented with peptic ulcer disease (PUD) during the study period, 96 patients underwent emergency laparotomy for perforated peptic ulcers. Of these, 8 patients were excluded from the study due to incomplete data and failure to meet the inclusion criteria. Thus, 84 patients were enrolled giving an average of 17 cases annually and represented 7.5% of cases. Of these, 18 (21.4%) patients were studied retrospectively and the remaining 66 (78.6%) patients were studied prospectively.

Socio-demographic characteristics

Forty-eight (57.1%) were males and females were 36 (42.9%) with a female ratio of 1.3:1. The patient's age ranged from 12 to 72 years with a median of 32.4 years. The peak incidence was in the 4th decade (31-40 years). The majority of patients, 52 (61.9%) were younger than 40 years. Most of patients, 64 (76.2%) had either primary or no formal education and more than three quarter of them were unemployed.

Clinical presentation

The duration of symptoms ranged from 1 to 12 days with a mean duration of 6.5 ± 2.3days. The median was 5.8 days. 24 (28.6%) presented within twenty-four hours of onset of symptoms, 25 (29.8%) between 24 and 48 hours and 30 (35.7%) over 48 hours afterwards. The duration of symptoms was not documented in 5 (5.9%) patients. The commonest presenting symptoms were sudden onset of severe epigastric pain in 82 (97.6%), abdominal distention in 64 (76.2%) and vomiting in 31

(36.9%) patients. Abdominal tenderness and classical signs of peritonitis were demonstrable in 74 (88.1%) and 56(66.7%) patients respectively (Table 1).

Fifty-eight (69.0%) patients reported no previous history of treatment for peptic ulcer disease. Patients with a previous history of peptic ulcer disease had had symptoms for durations ranging from six months to 14 years and all of them were not on regular anti-ulcer therapy. Three (3.6%) patients presented with re-perforation. Nine (10.7%) patients reported history of recent ingestion of non-steroidal anti-inflammatory drugs (NSAIDS) for joint and back pains. Other risk factors recorded included alcohol consumption and smoking in 72 (85.7%) and 54 (64.3%) patients respectively. Most patients who smoked also took alcohol.

In this study, six (7.1%) patients had associated premorbid illness namely osteoarthritis in 3 patients and hypertension, diabetes mellitus and sickle cell disease in 1 patient each respectively. Eight (9.5%) patients were HIV positive. Of these, 3 (37.5%) patients were known cases on ant-retroviral therapy (ARV) and the remaining 5 (62.5%) patients were newly diagnosed patients. CD4+ count distribution among HIV positive patients ranged from 56 cells/μl to 650 cells/μl with the mean of 236 cells/μl and standard deviation of 86 cells/μl. The median and the mode were 220 cells/μl and 160 cells/μl respectively. A total of two HIV patients (25.0%) had CD4+ count below 200 cells/μl and the remaining 6 patients (75.0%) had CD4+ count of ≥200 cells/μl. Of the eight patients with HIV infection, six (75.0%) patients reported to have risk factors for HIV infection. Of these, alcoholism [Odds Ratio 11.3, 95% C.I. (8.3-16.7), P = 0.021] and multiple sexual partners [Odds Ratio 10.8, 95% C.I. (6.7-14.9), P = 0.000] were found to be independently and significantly associated with increased risk to HIV infection

Radiological, operative and histopathological findings

Seventy-nine (94.0%) of the patients had plain abdominal and chest radiographs done, with free gas under the diaphragm (pneumoperitonium) demonstrated in 52 (65.8%) of them. All patients in this study underwent laparotomy. The time interval between the beginning of the symptoms of perforation and surgery ranged from12 to140 hours with the median of 72 hours. The majority of patients (76.2%) presented 48 hours or more after the onset of the symptoms of perforation. During operation, all the cases were opened through midline incision and after opening of the peritoneum, there was expulsion of gas in all cases. Most perforations were located on the duodenum {78, 92.9%), whereas in the remaining six (7.1%) patients had their ulcers located on the stomach. The duodenal to gastric ulcers ratio was 12.7: 1. The majority of patients, 82 (97.6%) had single perforation and the remaining 2 (2.4%) patients had both duodenal and gastric perforations. The mean age of the patients with gastric ulcers (56.4 ± 12.5) was significantly higher than that of those with duodenal ulcers (32.8 ± 14.4) (P = 0.002). The median size of the ulcer was 5.4 mm (2-20 mm). Seven (8.3%) of the perforations were found to be sealed. Thirteen (15.5%) of the perforations were of minimal size (≤5 mm) and sixty-four (76.2%) were massive (>10 mm). All perforations were found adhered with omentum and the nature of peritoneal fluid was serosanguineous in 34 (40.5%) patients, bilious in 28 (33.3%) patients and purulent in 14 (16.7%) patients. The amount of peritoneal fluid varied from 500 to 1000 mls with a median of 564 mls. The nature of peritoneal fluid was not documented in 8 (9.5%) patients. Histological examination of the biopsy specimens revealed no malignancy. All biopsies were not stained for *Helicobacter pylori.*

Table 1 Clinical presentation

Clinical presentation	Frequency	Percentage
Severe abdominal pain	82	97.6
Abdominal distention	64	76.2
Vomiting	31	36.9
Nausea	30	35.7
Severe dyspepsia	28	33.3
Constipation	25	29.8
Fever	18	21.4
Shock	28	33.3
Abdominal tenderness	74	88.1
Classical signs of peritonitis	56	66.7

Surgical treatment

The majority of patients, 70 (83.3%) had Graham's omental patch of the perforations with either a pedicled omental patch or a free graft of omentum. Those with sealed perforations had peritoneal lavage with warm saline and mass closure of the abdomen. One patient had truncal vagotomy and Roux-en-Y gastro-jejunostomy in addition to simple closure. One patient who had a large ulcer, which penetrated to the pancreas and caused pyloric obstruction, underwent subtotal gastrectomy.

Outcome of Treatment

Post-operative complications were recorded in 25 (29.8%) patients. Of these, surgical site infection (48.0%) was the most common post-operative complications (Table 2). The mean age of patients who developed complications was 52.4 ± 16.4 years, whereas the mean age of patients without complications was 32.6 ± 10.2 years. This age difference was statistically significant (P = 0.011). The complication rates for 0, 1, 2 and 3 Boey scores were 8.0%, 12.0%, 20.0% and 60.0%, respectively (P = 0.002, Pearson $\chi 2$ test)

Table 2 Post-operative complications (N = 25)

Complications	Frequency	Percentage
Surgical site infections	12	48.0
Post-operative pyrexia	9	36.0
Pulmonary infection	7	28.0
Intra-abdominal abscess	5	20.0
Wound dehiscence/burst abdomen	5	20.0
Re-perforation	4	16.0
Septic shock	3	12.0
Enterocutaneous fistula	3	12.0
Peritonitis	3	12.0
Incisional hernia	2	8.0
Cardiopulmonary arrest	2	8.0
Acute renal failure	1	4.0
Paralytic ileus	1	4.0

Table 3 shows predictors of complications according to univariate and multivariate logistic regression analysis. The overall length of hospital stay (LOS) ranged from 1 to 48 days with a median of 14 days. The median LOS for non-survivors was 3 days (range 1-8 days). Patients who developed complications stayed longer in the hospital and this was statistically significant (P = 0.005). In this study, nine patients died giving a mortality rate of 10.7%. The mortality rate increased progressively, with increasing numbers of Boey scores: 0%, 11.1%, 33.3%, and 56.6% for 0, 1, 2, and 3 factors, respectively (P < 0.001, Pearson $\chi 2$ test).

Table 4 shows predictors of mortality according to univariate and multivariate logistic regression analysis.

Table 3 Predictors of complications according to univariate and multivariate logistic regression analysis

Predictor(independent) variable	Complication N (%)	No complication n (%)	Univariate analysis		Multivariate analysis	
			O.R. 95% C.I.	p-value	O.R. 95% C.I.	p-value
Age (in years)						
<40	15 (28.8)	37 (71.2)				
≥40	10 (31.2)	22 (68.8)	3.91(0.94-5.23)	0.167	1.23(0.93-2.34)	0.786
Sex						
Male	14 (29.2)	36 (70.8)				
Female	11 (30.6)	25 (69.4)	1.87(0.22-4.88)	0.334	3.32(0.45-4.66)	0.937
Premorbid illness						
Yes	4 (66.7)	2(33.3)				
No	21(26.9)	57(73.1)	3.54(1.33-5.87)	0.012	5.28(2.39-6.82)	**0.007**
Previous PUD						
Yes	7(26.9)	19(73.1)				
No	18(31.0)	40(69.0)	0.21(0.11-1.78)	0.051	1.65(0.32-2.89)	0.786
NSAIDs use						
Yes	3(33.3)	6(66.7)				
No	22(29.3)	53(70.7)	1.98(0.99-3.91)	0.923	1.02(0.78-3.90)	0.123
Alcohol use						
Yes	22(30.6)	50(69.4)				
No	3(25.0)	9(75.0)	3.05(0.19-2.86)	0.054	0.45(0.22-5.21)	0.321
Cigarette smoking						
Yes	17(31.5)	37(68.5)				
No	8(26.7)	22(73.3)	3.11(0.44-5.23)	0.145	3.02(0.99-4.56)	0.334
Treatment delay						
< 48	18(90.0)	2(10.0)				
≥ 48	7(14.6)	41(85.4)	1.06(1.01-5.45)	0.021	0.23(0.11-0.95)	**0.003**
HIV status						
Positive	6(75.0)	2 (25.0)				
Negative	19(25.0)	57(75.0)	2.87(1.22-4.97)	0.023	1.92(1.31-4.22	**0.001**
CD4 count						
<200 cells/μl	1 (50.0)	1(50.0)				
≥ 200 cells/μl	1(16.7)	5(83.3)	4.05(3.27-5.01)	0.029	2,94(2.44-6.98)	**0.000**
Nature of perforation						
Acute	24(32.4)	50(67.6)				
Chronic	1(10.0)	9(90.0)	4.94(2.84-8.92)	0.009	2.95(1.11-6.98)	**0.018**

Table 4 Predictors of mortality according to univariate and multivariate logistic regression analysis

Predictor (independent) variable	Survivors N (%)	Non-survivors n (%)	Univariate analysis		Multivariate analysis	
			O.R. (95% C.I.)	p-value	(O.R. 95% C.I.)	p-value
Age						
< 40	51(98.1)	1 (1.9)				
≥40	24(75.0)	8 (25.0)	2.33(1.25-3.42)	0.032	4.61(2.72-7.91)	**0.002**
Sex						
Male	42 (87.5)	6 (12.5)				
Female	33 (91.7)	3 (8.3)	1.25 (0.32-3.56)	0.896	2.93 (0.94-3.81)	0.983
Premorbid illness						
Yes	2 (33.3)	4 (66.7)				
No	73 (93.6	5 (6.4)	6.21(1.49-7.01)	0.039	3.78(2.98-7.90)	**0.017**
Previous PUD						
Yes	23 (88.0)	3(12.0)				
No	52 (89.7)	6 (10.3)	1.75(0.76-4.34)	0.896	3.11(0.98-4.88)	0.345
HIV status						
Positive	1(12.5)	7 (87.5)				
Negative	74(97.4)	2 (2.6)	0.56(0.12-0.86)	0.005	1.74(1.21-4.98)	**0.001**
CD 4+ count						
< 200 cells/µl	1(50.0)	1 (50.0)				
≥ 200 cells/µl	4(66.7)	2 (33.3)	5.91(2.76-7.99)	0.001	1.65(1,22-7.43)	**0.000**
Duration of illness						
<24 hours	23 (92.0)	2 (8.0)				
≥24 hours	48 (87.3)	7 (12.7)	2.32(0.54-6.45)	0.986	0.09(0.02-1.11)	0.315
Shock on admission (SBP < 90 mmHg)						
Yes	28 (77.8)	8 (22.2)				
No	47 (87.9)	1(2.1)	7.9(3.98-9.88)	0.022	3,74(2,11-7.76)	**0.005**
Timing of surgical treatment						
<48 hours	19 (95.0)	1 (5.0)				
≥ 48 hours	56 (87.5)	8 (12.5%)	2.87(2.11-7.21)	0.044	2.91(1.22-6.66)	**0.028**
Amount of fluid (mls						
< 200	19 (95.0)	1 (5.0)				
≥200	56(87.5)	8 (12.5)	0.67(0.23-4.65)	0.982	1.61(0.89-2.73)	0.067
Site of perforation						
Duodenum	72 (93.4)	5 (6.6)				
Gastric	2 (33.3)	4 (66.7)	5.81(3.33-6.92)	0.012	1.35(1.11-3.86)	**0.018**
Size of ulcer						
Sealed	7 (100.0)	0(0)				
<5 mm	12 (92.3)	1(7.7)				
≥5 mm	56 (87.5)	8(12.5)	1.98(0.45-3.82)	0.987	3.13(0.99-4.89)	0.453
Complications						
Present	18 (72.0)	7(28.0)				
Absent	57(96.6)	2 (3.4)	1.98(1.54-7.93)	0.005	2.86(2.22-6.45)	**0.011**

Follow up of patients

Out of 75 survivors, 46 (61.3%) patients were followed up for 6 to 12 months after surgery. Depending upon their symptoms at each visit, patients were classified according to Visick grading system as follows: Visick grade I, 38 (82.6%) patients, Visick grade II, 4 (8.7%) patients, Visick grade III and IV, 2 (4.3%) patients each respectively. One of patients (2.2%) in Visick grade IV presented with re-perforation which necessitated re-operation.

Discussion

In this review, a total of 84 patients were enrolled over a five year period giving an average of 17 cases annually. This figure is similar to what was reported by Schein *et al* [19]. Mieny *et al* [20] in South Africa reported a low incidence of perforated PUD. These differences reflect differences in the rate of risk factors for perforated peptic ulcer disease from one country to another. The figures in our study may actually be an underestimate and the magnitude of the problem may not be apparent because of high number of patients excluded from this study.

In the present study, perforated peptic ulcer disease were found to be most common in the fourth decade of life and tended to affect more males than females, with a male to female ratio of 1.3:1 which is comparable with other studies in developing countries [3,21-23]. Our demographic profile is in sharp contrast to what is reported in developed countries where the majority of the patients are above 60 years and the incidence is higher in elderly females taking ulcerogenic medications [24]. Male predominance in this age group is attributed to excessive alcohol consumption and smoking among young males which is common in our environment. Alcohol consumption and smoking have been reported to be associated with increased risk for perforated peptic ulcer. Alcohol, as a noxious agent causes gastric mucosal damage, stimulates acid secretion and increases serum gastrin levels [25] and smoking inhibits pancreatic bicarbonate secretion, resulting in increased acidity in the duodenal bulb. It also inhibits the healing of duodenal ulcers [21,26].

The rate of H. pylori infection in patients with perforated peptic ulcers ranges from 50%-80% and *H. pylori* infection, as a risk factor for perforated PUD, appears to be more relevant in younger patients. This is in contrast to elderly patients, where NSAIDs may play a more significant etiologic role [27]. Determination of *Helicobacter Pylori* was not performed in our study due to lack of reagents.

Use of NSAID is an important cause of perforated peptic ulcer in the West. In our series, NSAID use as an offending cause could be attributable in only 10.7% patients. NSAID inhibit prostaglandin synthesis so further reducing gastric mucosal blood flow [27].

In agreement with other studies [3,24], more than sixty percent of patients had no past history suggestive of peptic ulcer disease and those with a known history of PUD were not on regular treatment. This is in sharp contrast to Nuhu *et al* in Nigeria who reported that 71% of cases had previous history of peptic ulcer disease [21]. It has been reported that in many developing countries, the diagnosis of PUD is first made in many instances after perforation [28]. The present study confirms this observation because more than sixty percent of the patients with perforation were not diagnosed previously as cases of PUD and therefore were not on treatment. Patients with no previous diagnosis of peptic ulcer have a higher risk of PUD perforation than patients with a known history of ulcer disease. This may be because preventative measures are more likely to have been taken in patients with a known history of ulcer. Furthermore, these patients are perhaps more likely to seek treatment earlier.

In this study, most of patients had either primary or no formal education and more than three quarter of them were unemployed. Similar occupational pattern was reported by others [21,22]. This observation has an implication on accessibility to health care facilities and awareness of the disease.

It has been reported that the interval between perforation and initiation of treatment is a better predictor of outcome. In the present study most of patients presented late more than 24 hours from the start of symptoms. This is in agreement with other studies in most developing countries [3,21-23,28]. Late presentation in our study may be attributed to lack of accessibility to health care facilities and lack of awareness of the disease. Hospital treatment is expensive and the patients may seek care only when the pain is unbearable. Patients may take medications in the pre-hospital period with hope that the symptom will abate. It is also possible that some clinicians managing the patients initially may not have considered perforation as a possible diagnosis.

More than 90% of our patients had classical presentation with sudden onset of sharp epigastric pain, as most of the studied patients were young aged in contradistinction to elderly patients in whom silent perforations usually occur [3,29].

As reported in other studies [5,9,30], associated premorbid illness was documented in 7.1% of cases. Associated premorbid illnesses have been reported to influence the outcome of patients with perforated peptic ulcers [5]. In the present study, associated premorbid illness predicted the outcome of patients with perforated peptic ulcers.

The prevalence of HIV infection among patients with perforated PUD in the present study was 9.5% that is higher than 6.5% [31] in the general population in Tanzania. This difference was statistically significant ($P < 0.001$). The high prevalence of HIV infection in our patients may be attributed to high percentage of the risk factors for HIV infection reported in the present study population. The overall HIV seroprevalence in our study may actually be an underestimate and the magnitude of the problem may not be apparent because many cases (8 patients) were excluded from the study due to failure to meet the inclusion criteria. We could not find any literature regarding the effect of HIV infection on the perforation rate and outcome in patient with perforated PUD. This calls for a need to research on this observation. In this study, HIV infection was found to be associated with high perforation rate and poor postoperative outcome. This observation calls for routine HIV screening in patients suspected to have perforated PUD.

In agreement with other studies [3,4,21,22,32], the diagnosis of perforated PUD in this study was made from history and identification of free air under the diaphragm in plain abdominal and chest radiographs, and the diagnosis was confirmed at laparotomy. The value of the radiological investigation has been compared with other writers and with current radiological techniques; 80-90% of cases are correctly diagnosed [4,33]. In case of perforated PUD ulcer, free intraperitoneal gas is less likely to be seen if the time interval between the perforation and radiological examination in short [4]. Recently, Computerized tomography (CT) scans with oral contrast are now considered the reliable method of detecting small pneumoperitonium before surgery and the gold standard for the diagnosis of a perforation [34,35]. Abdominal ultrasonography has also been found to be superior to plan radiographs in the diagnosis of free intra-peritoneal air [35]. None of these imaging studies were used in the diagnosis of free intra-peritoneal air in our study. We relied on plain radiographs of the abdominal/chest to establish the diagnosis of free intraperitoneal air which was demonstrated in 65.8% of cases. We could not establish, in our study, the reason for the low detection rate of free air under the diaphragm.

In our study, duodenal ulcer perforation was the most common type of perforation with a duodenal to gastric ulcer ratio of 12.7:1. This is comparable to a study in Kenya which reported a duodenal to gastric ulcer ratio of 11.5:1 [32]. A high duodenal to gastric ulcer ratio of 25:1 was reported in Sudan [36]. A study in Ghana reported high incidence of gastric ulcer perforations than duodenal ulcer perforation [37]. Low duodenal to gastric ulcer ratios of 3:1 to 4:1 have been reported from the western world [32,37]. Gastric ulcer is considered a rare disease in Africa being 6-30 times less common than duodenal ulcers [37,38]. There was no obvious explanation to account for these duodenal to gastric ulcer ratio differences.

In this study, Graham's omental patch of the perforations with either a pedicled omental patch or a free graft of omentum was the operation of choice in our centre. Similar surgical treatment pattern was reported in other studies [3,4,21,22]. This is a rapid, easy and life-serving surgical procedure that has been shown to be effective with acceptable mortality and morbidity [22,39]. Although this procedure has been associated with ulcer recurrence rates of up to 40% in some series, Graham's omental patch of PUD perforations remains a surgical procedure of choice in most centres and to avoid recurrence the procedure should be followed by eradication of *H. pylori* [22,40]. Simple closure of perforation with omental patch and the use of proton pump inhibitors have changed the traditional definitive peptic ulcer surgery of truncal vagotomy and drainage procedures [41]. Definitive surgery is indicated only for those who are reasonably fit and presented early to the hospital for surgery [22]. Definitive peptic ulcer surgery increases operative time, exposes the patient to prolonged anaesthesia and also increases the risk of postoperative complications. This is especially true in developing countries including Africa where patients often present late with severe generalized peritonitis [23]. In the present study, only one patient who presented early with stable haemodynamic state underwent definitive peptic ulcer surgery of truncal vagotomy and drainage. Recently, laparoscopic repair of perforated peptic ulcer has also been reported, [42] and this is believed to help reduce postoperative morbidity and mortality [43].

The laparoscopic technique in closure of perforated peptic ulcers is being practiced in several centres in developed countries [42,43], it has not yet been tried in any of our hospitals in this country.

Overall complications rate in this series was 29.8% which is comparable to what was reported by others [4,44]. High complications rate was reported by Montalvo-Javé *et al* [6]. This difference in complication rates can be explained by differences in antibiotic coverage, meticulous preoperative care and proper resuscitation of the patients before operation, improved anesthesia and somewhat better hospital environment. In keeping with other studies [21,22,39], surgical site infection was the most common complication. High rate of surgical site infection in the present study may be attributed to contamination of the laparotomy wound during the surgical procedure.

Perforated peptic ulcer is a serious condition with an overall reported mortality of 5%-25%, rising to as high as 50% with age [5-7,9,11,44]. In this study mortality rate was high in patients who had age ≥ 40 years, delayed presentation (>24 hrs), shock at admission (systolic BP < 90 mmHg), HIV positivity, low CD4 count (< 200 cells/μl) and concomitant diseases. Also gastric ulcers were associated with an increased mortality risk. Boey's score, which is a score based on scoring factors as shock on admission, confounding medical illness, and prolonged perforation, has been found to be a useful tool in predicting outcome [11]. In this study, Boey score was a good predictor of both mortality and postoperative complication and therefore should be used in our setting as a tool for predicting outcome in patients with perforated peptic ulcers.

Since tests for detecting *H. Pylori* was not possible in our patients due to logistic problems, we did not take this into consideration in our discussion. However the use of the 'triple regime' produced excellent results in 82.6% of our patients which is comparable to the results from recent studies [3. 4, 21, 22, 45] which have successfully used simple closure followed by eradication of *H-Pylori* as a treatment for perforated peptic ulcer. This is in contrast to the earlier studies [46,47] which reported emergency definitive surgery as a means to prevent recurrence and re-operation rates. These findings are extremely important for developing countries like Tanzania where delay in presentation often prevents any attempt at definitive surgery.

Before generalizing the results of our study several important issues need to be addressed. First, since all the subjects in the present study underwent pen repair, results from this study may not fully represent those after laparoscopic repair. Second, we did not study the association of *H. pylori* with the postoperative outcomes because of lack of necessary facilities at the study center. Third, data obtained retrospectively and failure to detect HIV infection during window period may have underestimated the prevalence of HIV infection. Fourth, since our duration of postoperative follow up was relatively short, we could not estimate the long term effect of Graham's omental patch.

Conclusion

Perforation of peptic ulcer remains a frequent clinical problem in our environment predominantly affecting young males not known to suffer from PUD. Simple closure with omental patch followed by *Helicobacter pylori* eradication was effective with excellent results in majority of cases despite patients' late presentation in our center.

Acknowledgements

The authors are grateful to our senior house officers (residents) in the Department of Surgery for their assistance in data collection and to all those who were involved in the care of our patients.

Author details

[1]Department of Surgery, Weill-Bugando University College of Health Sciences, Mwanza, Tanzania. [2]Department of Internal Medicine, Weill-Bugando University College of Health Sciences, Mwanza, Tanzania. [3]Department of Surgery, Muhimbili University of Health and Allied Sciences, Dar Es Salaam, Tanzania.

Authors' contributions

PLC - study design, literature search, data analysis, manuscript writing & editing and submission of the manuscript, JBM, MK, MDM, HMJ, RK, ABC participated in data analysis, manuscript writing & editing and JMG-supervised and coordinated the manuscript writing & editing. All the authors read and approved the final manuscript.

Competing interests

The authors declare that they have no competing interests. The study had no external funding. Operational costs were met by authors

References

1. Türkdoğan MK, Hekim H, Tuncer İ, Aksoy H: **The epidemiological and endoscopic aspects of peptic ulcer disease in Van region.** *Eastern Journal of Medicine* 1999, **4(1)**:6-9.
2. Isenberg JI, McQuaid KR, Laine L, Rubin W: **Acid-peptic disorders.** In *Textbook of Gastroenterology.* Edited by: Yamada T. J.B Lippincott comp., Philadelphia; 1991:1241-98, ch.61.
3. Elnagib E, Mahadi SE, Mohamed E, Ahmed ME: **Perforated peptic ulcer in Khartoum.** *Khartoum Medical Journal* 2008, **1(2)**:62-64.
4. Khan SH, Aziz SA, Ul-Haq MI: **Perforated peptic ulcers: A review of 36 cases.** *Professional Med J* 2011, **18(1)**:124-127.
5. Makela JT, Kiviniemi H, Ohtonen P, Laitinen SO: **Factors That Predict Morbidity and Mortality in Patients with Perforated Peptic Ulcers.** *Eur J Surg* 2002, **168**:446-451.
6. Montalvo-Javé EE, Corres-Sillas O, César Athié-Gutiérrez C: **Factors associated with postoperative complications and mortality in perforated peptic ulcer.** *Cir Cir* 2011, **79**:128-135.
7. Testini M, Portincasa P, Piccinni G, Lissidini G, Pellegrini F, Greco L: **Significant factors associated with fatal outcome in emergency open surgery for perforated peptic ulcer.** *World J Gastroenterol* 2003, **9**:2338-2340.
8. Soll AH: **Peptic ulcer and its complications.** In *Sleisinger & Fordtran's Gastrointestinal and Liver Disease: Pathophysiology, Diagnosis, Management..* 6 edition. Edited by: Feldman M, Scharschmidt BF, Sleisenger MH. Philadelphia, PA: W.B. Saunders; 1998:620-678.
9. Rajesh V, Sarathchandra S, Smile SR: **Risk factors predicting operative mortality in perforated peptic ulcer disease.** *Trop Gastroenterol* 2003, **24**:148-150.
10. Hermansson M, Von Holstein CS, Zilling T: **Surgical approach and prognostic factors after peptic ulcer perforation.** *Eur J Surg* 1999, **165**:566-572.
11. Boey J, Choi KY, Alagaratnam TT, Poon A: **Risk stratification in perforated duodenal ulcers. A prospective validation of predictive factors.** *Ann Surg* 1986, **205**:22-26.
12. Kudva MV, Thein-Htut T: **Profile of Peptic Ulcer Disease in Malaysia.** *Sing Med J* 1988, **29**:544-547.
13. Hill AG: **The management of perforated peptic ulcer in a resource poor environment.** *East Afr Med J* 2001, **78(8)**:346-348.
14. Windsor JA, Hill AG: **The management of perforated peptic ulcer.** *N Z Med J* 1995, 47-48.
15. Cuschieri A: **Disorders of stomach and duodenum.** In *Essential surgical practice..* 4 edition. Edited by: Cuschieri A, Steel RJC, Moosa AR. London: Arnold; 2002:261-319.
16. Mehboob M, Khan JA, Rehman Shafiq-ur, Saleem SM, Abdul Qayyum A: **Peptic duodenal perforation-an audit.** *JCPSP* 2000, **10**:101-3.
17. Gutierrez de La pena C, Merquez R, Fakih F, Dominguez-Adame E, Medina J: **Simple closure or vagotomy and pyloroplasty for the treatment of a perforated duodenal ulcer comparison of results.** *Dig surg* 2000, **17**:225.
18. Visick AH: **Measured radical gastrectomy. Review of operations for peptic ulcer.** *Lancet* 1948, **1**:505-510.
19. Schein M, Saadia R, Decker GA: **Perforated peptic ulcer at the J. G. Strijdom Hospital: A retrospective study of 99 patients.** *S Afr Med J* 1986, **70(5)**:21-23.
20. Mieny CJ, Kopelowitz W, Colsen P: **Management of perforated peptic ulcer.** *S Air] Surg* 1974, **12**:27-29.
21. Nuhu A, Madziga AG, Gali BM: **Acute perforated duodenal ulcer in Maiduguri.** *The Internet Journal of Surgery* 2009, **21**:1.
22. Nasio NA, Saidi H: **Perforated Peptic Ulcer Disease at Kenyatta National Hospital, Nairobi.** *East and Central African Journal of Surgery* 2009, **14(1)**:13-16.
23. Tessema E, Meskel Y, Kotiss B: **Perforated peptic ulcer in Tikur Anbessa Hospital.** *Ethiop Med Journal* 2005, **43(1)**:9-13.
24. Kang JY, Elders A, Majeed A: **Recent trend in hospital admission and mortality rate for peptic ulcer in Scotland 1982 - 2002.** *Aliment Pharmacol Ther* 2006, **24(1)**:65-79.
25. Türkdoğan MK, Hekim H, Tuncer I, Aksoy H: **The epidemiological and endoscopic aspects of peptic ulcer disease in Van region.** *Eastern Journal of Medicine* 1999, **4(1)**:6-9.

26. Stabile BE, Passaro EP: **Duodenal ulcer: a disease in evolution.** *Curr Probl Surg* 1984, **21**:1-79.
27. Collier DS, Pain JA: **Non-steroidal anti-inflammatory drugs and peptic ulcer perforation.** *Gut* 1985, **26**:359-363.
28. Ajao OG: **Perforated duodenal ulcer in a tropical African population.** *J Natl Med Assoc* 1979, **71**:272-3.
29. Jeffrey AN, Randal R, Alfred EC, Stephen FH, Robert WT: *'Surgery basic science and clinical evidence'* USA: Donnelley and Sons, Willard OH; 2001, 489-500.
30. Bas G, Eryilmaz R, Okan I, Sahin M: **Risk Factors of Morbidity and Mortality in Patients with Perforated Peptic Ulcer.** *Acta Chir Belg* 2008, **108**:424-427.
31. Urassa M, Isingo R, Kumogola Y, Mwidunda P, Helelwa M, Changulucha J, Mngara J, Zaba B, Calleja T, Slaymaker E: **Effect of PMTCT availability on choice of ANC in Mwanza and Magu districts and its impact on HIV sentinel surveillance.** *Report of ANC surveillance Mwanza and Magu Districts, Tanzania* 2007, (Unpubl.).
32. Kuremu RT: **Surgical management of peptic ulcer disease.** *East Afr Med J* 2002, **76(9)**:454-456.
33. Lee CW, Yip AW, Lam KH: **Pneumogastrogram in the diagnosis of perforated peptic ulcer.** *Aust N Z J-Surg* 1993, **63**:459-61.
34. Amela S, Serif B, Lidija L: **Early radiological diagnostics of gastrointestinal infection in the management of peptic ulcer perforation.** *Radiol Oncol* 2006, **40(2)**:67-72.
35. Chen SC, Yen ZS, Wang HP, Lin FY, Hsu CY, Chen WJ: **Ultrasonography is superior to plain radiography in the diagnosis of pneumoperitonium.** *Br J Surg* 2002, **89**:351-354.
36. Fedail S, Araba BMO, Homeda MM, Ghandour ZM: **Upper gastrointestinal endoscopy in Sudan: Analysis of 2500 endoscopies.** 1983, **2**:897-9.
37. Ohene-Yeboah M, Togbe B: **Perforated gastric and duodenal ulcers in an urban African population.** *West Afr J Med* 2006, **25(3)**:205-211.
38. Umerah BC, Singarayar J, Ramzan MK: **Incidence of peptic ulcer in the Zambian African- a radiological study.** *Med J Zambia* 1987, **12**:117-118.
39. Khalil AR, Yunas M, Qutbe AJ, Nisar W, Imran M: **Grahm's omentopexy in closure of perforated duodenal ulcer.** *J Med Sci* 2010, **18(2)**:87-90.
40. Sharma SS, Manju RM, Sharma SM, Kulkarni H: **A prospective cohort study of postoperative complications in the management of perforated peptic ulcer.** *BMC Surgery* 2006, **6**:8.
41. Gurleyik E: **Changing trend in emergency surgery for perforated duodenal ulcer.** *J Coll Physicians Surg Pak* 2003, **13**:708-10.
42. Beena B, Vaidya , Chaitanya : **Laparoscopic repair of perforated peptic ulcer with delayed Presentation.** *Journal of laparoendoscopic and advanced surgical technique* 2009, **19(2)**:153-156.
43. Song KY, Kim TH, Kim SN, Park CH: **Laparoscopic repair of perforated duodenal ulcer: the simple one - stitch suture with omental patch technique.** *Surg Endoscope* 2008, **22(7)**:1632-5.
44. Lee FY, Leung KL, Lai BS, Ng SS, Dexter S, Lau WY: **Predicting mortality and morbidity of patients operated on for perforated peptic ulcers.** *Arch Surg* 2001, **139**:90-94.
45. Gupta BS, Talukdar RN, Neupane HC: **Cases of Perforated Duodenal Ulcer treated in College of Medical Sciences, Bharatpur over a period of one year.** *Kathmandu University Medical Journal* 2003, **1(3)**:166-169.
46. Jordan GL, De Bakey ME: **Surgical Management of perforated peptic ulcer.** *Ann Surg* 1974, **179**:628-33.
47. Gray JG, Roberts AK: **Definitive emergency treatment of perforated duodenal ulcer.** *Surg Gynaecol Obstet* 1976, **143**:890-4.

12

Combined totally mini-invasive approach in necrotizing pancreatitis

Luca Sorrentino[1], Osvaldo Chiara[1*], Massimiliano Mutignani[2], Fabrizio Sammartano[1], Paolo Brioschi[3] and Stefania Cimbanassi[1]

Abstract

Background: Currently, both the step-up approach, combining percutaneous drainage (PD) and video-assisted retroperitoneal debridement (VARD), and endoscopic transgastric necrosectomy (ETN) are mini-invasive techniques for infected necrosis in severe acute pancreatitis. A combination of these approaches could maximize the management of necrotizing pancreatitis, conjugating the benefits from both the experiences. However, reporting of this combined strategy is anecdotal. This is the first reported case of severe necrotizing pancreatitis complicated by biliary fistula treated by a combination of ETN, PD, VARD, and endoscopic biliary stenting. Moreover, a systematic literature review of comparative studies on minimally invasive techniques in necrotizing pancreatitis has been provided.

Case presentation: A 59-year-old patient was referred to our center for acute necrotizing pancreatitis associated with multi-organ failure. No invasive procedures were attempted in the first month from the onset: enteral feeding by a naso-duodenal tube was started, and antibiotics were administered to control sepsis. After 4 weeks, CT scans showed a central walled-off pancreatic necrosis (WOPN) of pancreatic head communicating bilateral retroperitoneal collections. ETN was performed, and bile leakage was found at the right margin of the WOPN. Endoscopic retrograde cholangiopancreatography confirmed the presence of a choledocal fistula within the WOPN, and a biliary stent was placed. An ultrasound-guided PD was performed on the left retroperitoneal collection. Due to the subsequent repeated onset of septic shocks and the evidence of size increase of the right retroperitoneal collection, a VARD was decided. The CT scans documented the resolution of all the collections, and the patient promptly recovered from sepsis. After 6 months, the patient is in good clinical condition.

Conclusions: No mini-invasive technique has demonstrated significantly better outcomes over the others, and each technique has specific indications, advantages, and pitfalls. Indeed, ETN could be suitable for central WOPNs, while VARD or PD could be suggested for lateral collections. A combination of different approaches is feasible and could significantly optimize the clinical management in critically ill patients affected by complicated necrotizing pancreatitis.

Keywords: Severe pancreatitis, Step-up approach, Video-assisted retroperitoneal debridement, Endoscopic transgastric necrosectomy, Percutaneous drainage, Walled-off pancreatic necrosis

* Correspondence: osvaldo.chiara@ospedaleniguarda.it
[1]Trauma Team and Emergency Surgery, Niguarda Trauma Center, Niguarda Ca' Granda Hospital, Piazza Ospedale Maggiore 3, Milan 20162, Italy
Full list of author information is available at the end of the article

Background

Severe necrotizing pancreatitis is related to a high mortality rate, ranging from 20% in patients with sterile necrosis up to 40% in case of infected necrosis associated with multi-organ failure (MOF) [1, 2]. Therefore, occurrence of severe sepsis doubles the risk of death, and this mortality is even higher with increasing age [2, 3]. Early open surgery has been initially proposed for necrotizing pancreatitis, but poor outcomes were observed due to the high risk of bleeding and pancreatic or colonic fistula, leading to a peri-operative morbidity of 50–60% and a mortality rate equal to 20–25% [4, 5]. Since early open surgery could worsen prognosis, nowadays, other less invasive procedures, such as percutaneous drainage (PD), endoscopic transgastric necrosectomy (ETN), or video-assisted retroperitoneal debridement (VARD) are suggested [5, 6]. Therefore, open surgical necrosectomy with repeated laparotomies is considered the last choice whereas other therapeutic options have failed. Currently, the step-up approach, which includes PD possibly followed by VARD or endoscopic transluminal drainage followed by ETN, is proposed as a standard of care for necrotizing pancreatitis [6]. However, few trials have compared the step-up approach with open necrosectomy; therefore, a consensus on the best timing and management of these techniques is lacking [6, 7]. Moreover, the percutaneous step-up approach is certainly useful for lateral fluid or necrotic collections, but its role for medial collections (such as those posteriorly to the stomach) is much more controversial, and ETN could be more suitable in these cases [6]. Combined approaches could conjugate benefits from both endoscopic and percutaneous or minimally invasive drainages, thus representing a possible solution for severe necrotizing pancreatitis, but they are anecdotal and rarely reported in literature above all in case of pancreatitis-related complications [8]. Particularly, biliary fistula involving the common bile duct is a rare complication of acute necrotizing pancreatitis, its pathogenesis is supposed to be related to the necrotizing inflammatory process and its management is considered to be extremely difficult [9]. Here, we present the first case in our knowledge of a patient affected by severe necrotizing pancreatitis complicated by biliary fistula, successfully treated by a combined minimally invasive approach conjugating ETN, PD, VARD, and endoscopic retrograde cholangiopancreatography (ERCP) with biliary stenting.

Case presentation

A 59-year-old man was admitted to a community hospital for worsening abdominal pain in the upper quadrants with jaundice (total bilirubin 13.4 mg/dL) and evidence of highly elevated serum amylase (5400 U/L). An abdominal ultrasound showed cholelithiasis with common bile duct dilatation due to biliary sludge. Due to the presence of biliary obstruction, an ERCP was attempted but failed due to impossible cannulation of the papilla; therefore, the procedure was immediately interrupted. Moreover, 2 days after patient hospitalization in the primary hospital, his clinical conditions worsened by the development of MOF, since acute respiratory distress syndrome (ARDS) and acute renal failure with anuria occurred. Therefore, the patient underwent endotracheal intubation and was referred to the intensive care unit of our referral tertiary center. The patient had no relevant past history or medications. On admission at our hospital, the patient presented with elevated serum creatinine (4.26 mg/dL, normal range 0.7–1.2 mg/dL) and blood urea nitrogen (111 mg/dL, normal range 18–48 mg/dL). The serum amylase was equal to 233 U/L (normal range 28–100 U/L), and the total bilirubin was 8.33 mg/dL (normal range 0.25–1 mg/dL). A marked anemia was evident (hemoglobin 7.8 g/dL, hematocrit 23.6%) without leukocytosis. Arterial blood gas analysis revealed hypoxia without acidosis (pH 7.41, base excess −0.2, lactate 1 mmol/L). The APACHE II score at admission was 30. Enteral feeding was started immediately upon naso-duodenal tube placement, and continuous veno-venous hemofiltration (CVVH) was introduced for acute renal failure also considering the occurrence of hyperkalemia up to 6 mmol/L. Continuous vasopressor support was not necessary, as hemodynamic stability was maintained by fluid infusion.

However, several episodes of shock associated with hyperpyrexia up to 38.5 °C occurred and required short-course treatment with vasopressor. These episodes were hemodynamically consistent with septic shock, but blood cultures were initially negative, as well as skin and mucosal swabs. Only urine cultures were found positive for *Escherichia coli*; therefore, piperacillin/tazobactam therapy was started based on antibiograms. Due to persistent ARDS with PaO_2/FiO_2 ratio <100 mmHg, the patient needed prolonged artificial ventilation, and a percutaneous tracheostomy was performed. Several attempts of weaning from mechanical ventilation failed. Intra-abdominal pressure was monitored, being constantly equal to 12 mmHg. Abdominal ultrasound confirmed the presence of distended gallbladder with multiple gallstones and biliary sludge without signs of acute cholecystitis, but common bile duct diameter was normal, apparently with no more evidence of obstructing sludge into the biliary tree.

The patient underwent CT scan which showed acute necrosis of the cephalic portion of the pancreas, with reduced enhancement in pancreatic tail and a 11 × 5.5 cm fluid collection in the right retroperitoneal space (Fig. 1). Severe edema of peri-pancreatic adipose tissue was documented, with abdominal and pelvic effusion. Urine iodine excretion was negligible, and bilateral pleural effusion was documented. Weekly follow-up CT

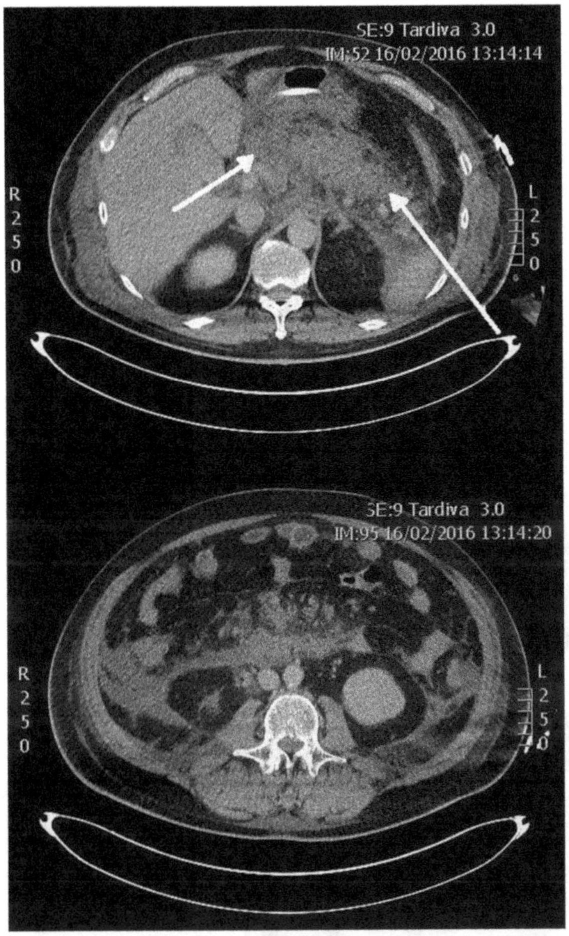

Fig. 1 First CT scans at admission. Acute pancreatic necrosis and edema of pancreatic tail and surrounding adipose tissue are visible (*arrows*)

scans demonstrated the appearance of a 13 × 9 cm highly dense retroperitoneal collection cranial to the pancreatic head communicating with another 6 × 5 cm collection near the left hepatic lobe. Head and neck of the pancreas were no more recognizable, and a significant compression was evident on portal vein. Moreover, a progressive increase in bilateral retroperitoneal fluid collections was detected, as well as a further 12 × 4 cm necrotic collection under the uncinate process.

Four weeks after the admission, these collections were in communication with a unique large 24 × 10 cm retroperitoneal collection characterized by a partially fluid content. Also, the necrotic collection cranial to the pancreatic head connected with the left hepatic lobe collection augmented, with a diameter of 15 × cm, and acquired features of walled-off pancreatic necrosis (WOPN) (Fig. 2). Due to the worsening of retro-gastric WOPN with gastroduodenal extrinsic compression and the clinical evidence of ongoing sepsis, the patient was subjected to ETN of the WOPN. A 1.6 × 2 cm metallic stent (Niti-S yo-yo stent, Taewoong, South Korea) was positioned, draining abundant necrotic and purulent material, and a 6-Fr naso-cystic tube was then positioned to guarantee continuous irrigation of the drained WOPN with 2 L saline/die (Fig. 3a). Cultures on purulent material revealed the presence of *Stenotrophomonas maltophilia* and blood cultures were positive for *E. coli*; therefore, antibiotics cefotaxime and sulfamethoxazole/trimethoprim were started targeted on antibiograms.

Endoscopic transgastric pancreatic necrosectomy was repeated two times over the following 2 weeks, and during the last endoscopy, a biliary leakage was encountered from an unspecified site on the right margin of the WOPN. Subsequently, the patient repeated abdominal CT scan which confirmed a significant reduction of the WOPN, being 5.6 × 4.3 cm, while the large right and left retroperitoneal collections increased in size (Fig. 3b, c). Then, an ultrasound-guided PD was performed of the left retroperitoneal collection, positioning a 10-Fr drainage tube (Fig. 3d). Due to size reduction of the WOPN and consequent less extrinsic compression on the duodenum, an ERCP became feasible. ERCP confirmed a biliary fistula from the distal third of the common bile duct to the WOPN cavity; therefore, sphincterotomy of papilla was performed and a 6 mm × 4 cm fully covered metallic biliary stent (Wallflex, Boston Scientific, Boston, MA, USA) was positioned (Fig. 4a). Endoscopic second-look documented almost complete debridement of the WOPN.

The following CT scans showed a progressive reduction of both the WOPN and the left retroperitoneal collection but only a modest decrease of the large right retroperitoneal necrotic collection which appeared only partially liquefied. Moreover, the patient remained febrile despite meropenem, colistin, and fluconazole were started after *Klebsiella pneumoniae* carbapenemase-producing bacteria and *Candida albicans* were isolated on pus collected from abdominal drainage and on blood cultures. Therefore, VARD was decided 2 weeks after the last ETN. The patient was positioned on the left flank; the right lower costal margin and the iliac crest were marked on the skin. Ultrasound was used to localize the necrotic retroperitoneal tissue underlying the skin between markings and a 5-cm incision was performed on this site, about 2 cm above the iliac crest. Once the access to the retroperitoneal space is completed, necrotic material was evacuated by aspiration. Then, a 10-mm laparoscope was inserted through the incision without gas insufflation, and the right retroperitoneal space was explored. Debridement of necrotic material was performed by forceps and with a laparoscopic jet irrigation/suction device, and a plentiful quantity of infected debris was evacuated. When the descending part of the duodenum was visualized frontally, with the inferior vena cava being visible inferiorly and the right mesocolon superiorly, the VARD was considered completed (Fig. 5a). The

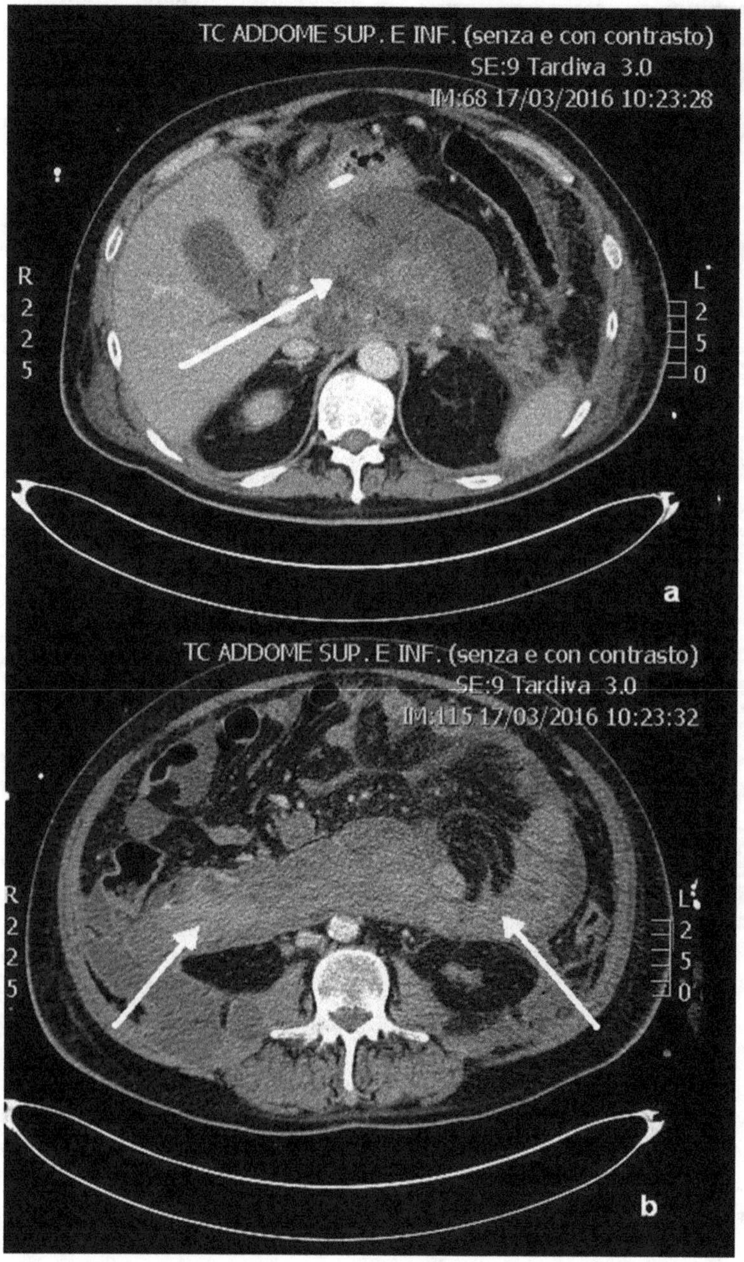

Fig. 2 CT scans after 4 weeks. Acute pancreatic necrosis is replaced by a central walled-off pancreatic necrosis (**a**, *arrow*) and lateral retroperitoneal fluid collections (**b**, *arrows*)

retroperitoneal space was then flushed with 4 L saline solution, and two 32-Fr drainages were positioned superiorly and inferiorly; the fascia and skin were closed (Fig. 5b). The procedure was uneventful, and no bleeding occurred intraoperatively or in the post-operative course. A continuous irrigation with 5 L saline solution was infused in 24 h via the superior drainage, and fluids were collected by the inferior drainage.

Subsequently, a gradual decrease of inflammatory markers was recorded together with an improvement of clinical conditions, and the patient became afebrile after 6 days from the VARD. The following CT scan demonstrated a significant reduction of all abdominal collections, being the right retroperitoneal collection sized 7.5 × 4 cm (Fig. 6). No biliary material was detected in drainages. Two weeks after VARD, all antibiotics were stopped, creatinine and serum electrolytes were in normal ranges, and CVVH was terminated. The patient was completely weaned from lung ventilation and fluid challenge, and tracheostomy was closed. Enteral feeding from naso-duodenal tube was continued; the patient was discharged from the intensive care unit and transferred

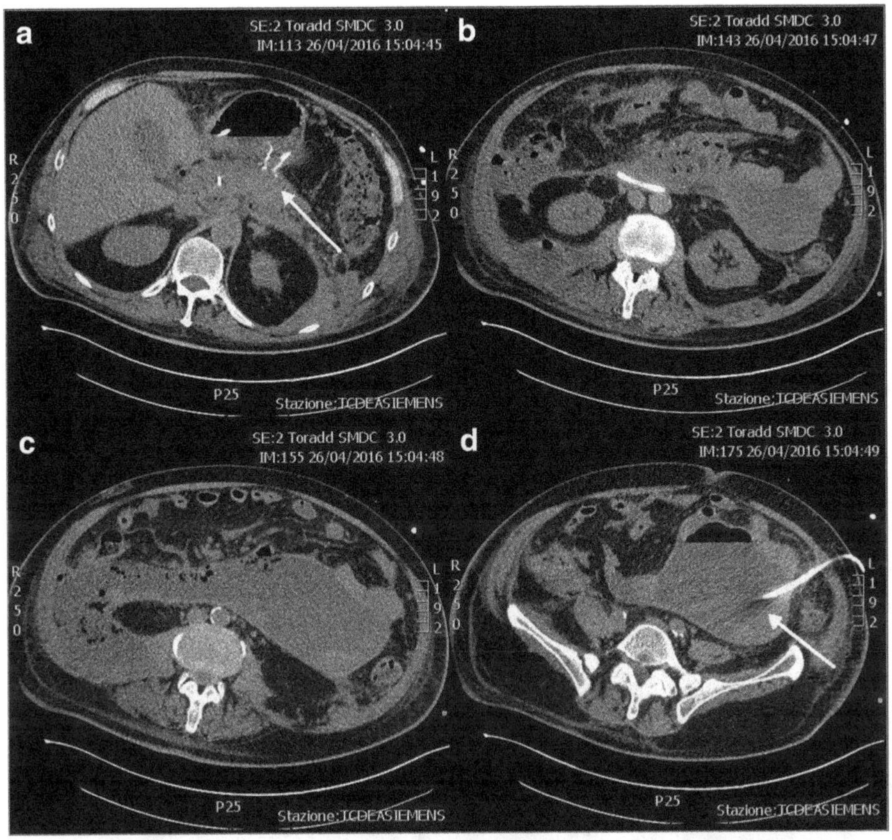

Fig. 3 a–d Transgastric necrosectomy and percutaneous drainage. The central necrotic collection has been almost completely solved after transgastric necrosectomy (**a**, *arrow*), and a percutaneous drainage was performed on the left retroperitoneal collection (**d**, *arrow*)

to the surgical ward. Subsequent CT scan showed further reduction of all intra-abdominal collections and the left drainage was removed, while only one right drainage positioned after VARD was left and continued to drain purulent material. The patient gradually started per os feeding and enteral feeding stopped. After 3 weeks, CT scan was repeated and documented reduction of the right retroperitoneal collection and the large right drainage was therefore replaced with a 10-Fr drainage which was removed after 2 weeks. The patient was discharged in good clinical conditions, and 1 month after discharge, a CT scan demonstrated resolution of the intra-abdominal collections. A subsequent ERCP was performed to remove the biliary stent but a common bile duct post-inflammatory stenosis was detected; therefore, a new 8 mm × 6 cm fully covered metallic biliary stent (Wallflex, Boston Scientific, Boston, MA, USA) was positioned (Fig. 4b). After 2 months, the transgastric metallic stent used for ETN and biliary stent were both removed, with no residual structure of the bile duct.

Literature review

A systematic review was performed by searching in PubMed the following keywords: "necrotizing pancreatitis" AND "necrosectomy" OR "VARD" OR "percutaneous drainage" OR "walled-off pancreatic necrosis". Only comparative studies or randomized clinical trials about interventions for necrotizing pancreatitis, from 2000 to 2017, were included. Sixty-eight studies were found and analyzed: 11 were excluded due to a single-arm design without a control group, 28 were excluded because they were not relevant or off-topic, 2 were excluded because outcomes were not properly reported, and 10 were excluded because they were not in English language. Therefore, a total of 18 studies were included in the systematic review (Table 1).

Since the open necrosectomy with lateral approach proposed by Fagniez for peri-pancreatic debridement through the retrocolic space, various mini-invasive techniques have been described to replace such a complicated surgery [4, 6]. Carter et al. initially described a novel technique of mini-invasive percutaneous necrosectomy by positioning under CT guidance an 8-F nephrostomy catheter into the necrotic cavity, by passing between the spleen and the splenic flexure of the colon on the left side, or through the gastrocolic omentum on the right side [10]. The path traced by this catheter was therefore gradually dilated by the surgeon to insert a

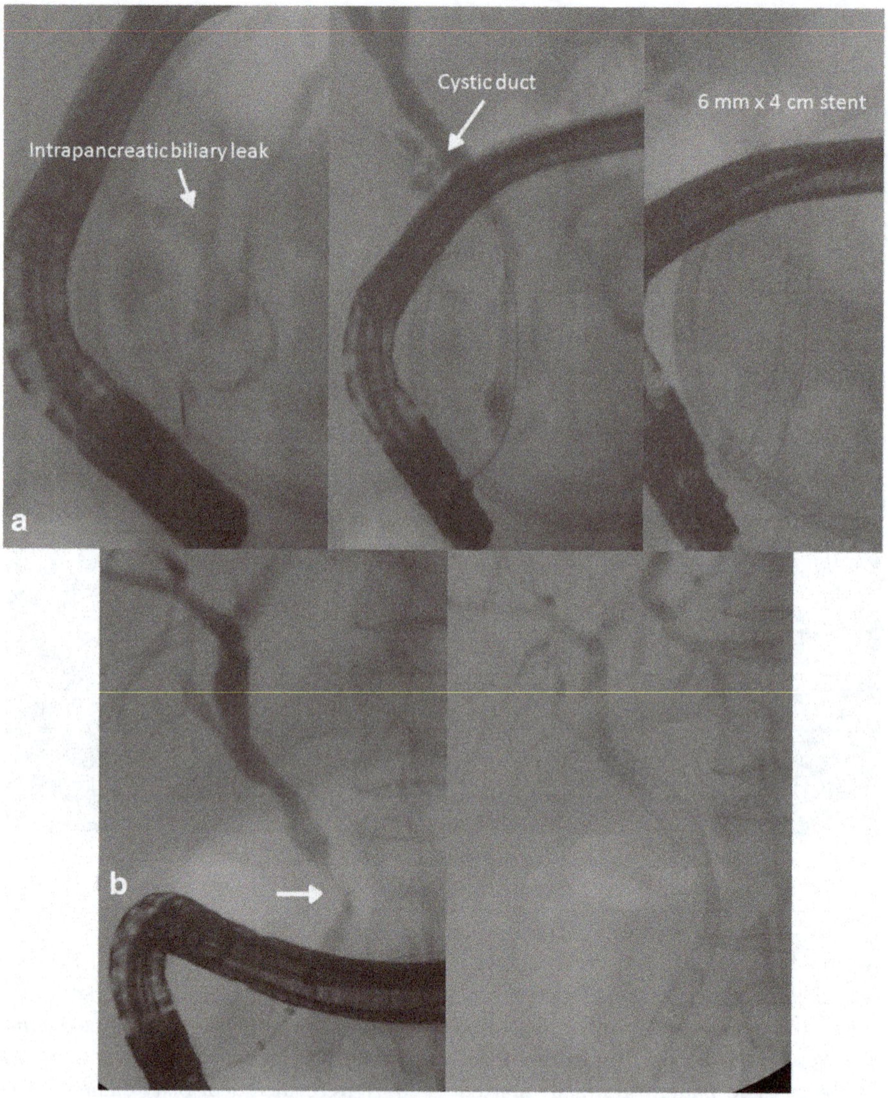

Fig. 4 ERCP and biliary stenting. Cholangiography confirmed an intrapancreatic biliary leak (*arrow*), and a 18 Fr × 4 cm biliary stent was positioned (**a**). ERCP after patient discharge demonstrated a common bile duct post-inflammatory stenosis (*arrow*), and a 24 Fr × 6 cm biliary stent was positioned (**b**)

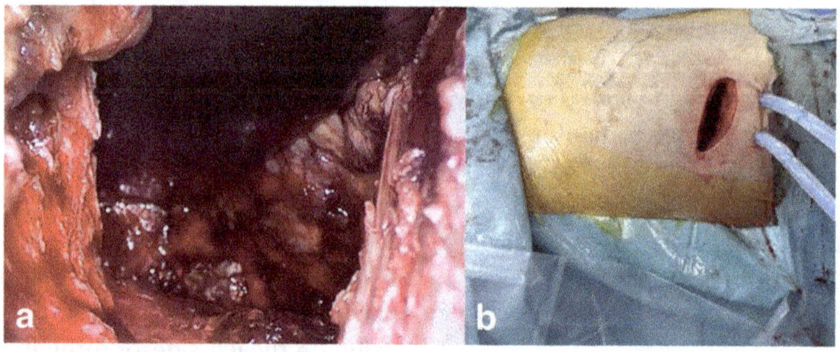

Fig. 5 Video-assisted retroperitoneal debridement. VARD was performed on the *right* retroperitoneal necrotic collection (**a**). Two large bore drains were *left* for lavage and drainage of the necrotic cavity (**b**)

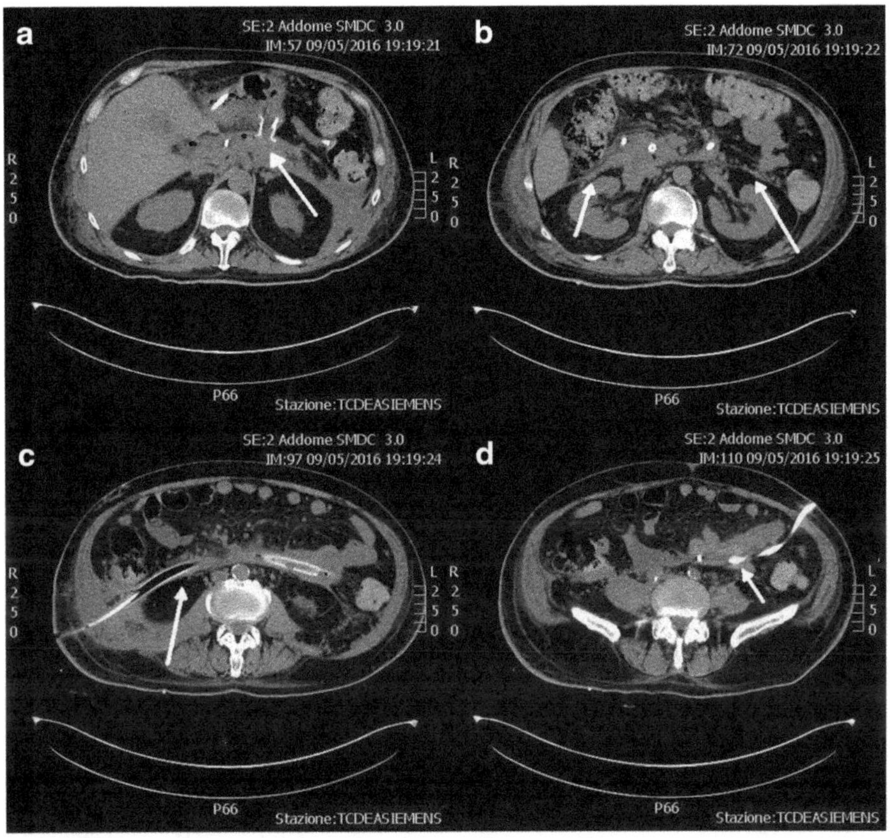

Fig. 6 a–d CT scans after VARD. After transgastric necrosectomy, VARD, and percutaneous drainage, all the retroperitoneal necrotic collections dramatically reduced (*arrows*)

30-F Amplatz, and necrosectomy was finally performed with the aid of an operative nephroscope. A post-operative continuous lavage was then allowed through positioned drains. In case of need to repeat necrosectomy, this was performed by sinus tract endoscopy using a flexible or rigid endoscope through the precedent percutaneous path, with the aid of endoscopic snares or forceps. Percutaneous necrosectomy performed after prior open surgery was compared to percutaneous necrosectomy as a first-line treatment in a comparative study on 14 patients affected by necrotizing pancreatitis: interestingly, in the latter group, open surgery was safely avoided in 80% of patients who were discharged after a median of 3 percutaneous procedures only [10]. Moreover, only 40% of these patients required post-operative intensive care unit (ICU). However, 20% mortality was reported with upfront percutaneous necrosectomy vs. 0% in patients previously treated with open necrosectomy.

After that initial experience, subsequent studies have systematically compared open necrosectomy to percutaneous necrosectomy or VARD, to assess if these minimally invasive retroperitoneal approaches were associated with better outcomes in terms of complications, mortality, and length of stay. van Santvoort and the Dutch Acute Pancreatitis Study Group have published in 2007 a comparative study on 30 patients with infected necrotizing pancreatitis: 15 patients who were treated by VARD were case-matched and compared to 15 patients subjected to standard open necrosectomy by laparotomy [11]. No significant differences were observed both in post-operative complications requiring re-intervention ($p = 1.000$) and in mortality rate ($p = 0.08$), but new-onset MOF occurred more frequently in the open necrosectomy group ($p = 0.008$). These results were encouraging and advocated the need of a randomized controlled trial on this topic.

Three years later, the same research group published the first randomized clinical trial on open necrosectomy vs. step-up approach with PD followed by VARD if necessary in a cohort of 88 patients affected by necrotizing pancreatitis, who were randomly assigned to the two treatment arms [7]. A significant reduction of new-onset MOF was confirmed with the step-up approach (12 vs. 40% with open necrosectomy, $p = 0.002$), as well as incisional hernias (7 vs. 24%, $p = 0.03$) and new-onset diabetes (16 vs. 38%, $p = 0.02$). Interestingly, major complications including visceral perforation, entero-cutaneous or pancreatic fistula, and bleeding occurred in

Table 1 Main studies assessing minimally invasive techniques for severe necrotizing pancreatitis

Study	Design	Number of cases	Outcomes	Limitations
van Santvoort et al. [7]	Open necrosectomy vs. PD ± VARD, randomized controlled trial	88 patients (45 open necrosectomy vs. 43 PD ± VARD)	Major complications occurred in 69% of open necrosectomy patients vs. 40% of PD ± VARD patients ($p = 0.006$); open necrosectomy was associated with more incisional hernias ($p = 0.03$) and new-onset diabetes ($p = 0.02$). Mortality was not different.	Trial not designed to assess differences in mortality.
Bakker et al. [22]	ETN vs. VARD or open necrosectomy, randomized controlled trial	20 patients (10 ETN vs. 10 VARD/ open necrosectomy)	ETN reduced both the proinflammatory response ($p < 0.004$) and major complications, multiple organ failure or death ($p = 0.03$)	Small number of patients
Bausch et al. [23]	VARD vs. ETN vs. open necrosectomy, retrospective study	32 patients (14 VARD vs. 18 ETN vs. 30 open necrosectomy)	Open necrosectomy had higher overall mortality ($p < 0.05$), ongoing sepsis rates and bleedings; ETN was complicated by gastric perforation in 28% of cases requiring immediate laparotomy	Small number of patients, retrospective study.
van Brunschot et al. [24]	Endoscopic transgastric drainage ± ETN vs. PD ± VARD, randomized controlled trial	98 patients	End-points are rates of major complications, need for re-interventions, quality of life, and cost-analysis between endoscopic step-up approach and surgical step-up approach. Results are still awaited.	Results still awaited
Kumar et al. [19]	ETN vs. PD ± open necrosectomy, matched cohort study	24 patients (12 ETN vs. 12 PD ± open necrosectomy)	ETN was superior in clinical remission rate ($p < 0.01$) and reduced major complications, length of stay, and post-operative health care utilization ($p < 0.01$).	Small number of patients.
Rasch et al. [25]	Open necrosectomy vs. endoscopic transgastric drainage ± ETN ± PD, retrospective multicenter study	220 patients (30 open necrosectomy vs. 190 step-up approach)	Lower complication rate (44.7 vs. 73.3%, $p < 0.001$), lower mortality (10.5 vs. 33.3%, $p = 0.002$), and lower incidence of diabetes (4.7 vs. 33.3%, $p < 0.001$) was demonstrated with step-up approach compared to open necrosectomy; 18.9% of step-up approach patients required open necrosectomy.	Retrospective study
Carter et al.[10]	Open necrosectomy + percutaneous necrosectomy vs. upfront percutaneous necrosectomy, case series	14 patients (4 open necrosectomy vs. 10 percutaneous necrosectomy)	Upfront percutaneous necrosectomy by sinus tract endoscopy had 20% mortality vs. 0% with open necrosectomy, but only 40% of patients required ICU (vs. 100%).	Retrospective case series, small number of patients
Gardner et al. [18]	Endoscopic transgastric drainage vs. ETN, retrospective study	45 patients (25 ETN vs. 20 endoscopic transgastric drainage)	Walled-off pancreatic necrosis successfully resolved in 88% of patients treated with ETN vs. 45% with endoscopic drainage ($p < 0.01$).	Retrospective study, referral center bias
Raraty et al. [12]	Open necrosectomy vs. VARD, retrospective study	189 patients (52 open necrosectomy vs. 137 VARD)	Organ failure in 31% of patients treated by VARD vs. 56% with open necrosectomy ($p < 0.0001$); 43 vs. 77% respectively required ICU support. Mortality rate was 19% with VARD vs. 38% with open necrosectomy ($p = 0.009$).	Retrospective study, referral center bias
Guo et al. [14]	Open necrosectomy vs. retroperitoneal necrosectomy, retrospective study	412 patients (108 retroperitoneal necrosectomy vs. 304 open necrosectomy)	Mortality rate was 8.3% with retroperitoneal necrosectomy vs. 20.4% with open necrosectomy ($p = 0.004$); complications rate and mean ICU stay were significantly lower.	Retrospective study
Tan et al. [20]	Open necrosectomy vs. ETN, multicentric retrospective study	32 patients (21 open necrosectomy vs. 11 ETN)	Acute complications rate was 86% in open necrosectomy vs. 27% with ETN ($p = 0.002$),	Clinical severity scores were unbalanced between groups,

Table 1 Main studies assessing minimally invasive techniques for severe necrotizing pancreatitis *(Continued)*

			ICU stay and hospitalization were significantly reduced with ETN.	retrospective study, small number of patients
Bang et al. [26]	Endoscopic transgastric drainage ± ETN vs. "algorithmic approach" including endoscopic drainage, ETN, PD, percutaneous necrosectomy, open necrosectomy, observational study	100 patients (47 endoscopic transgastric drainage ± ETN vs. 53 "algorithmic approach")	Treatment success rate equal to 91% with "algorithmic approach" vs. 60% with endoscopic drainage ± ETN ($p < 0.001$).	Observational study without randomization, unbalanced gender and race between groups
van Santvoort et al. [11]	Open necrosectomy vs. VARD, case-matched retrospective study	30 patients (15 open necrosectomy vs. 15 VARD)	Post-operative multiple organ failure occurred in 2 patients in VARD group vs. 10 patients treated by open necrosectomy ($p = 0.0008$). Complications and mortality rates were equal between groups.	Retrospective study, small number of patients
Senthil Kumar et al. [15]	Open necrosectomy vs. VARD, case-matched retrospective study	30 patients (15 open necrosectomy vs. 15 VARD)	Post-operative complications in 26.6% of patients treated by VARD vs. 53.3% of patients treated by open necrosectomy ($p = 0.248$). Re-interventions, ICU stay, and hospitalization were similar.	Retrospective study, small number of patients
Pupelis et al. [16]	Open necrosectomy vs. ultrasound-focused necrosectomy, prospective study	58 patients (36 necrosectomy vs. 22 focused necrosectomy)	Resolution of sepsis was earlier with focused necrosectomy; ICU stay longer with open necrosectomy ($p = 0.024$).	Mini-invasive transgastric or percutaneous techniques not considered.
Tu et al. [13]	Open necrosectomy vs. VARD, retrospective study	50 patients (32 open necrosectomy vs. 18 VARD)	VARD was associated with shorter operative time (130 vs. 148 min, $p = 0.007$) and shorter hospitalization (40.8 vs. 55.9 days, $p = 0.053$) compared to open necrosectomy. Fewer complications with VARD (43.8 vs. 27.8%).	Retrospective study
Gluck et al. [17]	Endoscopic transgastric drainage + PD vs. PD only, retrospective study	95 patients (49 endoscopic drainage + PD vs. 46 PD only)	Endoscopic drainage + PD significantly reduced hospitalization, CT scans, and ERCPs ($p < 0.05$) compared to PD only.	Retrospective study
Woo et al. [21]	Endoscopic transgastric drainage or ETN vs. open necrosectomy vs. PD	30 patients (12 endoscopic treatment vs. 8 PD vs. 10 open necrosectomy)	Mean hospitalization time was 62 days with endoscopic treatment vs. 101 days with PD and 91 days with open necrosectomy ($p = 0.046$). Pancreatic fistula and new-onsetdiabetes were more frequent with open necrosectomy ($p = 0.04$, $p = 0.012$).	Retrospective study, small number of patients

***PD*, percutaneous drainage, *ETN* endoscopic transgastric necrosectomy, *VARD* video-assisted retroperitoneal debridement**

40% of patients treated by the step-up approach vs. 69% of patients treated by open necrosectomy ($p = 0.006$). However, mortality was equal between groups and the study was not designed to assess a difference in mortality. Notably, up to 35% of patients in the step-up approach group were successfully treated with PD only without the need of subsequent VARD, suggesting that aggressive necrosectomy could be spared in favor of simple drainage of infected fluid in a substantial proportion of patients.

According to these findings, a large retrospective study on 189 patients treated in a tertiary referral center demonstrated a significant benefit of VARD over open necrosectomy in terms of needed ICU support ($p < 0.0001$) and complications (55 vs. 81%, $p = 0.001$) [12]. Moreover, this study demonstrated also a significant reduction in mortality with VARD (19 vs. 38%, $p = 0.016$), being the use of a minimally invasive necrosectomy an independent predictor of mortality together with age and preoperative status of MOF. Other advantages associated with VARD and globally to retroperitoneal approaches compared to open necrosectomy with anterior laparotomy were shorter operative times and shorter hospitalization in two more recent large-population retrospective study [13, 14]. Conversely to these evidence, Senthil Kumar et al. reported that post-operative complications were fewer but not significantly different with VARD compared to open necrosectomy, being re-intervention rate, ICU stay, and overall hospital stay similar between groups [15]. This study was case-matched, but its retrospective design and the small size of cohort could explain those controversial findings.

Interestingly, retroperitoneal debridement could be further improved by ultrasound-guided navigation and positioning of percutaneous catheters. Pupelis et al. demonstrated an earlier resolution of sepsis and a shorter ICU stay with ultrasound-guided focused necrosectomy compared to conventional open necrosectomy in a cohort of 58 patients [16]. Minimally invasive retroperitoneal necrosectomy and PD are particularly suitable in case of lateral necrotic collections extended in the retroperitoneal gutters, but central WOPN are much less manageable with these approaches. Endoscopic transgastric routes could represent a better indication for such collections. Recently, Gluck et al. have retrospectively evaluated the clinical impact of adding endoscopic transgastric drainage to PD compared to PD alone on 95 cases of necrotizing pancreatitis [17]. Endoscopic drainage led to shorter length of stay, fewer CT scans, and reduced use of ERCP ($p < 0.05$), although mortality did not vary between cohorts.

However, endoscopic drainage can easily resolve fluid collections, while it could be less effective for mostly solid WOPN. Indeed, in 2009, Gardner and colleagues investigated the use of endoscopic transgastric drainage vs. ETN and found that WOPN successfully resolved in 88% of patients treated by ETN vs. 45% of patients treated by endoscopic drainage only, with the same number of procedures ($p < 0.01$) [18]. Subsequently, two studies have explored the clinical benefit of ETN vs. PD or open necrosectomy: ETN was found to be superior in clinical remission rate, reduced complications, shorter hospitalization, and ICU stay [19, 20]. In particular, major complications were recorded in 86% of open necrosectomy patients vs. 27% only in ETN patients [20]. More recently, Woo et al. retrospectively compared ETN, PD, and open necrosectomy on 30 patients: the mean hospitalization time was 62 days with ETN, 91 days with open necrosectomy, and 101 days with PD ($p = 0.046$), but pancreatic fistula and new-onset diabetes were more frequent with open necrosectomy [21].

Then, literature review demonstrated that both retroperitoneal and endoscopic transgastric mini-invasive techniques are associated with less complications compared to open necrosectomy in management of infected or unsolving or symptomatic WOPN. However, few clinical trials have compared the alternative use of these minimally invasive procedures, and fewer studies have investigated and reported their combination. The PENGUIN trial investigated the use of ETN in 10 patients compared to open necrosectomy or VARD in 10 patients and demonstrated superiority of the former technique in terms of reduced global morbidity and mortality rate, from 80 to 20% [22]. These results should be prudently considered, but certainly, a noninferiority of ETN versus VARD could be inferred. Conversely, a retrospective study on 62 patients comparing open necrosectomy vs. VARD and vs. ETN showed a significant reduction both in complications and in mortality with the mini-invasive approaches compared to open necrosectomy [23]. Notably, both VARD and ETN were superior to open surgery, but the two mini-invasive techniques themselves had almost equivalent outcomes. Interestingly, the rate of re-laparotomy was higher in the ETN group because of free gastric perforation, a specific complication of the technique which occurred in 28% of cases, particularly when a proper transgastric window for the procedure with a large contact between gastric wall and WOPN is not present.

More recently, the TENSION trial has been designed to compare the surgical step-up approach (PD followed by VARD) versus the endoscopic step-up approach (endoscopic transgastric drainage followed by ETN); results of the TENSION trial are intensely expected [24]. However, again the two pathways have been considered as separate alternatives and not as possibly combined procedures. Conjugation of the two techniques has been recently reported in literature for the first time on a patient with severe acute pancreatitis complicated by infected WOPN extended laterally to the retroperitoneal spaces, similarly to our patient [8]. In this case report, the WOPN was complicated by multiple enteric fistulae, and endoscopic transgastric drainage was necessarily completed by VARD for a proper control of retroperitoneal collections, suggesting that a mini-invasive approach combining all the abovementioned techniques could maximize the clinical benefit in the critically ill patient [8].

Indeed, as previously stated, ETN is preferable for management of pancreatic or peri-pancreatic WOPN, while lateral collections are preferentially treated by PD or VARD based on the proportion of fluid and solid necrosis. Moreover, lateral collections could spread not only from a medial WOPN as a result of necrosis extension but also if retroperitoneal compartmentalization is lost after transgastric necrosectomy and lavage through a naso-cystic tube, with subsequent spread of necrotic fluids in communicating recesses and cavities. In these cases, PD for fluid collections and VARD for more solid collections may be taken in consideration.

A large retrospective study has compared open necrosectomy vs. a step-up approach consisting in transgastric drainage and/or ETN and/or PD in 220 patients affected by severe necrotizing pancreatitis [25]. Interestingly, this study assessed the usefulness of combination of transgastric and percutaneous routes to control infected necrosis, although the use of VARD was not reported. The study showed a markedly reduced complications rate with the step-up approach (44.7 vs. 73.3%, $p < 0.001$), together with lower mortality (10.5 vs. 33.3%, $p = 0.002$) and lower incidence of diabetes (4.7 vs. 33.3%, $p < 0.001$) compared to open necrosectomy. However, 18.9% of step-up approach patients later required open necrosectomy [25].

Finally, an observational study without randomization on 100 patients has compared upfront endoscopic transgastric drainage with or without ETN vs. a so-called algorithmic approach which consisted of a stepwise combined approach based on size and location of WOPN [26]. If WOPN was central and <12 cm in diameter, endoscopic transgastric drainage was performed as a first-line treatment. In case of WOPN >12 cm or extended to the retroperitoneal gutters or not responding after endoscopic transgastric drainage, ETN was performed by creating multiple transgastric conduits (multiple transluminal gateway technique). Suboptimal response after four procedures was probably related to the prevalent lateral extension of WOPN into the retroperitoneum; therefore, a percutaneous sinus tract endoscopic necrosectomy was subsequently performed. In case of failure of the abovementioned techniques, open necrosectomy was considered. Interestingly, treatment success rate was significantly higher for "algorithmic approach" compared to upfront endoscopic drainage or ETN (91 vs. 60%, $p < 0.001$) [26]. Moreover, using the algorithmic approach was the only independent predictor of successful treatment, although open necrosectomy was included among treatments. This study was not designed as a randomized trial and VARD was not used; therefore, its findings should be cautiously considered. However, it suggests that even open necrosectomy could still be a proper indication as a last chance in selected patients, if a wise and thoughtful combination of minimally invasive approaches is used. The key for success for WOPN management could rely in a proper timing of multiple adequate treatments, rather than in type of treatment itself.

Discussion

The step-up approach is becoming a treatment option for necrotizing acute pancreatitis instead of early surgery. Its philosophy is expressed by the "3D" concept: delay, drain, and debride [27]. It means that the optimal management should include a first step of intensive care treatment for recovery from challenging clinical conditions, waiting the formation of WOPN. Generally, this step should last 4 weeks at least, when a well-defined walled-off necrosis or pseudocyst is expected. Then, a second step for percutaneous or endoscopic drainage should follow, eventually completed by the third step which consists of minimally invasive surgery if debridement is needed [6, 27].

In the presented case, 6 weeks were necessary before a well-defined, although not capsulated, necrotic collection near the pancreatic head was visible. Since the worsening of clinical conditions notwithstanding maximal intensive care support, an ETN was first attempted for central WOPN, while PD was preferred on the left retroperitoneal collection since it was mostly fluid and in a lateral position, easily approachable by ultrasound exploiting the lumbar window. However, despite a significant reduction in size of these infected collections after repeated ETN with a proper antibiotic therapy, sepsis control was still not achieved and the right retroperitoneal collection progressively increased. The VARD was chosen instead of PD because of the semi-solid nature of the right collection. VARD allowed a prompt and extensive debridement of most of the right retroperitoneal infected necrosis, with a fast resolution of severe sepsis.

Most of the abovementioned studies have demonstrated a better clinical outcome with minimally invasive techniques compared to open necrosectomy. However, due to the heterogeneity of these studies and between each case of necrotizing pancreatitis, definitive evidence-based conclusions about the best surgical approach are currently difficult to be drawn. Only few randomized clinical trials are available on this topic, but these evidence could be biased by small number of patients or a study design not suitable to assess differences in mortality, which should be a main endpoint. Several other studies were based on retrospectively reviewed cohorts of patients treated in different centers or in the same hospital but by different surgeons with different approaches and different timings. Therefore, the differences in outcomes between open necrosectomy and minimally invasive techniques could be also explained by the delayed time often occurred before the use of ETN or PD or VARD compared to open necrosectomy and not only by significant morbidity associated with surgical necrosectomy itself [28]. Moreover, other variables could have impacted on outcomes, such as the preferential use of early enteral feeding or the possible clinical stabilization in ICU before any invasive procedure. This point was endorsed by the recent work by Bang and colleagues, which demonstrated that a step-by-step approach even including open necrosectomy could be associated with a significantly higher success rate than endoscopic debridement as a stand-alone therapy [26]. These data suggest that probably, it is not the specific technique itself to determine the outcome, but a wise multi-staged combined approach with adequate timing, possibly including surgical necrosectomy if indicated.

Furthermore, minimally invasive techniques are not free from severe complications. Severe hemorrhage is widely reported, occurring in up to 20% of patients after VARD [7, 23]. A mortality rate up to 30–40% is observed in case of procedure-related hemorrhage, being this risk particularly high in early procedures due to the intensively vascularized inflammatory collections and the frequent impairment in coagulation [6]. Therefore, a hybrid room should be available 24/24 for emergency hemorrhage control, both intravascular and/or surgical, in case of life-threatening bleeding.

Also, colonic perforation is reported as a complication of VARD in 15% of patients, but it is unusual if necrosectomy is avoided in the first weeks, thanks to the easier feasibility after procedure delay [29, 30]. Therefore, avoiding necrosectomy in the first weeks after necrotizing pancreatitis facilitates procedures on necrotic collections and improves the outcome, as what occurred in our case.

A specific complication of ETN could be gastric perforation. In the trial by Bausch et al., ETN was associated with gastric perforation in about one third of patients, who required immediate laparotomy [23]. Moreover, extended or repeated ETN could lead to iatrogenic injuries to the common bile duct or pancreas, with subsequent biliary or pancreatic fistula. In our case, a biliary leakage became evident in the third ETN, suggesting biliary fistulization with the WOPN. Biliary fistula secondary to acute pancreatitis has been rarely reported, and its pathogenesis could be related to the peri-pancreatic necrotic erosion of the common bile duct as well as direct necrosis or autodigestion of the extrahepatic biliary system, or possible iatrogenic injury during necrosectomy [31–33].

In our case, biliary fistula was not evident on CT scan since classical signs such as air into the biliary tree or interruption of choledocal wall opening into the WOPN were not visible; however, the appearance of bile in the WOPN cavity during necrosectomy may be considered a direct sign of biliary fistula [32]. ERCP confirmed the presence of biliary fistula involving distal common bile duct. Management options include primary reconstruction of bile duct with or without Kehr tube, biliary diversion, and in extremis, pancreaticoduodenectomy [9, 32–34]. Since the biliary lesion appeared to be small, a stenting was decided with resolution of the leak. Bilio-pancreatic endoscopy and stenting still has not a clear role in severe necrotizing pancreatitis complicated by biliary fistula, while its role in case of fistulization to pseudocyst is much more practiced [35, 36].

Our case suggests that the evident advantages of minimally invasive techniques should be always cautiously considered together with their potential drawbacks. Maybe treating our patient with delayed open necrosectomy without ETN would have spared a biliary complication to the patient, shortening the clinical course with a better clinical outcome. A priori exclusion of open necrosectomy, if indicated, should be discouraged. Moreover, a delayed VARD was necessary due to ongoing sepsis and extended WOPN after several weeks from admission, probably because endoscopic necrosectomy was not sufficient to achieve an adequate local control of the WOPN. Therefore, a single minimally invasive technique could be inadequate to provide a resolution in such cases of necrotizing pancreatitis. A persistent repetition of a single treatment, even if minimally invasive, could lead to further complications beyond those directly related to the disease itself and should be discouraged.

Conclusions

To the best of our knowledge, the case presented is the first one of severe necrotizing pancreatitis complicated by biliary fistula treated by a combination of ETN, PD, VARD, and ERCP with biliary stenting. Delay of any procedure after 4–6 weeks from the onset of pancreatitis could be helpful for patient stabilization. ETN, VARD, and PD should be tailored on localization (medial vs. lateral, retroperitoneal vs. intraperitoneal) and on quality (mostly fluid vs. mostly solid) of the collections. A combination of different approaches, even including open necrosectomy when indicated, could significantly optimize the clinical management in critically ill patients affected by complicated necrotizing pancreatitis. Recent literature supports that mini-invasive approaches are associated with better outcomes over early open necrosectomy. However, minimally invasive techniques are not free from complications, and surgical necrosectomy should not be excluded a priori and could still have an indication in some cases of necrotizing pancreatitis.

Abbreviations

ARDS: Acute respiratory distress syndrome; CVVH: Continuous veno-venous hemofiltration; ERCP: Endoscopic retrograde cholangiopancreatography; ETN: Endoscopic transgastric necrosectomy; MOF: Multi-organ failure; PD: Percutaneous drainage; VARD: Video-assisted retroperitoneal debridement; WOPN: Walled-off pancreatic necrosis

Acknowledgements

Not applicable.

Funding

No funding was provided for this study.

Authors' contributions

LS, OC, FS, and SC contributed to the design and drafting of the manuscript and performed and described the surgical procedure. MM performed and described the endoscopic procedures. PB followed and described the management of the patient in the intensive care unit. All authors edited, read, and approved the final manuscript.

Competing interests

The authors declare that they have no competing interests.

Author details

[1]Trauma Team and Emergency Surgery, Niguarda Trauma Center, Niguarda Ca' Granda Hospital, Piazza Ospedale Maggiore 3, Milan 20162, Italy. [2]Digestive Endoscopy Service, Niguarda Ca' Granda Hospital, Piazza Ospedale Maggiore 3, Milan 20162, Italy. [3]Intensive Care Unit, Niguarda Trauma Center, Niguarda Ca' Granda Hospital, Piazza Ospedale Maggiore 3, Milan 20162, Italy.

References

1. Trikudanathan G, Attam R, Arain MA, Mallery S, Freeman ML. Endoscopic interventions for necrotizing pancreatitis. Am J Gastroenterol. 2014;109(7):969–81.
2. Werge M, Novovic S, Schmidt PN, Gluud LL. Infection increases mortality in necrotizing pancreatitis: a systematic review and meta-analysis. Pancreatology. 2016; Jul 9 [Epub ahead of print].
3. Larvin M, McMahon MJ. APACHE-II score for assessment and monitoring of acute pancreatitis. Lancet. 1989;2(8656):201–5.
4. Fagniez PL, Panis Y. Surgical treatment of acute pancreatitis. Rev Prat. 1996; 46(6):704–8.
5. Hackert T, Büchler MW. Decision making in necrotizing pancreatitis. Dig Dis. 2016;34(5):517–24.
6. Logue JA, Carter CR. Minimally invasive necrosectomy techniques in severe acute pancreatitis: role of percutaneous necrosectomy and video-assisted retroperitoneal debridement. Gastroenterol Res Pract. 2015;2015:693040.
7. van Santvoort HC, Besselink MG, Bakker OJ, Hofker HS, Boermeester MA, Dejong CH, van Goor H, Schaapherder AF, van Eijck CH, Bollen TL, van Ramshorst B, Nieuwenhuijs VB, Timmer R, Laméris JS, Kruyt PM, Manusama ER, van der Harst E, van der Schelling GP, Karsten T, Hesselink EJ, van Laarhoven CJ, Rosman C, Bosscha K, de Wit RJ, Houdijk AP, van Leeuwen MS, Buskens E, Gooszen HG, Dutch Pancreatitis Study Group. A step-up approach or open necrosectomy for necrotizing pancreatitis. N Engl J Med. 2010;362(16):1491–502.
8. Fagenholz PJ, Thabet A, Mueller PR, Forcione DG. Combined endoscopic trangastric drainage and video assisted retroperitoneal pancreatic debridement—the best of both worlds for extensive pancreatic necrosis with enteric fistulae. Pancreatology 2016; Jun 19 [Epub ahead of print].
9. Chaudhary A, Sachdev A, Negi S. Biliary complications of pancreatic necrosis. Int J Pancreatol. 2001;29(3):129–31.
10. Carter CR, McKay CJ, Imrie CW. Percutaneous necrosectomy and sinus tract endoscopy in the management of infected pancreatic necrosis: an initial experience. Ann Surg. 2000;232(2):175–80.
11. van Santvoort HC, Besselink MG, Bollen TL, Buskens E, van Ramshorst B, Gooszen HG, Dutch Acute Pancreatitis Study Group. Case-matched comparison of the retroperitoneal approach with laparotomy for necrotizing pancreatitis. World J Surg. 2007;31(8):1635–42.
12. Raraty MG, Halloran CM, Dodd S, Ghaneh P, Connor S, Evans J, Sutton R, Neoptolemos JP. Minimal access retroperitoneal pancreatic necrosectomy: improvement in morbidity and mortality with a less invasive approach. Ann Surg. 2010;251(5):787–93.
13. Tu Y, Jiao H, Tan X, Sun L, Zhang W. Laparotomy versus retroperitoneal laparoscopy in debridement and drainage of retroperitoneal infected necrosis in severe acute pancreatitis. Surg Endosc. 2013;27(11):4217–23.
14. Guo Q, Lu H, Hu W, Zhang Z. A retroperitoneal approach for infected pancreatic necrosis. Scand J Gastroenterol. 2013;48(2):225–30.
15. Senthil Kumar P, Ravichandran P, Jeswanth S. Case matched comparison study of the necrosectomy by retroperitoneal approach with transperitoneal approach for necrotizing pancreatitis in patients with CT severity score of 7 and above. Int J Surg. 2012;10(10):587–92.
16. Pupelis G, Fokin V, Zeiza K, Plaudis H, Suhova A, Drozdova N, Boka V. Focused open necrosectomy in necrotizing pancreatitis. HPB (Oxford). 2013;15(7):535–40.
17. Gluck M, Ross A, Irani S, Lin O, Gan SI, Fotoohi M, Hauptmann E, Crane R, Siegal J, Robinson DH, Traverso LW, Kozarek RA. Dual modality drainage for symptomatic walled-off pancreatic necrosis reduces length of hospitalization, radiological procedures, and number of endoscopies compared to standard percutaneous drainage. J Gastrointest Surg. 2012;16(2):248–56.
18. Gardner TB, Chahal P, Papachristou GI, Vege SS, Petersen BT, Gostout CJ, Topazian MD, Takahashi N, Sarr MG, Baron TH. A comparison of direct endoscopic necrosectomy with transmural endoscopic drainage for the treatment of walled-off pancreatic necrosis. Gastrointest Endosc. 2009;69(6):1085–94.
19. Kumar N, Conwell DL, Thompson CC. Direct endoscopic necrosectomy versus step-up approach for walled-off pancreatic necrosis: comparison of clinical outcome and health care utilization. Pancreas. 2014;43(8):1334–9.
20. Tan V, Charachon A, Lescot T, Chafaï N, Le Baleur Y, Delchier JC, Paye F. Endoscopic transgastric versus surgical necrosectomy in infected pancreatic necrosis. Clin Res Hepatol Gastroenterol. 2014;38(6):770–6.
21. Woo S, Walklin R, Wewelwala C, Berry R, Devonshire D, Croagh D. Interventional management of necrotizing pancreatitis: an Australian experience. ANZ J Surg. 2015 Nov 24 [Epub ahead of print]
22. Bakker OJ, van Santvoort HC, van Brunschot S, Geskus RB, Besselink MG, Bollen TL, van Eijck CH, Fockens P, Hazebroek EJ, Nijmeijer RM, Poley JW, van Ramshorst B, Vleggaar FP, Boermeester MA, Gooszen HG, Weusten BL, Timmer R, Dutch Pancreatitis Study Group. Endoscopic transgastric vs surgical necrosectomy for infected necrotizing pancreatitis: a randomized trial. JAMA. 2012;307(10):1053–61.
23. Bausch D, Wellner U, Kahl S, Kuesters S, Richter-Schrag HJ, Utzolino S, Hopt UT, Keck T, Fischer A. Minimally invasive operations for acute necrotizing pancreatitis: comparison of minimally invasive retroperitoneal necrosectomy with ETN. Surgery. 2012;152(3):S128–34.

24. van Brunschot S, van Grinsven J, Voermans RP, Bakker OJ, Besselink MG, Boermeester MA, Bollen TL, Bosscha K, Bouwense SA, Bruno MJ, Cappendijk VC, Consten EC, Dejong CH, Dijkgraaf MG, van Eijck CH, Erkelens GW, van Goor H, Hadithi M, Haveman JW, Hofker SH, Jansen JJ, Laméris JS, van Lienden KP, Manusama ER, Meijssen MA, Mulder CJ, Nieuwenhuis VB, Poley JW, de Ridder RJ, Rosman C, Schaapherder AF, Scheepers JJ, Schoon EJ, Seerden T, Spanier BW, Straathof JW, Timmer R, Venneman NG, Vleggaar FP, Witteman BJ, Gooszen HG, van Santvoort HC, Fockens P, Dutch Pancreatitis Study Group. Transluminal endoscopic step-up approach versus minimally invasive surgical step-up approach in patients with infected necrotising pancreatitis (TENSION trial): design and rationale of a randomised controlled multicenter trial [ISRCTN09186711]. BMC Gastroenterol. 2013;13:161.
25. Rasch S, Phillip V, Reichel S, Rau B, Zapf C, Rosendahl J, Halm U, Zachäus M, Müller M, Kleger A, Neesse A, Hampe J, Ellrichmann M, Rückert F, Strauß P, Arlt A, Ellenrieder V, Gress TM, Hartwig W, Klar E, Mössner J, Post S, Schmid RM, Seufferlein T, Siech M, Werner J, Will U, Algül H. Open surgical versus minimal invasive necrosectomy of the pancreas—a retrospective multicenter analysis of the German Pancreatitis Study Group. PLoS One. 2016;11(9):e0163651.
26. Bang JY, Holt BA, Hawes RH, Hasan MK, Arnoletti JP, Christein JD, Wilcox CM, Varadarajulu S. Outcomes after implementing a tailored endoscopic step-up approach to walled-off necrosis in acute pancreatitis. Br J Surg. 2014;101(13):1729–38.
27. Besselink MG. The 'step-up approach" to infected necrotizing pancreatitis: delay, drain, debride. Dig Liver Dis. 2011;43(6):421–2.
28. Doctor N, Philip S, Gandhi V, Hussain M, Barreto SG. Analysis of the delayed approach to the management of infected pancreatic necrosis. World J Gastroenterol. 2011;17(3):366–71.
29. Ulagendra Perumal S, Pillai SA, Perumal S, Sathyanesan J, Palaniappan R. Outcome of video-assisted translumbar retroperitoneal necrosectomy and closed lavage for severe necrotizing pancreatitis. ANZ J Surg. 2014;84(4):270–4.
30. Besselink MG, van Santvoort HC, Nieuwenhuijs VB, Boermeester MA, Bollen TL, Buskens E, Dejong CH, van Eijck CH, van Goor H, Hofker SS, Lameris JS, van Leeuwen MS, Ploeg RJ, van Ramshorst B, Schaapherder AF, Cuesta MA, Consten EC, Gouma DJ, van der Harst E, Hesselink EJ, Houdijk LP, Karsten TM, van Laarhoven CJ, Pierie JP, Rosman C, Bilgen EJ, Timmer R, van der Tweel I, de Wit RJ, Witteman BJ, Gooszen HG, Dutch Acute Pancreatitis Study Group. Minimally invasive 'step-up approach' versus maximal necrosectomy in patients with acute necrotising pancreatitis (PANTER trial): design and rationale of a randomised controlled multicenter trial [ISRCTN13975868]. BMC Surg. 2006;6:6.
31. Sakorafas GH, Sarr MG, Farnell MB. Pancreaticobiliary fistula: an unusual complication of necrotising pancreatitis. Eur J Surg. 2001;167(2):151–3.
32. Brar R, Singh I, Brar P, Prasad A, Doley RP, Wig JD. Pancreatic choledochal fistula complicating acute pancreatitis. Am J Case Rep. 2012;13:47–50.
33. Dhall JC, Marwah S, Singh RB, Marwah N, Mathur SK. Extra-hepatic biliary-ductal necrosis in acute pancreatitis: a rare complication. Pediatr Surg Int. 2000;16(3):209–10.
34. Miller BM, Traverso LW, Freeny PC. Intrapancreatic communication of bile and pancreatic ducts secondary to pancreatic necrosis. Arch Surg. 1988;123(8):1000–3.
35. Al Ali JA, Chung H, Munk PL, Byrne MF. Pancreatic pseudocyst with fistula to the common bile duct resolved by combined biliary and pancreatic stenting—a case report and literature review. Can J Gastroenterol. 2009;23(8):557–9.
36. Wysocki AP, McKay CJ, Carter CR. Infected pancreatic necrosis: minimizing the cut. ANZ J Surg. 2010;80(1-2):58–70.

13

Bologna guidelines for diagnosis and management of adhesive small bowel obstruction (ASBO): 2013 update of the evidence-based guidelines from the world society of emergency surgery ASBO working group

Salomone Di Saverio[1†], Federico Coccolini[5], Marica Galati[1], Nazareno Smerieri[1], Walter L Biffl[4], Luca Ansaloni[5], Gregorio Tugnoli[1], George C Velmahos[7], Massimo Sartelli[8], Cino Bendinelli[13], Gustavo Pereira Fraga[17], Michael D Kelly[3], Frederick A Moore[11], Vincenzo Mandalà[6], Stefano Mandalà[6], Michele Masetti[1], Elio Jovine[1], Antonio D Pinna[2], Andrew B Peitzman[16], Ari Leppaniemi[15], Paul H Sugarbaker[9], Harry Van Goor[10], Ernest E Moore[4], Johannes Jeekel[12] and Fausto Catena[2,14*†]

Abstract

Background: In 2013 Guidelines on diagnosis and management of ASBO have been revised and updated by the WSES Working Group on ASBO to develop current evidence-based algorithms and focus indications and safety of conservative treatment, timing of surgery and indications for laparoscopy.

Recommendations: In absence of signs of strangulation and history of persistent vomiting or combined CT-scan signs (free fluid, mesenteric edema, small-bowel feces sign, devascularization) patients with partial ASBO can be managed safely with NOM and tube decompression should be attempted. These patients are good candidates for Water-Soluble-Contrast-Medium (WSCM) with both diagnostic and therapeutic purposes. The radiologic appearance of WSCM in the colon within 24 hours from administration predicts resolution. WSCM maybe administered either orally or via NGT both immediately at admission or after failed conservative treatment for 48 hours. The use of WSCM is safe and reduces need for surgery, time to resolution and hospital stay.

NOM, in absence of signs of strangulation or peritonitis, can be prolonged up to 72 hours. After 72 hours of NOM without resolution, surgery is recommended.

Patients treated non-operatively have shorter hospital stay, but higher recurrence rate and shorter time to re-admission, although the risk of new surgically treated episodes of ASBO is unchanged. Risk factors for recurrences are age <40 years and matted adhesions. WSCM does not decrease recurrence rates or recurrences needing surgery.

Open surgery is often used for strangulating ASBO as well as after failed conservative management. In selected patients and with appropriate skills, laparoscopic approach is advisable using open access technique. Access in left

(Continued on next page)

* Correspondence: faustocatena@gmail.com
†Equal contributors
[2]Emergency Surgery Unit, Department of General and Multivisceral Transplant Surgery, S Orsola Malpighi University Hospital, Bologna, Italy
[14]Department of Emergency and Trauma Surgery, Maggiore Hospital of Parma, Parma, Italy
Full list of author information is available at the end of the article

(Continued from previous page)
upper quadrant or left flank is the safest and only completely obstructing adhesions should be identified and lysed with cold scissors. Laparoscopic adhesiolysis should be attempted preferably if first episode of SBO and/or anticipated single band. A low threshold for open conversion should be maintained.
Peritoneal adhesions should be prevented. Hyaluronic acid-carboxycellulose membrane and icodextrin decrease incidence of adhesions. Icodextrin may reduce the risk of re-obstruction. HA cannot reduce need of surgery.
Adhesions quantification and scoring maybe useful for achieving standardized assessment of adhesions severity and for further research in diagnosis and treatment of ASBO.

Background of WSES guidelines

Adhesive small bowel obstruction requires appropriate management with a proper diagnostic and therapeutic pathway. Indication and length of Non Operative treatment and appropriate timing for surgery may represent an insidious issue.

Delay in surgical treatment may cause a substantial increase of morbidity and mortality. However repeated laparotomy and adhesiolysis may worsen the process of adhesion formation and their severity. Furthermore the introduction and widespread of laparoscopy has raised the question of selection of appropriate patients with ASBO good candidate for laparoscopic approach. On the other hand, several adjuncts for improving the success rate of NOM and clarifying indications and timing for surgery are currently available, such as hyperosmolar water soluble contrast medium.

No consensus has been reached in diagnosing and managing the patients with ASBO and specific and updated guidelines are lacking.

We carried out an extensive review of the English-language literature and found that there was little high-level evidence in this field, and no systematically described practical manual for the field. Most importantly, there are no standardized diagnostic criteria and therapeutic management guidelines for ASBO, therefore, we would like to establish standards for these items. The Bologna Guidelines include evidence-based medicine and reflect the international consensus obtained through earnest discussions among professionals in the field on 1–3 July, 2010, at the Belmeloro Convention Center, Bologna, Italy.

We aimed to validate and refine the first version of the guidelines, hypothesizing that a model, incorporated in a treatment algorithm, would be predictive, would prevent delayed management of strangulation and would be successfully improved.

Therefore in 2013 the guidelines have been revised and updated by the WSES Working Group on ASBO with the development of diagnosis and treatment evidence-based algorithms (Figure 1, Figure 2).

Furthermore a customary management can help to standardize care throughout a district, a region, or a state satisfying the corporate governance requirements of "clinical efficacy" and "economic efficiency" with the results of improved outcomes and decreased costs.

Improvement of performance is a mainstay of any practice management guideline.

Notes on the use of the guidelines

The Guidelines are evidence-based, with the grade of recommendation also based on the evidence. The Guidelines present the diagnostic and therapeutic methods for optimal management and prevention of ASBO.

The practice Guidelines promulgated in this work do not represent a standard of practice. They are suggested plans of care, based on best available evidence and the consensus of experts, but they do not exclude other approaches as being within the standard of practice. For example, they should not be used to compel adherence to a given method of medical management, which method should be finally determined after taking account of the conditions at the relevant medical institution (staff levels, experience, equipment, etc.) and the characteristics of the individual patient. However, responsibility for the results of treatment rests with those who are directly engaged therein, and not with the consensus group.

Definition

Abdominal adhesions, which can begin forming within a few hours after an operation, represent the most common cause of intestinal obstruction being responsible for 60% to 70% of SBO [1,2]. Adhesional postoperative small bowel obstruction is characterized by the presence of abdominal pain, vomiting, distention, and obstipation, in conjunction of confirmatory imaging.

Risk factors

Patients with ASBO treated nonsurgically have shorter hospital stay, however they have an higher recurrence rate, shorter time to re-admission, although the risk of new surgically treated episodes of ASBO is the same (Level of Evidence 2b).

SBO can be classified according to completeness: Partial vs. Complete (or high grade vs. low grade), according to etiology: Adhesional vs. Non-adhesional, according to timing: Early vs. Late (>30 days after surgery).

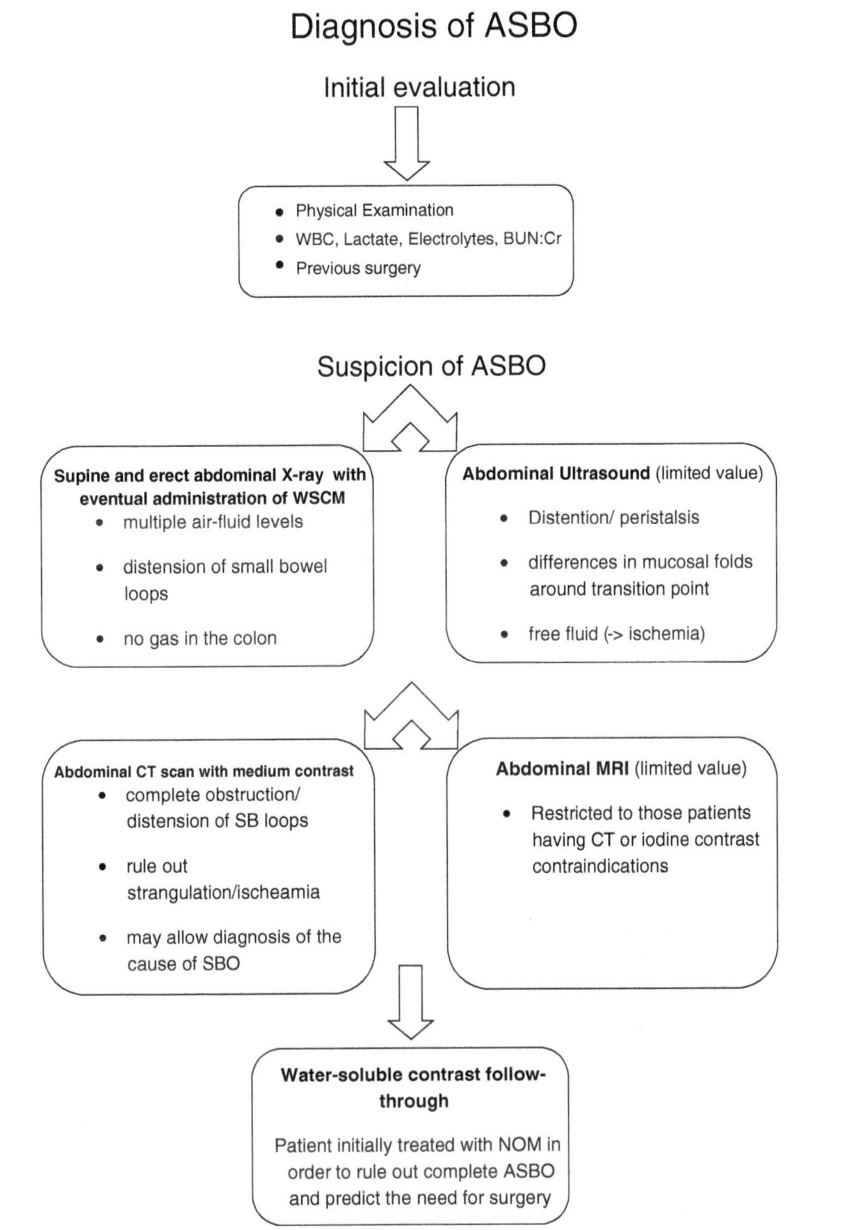

Figure 1 **Evidence-based Algorithm for Diagnosis and Assessment of ASBO.**

Even if Zielinski and Bannon proposed to switch the traditional focus of differentiating SBO to one of predicting failure of NOM with the goal of exploring patients with expected failure as soon as possible [3].

The most important risk factor for adhesive SBO is the type of surgery and extent of peritoneal damage.

The technique of the procedure (open VS laparoscopic) play an important role in the development of adhesion related morbidity. In a retrospective review of 446.331 abdominal operation, Galinos et al. noticed that the incidence was 7.1% in open cholecystectomies vs 0.2% in laparoscopic; 15.6 in open total abdominal hysterectomies vs 0.0% in laparoscopic; 23.9% in open adnexal operations vs 0.0% in laparoscopic and there was no significant difference between open and laparoscopic appendectomies (1.4% vs 1.3%) [4].

In a further recent paper Reshef et al. compared the risk of ASBO in 205 patients who underwent laparoscopic colorectal surgery and 205 who underwent similar open operations, both without any previous history of open surgery. After a mean follow-up of 41 months the authors found that although the rate of admission for ASBO was similar (9% vs 13%, $p = 0.3$ for the laparoscopic and the open group), the need for operative

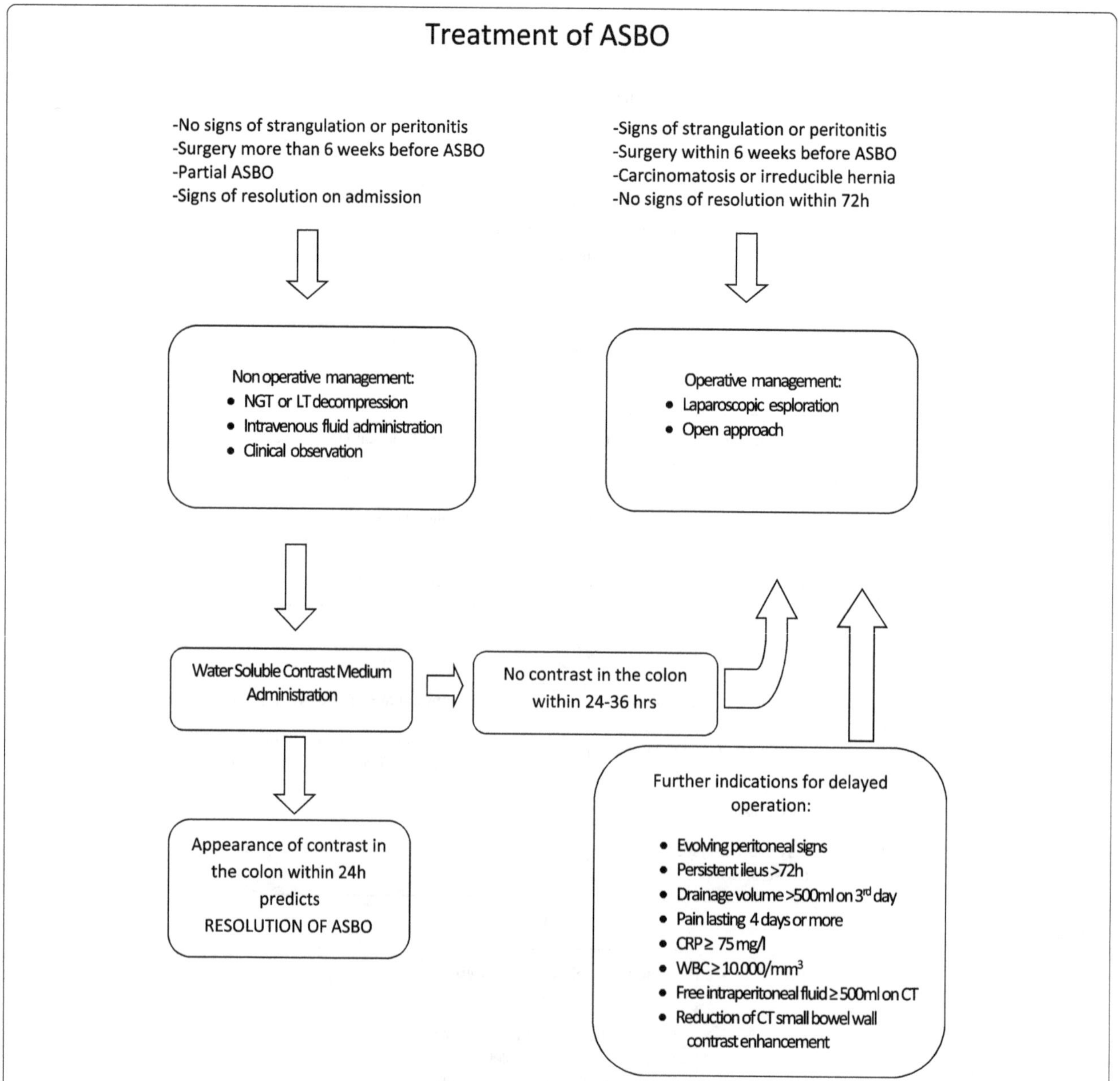

Figure 2 Evidence-based Algorithm for Management and Treatment of ASBO.

intervention for ASBO was significantly lower after laparoscopic operations (2% vs 8%, $p = 0.006$). These data suggest that the lower incidence of adhesions expected after laparoscopic surgery likely translates into long-term benefits in terms of reduced SBO [5].

Other well-known risk factors include surgeries of the colon and rectum (i.e. total colectomy with ileal pouch-anal anastomosis), gynecologic surgeries, age younger than 60 years, previous laparotomy within 5 years, peritonitis, multiple laparotomies, emergency surgery, omental resection, and penetrating abdominal trauma, especially gunshot wounds, a high number of prior episodes of ASBO [1-10].

Initial evaluation

After an accurate physical examination and the evaluation of WBC, Lactate, Electrolytes, BUN/Creat; first step of diagnostic work up for ASBO is supine and erect plain abdominal X-ray which can show multiple air-fluid levels, distension of small bowel loops and the absence of gas in the colonic section [11].

All patients being evaluated for small bowel obstruction should have plain films (Level of Evidence 2b GoR C).

Secondary evaluation

CT scan is highly diagnostic in SBO and has a great value in all patients with inconclusive plain films for complete or high grade SBO [12]. However CT-scans should not be routinely performed in the decision-making process except when clinical history, physical examination, and plain film are not conclusive for small bowel obstruction diagnosis [13] (Level of Evidence 2b GoR B).

CT scan often allows to confirm the presence of complete obstruction, to reach the diagnosis of the cause of SBO, it also exclude a non-adhesional pathology and assess the occurrence of strangulation with a sensitivity and specificity higher than 90% and a NPV of nearly 100% [14].

The association of CT scan signs of bowel ischemia should lead a low threshold for surgical intervention (Level of Evidence 2a GoR B).

Ultrasound has a limited value in bowel obstruction or in patients with distended bowel, because the air may obscure the underlying findings. Usual US findings are: distention, peristalsis (differential diagnosis of ileus vs. mechanical SBO), differences in mucosal folds around transition point, free fluid (sign of ischemia) [15].

MRI use should be restricted to those patients having CT or iodine contrast contraindications (Level of Evidence 2c GoR C).

Water-soluble contrast follow-through is valuable in patients undergoing initial non operative conservative management in order to rule out complete ASBO and predict the need for surgery [16] (Level of Evidence 1b GoR A). Water-soluble contrast administration has both diagnostic and therapeutic value [17,18].

This investigation is safer than barium in cases of perforation and peritoneal spread and has possible therapeutic value in the case of adhesive small intestine obstruction [19].

Conservative treatment and timing for surgery

The management of ASBO is controversial because surgery can induce new adhesions, whereas conservative treatment does not remove the cause of the obstruction [20]. Conservative treatment involves nasogastric intubation, intravenous fluid administration, and clinical observation. Strangulation of the bowel requires immediate surgery, but intestinal ischemia can be difficult to determine clinically.

Potentially, acute care surgery (ACS) model may adversely affect patients who present with SBO because they may be handed over from surgeon to surgeon without definitive care. These patients may not require an operation initially but may require one subsequently because of the development of complications or if the SBO does not resolve with conservative treatment.

In an Australian retrospective study Lien et al. observed that, in the ACS period, there was no significant difference in complication rates or length of hospital stay in those who were not handed over and those who were, both in the pre-ACS and ACS period.

The authors suggested that clinical handover may provide an 'audit-point' for patient management and opportunity for collaborative input. Moreover, participation of doctors with greater clinical experience may minimize errors in information transfer due to increased acumen in recognizing potential complications [21].

A delay in operation for SBO places patients at higher risk for bowel resection. In a retrospective review Leung and coll find that younger patients ($P = 0.001$), no previous operation ($P < 0.001$), and absence of adhesive disease ($P < 0.001$) were more likely to go to operation. Acquiring a CT scan ($P = 0.029$) or radiograph ($P < 0.001$) were factors that increased time to the operating room (OR). In the group with time to OR less than 24 hours, 12% of patients had bowel resection versus time to OR greater than 24 hours, 29% of them required bowel resection [22].

Several issues are raised when managing patients with ASBO.

Operative management VS Non operative management

Patients without the signs of strangulation or peritonitis or history of persistent vomiting or combination of CT scan signs (free fluid, mesenteric edema, lack of feces signs, devascularized bowel) and partial ASBO can safely undergo non-operative management (LoE 1a GoR A). In these patients tube decompression should be attempted (Level of Evidence 1b GoR A), either with NGT or LT [23].

In conservatively treated patients with ASBO, the drainage volume through the long tube on day 3 (cut-off value; 500 mL) was the indicator for surgery [24].

Also in patients with repeated episodes and many prior laparotomies for adhesions, prolonged conservative treatment (including parenteral nutritional support) may be prudent and often avoid a complex high-risk procedure [25], but the use of supplementary diagnostic tools might be desirable to find the patients who will need early operative treatment [26].

Patients who had surgery within the six weeks before the episode of small bowel obstruction, patients with signs of strangulation or peritonitis (fever, tachycardia and leucocytosis, metabolic acidosis and continuous pain), patients with irreducible hernia and patients who started to have signs of resolution at the time of admission are NOT candidate for conservative treatment +/− WSCA administration (Level of Evidence 1a GoR A) [27,28].

Complete SBO (no evidence of air within the large bowel) and increased serum creatine phosphokinase predicts NOM failure (Level of Evidence 2b GoR C). Free intraperitoneal fluid, mesenteric edema, lack of the "small bowel feces sign" at CT, and history of vomiting, severe abdominal pain ($VAS > 4$), abdominal guarding, raised WCC and devascularized bowel at CT predict the need for emergent laparotomy at the time of admission (Level of Evidence 2c GoR C).

The appearance of water-soluble contrast in the colon on abdominal X ray within 24 hours of its administration predicts resolution of ASBO (Level of Evidence 1a GoR A). Among patients with ASBO initially managed with a conservative strategy, predicting risk of operation is difficult.

Tachycardia, fever, focal tenderness, increased white blood cell counts, and elevated lactate levels can indicate intestinal ischemia, but these indicators are not very specific [29]. When intestinal ischemia is unlikely, a conservative approach can be followed for 24–48 h.

Zielinski and Bannon in a recent review suggest to combine data from oral contrast meal with their predictive model which identifies patients with mesenteric edema, lack of the small bowel feces signs and obstipation from 12 hours at high risk. The authors recommend urgent exploration for any patient presenting with signs of strangulation or all three of the new model features on admission and without contrast in the colon within 8 hours of administration [3].

Moreover Schraufnagel et al. in n univariate analyses shown that complications, resection, prolonged length of stay and death are more likely in patients admitted for ASBO and operated on the fourth day or later [30].

Non operative management

There are no advantages with the use of long tube decompression compared with the use of nasogastric tubes (Level of Evidence 1b GoR A) [23,31].

However early tube decompression, either with long or nasogastric tube, may be beneficial (Level of Evidence 2b GoR C) in the initial management of non strangulating ASBO, in adjunct with fluid resuscitation and electrolytes imbalances correction. For challenging cases of ASBO, the long tube should be placed as soon as possible [24] more advisable by endoscopy, rather than by fluoroscopic guide [32].

The use of Gastrografin in ASBO is safe (in terms of morbidity and mortality) and reduces the need for surgery, the time to resolution of obstruction and the hospital stay (Level of Evidence 1a GoR A) [16,19,33-35]. Nevertheless anaphylactoid reaction and lethal aspiration have been described [36].

Gastrografin may be administered on the dosage of 50–150 ml, either orally or via NGT and can be given both at immediately admission or after an attempt of initial traditional conservative treatment of 48 hours (Level of Evidence 1b GoR A).

Regarding the therapeutic value of Gastrografin, some authors affirmed that water-soluble contrast reduces the hospital stay but does not reduce the need for surgery [27,37,38], others has proven that is effective in both reducing the need for surgery and shortening hospital stay, without differences in complications and mortality [28].

As further adjuncts needs to be mentioned that oral therapy with magnesium oxide, L. acidophilus and simethicone may hasten the resolution of conservatively treated partial ASBO and shorten the hospital stay (Level of Evidence 1b GoR A) [39].

To be thorough it has to be mentioned Hyperbaric oxygen (HBO) therapy, that appears to be beneficial in older patients with high anesthesiologic risk (Level of Evidence 2b GoR B). HBO therapy may be an option in the management of patients for whom surgery should be avoided [40].

Indication for delayed operation

Usually NOM, in absence of signs of strangulation or peritonitis, can be prolonged up to 72 hours of adhesive SBO (Level of Evidence 2b GoR C) [41].

After 3 days without resolution, WSCA study or surgery is recommended (Level of Evidence 2b GoR C) [31].

If ileus persists more than 3 days and the drainage volume on day 3 is > 500 ml, surgery for ASBO is recommended (Level of Evidence 2b GoR C) [24].

With closely monitoring and in the absence of signs suggestive of complications, an observation period even longer than 10 days before proceeding to surgical intervention appears to be safe [42].

However at any time, if onset of fever and leukocytosis greater than 15 000/mm3 (predictors of intestinal complications) are observed, then NOM should be discontinued and surgery is recommended.

The patients non responders to the long-tube and conservative treatment within 72 hours have a considerable risk of recurrent ASBO (Level of Evidence 2b GoR C).

Risk factors for recurrences are age <40 years, matted adhesion (Level of Evidence 1b GoR A) and postoperative surgical complications [43].

Gastrografin use does not affect the recurrences rates or recurrences needing surgery when compared to traditionally conservatively treated patients (Level of Evidence 1b GoR A) [19].

Surgical treatment: open VS laparoscopic approach

Open surgery is the preferred method for the surgical treatment of strangulating ASBO and after failed conservative management (LOE 2c GOR C).

In highly selected group of patients the laparoscopic can be attempted using an open access technique (LOE 2c GOR C).

The access in the left upper quadrant should be safe (LOE 4 GOR C).

Laparoscopic lysis of adhesions should be attempted preferably in case of first episode of SBO and/or anticipated single band adhesion (i.e. SBO after appendectomy or hysterectomy) (LOE 3b GOR C).

A low threshold for open conversion should be maintained if extensive adhesions are found (LOE 2c GOR C).

Conversion to laparoscopic-assisted adhesiolysis (mini-laparotomy with an incision less than 4 cm long) or laparotomy should be considered in those patients presenting with dense or pelvic adhesion (LOE 3b GOR C).

The extent of adhesiolysis is a matter still under debate. The approaches to adhesiolysis for bowel obstruction among general surgeons in the United Kingdom were established in 1993 [44]. Half of all surgeons divided all adhesions to prevent recurrence of bowel obstruction, whereas the other half limited adhesiolysis to only the adhesions responsible for the obstruction.

The risk of anterior abdominal wall adhesions increases with the number of previous laparotomies although this relationship is not as evident as the relationship between previous laparotomies and adhesiolysis-induced enterotomy [45,46].

Higher age and higher number of previous laparotomies appeared to be predictors of the occurrence of inadvertent enterotomy [46]. Patients with three or more previous laparotomies had a 10-fold increase in enterotomy compared with patients with one or two previous laparotomies strongly suggesting more dense adhesion reformation after each reoperation.

Historically, laparotomy and open adhesiolysis have been the treatment for patients requiring surgery for small bowel obstruction. Unfortunately, this often leads to further formation of intraabdominal adhesions with approximately 10% to 30% of patients requiring another laparotomy for recurrent bowel obstruction [29].

In animal models laparoscopy has been shown to decrease the incidence, extent, and severity of intraabdominal adhesions when compared with open surgery, thus potentially decreasing the recurrence rate for adhesive small bowel obstruction [47].

Tolutope and Scott administered a questionnaire to all the general surgeons registered in the state of Connecticut, trying to know their opinions about the use of laparoscopic lysis of adhesions (LLA) to manage adhesive small bowel obstruction compared with open lysis of adhesions (OLA) in terms of safety, contraindications, and outcomes.

According to their self-reports, 60% of the respondents used LLA in their practice, with 38% of this group using LLA for less than 15% of their adhesive SBO cases. Compared with surgeons out of training more than 15 years, a greater number of surgeons out of training less than 15 years considered LLA to be safer (P = 0.03) and to have better outcomes (P = 0.04) than OLA. More surgeons in academic/teaching hospitals considered LLA to be safe than did surgeons in nonacademic/nonteaching settings (P = 0.04), and more members of the Society of American Gastrointestinal and Endoscopic Surgeons/ Society of Laparoendoscopic Surgeons, considered LLA to be safe than nonmembers (P = 0.001).

These data suggest that recent training and interest or membership in minimally invasive surgery associations influence surgeons' choice for laparoscopic lysis of adhesions [48].

Laparoscopy seems to have an advantage above laparotomy in terms of adhesion formation to the abdominal wall and to the operative site [49,50], both because of no further scar on anterior parietal peritoneum and because usually the exploration of the ileum is limited to solve the cause of obstruction, extending the dissection until the ligament of Treitz only when the cause of obstruction is not be detected [51].

Laparoscopic adhesiolysis for small bowel obstruction has a number of potential advantages: (1) less postoperative pain, (2) faster return of intestinal function, (3) shorter hospital stay, (4) reduced recovery time, allowing an earlier return to full activity, (5) decreased wound complications, and (6) decreased postoperative adhesion formation [52,53].

These data have been validated in a meta-analysis in which Ming-Zhe Li et al. found that there was no statistically significant difference between open versus laparoscopic adhesiolysis in the number of intraoperative bowel injuries, nor for wound infections, neither with respect to the overall mortality. Conversely there was a statistically significant difference concerning pulmonary complications and a considerable reduction in prolonged ileus in the laparoscopic group compared with the open group. The authors sustain that laparoscopic approach is safer than the open procedure, but in the hands of experienced laparoscopic surgeons in selected patients [54].

Besides Stephanian et al. observed that minimal trauma, short duration of the operation, good cosmetic results and uncomplicated course of postoperative period witness the efficacy of laparoscopic approach [55].

In a consensus conference on laparoscopic adhesiolysis, an italian panel of experts recommended intraoperative selection of patients after esploratory laparoscopy, because this approach allows as many patients as possible to benefit from this mini-invasive procedure. They agree that the only absolute exclusion criteria for laparoscopic adhesiolysis in SBO are those related to pneumoperitoneum (i.e. hemodynamic instability or cardiopulmonary impairment); all other contraindication are relative and shoud be judjed on a case-to-case basis, depending on the laparoscopic skills of the surgeon. Moreover non resolving partial incomplete SBO(after a negative Gastrografin test) and chronic obstructive symptoms are the ideal application for laparoscopic adhesiolysis with rates of conversion as low as 8.7% [56].

However no randomized controlled trial comparing open to laparoscopic adhesiolysis exists up to date, and both the precise indications and specific outcomes of laparoscopic adhesiolysis for adhesive SBO remain poorly understood. The only RCT on laparoscopic adhesiolysis assessed the incidence of chronic abdominal pain after randomization to laparoscopic adhesiolysis or no treatment during diagnostic laparoscopy and it failed to demonstrate any significant differences in terms of pain or discomfort [57].

Although data from a retrospective clinical controlled trial suggest that laparoscopy seems feasible and better in terms of hospital stay and mortality reduction [58].

In a retrospective analiysis Grafen et al. compared the outcomes of laparoscopic management of ASBO to both exploratory laparotomy and secondary conversion to open surgery. 93 patients were divided into successful laparoscopy (71%), secondary conversion (26%) and primary laparotomy (3%). The first group had more simple adhesions, fewer prior operations, lower ASA score, shortest operative time, as was the duration of both intensive care unit and hospital stay; moreover they were younger and had a shorter duration of SBO prior to their operation. Despite that mortality was 6%, regardless of operative technique. The authors, moreover, found that patients who only had prior appendectomy or cholecystectomy could all be managed laparoscopically without need for secondary conversion; on the other hand a prolonged ileus (mean 4.3 days) with progressive abdominal distension and a higher number or more demanding previous operations address to a primary laparotomy. Finally the reasons for converting to open adhesiolysis were: inadequate laparoscopic control due to intestinal distension, extensive adhesions, iatrogenic perforations and resection of necrotic segments [59].

When deciding between an open or laparoscopic approach, the first consideration is that the surgeon be trained and capable of performing advanced laparoscopy.

With regards to patient selection, individuals with an acute small bowel obstruction and peritonitis, free air or gangrenous bowel requiring an emergent operation are best managed with a laparotomy. Patients without peritonitis who do not resolve with nonoperative management should be considered for laparoscopic adhesiolysis. In these cases, it is important to consider the bowel diameter, degree of abdominal distention, and location of the obstruction (ie, proximal or distal). Suter et al. [60] found that a bowel diameter exceeding 4 cm was associated with an increased rate of conversion: 55% versus 32%. Patients with a distal and complete small bowel obstruction have an increased incidence of intraoperative complications and increased risk of conversion. Patients with persistent abdominal distention after nasogastric intubation are also unlikely to be treated successfully with laparoscopy.

The influence of dense adhesions and the number of previous operations on the success of laparoscopic adhesiolysis is controversial. León et al. state that a documented history of severe or extensive dense adhesions is a contraindication to laparoscopy [61]. In contrast, Suter et al. found no correlation between the number and or type of previous surgeries and the chance of a successful laparoscopic surgery [60]. Other factors such as an elevated white blood cell count or a fever have not been demonstrated to correlate with an increased conversion rate. One group of patients who are good candidates for laparoscopic adhesiolysis are those with a nonresolving, partial small bowel obstruction or a recurrent, chronic small bowel obstruction demonstrated on contrast study [61,62].

In an Irish systematic review of over 2000 cases of ASBO, 1284 (64%) were successfully treated with a laparoscopic approach, 6.7% were lap-assisted, and 0.3% were converted to hernia repair; the overall conversion rate to midline laparotomy was 29%. Dense adhesions, bowel resection, unidentified pathology and iatrogenic injury accounted for the majority of conversions. When the etiology was attributed to a single-band adhesion, the success rate was 73.4%. Morbidity and mortality were respectively 14.8% and 1.5%. The inadvertent enterotomy rate was 6.6%. In this perspective laparoscopy seems to be feasible and effective treatment for ASBO with acceptable morbidity [63].

Navez et al. reported that when the cause of obstruction was a single band, laparoscopic adhesiolysis was successful 100% of the time [64].

When other etiologies are found, such as internal hernia, inguinal hernia, neoplasm, inflammatory bowel disease, intussusception, and gallstone ileus, conversion to a minilaparotomy or a formal laparotomy is often required.

Inadvertent enterotomy during reopening of the abdomen or subsequent adhesion dissection is a feared complication of surgery after previous laparotomy. The incidence can be as high as 20% in open surgery and between 1% and 100% in laparoscopy [65].

The incidence of intraoperative enterotomies during laparoscopic adhesiolysis ranges from 3% to 17.6%, with most authors reporting an incidence of about 10% [66,67].

One of the most dreaded complications of surgery is a missed enterotomy. Although a missed enterotomy can occur after laparotomy, the incidence is higher after laparoscopic surgery.

The long-term results regarding recurrence are limited, with most series reporting a mean follow-up between 12 and 24 months.

Feasibility of diagnostic laparoscopy is ranging from 60% to 100% whilst therapeutic effectiveness of the laparoscopic approach is lower (40-88%). Predictive factors for successful laparoscopic adhesiolysis are: number of previous laparotomies ≤2, non-median previous laparotomy, appendectomy as previous surgical treatment causing adherences, unique band adhesion as pathogenetic mechanism of small bowel obstruction, early laparoscopic management within 24 hours from the onset of symptoms, no signs of peritonitis on physical examination, experience of the surgeon [68,69].

Surgical operating time is greater in patients who underwent laparoscopic surgery compared to patients who underwent a laparotomy [70,71].

Postoperative morbidity is lower in patients who underwent laparoscopic adhesiolysis compared to those who underwent the laparotomic approach. Furthermore a greater rate of morbidity is present in patients who underwent laparotomic conversion; whereas mortality is comparable in the two groups (0-4%). Finally the laparoscopic adhesiolysis can avoid laparotomy, which is itself a cause of new adhesions and bowel obstruction, although some authors noticed a greater incidence of recurrent small bowel obstructions in patients who underwent laparoscopy compared to those in which a laparotomy was performed [72,73].

Operative technique has a capital role for a successful laparoscopic treatment [52]. The initial trocar should be placed away (alternative site technique) from the scars in an attempt to avoid adhesions. Some investigators have recommended the use of computed tomography scan or ultrasonography to help determine a safe site for the initial trocar insertion.

The left upper quadrant or the left flank are usually the safest safe place to gain access to the abdominal cavity. Alternatively a 10 mm port can be inserted in the left flank with two additional 5 mm ports in the left upper and lower quadrant (or 10 mm and 5 mm respectively) [74]. Therefore, by triangulating 3 ports aimed at the right lower quadrant, a good exposure and access to the right iliac fossa can be obtained and a technique running the small bowel in a retrograde fashion, starting from the ileocecal valve (decompressed intestine) proximally towards the transition point between collapsed and dilated loops.

The open (Hasson) approach under direct vision is the more prudent. Once safe access is obtained, the next goal is to provide adequate visualization in order to insert the remaining trocars. This often requires some degree of adhesiolysis along the anterior abdominal wall. Numerous techniques are available, including finger dissection through the initial trocar site and using the camera to bluntly dissect the adhesions. Sometimes, gentle retraction on the adhesions will separate the tissue planes. Most often sharp adhesiolysis is required. The use of cautery and ultrasound dissection should be limited or possibly avoided in order to prevent thermal tissue damage and bowel injury [74].

The risk of enterotomy can be reduced if meticulous care is taken in the use of atraumatic graspers only and if the manipulation of friable, distended bowel is minimized by handling the mesentery of the bowel whenever possible [74]. In fact to handle dilated and edematous bowel during adhesiolysis is dangerous and the risk increases with a long lasting obstruction; this is the reason why early operation is advisable as one multicenter study showed: the success rate for early laparoscopic intervention for acute SBO is significantly higher after a shorter duration of symptoms (24 h vs 48 h) [75].

After trocar placement, the initial goal is to expose the collapsed distal bowel [74]. This is facilitated with the use of angled telescopes and maximal tilting/rotating of the surgical table. It may also be necessary to move the laparoscope to different trocars to improve visualization. Only pathologic adhesions should be lysed. Additional adhesiolysis only adds to the operative time and to the risks of surgery without benefit. The area lysed should be thoroughly inspected for possible bleeding and bowel injury.

In conclusion, careful selection criteria for laparoscopy [76] may be: (1) Hemodynamic stability and patient not in shock, (2) absence of peritonitis or severe intra-abdominal sepsis, (3) proximal i.e. SB obstruction, (4) localized distension on radiography, and/or (5) absence of severe abdominal distension, (6) anticipated single band, (7) low or intermediate predicted PAI score in < = 3 abdominal quadrants, and last but not least (8) the experience and laparoscopic skills of the surgeon. A partial obstruction is better first approached with a non-operative challenge with hyperosmolar water soluble contrast medium with both therapeutic and diagnostic purposes. A complete SB obstruction should no longer be considered an exclusion criteria for laparoscopic approach.

The experts panel also agreed, as from the cited studies, that laparoscopic lysis of adhesions should be attempted preferably in case of first episode of SBO and/or anticipated single band adhesion (i.e. SBO after appendectomy or hysterectomy). Previous midline incision is not an absolute exclusion criteria for laparoscopic approach.

A multicenter series of 103 patients from the WSES - Iitalian Working Group on peritoneal adhesions and ASBO management, presented at the 2013 Clinical Congress of American College of Surgeons [77], described a safe and effective surgical technique for laparoscopic approach to ASBO and confirmed that laparoscopy should be attempted preferably in case of first episode of SBO and/or anticipated single band adhesion (i.e. SBO after appendectomy or hysterectomy). A low threshold for open conversion should be maintained if extensive adhesions are found, as often occurs in patients with previous midline laparotomy and multiple surgeries. Previous midline laparotomy incision and multiple previous episodes of ASBO with estimated PAI score of > =2 in more than 3 abdominal regions, were significantly associated in this series with increased risk of conversion and longer operative times.

Prevention

We do need to prevent ASBO (LOE 2b GoR B).

In view of the incidence of adhesions and recurrence rates of ASBO as well as of the magnitude of the medical problems and financial burden related to adhesions, prevention or reduction of postoperative adhesions in an important priority. Hyaluronic acid-carboxycellulose membrane and icodextrin are able to reduce adhesions (respectively LOE 1a GOR A and LOE 1b GOR A).

Icodextrin may reduce the risk of re-obstruction for ASBO (LOE 1 b GOR A).

Hyaluronic acid-carboxycellulose can not reduce the need of surgery for ASBO (LOE 1a GOR A).

Most of the available literature is based on gynecologic patients. For general surgical patients no recommendations or guidelines exist.

Any prevention strategy should be safe, effective, practical, and cost effective. A combination of prevention strategies might be more effective [78].

In the same review the authors recommend a laparoscopic approach if possible, the use of bioabsorbable barriers, a meticulous hemostasis, avoiding excessive tissue dissection and ischemia and reducing remaining surgical material [78].

In the long term follow up study from Fevang et al. [79] the surgical treatment itself decreased the risk of future admissions for ASBO, even though the risk of new surgically treated ASBO episodes was the same regardless of the method of treatment (surgical vs conservative).

Intraoperative techniques such as avoiding unnecessary peritoneal dissection, avoiding spillage of intestinal contents or gallstones [80], and the use of starch-free gloves [81-83] are basic principles that should be applied to all patients.

In most abdominal procedures the laparoscopic approach is associated with a significantly lower incidence of adhesive SBO or adhesion-related re-admission [79,83].

There is some class I evidence in obstetrics supporting the theory that suturing the peritoneum increases the risk of adhesions [84].

Concerning mechanical barriers no progresses has been made in the last 6 years. The authors remain convinced that the absorbable adhesion barrier Interceed reduces the

PERITONEAL ADHESION INDEX:

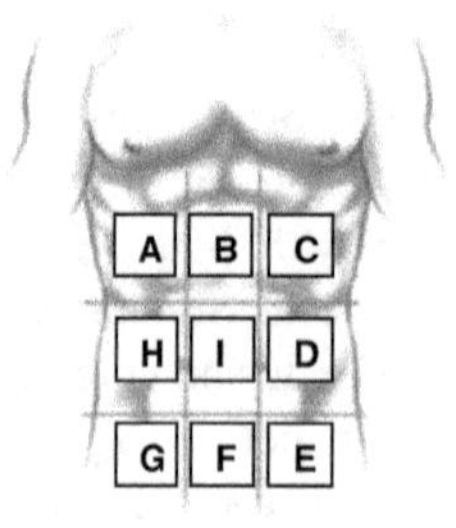

Regions:	Adhesion grade:
A Right upper	___
B Epigastrium	___
C Left upper	___
D Left flank	___
E Left lower	___
F Pelvis	___
G Right lower	___
H Right flank	___
I Central	___
L Bowel to bowel	___

Adhesion grade score:

0 No adhesions

1 Filmy adhesions, blunt dissection

2 Strong adhesions, sharp dissection

3 Very strong vascularized adhesions, sharp dissection, damage hardly preventable

PAI ☐

Figure 3 Peritoneal adhesion index: by ascribing to each abdomen area an adhesion related score as indicated, the sum of the scores will result in the PAI.

incidence of adhesion formation following laparoscopy and laparotomy [85-90]. Gore-Tex may be superior to Interceed in preventing adhesion formation but its usefulness is limited by the need for suturing and later removal [91]. There was no evidence of effectiveness of Seprafilm and Fibrin sheet in preventing adhesion formation [92-99].

Chemical/fluid agents have the theoretical advantage of covering more potential sites of adhesion formation than mechanical barriers.

In the newest P.O.P.A. study Catena et al. randomized 91 patients to have 2000 cc of icodextrin 4% and 90 to have the traditional treatment. The authors noted no significant difference in the incidence of small bowel leakage or anastomotic breakdown; operative times, blood losses, incidence of small bowel resections, return of bowel function, LOS, early and late morbility and mortality was comparable. After a mean follow-up of 41.4 months, there have been 2 cases of ASBO recurrence in the icodextrin group and 10 cases in the control group ($p < 0.05$). Only one patient in the first group was submitted to surgery showing an Adhesion Severity Score = 2, whereas three patients in the latter group were operated, and the ASS was respectively 3,2 and 3. In accordance with this data, the use of icodextrin 4% solution seems to be safe and effective to prevent intra-abdominal adhesion formation and the risk of re-obstruction [100].

Intergel solution (Lifecore Biomedical, Inc, Chaska, MN), which contains .5% ferric hyaluronate, is another product used for adhesion prevention. In preliminary studies it has been shown to reduce the number, severity, and extent of adhesions in peritoneal surgery [101]. However, the use of Intergel in abdominal surgery in which the gastrointestinal tract was opened still led to an unacceptably high rate of postoperative complications [102].

An interesting experimental finding is the reduction of both number and type of adhesions after postoperative stimulation of gastrointestinal motility by a prokinetic agent [103].

Finally merits mention that peritoneal infusion with cold saline has shown to decrease the degree of postoperative intra-abdominal adhesion formation in an animal model [104].

Adhesions quantification

Among the different adhesions scoring systems which have been proposed mainly by gynecologists, the more complete and easy to use one is the PAI score proposed by Coccolini et al. [105]. In fact, specific attention should be paid to uniformity of measurement. We therefore suggest a regimented classification system for adhesions in an effort to standardize their definition and subsequent analysis. In this way, different surgeons in different treatment centers can more effectively evaluate patients and compare their conditions to past evaluations using a universal classification system (Figure 3). This classification is based on the macroscopic appearance of adhesions and their extent to the different regions of the abdomen. Using specific scoring criteria, clinicians can assign a peritoneal adhesion index (PAI) ranging from 0 to 30, thereby giving a precise description of the intra-abdominal condition [105].

Conclusions

ASBO is a common disease. Non operative management should be attempted in absence of signs of peritonitis or strangulation. WSCM is safe and has a definite role in diagnosis (for predicting the resolution or need for surgery) and therapy (for reducing the operative rate and shortening time to resolution of symptoms and hospital stay). Open surgery for several surgeons still remains the safest and most effective operative approach, although laparoscopic approach appears to be safe and feasible in the hands of experienced laparoscopic surgeons and in selected patients, because there are less overall complications, prolonged ileus rates and pulmonary complication associated with its use. Prevention with hyaluronic acid-carboxycellulose membrane or icodextrin, has actually gained a capital relevance. Adhesions quantification and scoring is a promising development tool for further research towards diagnosis and management of ASBO and peritoneal adhesions prevention.

Competing interests
The authors declare that they have no competing interests.

Authors' contributions
FC, SDS: conception and design of the study; organised the consensus conference; preparation of the draft; merged the committee preliminary statements with the observations and recommendations from the panel, summarised the discussion on standards of diagnosis and treatment for ASBO SDS, FC, MG, FeCo manuscript writing, drafting and review. FC, SDS, MDK, JJ organised the consensus conference, merged the committee preliminary statements with the observations and recommendations from the panel, critically contributed to the consensus statements. MDK, WLB, LA, VM, HVG, EEM, JJ contributed to critical discussion of the draft. All authors read and approved the final manuscript.

Author details
[1]Emergency and Trauma Surgery Unit, Departments of Emergency and Surgery, Maggiore Hospital Trauma Center, Bologna, Italy. [2]Emergency Surgery Unit, Department of General and Multivisceral Transplant Surgery, S Orsola Malpighi University Hospital, Bologna, Italy. [3]Upper GI Unit, Department of Surgery, Frenchay Hospital, North Bristol, NHS Trust, Bristol, UK. [4]Department of Surgery, Denver Health, University of Colorado Health Sciences Denver, Denver Health Medical Center, 777 Bannock Street, Denver CO 80204, USA. [5]General Surgery I, Ospedali Riuniti di Bergamo, Bergamo, Italy. [6]Department of General and Emergency Surgery, Associated Hospitals "Villa Sofia - Cervello", Palermo, Italy. [7]Department of Surgery, Massachusetts General Hospital, Harvard Medical School, Boston, MA, USA. [8]Department of Surgery, Macerata Hospital, Via Santa Lucia 2, 62100, Macerata, Italy. [9]Washington Cancer Institute, Washington Hospital Center, Washington, DC 20010, USA. [10]Department of Surgery, Radboud University Nijmegen Medical Centre, P.O. Box 91016500HB, Nijmegen, The Netherlands. [11]Department of Surgery, University of Florida, Gainesville, FL 32610-0254, USA. [12]Department of Surgery, Erasmus University Medical Center, PO Box 20403000CA, Rotterdam, The Netherlands. [13]Department of Surgery, John Hunter Hospital and University of Newcastle, Locke Bag 1 Hunter Region Maile Centre, Newcastle, NSW 2310, Australia. [14]Department of Emergency and Trauma

Surgery, Maggiore Hospital of Parma, Parma, Italy. [15]Emergency Surgery, Department of Abdominal Surgery, Meilahti Hospital, University of Helsinki, Haartmaninkatu 4, 340, Helsinki FIN-00029HUS, Finland. [16]Division of General Surgery, University of Pittsburgh Physicians, Pittsburgh 15213PA, USA. [17]Division of Trauma Surgery, University of Campinas, Campinas, SP, Brazil.

References:

1. Parker C, Ellis H, Moran BJ, *et al*: **Postoperative adhesions: ten-year followup of 12,584 patients undergoing lower abdominal surgery.** *Dis Colon Rectum* 2001, **44:**822–830.
2. Ellis: **The magnitude of adhesion related problems.** *Ann Chir Gynaecol* 1998, **87:**9–11.
3. Zielinski MD, Bannon MP: **Current management of small bowel obstruction.** *Adv in Surg* 2011, **45:**1–29.
4. Galinos B, Branco BC, Beat S, Lydia L, Kenji I, Demetrios D: **The incidence and risk factors of post-laparotomy adhesive small bowel obstruction.** *J Gastrointest Surg* 2010, **14:**1619–1628. doi:10.1007/s11605-010-1189-8.
5. Reschef A, Hull TL, Kiran RP: **Risk of adhesive obstruction after colorectal surgery: the benefits of the minimally invasive approach may extend well beyond the perioperative period.** *Surg Endosc* 2013, **27:**1717–1720. doi:10.1007/s00464-012-2663-z.
6. Parker C, Wilson MS, Menzies D, *et al*: **The SCAR-3 study: 5-year adhesionrelated readmission risk following lower abdominal surgical procedures.** *Colorectal Dis* 2005, **7:**551–558.
7. Stewart RM, Page CP, Brender J, *et al*: **The incidence and risk of early postoperative small bowel obstruction: a cohort study.** *Am J Surg* 1987, **154:**643–647.
8. Howard B, Steven W, Ozeran S: **Factors predicting the recurrence of adhesive small-bowel obstruction.** *Am J Surg* 1995, **170**(4):361–365.
9. Barkan Webster S, Ozeran S: **Factors predicting the recurrence of adhesive small-bowel obstruction.** *Am J Surg* 1995, **170:**361–365.
10. Miller G, Boman J, Shrier I, Gordon PH: **Natural history of patients with adhesive small bowel obstruction.** *Br J Surg* 2000, **87**(9):1240–1247.
11. Di Saverio S, Tugnoli G, Orlandi PE, Catena F, *et al*: **A 73-year-old man with long-term immobility presenting with abdominal pain.** *PLoS Med* 2009, **6:**e1000092.
12. Obuz F, Terzi C, Sokmen S, Yilmaz E, Yildiz D, Fuzun M: **The efficacy of helical CT in the diagnosis of small bowel obstruction.** *Eur J Radiol* 2003, **48**(3):299–304.
13. Trésallet C, Lebreton N, Royer B, Leyre P, Godiris-Petit G, Menegaux F: **Improving the management of acute adhesive small bowel obstruction with CT-scan and water-soluble contrast medium: a prospective study.** *Dis Colon Rectum* 2009, **52**(11):1869–1876.
14. Zalcman M, Sy M, Donckier V, Closset J, Gansbeke DV: **Helical CT signs in the diagnosis of intestinal ischemia in small-bowel obstruction.** *AJR Am J Roentgenol* 2000, **175**(6):1601–1607.
15. Grassi R, Romano S, D'Amario F, *et al*: **The relevance of free fluid between intestinal loops detected by sonography in the clinical assessment of small bowel obstruction in adults.** *Eur J Radiol* 2004, **50**(1):5–14.
16. Choi HK, Chu KW, Law WL: **Therapeutic value of gastrografin in adhesive small bowel obstruction after unsuccessful conservative treatment: a prospective randomized trial.** *Ann Surg* 2002, **236:**1–6.
17. Srinivasa S, Thakore N, Abbas S, Mahmood M, Kahokehr AA, Hill AG: **Impact of Gastrografin in clinical practice in the management of adhesive small bowel obstruction.** *Can J Surg* 2011, **54**(2).
18. Wadani HAI, Al Awad NI, Hassan KA, Zakaria HM, Al Mulhim AA, Alaqeel FO: **Role of water soluble contrast agents in assigning patients to a non-operative course in adhesive small bowel obstruction.** *Oman Med J* 2011, **26**(6):454–456. doi:10.5001/omj.2011.116.
19. Di Saverio S, Catena F, Ansaloni L, Gavioli M, Valentino M, Pinna AD: **Watersoluble contrast medium (gastrografin) value in adhesive small intestine obstruction (ASIO): a prospective, randomized, controlled, clinical trial.** *World J Surg* 2008, **32**(10):2293–2304.
20. Barkan H, Webster S, Ozeran S: **Factors predicting the recurrence of adhesive small-bowel obstruction.** *Am J Surg* 1995, **70:**361–365.
21. Ivy L, Shing W, Wong P, Malouf P, Truskett G: **Effect of handover on the outcomes of small bowel obstruction in an acute care surgery model.** *ANZ J Surg* 2012. 10.1111/j.1445-2197.2012.06248.x.
22. Leung AM, Vu H: **Factors predicting need for and delay in surgery in small bowel obstruction.** *Am Surg* 2012, **78**(4):403–407.
23. Fleshner PR, Siegman MG, Slater GI, Brolin RE, Chandler JC, Aufses AH Jr: **A prospective, randomized trial of short versus long tubes in adhesive small-bowel obstruction.** *Am J Surg* 1995, **170**(4):366–370.
24. Sakakibara T, Harada A, Yaguchi T, Koike M, Fujiwara M, Kodera Y, Nakao A: **The indicator for surgery in adhesive small bowel obstruction patient managed with long tube.** *Hepatogastroenterology* 2007, **54**(75):787–790.
25. Moran BJ: **Adhesion-related small bowel obstruction.** *Colorectal Dis* 2007, **9**(Suppl 2):39–44.
26. Fevang BT, Jensen D, Svanes K, Viste A: **Early operation or conservative management of patients with small bowel obstruction?** *Eur J Surg* 2002, **168**(8–9):475–481.
27. Abbas S, Bissett IP, Parry BR: **Oral water soluble contrast for the management of adhesive small bowel obstruction.** *Cochrane Database Syst Rev* 2007, **18**(3), CD004651.
28. Branco BC, Barmparas G, Schnüriger B, Inaba K, Chan LS, Demetriades D: **Systematic review and meta-analysis of the diagnostic and therapeutic role of water-soluble contrast agent in adhesive small bowel obstruction.** *Br J Surg* 2010, **97**(4):470–478.
29. Landercasper J, Cogbill TH, Merry WH, Stolee RT, Strutt PJ: **Long-term outcome after hospitalization for small-bowel obstruction.** *Arch Surg* 1993, **128:**765–770.
30. Schraufnagel D, Rajaee S, Millham FH: **How many sunsets?Timing of surgery in adhesive small bowel obstruction: A study of the Nationwide Inpatient Sample.** *J Trauma Acute Care Surg* 2013, **74**(1):181–187. doi:10.1097/TA.0b013e31827891a1. discussion 187–9.
31. Diaz JJ Jr, Bokhari F, Mowery NT, Acosta JA, Block EF, Bromberg WJ, Collier BR, Cullinane DC, Dwyer KM, Griffen MM, Mayberry JC, Jerome R: **Guidelines for management of small bowel obstruction.** *J Trauma* 2008, **64**(6):1651–1664.
32. Guo S-B, Duan Z-J: **Decompression of the small bowel by endoscopic long-tube placement.** *World J Gastroenterol* 2012, **18**(15):1822–1826. doi:10.3748/wjg.v18.i15.1822.
33. Assalia A, Kopelman D, Bahous H, Klein Y, Hashmonai M: **Gastrografin for mechanical partial, small bowel obstruction due to adhesions.** *Harefuah* 1997, **132**(9):629–633.
34. Choi HK, Law WL, Ho JW, Chu KW: **Value of gastrografin in adhesive small bowel obstruction after unsuccessful conservative treatment: a prospective evaluation.** *World J Gastroenterol* 2005, **11**(24):3742–3745.
35. Burge J, Abbas SM, Roadley G, Donald J, Connolly A, Bissett IP, Hill AG: **Randomized controlled trial of Gastrografin in adhesive small bowel obstruction.** *ANZ J Surg* 2005, **75**(8):672–674.
36. Wadani HAI, Awad NIA, Hassan KA, Zakaria HM, Abdulmohsen Al Mulhim A, Alaqeel FO: **Role of water soluble contrast agents in assigning patients to a Non-operative course in adhesive small bowel obstruction.** *Oman Medical Journal* 2011, **26**(6):454–456. doi:10.5001/omj2011.116.
37. Biondo S, Parés D, Mora L, Martí Ragué J, Kreisler E, Jaurrieta E: **Randomized clinical study of Gastrografin administration in patients with adhesive small bowel obstruction.** *J Surg* 2003, **90**(5):542–546.
38. Abbas SM, Bissett IP, Parry BR: **Meta-analysis of oral water-soluble contrast agent in the management of adhesive small bowel obstruction.** *Br J Surg* 2007, **94**(4):404–411.
39. Chen SC, Yen ZS, Lee CC, Liu YP, Chen WJ, Lai HS, Lin FY, Chen WJ: **Nonsurgical management of partial adhesive small-bowel obstruction with oral therapy: a randomized controlled trial.** *CMAJ* 2005, **173**(10):1165–1169.
40. Ambiru S, Furuyama N, Kimura F, Shimizu H, Yoshidome H, Miyazaki M, Ochiai T: **Effect of hyperbaric oxygen therapy on patients with adhesive intestinal obstruction associated with abdominal surgery who have failed to respond to more than 7 days of conservative treatment.** *Hepatogastroenterology* 2008, **55**(82–83):491–495.
41. Cox MR, Gunn IF, Eastman MC, Hunt RF, Heinz AW: **The safety and duration of non-operative treatment for adhesive small bowel obstruction.** *Aust N Z J Surg* 1993, **63**(5):367–371.
42. Shou-Chuan S, Kuo-Shyang J, Lin S-C, *et al*: **Adhesive small bowel obstruction: How long can patients tolerate conservative treatment?** *World J Gastroenterol* 2003, **9**(3):603–605.
43. Duron JJ, Silva NJ, du Montcel ST, Berger A, Muscari F, Hennet H, Veyrieres M, Hay JM: **Adhesive postoperative small bowel obstruction: incidence**

and risk factors of recurrence after surgical treatment: a multicenter prospective study. *Ann Surg* 2006, **244**(5):750–757.

44. Scott-Coombes DM, Vipond MN, Thompson JM: **General surgeons attitudes to the treatment and prevention of abdominal adhesions.** *Ann R Coll Surg Engl* 1993, **75**:123–128.
45. Levrant SG, Bieber E, Barnes R: **Risk of anterior abdominal wall adhesions increases with number and type of previous laparotomy.** *J Am Assoc Gynecol Laparosc* 1994, **1**(4):S19.
46. Van Der Krabben AA, Dijkstra FR, Nieuwenhuijzen M, *et al*: **Morbidity and mortality of inadvertent enterotomy during adhesiolysis.** *Br J Surg* 2000, **87**:467–471.
47. Tittel A, Treutner KH, Titkova S, *et al*: **Comparison of adhesion reformation after laparoscopic and conventional adhesiolysis in an animal model.** *Langenbeck's Arch Surg* 2001, **386**:141–145.
48. Tolutope O, Scott W: **Helton. Survey opinions on operative management of adhesive small bowel obstruction: laparoscopy versus laparotomy in the state of Connecticut.** *Surg Endosc* 2011, **25**:2516–2521.
49. Gamal EM, Metzger P, Szabo G, *et al*: **The influence of intraoperative complications on adhesion formation during laparoscopic and conventional cholecystectomy in an animal model.** *Surg Endosc* 2001, **15**:873–877.
50. Gadallah MF, Torres-Rivera C, Ramdeen G, Myrick S, Habashi S, Andrews G: **Relationship between intraperitoneal bleeding, adhesions, and peritoneal dialysis catheter failure: a method of prevention.** *Adv Perit Dial* 2001, **17**:127–129.
51. Agresta F, Ansaloni L, Baiocchi GL, Bergamini C, Campanile FC, Carlucci M, Cocorullo G, Corradi A, Franzato B, Lupo M, Mandalà V, Mirabella A, Pernazza G, Piccoli M, Staudacher C, Vettoretto N, Zago M, Lettieri E, Levati A, Pietrini D, Scaglione M, De Masi S, De Placido G, Francucci M, Rasi M, Fingerhut A, Uranüs S, Garattini S: **Laparoscopic approach to acute abdomen from the Consensus Development Conference of the Società Italiana di Chirurgia Endoscopica e nuove tecnologie (SICE), Associazione Chirurghi Ospedalieri Italiani (ACOI), Società Italiana di Chirurgia (SIC), Società Italiana di Chirurgia d'Urgenza e del Trauma (SICUT), Società Italiana di Chirurgia nell'Ospedalità Privata (SICOP), and the European Association for Endoscopic Surgery (EAES).** *Surg Endosc* 2012, **26**(8):2134–2164. doi:10.1007/s00464-012-2331-3.
52. Nagle A, Ujiki M, Denham W, Murayama K: **Laparoscopic adhesiolysis for small bowel obstruction.** *Am J Surg* 2004, **187**(4):464–470.
53. Szomstein S, Lo Menzo E, Simpfendorfer C, *et al*: **Laparoscopic lysis of adhesions.** *World J Surg* 2006, **30**:535–540.
54. Ming-Zhe L, Lei L, Long-bin X, Wen-hui W, Yu-long H, Xin-ming S: **Laparoscopic versus open adhesiolysis in patients with adhesive small bowel obstruction: a systematic review and meta-analysis.** *Am J Surg* 2012, **204**(5).
55. Stephanian SA, Apoian VT, Abramian RA, Drampian AF, Eiramdhzian KT: **Laparoscopic adhesiolysis in the treatment of acute adhesive obstruction of the small intestine.** *Klin Khir* 2011, **7**:11–14.
56. Vettoretto N, Carrara A, Corradi A, De Vivo G, Lazzaro L, Ricciardelli L, Agresta F, Amodio C, Bergamini C, Catani M, Cavaliere D, Cirocchi R, Gemini S, Mirabella A, Palasciano N, Piazza D, Piccoli M, Rigamonti M, Scatizzi M, Tamborrino E, Zago M: **Laparoscopic adhesiolysis: consensus conference guidelines. Colorectal diseases.** *The Association of Coloproctology of great Britain and Ireland* 2012, **14**:e208–e2015.
57. Swank DJ, Swank-Bordewijk SC, Hop WC, van Erp WF, Janssen IM, Bonjer HJ, Jeekel J: **Laparoscopic adhesiolysis in patients with chronic abdominal pain: a blinded randomised controlled multi-centre trial.** *Lancet* 2003, **361**(9365):1247–1251.
58. Cirocchi R, Abraha I, Farinella E, Montedori A, Sciannameo F: **Laparoscopic versus open surgery in small bowel obstruction.** *Cochrane Database Syst Rev* 2010, **17**(2):CD007511. Review.
59. Grafen FC, Neuhaus V, Schöb O, Turina M: **Management of acute small bowel obstruction from intestinal adhesions: indications for laparoscopic surgery in a community teaching hospital.** *Langenbecks Arch Surg* 2010, **395**:57–63.
60. Suter M, Zermatten P, Hakic N, *et al*: **Laparoscopic management of mechanical small bowel obstruction: are there predictors of success or failure?** *Surg Endosc* 2000, **14**:478–484.
61. León EL, Metzger A, Tsiotos GG, *et al*: **Laparoscopic management of small bowel obstruction: indications and outcomes.** *J Gastrointest Surg* 1998, **2**:132–140.
62. Pekmezci S, Altinli E, Saribeyoglu K, *et al*: **Enteroclysis-guided laparoscopic adhesiolysis in recurrent adhesive small bowel obstructions.** *Surg Laparosc Endosc Percutan Tech* 2001, **12**:165–170.
63. O'Connor DB, Winter DC: **The role of laparoscopy in the management of acute small bowel obstruction: a review of over 2000 cases.** *Surg Endosc* 2012, **26**(1):12–17. doi:10.1007/s00464-011-1885-9.
64. Navez B, Arimont JM, Guit P: **Laparoscopic approach in acute small bowel obstruction. A review of 68 patients.** *Hepatogastroenterology* 1998, **45**:2146–2150.
65. Van Goor H: **Consequences and complications of peritoneal adhesions.** *Colorectal Dis* 2007, **9**(Suppl 2):25–34.
66. Sato Y, Ido K, Kumagai M, *et al*: **Laparoscopic adhesiolysis for recurrent small bowel obstruction: long-term follow-up.** *Gastrointest Endosc* 2001, **54**:476–479.
67. Chosidow D, Johanet H, Montario T, *et al*: **Laparoscopy for acute smallbowel obstruction secondary to adhesions.** *J Laparoendosc Adv Surg Tech* 2000, **10**:155–159.
68. Farinella E, Cirocchi R, La Mura F, Morelli U, Cattorini L, Delmonaco P, Migliaccio C, De Sol AA, Cozzaglio L: **Sciannameo F Feasibility of laparoscopy for small bowel obstruction.** *World J Emerg Surg* 2009, **4**:3.
69. Levard H, Boudet MJ, Msika S, *et al*: **Laparoscopic treatment of acute small bowel obstruction: a multicentre retrospective study.** *A N Z J Surg* 2001, **71**:641–646.
70. Wullstein C, Gross E: **Laparoscopic compared with conventional treatment of acute adhesive small bowel obstruction.** *Br J Surg* 2003, **90**:1147–1151.
71. Khaikin M, Schneidereit N, Cera S, Sands D, Efron J, Weiss G, Nogueras JJ, Vernava AM, Wexner SD: **Laparoscopic vs. open surgery for acute adhesive small-bowel obstruction: patient' outcome and costeffextiveness.** *Surg Endosc* 2007, **21**:742–746.
72. Peschaud F, Alves A, Berdah S, Kianmanesh R, Lurent C, Ma Brut JY, Mariette C, Meurette G, Pirro N, Veryrie N, Slim K: **Indicazioni alla laparoscopia in chirurgia generale e digestiva.** *J Chir* 2006, **6**:65–79.
73. Franklin ME, Gonzales JJ, Miter DB, Glass JL, Paulson D: **Laparoscopic diagnosis and treatment of intestinal obstruction.** *Surg Endosc* 2004, **18**:26–30.
74. Catena F, Di Saverio S, Ansaloni L, *et al*: **CHAPTER 7 Adhesive Small Bowel Obstruction.** In *Updates in Surgery: The Role of Laparoscopy in Emergency Abdominal Surgery*. Edited by Mandalà V. Verlag Italia: Springer; 2012:89–104. 10.1007/978-88-470-2327-7. ISBN 978-88-470-2326-0.
75. Levard H, Boudet MJ, Msika S, Molkhou JM, Hay JM, Laborde Y, *et al*: **French association for surgical research. Laparoscopic treatment of acute small bowel obstruction: a multicentre retrospective study.** *Aust N Z J Surg* 2001, **71**:641–646.
76. Duh QY: **Small bowel obstruction**. In *Endosurgery*. Edited by Toouli J, Gossot D, Hunter JG. New York: Churchill Livingstone; 1998:425–431.
77. Di Saverio S, Vettoretto N, Catena F, Italian Working Group on Peritoneal Adhesions and Asbo Management, *et al*: **Elasbo study: emergency laparoscopy for relief of adhesive small-bowel obstruction: indications, technique, and results in 103 cases from a multicenter study of the WSES.** *Clin Congr Am Coll Surg, Oral Free paper Sess Gen Surg*. ISP062013.
78. Schnüriger B, Barmparas G, Branco BC, Lustenberger T, Inaba K, Demetriades D: **Prevention of Postoperative peritoneal adhesions: a review of the literature.** *Am J Surg*, **201**(1):111–121.
79. Fevang BT, Fevang J, Lie SA, Søreide O, Svanes K, Viste A: **Long-term prognosis after operation for adhesive small bowel obstruction.** *Ann Surg* 2004, **240**(2):193–201.
80. Soybir GR, Koksoy F, Polat C, *et al*: **The effects of sterile or infected bile and dropped gallstones in abdominal adhesions and abscess formation.** *Surg Endosc* 1997, **11**:711–713.
81. Van den Tol P, Haverlag R, van Rossen ME, *et al*: **Glove powder promotes adhesion formation and facilitates tumour cell adhesion and growth.** *Br J Surg* 2001, **88**:1258–1263.
82. Cooke A, Hamilton DG: **The significance of starch powder contamination in the aetiology of peritoneal adhesions.** *Br J Surg* 1977, **64**:410–412.
83. Barmparas G, Branco BC, Schnüriger B, Lam L, Inaba K, Demetriades D: **The incidence and risk factors of post-laparotomy adhesive small bowel obstruction.** *J Gastrointest Surg* 2010, **14**(10):1619–1628.
84. Malvasi A, Tinelli A, Farine D, *et al*: **Effects of visceral peritoneal closure on scar formation at cesarean delivery.** *Int J Gynecol Obstet* 2009, **105**:131–135.
85. Adhesion Barrier Study Group: **Prevention of postsurgical adhesions by INTERCEED(TC7), an absorbable adhesion barrier: a prospective**

randomized multicenter clinical study. INTERCEED(TC7). *Fertil Steril* 1989, **51**(6):933–938.

86. Saravelos H, Li TC: **Post-operative adhesions after laparoscopic electrosurgical treatment for polycystic ovarian syndrome with the application of Interceed to one ovary: a prospective randomized controlled study.** *Hum Reprod* 1996, **11**(5):992–997.
87. Azziz R, Adhesion Barrier Study Group: **Microsurgery alone or with INTERCEED absorbable adhesion barrier for pelvic sidewall adhesion re-formation: The INTERCEED (TC7). II.** *Surg Gynecol Obstet* 1993, **177**:135–139.
88. Nordic Adhesion Prevention Study Group: **The efficacy of Interceed (TC7)* for prevention of reformation of postoperative adhesions on ovaries, fallopian tubes, and fimbriae in microsurgical operations for fertility: a multicenter study.** *Fertil Steril* 1995, **63**:709–714.
89. Wiseman DM, Trout JR, Franklin RR, *et al*: **Metaanalysis of the safety and efficacy of an adhesion barrier (Interceed TC7) in laparotomy.** *J Reprod Med* 1999, **44**:325–331.
90. Ahmad G, Duffy JM, Farquhar C, *et al*: **Barrier agents for adhesion prevention after gynaecological surgery.** *Cochrane Database Syst Rev* 2008, **16**, CD000475.
91. Montz FJ, Monk BJ, Lacy SM: **The gore-Tex surgical membrane: effectiveness as a barrier to inhibit postradical pelvic surgery adhesions in a porcine model.** *Gynecol Oncol* 1992, **45**:290–293.
92. Beck DE, Cohen Z, Fleshman JW, *et al*: **A prospective, randomized, multicenter, controlled study of the safety of Seprafilm adhesion barrier in abdominopelvic surgery of the intestine.** *Dis Colon Rectum* 2003, **46**:1310–1319.
93. Becker M, Dayton MT, Fazio VW, *et al*: **Prevention of postoperative abdominal adhesions by a sodium hyaluronate-based bioresorbable membrane: a prospective, randomized, double-blind multicenter study.** *J Am Coll Surg* 1996, **183**:297–306.
94. Vrijland WW, Tseng LN, Eijkman HJ, *et al*: **Fewer intraperitoneal adhesions with use of hyaluronic acid-carboxymethylcellulose membrane: a randomized clinical trial.** *Ann Surg* 2002, **235**:193–199.
95. Cohen Z, Senagore AJ, Dayton MT, *et al*: **Prevention of postoperative abdominal adhesions by a novel, glycerol/sodium hyaluronate/ carboxymethylcellulose-based bioresorbable membrane: a prospective, randomized, evaluator-blinded multicenter study.** *Dis Colon Rectum* 2005, **48**:1130–1139.
96. Kumar S, Wong PF, Leaper DJ: **Intra-peritoneal prophylactic agents for preventing adhesions and adhesive intestinal obstruction after nongynaecological abdominal surgery.** *Cochrane Database Syst Rev* 2009, **1**, CD005080.
97. Fazio VW, Cohen Z, Fleshman JW, *et al*: **Reduction in adhesive smallbowel obstruction by Seprafilm adhesion barrier after intestinal resection.** *Dis Colon Rectum* 2006, **49**:1–11.
98. Kudo FA, Nishibe T, Miyazaki K, *et al*: **Use of bioresorbable membrane to prevent postoperative small bowel obstruction in transabdominal aortic aneurysm surgery.** *Surg Today* 2004, **34**:648–651.
99. Zeng Q, Yu Z, You J, Zhang Q: **Efficacy and safety of Seprafilm for preventing postoperative abdominal adhesion: systematic review and meta-analysis.** *World J Surg* 2007, **31**(11):2125–2131.
100. Catena F, Ansaloni L, Di Saverio S, Pinna AD, P.O.P.A. Study: **Prevention of postoperative abdominal adhesions by icodextrin 4% solution after laparotomy for adhesive small bowel obstruction. A prospective randomized controlled trial.** *J Gastrointest Surg* 2012, **16**:382–388.
101. Johns DA, Ferland R, Dunn R: **Initial feasibility study of a sprayable hydrogel adhesion barrier system in patients undergoing laparoscopic ovarian surgery.** *J Am Assoc Gynecol Laparosc* 2003, **10**:334–338.
102. Tang CL, Jayne DG, Seow-Choen F, *et al*: **A randomized controlled trial of.5% ferric hyaluronate gel (Intergel) in the prevention of adhesions following abdominal surgery.** *Ann Surg* 2006, **243**:449–455.
103. Sparnon AL, Spitz L: **Pharmacological manipulation of postoperative intestinal adhesions.** *Aust N Z J Surg* 1989, **59**:725–729.
104. Fang CC, Chou TH, Lin GS, Yen ZS, Lee CC, Chen SC: **Peritoneal infusion with cold saline decreased postoperative intra-abdominal adhesion formation.** *World J Surg* 2010, **34**(4):721–727.
105. Coccolini F, Ansaloni L, Manfredi R, Campanati L, Poiasina E, Bertoli P, Capponi MG, Sartelli M, Di Saverio S, Cucchi M, Lazzareschi D, Pisano M, Catena F: **Peritoneal adhesion index (PAI): proposal of a score for the "ignored iceberg" of medicine and surgery.** *World J Emerg Surg* 2013, **8**(1):6.

14

Necrotizing fasciitis: literature review of contemporary strategies for diagnosing and management with three case reports: torso, abdominal wall, upper and lower limbs

Zdravko Roje[1*], Željka Roje[2], Dario Matić[3], Davor Librenjak[4], Stjepan Dokuzović[5] and Josip Varvodić[6]

Abstract

Necrotizing fasciitis (NF) is an uncommon soft tissue infection, usually caused by toxin-producing virulent bacteria. It is characterized by widespread fascial necrosis primarily caused by *Streptococcus hemolyticus*. Shortly after the onset of the disease, patients become colonized with their own aerobic and anaerobic microflora from the gastrointestinal and/or urogenital tracts. Early diagnosis with aggressive multidisciplinary treatment is mandatory. We describe three clinical cases with NF. The first is a 69 years old man with diabetes mellitus type II, who presented with NF on the posterior chest wall, shoulder and arm. He was admitted to the intensive care unit (ICU) with a clinical picture of severe sepsis. Outpatient treatment and early surgical debridement of the affected zones (inside 3 hours after admittance) and critical care therapy were performed. The second case is of a 63 years old paraplegic man with diabetes mellitus type I. Pressure sores and perineal abscesses progressed to Fournier's gangrene of the perineum and scrotum. He had NF of the anterior abdominal wall and the right thigh. Outpatient treatment and early surgical debridement of the affected zones (inside 6 hour after admittance) and critical care therapy were performed. The third patient was a 56 year old man who had NF of the anterior abdominal wall, flank and retroperitoneal space. He had an operation of the direct inguinal hernia, which was complicated with a bowel perforation and secondary peritonitis. After establishing the diagnosis of NF of the abdominal wall and retroperitoneal space (RS), he was transferred to the ICU. There he first received intensive care therapy, after which emergency surgical debridement of the abdominal wall, left colectomy, and extensive debridement of the RS were done (72 hours after operation of inquinal hernia). On average, 4 serial debridements were performed in each patient. The median of serial debridement in all three cases was four times. Other intensive care therapy with a combination of antibiotics and adjuvant hyperbaric oxygen therapy (HBOT) was applied during the treatment. After stabilization of soft tissue wounds and the formation of fresh granulation tissue, soft tissue defect were reconstructed using simple to complex reconstructive methods.

Background

Necrotizing soft tissue infection (NSTI) is a rare but potentially fatal infection involving skin, subcutaneous tissue and muscle [1]. It is usually accompanied by the systemic inflammatory response syndrome (SIRS) and needs prolonged intensive care treatment [2]. Necrotizing fasciitis is characterized by widespread necrosis of the subcutaneous tissue and fasciae. However NF as a soft tissue infection *"per se"* typically does not cause myonecrosis, but does invade the deep fascia and muscle [3]. Its rapid and destructive clinical course is assumed to be caused by polymicrobial symbiosis and synergy [1,2]. Monomicrobial infection is usually associated with immunocompromised patients (cancer, diabetes mellitus, vascular insufficiencies, organ transplantation or alcohol abusers) [4]. Many aerobic and anaerobic pathogens may be involved, including *Bacteroides, Clostridium, Peptostreptococcus, Enterobacteriaciae, Proteus, Pseudomonas,*

* Correspondence: zdroje@kbsplit.hr
[1]Division of Plastic Surgery and Burns, University Hospital Centre Split, Croatia
Full list of author information is available at the end of the article

and Klebsiella, but group A hemolytic streptococcus and *Staphylococcus aureus*, alone or in synergism, are the initiating infecting bacteria [5]. Typical sites of the infection are the extremities, (primarily the lower extremities), abdomen, and perineum [1]. In most NSTI cases anaerobic bacteria are present, usually in combination with aerobic gram-negative organisms. They proliferate in an environment of local tissue hypoxia. Because of lower oxidation-reduction potential, they produce gases such as hydrogen, nitrogen, hydrogen sulfide and methane, which accumulate in soft tissue spaces because of reduced solubility in water [6]. Establishing the diagnosis of NF (as the most common type of NSTI) can be challenging. Clinical findings may include swelling, pain, fever, erythema, induration, crepitations, sloughing off of the skin, or a blistering and purulent collection. The need for more rapid and scientific methods of NF diagnosis led to the development of a clinical scoring systems, like the LRINEC scoring system (The Laboratory Risk Indicator for Necrotizing Fasciitis) or the APACHE II scoring system (The Acute Physiology and Chronic Health Evaluation) [6,7]. Unfortunately, still the hallmark NF symptoms are intense pain and tenderness over the involved skin and underlying muscle [6]. Because NF is a surgical emergency and a life-threatening condition, the patient must be admitted to an ICU, where start IC therapy and where immediate and aggressive surgical debridement must be performed [8]. The purpose of this review is to present the basic concept of the diagnosis and treatment of NF during the last few decades, as well as the contemporary strategies for diagnosing and management.

Cases reports

Case I

A 69 years old, diabetic (type II) male was admitted to the Emergency department (ED) because of a four day history of fever, vomiting and nausea (Table 1). We found abscesses on the posterior chest wall (CW), the right shoulder and arm. His diabetes mellitus was treated with oral anti-diabetic drugs. He had swelling and erythema of the affected skin and was warm to palpations. In the central zone there was sloughed off skin with a big circle of necrosis and crepitations. He had strong pain in the abdomen which appeared bloated, with strong peristaltic action and diarrhea. Oliguria with dark urine was also present. His laboratory blood values showed a non-regulated diabetes mellitus with hyperglycemia of 32 mmol/L, white blood cell count of 18×10^9/L with 81.6% polymorphonuclear cells (PMNs), elevated C-reactive protein (CRP), hemoglobin, sodium and creatinine. His clinical picture indicated a state of bacterial sepsis and systemic toxemia. Ultrasonography showed reactive lymph nodes in both axillary regions and fluid collections on the posterior CW and the right arm. Anteroposterior chest x-ray revealed lung a shadow suggestive of inflammation in the basal level on the right side.

Because of progress of systemic signs of soft tissue bacterial infections with septicemia and SIRS, early fluid resuscitation was started in the Emergency department. The metabolic changes, such as hyperglycemia and ketoacidosis, were also treated, and intravenous antimicrobial therapy (Penicilin G, Clindamycin, Imipenem, Teicoplanin) was begun. Surgical treatment was performed shortly after admittance in ICU. We applied an immediate and aggressive surgical debridement of the posterior CW, right shoulder, and right arm, with extensive fasciotomy on the arm. All infected and necrotic skin and subcutaneous tissue were radically excised up to bleeding healthy edges. Tissue cultures and fluid aspirate were sent for immediate gram-stain and culture. All opened wounds were copiously irrigated with hydrogen peroxide, saline and an antibiotic dressing of 1% povidone iodine solution was used to cover the wound. Next, exploration was performed after 24 hours, and all ongoing infected tissue was excised. Wounds were monitored during the next 72 hours with twice daily dressing changes. During the next five days, adjuvant HBO therapy in a hyperbaric chamber was applied. On the first day, the patient received two treatments of HBO therapy, and subsequently one treatment daily during the next four days. HBO was given at 2.8 atmospheres absolute pressure (ATA) for 90 minutes per day. We performed two additional debridements and one necrectomy for wound stabilization. After four days, microbiological analysis indicated a necrotizing infection with mixed aerobes and anaerobes. The dominant flora was *Peptostreptococus spp, Bacteroides spp and Fusobacterium spp*, though *Streptococcus pyogenes* and *Staphylococcus aureus* were also found. Blood culture was positive for methicillin-resistant *Staphylococcus aureus (MRSA)*. The wound stabilized and fresh granulation tissue appeared after seven days, at which point a second defect reconstruction was performed using skin flaps, skin grafts, and topical negative pressure therapy with skin grafts. The patient made an encouraging recovery from a NF affecting such a large area of the body. We believe that this was possible because of the multidisciplinary team approach involving a general practitioner, general and plastic surgeons, radiologist, microbiologist, physiotherapist and nutritionist. The patient was discharged after 32 days of hospital stay. Five months later he had regulated diabetes, and sufficient CW movement with good respiration rate, and normal range of motion in the shoulder joint and arm.

Case II

A 63 years old, paraplegic and diabetic (type I) male patient was admitted to the Emergency department

Table 1 Clinical findings in three case reports

Clinical findings	First case: 69 yr/M DM-type II, with NF of CW, shoulder, and arm	Secound case: 63 yr/M DM-type I, paraplegic with Fournier's gangrene	Third case: 56 yr/M with inquinal hernia repair and NF of AW and RP space
Preexisting medical conditions	DM type-II, hypertension, alcohol abuse, heart disease, peripheral vascular and pulmonary disease, malnutrition, chronic wound (pressure sores, diabetes and venous ulcer)	DM type I, hypertension, paraplegia, obesity, heart disease, peripheral. vascular and pulmonary disease, immune deficiency, pressure sores	hypertension, alcohol abuse, peripheral vascular disease
Physical findings	swelling, erythema, redness, induration, crepitus, pain, fever, warm skin, blisters, skin discoloration, numbness, soft tissue emphysema, confusion, weakness, skin sloughing/necrosis	induration, pain, crepitus, fever, warm skin, blisters, skin discoloration, soft tissue emphysema, paraplegia confusion, numbness	swelling, erythema, redness, induration, crepitus, pain, fever, warm skin, blisters, soft tissue emphysema, confusion, weakness, skin sloughing/necrosis
Vital sings and laboratory valves	SIRS and signs of systemic toxicity, positive LRINEC scour system.	SIRS and signs of systemic toxicity, positive LRINEC scour system.	SIRS and signs of systemic toxicity, positive LRINEC scour system
Source of infection	skin abscess/furunculosis	perineal abscesses, Fournier's gangrene	inguinal hernia repair, bowel perforation.
Microbiology findings	aerobes and anaerobes	aerobes and anaerobes	aerobes and anaerobes
Treatment modalities:			
primary debridement	yes	yes	yes
operative intervals (days):			
admission to first debridment	3 hours	6 hours	72 hours
first to last debridment	2	5	5
first debridement. to final closure	14 days	12 days	12 days
days to granulation tissue formation	7 days	10 days	10 days
hydrofiber dressing	yes	yes	yes
Adjuvant HBO therapy	yes	yes	yes
HBO sessions	4 sessions	11 sessions	11 sessions
Combination of antibiotics used	Penincillin G, Clindamycin, Imipenem, Teicoplanin	Penicilin G, Gentamycin, Clyndamicin	Penicilin G, Gentamycin, Clyndamicin, Metronidazol
Outpatient treatment	oral anti-diabetic drugs, antihypertensive drugs, cardiotonics	Insulin therapy, antihypertensive drugs, cardiotonics, different types of peroral antibiotics for 2 months	antihypertensive drugs, cardiotonics,
ICU therapy	dominantly mechanical ventilation, nutritional support, whole blood, fresh frozen plasma, erythrocyte concentrate, combination of 4 antibiotics (AB) which depending on wound culture or blood culture (administered for 10 days and target AB for 18 days)	dominantly dialysis, nutritional support, blood whole blood, fresh frozen plasma, erythrocyte concentrate combination of 3 antibiotics which depending on wound culture or blood culture (administered for 10 days and target AB for 11 days)	dominantly nutritional support whole blood, fresh frozen plasma, erythrocyte concentrate combination of 4 antibiotics which depending on wound culture or blood culture (administered for 14 days)
Main complications	delay in diagnosis and first debridement, inadequate serial debridement's, bacteriemia, sepsis, wound infection (MRSA), pressure sores, skin graft lysis	delay in diagnosis and first debridement, inadequate serial debridement, bacteriemia, sepsis, MODS, wound infection-MRSA, skin graft lysis, diverting colostomy, pressure sores	delay in diagnosis and first debridement, inadequate serial debridement, bowel perforation, bacteriemia, sepsis, secondary peritonitis, MODS, wound infection(MRSA), diverting colostomy, pressure sores
Reconstruction	skin grafts (SG), local flaps, topical negative pressure therapy with SG	skin grafts, local flaps, topical negative pressure therapy with SG, component separation technique with biological mesh	direct sutures, local flaps, component separation technique with biological mesh

because of a two week history of high fever, perirectal pain, purulent drainage and a clinical picture of bacterial sepsis (Table 1). His diabetes mellitus was treated with insulin injections. He had pressure sores on the greater trochanter of right leg and sacral region which were treated with serial debridements and drainages on an outpatient basis by his family doctor during the previous two months. In his acute clinical status we found perianal induration with perianal abscesses and large grade III/IV sacral and trochanteric pressure sores, with multiple drainage sinuses. In both inguinal regions the patient had erythema and crepitations, stronger on the left side. The scrotal skin region was painful, edematous, and pruritic. On the left knee region there was an additional pressure sore with edema, fluid collections and lymphangitis in the ipsilateral inguinal region. His laboratory blood values showed signs and symptoms of SIRS with hyperglycemia of 21 mmol/L, a total leukocyte count of 6.35×10^9 with 78% of PMNs, 17% bands, 11% lymphocytes, and 120×10^9/L platelets, hemoglobin of 78 g/L, albumin 29 g/L, protein 61 g/L CRP of 69,1 mg/L, and creatinin 216 mmol/L. The patient was febrile, with symptoms of systemic toxicity. In his local status he had scrotal gangrene, fulminating perineal abscesses and a fluid collection with crepitations on the left thigh. The plain film radiography of the pelvic region showed the presence of gas in the perineum. CT scan of the left thigh revealed suspected septic arthritis secondary to the pressure sore in the knee region, and low attenuation in vastus lateralis muscle, and gas in both perineal regions. The diagnosis of Fournier's gangrene was reached based on clinical examination and laboratory findings.

After admittance to the Emergency department, we started treatment with aggressive fluid resuscitation, correction of laboratory parameters, hyperglycemia, metabolic acidosis, adding an empirical combination of antibiotics-Penicillin G, Gentamycin, and Clindamycin. The first debridement was performed on the perineum area and continued to the scrotum, inguinal regions, and the lower abdominal wall (AW). We also performed an endoscopic lavage of the knee joint and fasciotomy, with radical debridement, of the thigh anterior compartment of the left thigh. The anterior compartment was opened from inguinal ligament to just above the knee joint. All opened wounds were copiously irrigated with hydrogen peroxide, 0,9% physiologic solution and dressed with 1% povidone iodine solution. After the initial debridement, the wounds were carefully monitored during the next 24 to 72 hours and dressing changes were done twice daily. Adjuvant HBO therapy was applied over the course of the next seven days. On the first day, the patient received two treatments of HBO therapy, followed afterwards by one treatment daily. HBO was given at 2.8 ATA for 90 minutes per day. We performed three additional debridement and necrectomy procedures to stabilize the wound. The fecal incontinence was treated with a diverting colostomy. The results of microbiological analysis of the perineum and thigh cultures showed a polymicrobial infection with *Escerichia coli*, *Psudomonas aeruginosa*, and *Streptococcus pyogenes*, and the presence of mixed anaerobes, including *Bacteroides fragilis*. Blood cultures were positive for *Pseudomonas aeruginosa*. Debridement and necrectomy was done with large skin defect on the left thigh and the lower AW. In the course of next ten days, the wound stabilized and fresh granulation tissue formed. At this point, a second defect reconstruction was performed using local flaps, skin grafts, topical negative pressure therapy with skin grafts and the technique of component separation with a biological mesh for ventral hernia repair. The temporary diverting colostomy helped in the healing of skin grafts which were used to cover soft tissue defects. The paraplegia was an additional daily problem for the patient's hygiene. Pressure sores on the sacral and trochanter region were treated longer than other skin defects. Six months later the patient had regulated diabetes. All defects were closed secondarily except for the sacral pressure sore which was treated as a chronic wound.

Case III

A 56 years old healthy male patient was admitted to the Urology department for elective right inguinal hernia reparation (Table 1). The urologists performed a standard operation of a sliding inguinal hernia on the right side. Due to the weakness of the lower AW, the urologist reinforced the inguinal wall with synthetic Prolene mesh. Postoperatively, the patient showed a clinical picture of an acute abdomen. At this point, the urologists performed a revision surgery of the operated inguinal hernia, during which they found only a hematoma, removed the Prolen mesh and performed adequate haemostasis. Unfortunately they did not notice the bowel perforation and did not perform an explorative laparotomy at that time. During the next 24 hours, signs of septic shock with crepitations on the AW and right flank region appeared in the clinical picture. Through the suture line of the inguinal canal a fecal collection was drained. Postoperatively, the patient received a combination of Penicillin G, Clindamycin, Metronidazol and Gentamycin. The native abdomen x-ray showed air under the diaphragm. Magnetic resonance images provided dramatic evidence of an inflammatory process infiltrating the deep fascial plane of the anterior AW. Systemic manifestations of SIRS with body temperature more than 39°C, heart rate more than 100 beats per minute, breaths less than 30 per minute, $PaCO_2$ less than 32 mmHg and WBC account more than 18×10^9/L with a high number of immature forms, hypotension, hypoperfusion with a high level lactic acidosis, oliguria, and alteration of mental status and consciousness were indicators of severe sepsis and septic shock. The anesthesiologist introduced a central venous catheter and started intensive resuscitation.

The abdominal rigidity suggested a persisting peritonitis and an urgent laparotomy was done. Through a long midline incision we found a perforation of the caecum, necrosis of a great part of ascending colon, diffuse fecal peritonitis and signs of retroperitoneal NF. The surgical team executed extensive debridement, fasciectomy of the deep fascia on the AW, right orciectomy, right hemicolectomy, diverting colostomy on the descending colon and extensive debridement of the RS. The abdominal cavity and RS were extensively irrigated with hydrogen peroxide, saline and a solution of 1% povidone iodine, and drained on both sides. The structural and functional continuity of musculofascial system of the AW was obtained by component separation techniques (cite) and biological mesh. The wound was dressed with 1% povidone iodine solution. Dressing was controlled every 24 hours and serial debridements were performed. On the second postoperative day, the surgical team ordered adjuvant HBO therapy during the next 10 days. On the first day, the patient received two treatments of HBO therapy, followed by one treatment per day. HBO was given at 2.8 ATA for 90 minutes per day. In this case we needed five serial debridements to stabilize the wound. The results of microbiological analysis of the lower AW and retroperitoneal space showed a polymicrobial infection with *Escerichia coli, Psudomonas aeruginosa*, and *Streptococcus fecalis, Streptococcus pyogenes*, and the presence of mixed anaerobes, including *Bacteroides fragilis and Clostridum spp.* Blood cultures were positive for *Escerichia coli* and *Pseudomonas* aeruginosa. Methicillin-resistant *Staphylococcus aureus (MRSA)* was present in the second blood culture. Two weeks after the initial operation, the AW became stable and fresh granulation tissue appeared. At that point, we started closing the defects by using local advancement flaps, regenerative tissue matrix, and skin grafts. The closure of the diverting colostomy was performed three months postoperatively when the anterior abdominal has been strongly reinforced with a dermal matrix that was incorporated under the skin flaps. During long term follow up the colostomy was completely closed and regular bowel function was restored.

Incidence and classification

Necrotizing fasciitis, the most complicated and life threatening NSTI, has a progressive and rapidly advancing clinical course [1]. Although occurring in all age groups, NF is slightly more common in older age groups (> 50 years of age) [2]. The infection usually affects the deep fascial plane, with secondary necrosis of subcutaneous tissue and skin caused by the thrombosis of the subcutaneous and perforators vessels. The incidence of NF has been reported to be 0.40 cases per 100 000 adults [3]. There is a male to female ratio of 3:1 in all cases of NSTI, which relates predominately to the incidence of Fournier's gangrene of the perineum [3]. The terminology used for infections of skin and skin structures is often confusing. Skin and soft tissue infections (SSTIs) are best classified according to the anatomical site of infection, depth of infection, microbial source of infection, or by severity (minor superficial lesion to invasive, fulminant and even lethal infections) (Table 2.). The Infection Disease Society of America made practical classification of SSTIs into three groups: superficial, uncomplicated infection (includes impetigo, erysipelas and cellulitis), necrotizing infection; infections associated with bites and animal contact; surgical site infections and infections in the immunocompromised host [3]. The recent clinical classification distinguished four NF types: Type I (70-80%, polymicrobial/synergistic), type II (20% of cases; usually monomicrobial), type III (gram-negative monomicrobial, including marine-related organisms) and type IV (fungal) [1]. Although NF is rare, its mortality rate is high, ranging from 6% to 76%, although it is much lower in recent studies (approximately 26%) [5]. Establishing the diagnosis can be challenging. Every physician must know the answers to four main questions: "What is the clinical course of NSTIs, especially of NF?", "Which types of organisms are responsible for the infection?", "What is the depth of the infection?", and "Is NF a life or limb threatening disease?". The first answer ensures early diagnosis of NSTI/NF, the second determines the empirical spectrum of antimicrobial therapy, and the last two answers point out the timing and the extent of surgical intervention.

The causes of NF on the extremities are usually related to trauma, chronic wound infections, diabetes and vascular insufficiency, venous, diabetic and pressure sores, obesity, alcoholism, smoking, chronic liver disease, immune-suppression, or extravasation of drugs. This condition very often has a fatal outcome and many cases require amputation of an extremity rather than excision of the affected tissue to prevent proximal spread [6-9]. Delay in treatment of more than 6 to 12 hours or inadequate primary surgical debridement contribute to morbidity and mortality. The infection usually spreads rapidly along the fascial planes, accompanied by the production of particularly destructive bacterial enzymes that cause necrosis and liquefaction of the surrounding tissues. Crepitations and gas bubbles in soft tissue may be present. Published mortality reports with this conditions range between 8.7% and 73% (mean 32.2%) [3]. Unfavorable prognostic factors include old age, peripheral vascular insufficiency, and diabetes

Table 2 Classification scheme of skin and soft tissue infections (SSTIs) according to Sarani et al.[5]

Classification characteristic	Most common disease (underline) Incidence (%)
Anatomic localization	Fournier's gangrene of perineum and scrotum
Depth of infection	Necrotizing adiposities fasciitis, myonecrosis
Microbial cause	Type I: polymicrobial/synergistic/70-80% of cases Type II: monomicrobial (*Staphylococcus, Streptococcus, Clostridia spp*)/20% of cases Type III: marine related organisms Type IV: fungal
Severity of infection	
Uncomplicated infections	Superficial: impetigo, ecthyma Deeper: erysipelas, cellulitis Hair follicle associated: folliculitis, furunculosis Abscess: carbuncle, other cutaneous abscesses
Complicated infections	Secondary skin infections Acute wound infection (traumatic, bite related, postoperative) Chronic wound infections (diabetic wound infection, venous stasis ulcers, pressure sores) Perineal cellulitis with/without abscess
Necrotizing fasciitis	
Polymicrobial fasciitis (Type I)	Fournier's gangrene, synergistic necrotizing cellulitis with fasciitis and myositis Streptococcal gangrene
Monomicrobial fasciitis (Type II)	Marine-related organisms-*Vibrio vulneriformis* and other *Vibrio spp* Fungal spp
Myonecrosis	
Crepitant myonecrosis	Clostridial myonecrosis (traumatic gas gangrene and atraumatic gas gangrene-*Clostridium perfrigens and other Clostridial spp)* Synergistic necrotizing cellulitis with fasciitis and myositis
Non-crepitant myonecrosis	Streptococcal gangrene with myonecrosis-*Aeromonas hydrophila* myonecrosis

(Table 3.). Patients with diabetes appear to be particularly at great risk, representing over 70% of cases in one large review [10].

The causes of NF on the CW are usually related to some form of trauma, tumor resection, irradiation or surgical procedure. The incidence of sternal wound infection with osteomyelitis after median sternotomy is 0.4% to 5.9%, and mortality is as high as 70% in infected patients [11]. Tube thoracostomy for empyema is a particularly noteworthy cause where the mortality is about 89%, which is approximately twice as high t as that reported for other anatomic sites [4,12]. Delay or inadequate surgical debridement and severity of the underlying thoracic condition, are responsible for the high mortality rates. The importance of early, aggressive and often serial surgical debridements with removal of one or more ribs cannot be overemphasized [11].

Fournier's gangrene in elderly patients and diabetics is usually described as a fulminating infection of the inguinal region and the lower AW and the perineum along with the scrotum and penis in men, and the vulva in women. Fournier originally reported a disease that was idiopathic in nature, but many recent studies suggest a polymicrobial etiology of this disease. The idiopathic causes are seen very often in younger populations [13]. The main sources of infection are elective skin operations, skin abscesses and pressure sores. The frequent colorectal disease includes anorectal infections, ischiorectal abcesses, colon perforations, and some elective anorectal diagnostic procedures e.g., rectal biopsy, anal dilatation, or hemorrhoidal banding. A genitourologic cause of the disease includes urethral stricture, trauma from an indwelling Foley catheter and prostate biopsy. In women, Bartholin abscesses and vulval skin infections are the most common causes of NF. Surgical management includes wide incision and debridement of all involved areas. As the involvement of deep fascia and muscles is rare with this syndrome, it is not necessary to continue the debridement into the healthy-looking tissue. The mortality ranges from 11% to 45% despite the improvement in critical care, usage of broad-spectrum antibiotics and aggressive surgical debridement [13].

The types of necrotizing infections on the AW are numerous and the indication for AW reconstruction after serial surgical debridements and necrectomies

Table 3 Risk factors for development of NSTI and the LRINEC scoring system for prediction of NSTI

Risk factors	LRINEC scoring system		
	Variable	Values	Score
Preexisting conditions	C-reactive protein	≤150 mg/L	0
diabetes, immunosupression		> 150 mg/L	4
alcoholism, peripheral vascular disease, IV drug abuse, hypertension, corticosteroids, HIV, age < 50 years, GI malignance, malnutrition, major trauma, surgery, perforated viscera, chronic live disease, chronic renal insufficiency, obesity	White blood cell count	< 15 per mm^2	0
		15-25 per mm^2	1
		> 25 per mm^2	2
	Hemoglobin	≤13,5 g/dL	0
		11-13,5 g/dL	1
		< 11 g/dL	2
	Sodium	≥ 135 mmol/L	0
		> 135 mmol/L	2
Existing illness and injuries	Creatinine	< 141 µmol/L	0
Varicella with bacterial superinfection, fractures, liposuction, seawater-seafood, surgery, spider bite and other bites, Cesarean section, burns		> 141 µmol/≤L	2
	Glucose	≤10 mmol/L	0
		> 10 mmol/L	1

NSTI-necrotizing soft tissue infection; GI-gastrointestinal; HIV-human immunodeficiency virus;
LRINEC-Laboratory Risk Indicator for Necrotizing Fasciitis: A score of ≥ 6 is suspicious for NSTI, a score of ≥8 is highly predictive of NSTI

depends on the etiology, size and site of the defects. Complicated intra-abdominal infections such as appendicitis with perforation, infections after complex hernia repairing, perforated diverticulitis, cholecystitis, gastroduodenal perforations, small bowel perforations, obstructive colon cancer with perforation and complex trauma of the AW, are the main sources of NF in the AW and RS. Severe sepsis and septic shock can lead to multiple organ dysfunction syndromes (MODS). The defects of any size on the anterior AW may allow herniation of the viscera, which can lead into incarceration, and ultimately, strangulation. Any surgical incision can potentially result in ventral hernia, especially if a history of infection in that area is already present. Intra-abdominal infections "per se" include many pathological conditions, ranging from uncomplicated appendicitis to complicated fecal peritonitis [14,15]. Generally speaking, the choice of the surgical procedure depends on the anatomical source of infection, the degree of peritoneal and retroperitoneal inflammation, generalized septic response and patient's general conditions.

Retroperitoneal phlegmon with necrotizing fasciitis is an uncommon soft tissue infection that may become fatal. It usually ensues in cases of immunocompromised patients or advanced neoplastic disease. The infection spreads quickly and any delay in surgical intervention is associated with increased mortality. Necrotizing fasciitis of the anterior AW or perineum usually manifests with erythema and induration of the overlying skin. Nevertheless, when the retroperitoneum is involved, excision may be delayed due to the lack of clinical symptoms. Although the mortality rate of this infection is very high, survival is possible owing to the prompt and repeated wide surgical debridements and extensive necrectomy with proper broad spectrum antibiotic therapy [15,16].

Risk factors

The most common risk factor for the development of NSTI is diabetes mellitus, with an occurrence of 56% in all cases [7,17] (Table 3). The other co-morbidities include obesity, alcohol abuse, immunodeficiency, chronic renal failure, liver cirrhosis, hypertension, peripheral vascular disease, and age above 60 years. When such conditions occur simultaneously, the mortality rate increases remarkably on average 64,7%. [17,18]. According to this, the incidence of these infections is rising because of an increase in the number of immunocompromised patients, diabetes, cancer, alcoholism, vascular insufficiencies and organ transplants. Almost half of these infections are idiopathic, because we are not able to identify any underlying lesion at the site of the NSTI [7]. The best examples of such cases are scrotal or penile NF. Causative organisms are numerous and often may be polymicrobial (Table 3) [18,19].

There is no age or sex predilection for infection [18]. Because of the accompanying systemic illness and profound tissue inflammation, these patients are usually critically ill and have prolonged ICU stay. They need critical care therapy and complex surgical management, and can be treated in a specialized facility such as a burn center or a burn unit [7]. Laboratory based scoring systems as LRINEC score test (The Laboratory Risk Indicator for Necrotizing Fasciitis) [20] (Table 3.) or APACHE II score test (The Acute Physiology and Chronic Health Evaluation) may help in the early diagnosis of NF [21]. Both scoring tests are not NSTI specific, but are accurate predictors of mortality rates in most NF cases.

Pathophysiology and microbiological findings

According to the updated consensus for NSTIs (1,2), microbial invasion of skin and subcutaneous tissue occurs either through external trauma and surgical wounds, or directly through bacterial invasion from a perforated viscus. Table 4 present potential antibiotic therapeutic regimens for certain pathogenic organisms and predisposing factors. Microorganisms appearing in the skin and subcutaneous tissue spaces produce various endo- and exotoxins that cause prolonged vasoconstriction in the dermal capillary network. When these toxins are released into the systemic circulation, they produce the SIRS, which can progress into septic shock, MODS and finally, death [1,2,14]. The central pathohistological point in the pathogenesis of NSTIs is the thrombosis of perforating vessels of the skin and subcutis [17]. As the spread and extent of infection do not correspond with overlying skin changes, an inexperienced surgeon might not clearly determine the seriousness and extent of infection that takes place under the skin surfaces and in the subcutaneous space. In case of fulminating NF, MODS will develop within the first 24 hours of infection. In this case the disease will very often become fatal if not promptly recognized and treated with extensive surgical debridement, appropriate a combination of the antibiotics, and intensive care resuscitation [21].

From the clinical point of view, NF is usually a polymicrobial (Type-I) rather than a monomicrobial infection (Type-II) [18]. The analysis of our cases, during the *follow up* period of 15 years (36), point out that the most common bacterial species involved are: group A beta-hemolytic *Streptococcus pyogenes*, anaerobes (*Bacteroides, Clostridium, Peptostreptococcus*), group B *Streptococcus, Pneumococcus* and other *Streptococcus* species, *Staphylococcus aureus*, including hospital acquired *MRSA* and gram-negative enterobacteriaceae (*Escherichia coli, Acinetobacter species, Psudomonas, Serratia, and Klebsiella pneumniae*). In the retrospective study by Elliot et al. [17] they reviewed 198 patients with documented NSTI. These 182 patients grew an average of 4.4 types of microbes from original wound cultures, although a single pathogen was responsible in 28 patients. Eighty five patients had combined aerobic and anaerobic growth, the most common organisms being, *Bacteroides species*, aerobic streptococci, staphylococci, enterococci, *Escherihia coli*, and other gram-negative rods. Clostridial growth was common but did not affect mortality unless associated with pure clostridial myonecrosis. Mortality was affected by the presence of bacteriemia, delayed or inadequate surgery, and degree of MODS on admission. Monomicrobial cases are usually caused by Group A *Streptococcus pyogenes* and *Staphylococcus aureus*. They occur in otherwise healthy, young, immunocompetent patients and are most usually located on the extremities. In the study by Anderson et al. [22] more that 71% of cases had a polymicrobial source of infection. A polymicrobial infection is often diagnosed in immunocompromised patients and usually occurs in the perineum and trunk area [23]. Toxic shock syndrome is the most often accompanying syndrome of Streptococcal sepsis [24].

Clinical findings

The most representative clinical picture present with abscesses, infected traumatic and surgical wounds, intravenous drug abuse, pressure sores burns, perforated viscera (particular colon, rectum, and anus), recently performed liposuction, infected vascular prostheses and grafts, and invasive cancer [18,19]. Early clinical suspicion and surgery are the keys to improving survival, and patients with necrotizing infections need an integrated multidisciplinary approach to management. It is adjusting with the infecting organism(s), the site of infection, and the effects from any toxins produced, and incorporate various clinical and laboratory parameters In everyday clinical practice a universal clinical guideline that should be used in the diagnosis and treatment of all types of NSTI/NF does not exist (Table 2, 4, 5).

The clinical findings important for establishing the early NF diagnosis can be divided into two groups, early and advanced symptoms [25]. Primary or idiopathic NF usually occurs in the absence of a known causative factor or entry site for bacteria spreading. On the other side, secondary NF is the result of a known etiology and takes place through laceration of skin, cut, abrasion, contusion, burns, bite, subcutaneous injection or operative incision. The most common early signs are erythema, local warmth, skin induration and edema. In the disease's fulminant form, the patient is critically ill with signs and symptoms of severe septic shock and MODS, and extensive spreading of soft tissue necrosis. The clinical picture worsens very quickly, practically during only a few hours [25,26]. The acute form of the infection spreads for a few days and it first begins with severe pain before the cutaneous manifestations appear. The subacute NF form has an indolent clinical course, which progresses slowly over days or weeks [25].

Table 4 Suggested potential antibiotics therapeutic regimens depending on pathogens organisms, clinical conditions, predisposing factors, and antimicrobial choices

Pathogens and clinical condition	Predisposing factors	Antimicrobial choices
Gram-positive organisms		
Group A streptococcus (*S. pyogenes*) Erysipelas	Minor skin trauma or skin break	penicillins or cephalosporins, or alternative therapy: clindamycin, macrolides, glycopeptidescephalosporins, semi-synthetic resistant penicillin or
Cellulitis	Minor skin trauma or break	alternative therapy: clindamycin, macrolides, glycopeptides
Necrotizing fasciitis with/without myonecrosis	Minor skin trauma or skin break, superinfection of varicella lesion, DM, non-steroid anti-inflammatory drugs	high dose penicillin G, clindamycin or alternative therapy: clindamycin
Group β streptococcus (*S. agalactiae*) Necrotizing fasciitis	DM, premature neonates	high dose penicillin G, clindamycin or alternative therapy: clindamycin
Community-acquired meticillin resistant; *Staphilococcus aureus (CO-MRSA)*	No specific risk factors	glycopeptides or clindamycin, or alternative therapy: linezolidin, sulfomethoxazole, clindamycin
	Nasocomial MRSA in health care facilities is the major risk factor	high dose penicillin G, clindamycin or alternative therapy: clindamycin, metronidazole
Clostridium spp	Gross tidy and contaminated wounds	
	(*C. perfrigens*)	
	Colonic contamination (*C. septicum*)	
	IV drug use (C sordellil, C nayvi)	
Gram-negative organisms		
Pasteurella spp	Dog bites (P canis) Cat bites (P multocida)	amoxicillin, clavulanate piperacillin, tazobactam, III-generation cephalosporin metronidasole or alternative therapy: clindamycin, flouroquinolone, trimoxasole
Aeromonas spp (A. hydrophilia)	Freshwater exposure, medical leeches	fluoroquinolones or alternative therapy: trimoxasole, cephalsporins, aminolgycosides
Vibrio spp (V. vulnificus)	Chronic liver disease, DM	minocycline, cephalosporine or alternative therapy: ciprofloxacin
Klebsiella pneumonia	Chronic liver disease, DM	cephalosporines, amoxicillin, carbapenems, flouroquinolones, or alternative therapy: amynoglycosides
Escherichia coli	Cirrhosis	cephalosporines, amoxicillin, carbapenems, flouroquinolones, or alternative therapy: amynoglycosides
Serratia marcescens	Chronic renal failure, DM	cephalosporines, amoxicillin, piperacillin, tazobactam, carbapenems, flouroquinolones, or alternative therapy: amynoglycosides
Pseudomonas aeruginosa	Neutropenia, haematological malignancy, burns, HIV infection, injection drug use	amoxicilin, aminoglycosides, or alternative therapy: flouroquinolones

Early clinical status during the first 24 hours usually includes minor trauma, skin infection like folliculitis or abscess, gangrene on the extremities, pressure sore(s), or a complicated surgical incision like hernia repair. The external signs on the skin may be erythema or induration. The patient usually feels pain on the site of the injury. There is a disproportion between the character of the injury and intensity of the pain. Pain out of proportion with the apparent lesion severity should suggest a possible NF diagnosis [1,2].

During the next 2-4 days, the pain becomes more intense. In the clinical status we find many symptoms of general toxicity like fever, dehydration, confusion, dizziness, diarrhea, nausea, vomiting, weakness and malaise. If the patient is not admitted to an ICU or the diagnosis is established late in its course, more serious clinical symptoms ensue. The limbs and the area of body where the patient felt pain begin to swell, and may show a purplish rash or blisters with "dish-wash" purulent or haemorrhagic fluid. Cutaneous changes may be minimal, or may progress to blisters and bullae, and then to circumscribed necrosis of skin. Also, emphysema and gas formations with crepitations in overlying skin may appear. The pain grows, but remains an disproportionate to the clinical picture [1,5,6].

In the late phase within 4-6 days, symptoms of septic shock or MODS usually appear. Those symptoms may include cardiac shock with tachycardia, hypotension and decreased cardiac minute output, an elevated white blood cell count, metabolic acidosis, coagulopathy, changes in mental status and weakness. The patient in the late stage of NF appears apathetic and indifferent. If

Table 5 Treatment options classified by type of infection and clinical picture

Type of NSTI	Depth of involvement	Usual pathogens	Predisposing factors	Time of incubation and rate of progression	The main clinical signs	Treatment options
Polymicrobial NF-type I	fascia and muscle	obligate and facultative anaerobes	different type of wounds	long (48-96 h) Hour to days	foul- smelling drainage	ICU stay critical care therapy surgery antibiotics ev. HBO
Monomicrobial NF-type II (Steptococcal gangrene)	skin, fascia and muscle	Streptococci -groups A, C, G, and B; (B is more common)	excoriation or cut wound	short (6-48 h) A few hour	distinct margins	ICU stay critical care therapy surgery antibiotics ev. HBO
Gas gangrene (Clostridial myonecrosis)	muscle	C. perfirngens (C. perfirngens more common) and C. novyi	tidy wounds	short (6-48 h) A few hour	extreme system toxicity	ICU stay critical care therapy surgery antibiotics HBO
		C. septicum	gastrointestinal lesion			
Non-Clostridial myonecrosis	muscle and fascia	obligate and facultative anaerobes or *A. hydrophila*	different type of wounds	variable (12-96 h) Hour to days	gas in soft tissue	ICU stay critical care therapy surgery antibiotics HBO

the patient has an accompanying illness like diabetes, obesity, alcoholism, malignancy, malnutrition or immune deficiency, the general status is compromised with additional symptoms of these illnesses [2,15].

As early clinical findings, in the course of our clinical cases, we especially emphasize tenderness, swelling, erythema, and pain [2]. Those clinical symptoms and signs are similar to the course of superficial cellulitis, and it is very difficult to establish an early diagnose of NF at that moment. Nevertheless, a high suspicion must be present in all cases of rapidly progressive cellulitis, associated with severe progressive pain [6]. The hallmark symptoms of NF on the perineum, extremities and posterior CW include intense pain and tenderness over the involved skin and underlying muscle [5,6,27]. Over the next several hours and days, local pain can progresses to anesthesia because all cutaneous nerves are destroyed, which depends on the extent of tissue necrosis.

It is particularly difficult to establish the diagnosis of NSTI in outpatient facilities, because many of concomitant co-morbidities are able to cover the true clinical picture of necrotizing infections. Misdiagnosing NF is particularly common in children, and usually associated with recent varicella-zoster infection [5,28]. The surgical exploration of the suspected infection site, combined with microbiological and histopathological analysis of 1 cm^3 of soft tissue, is the gold standard for establishing an early NF diagnosis [5].

Necrotizing infection of the AW with concomitant secondary peritonitis always presents a very challenging issue, especially when it appears after an unrecognized bowel perforation during inguinal hernia repair. The mortality rate associated with acute pancreatitis and concomitant retroperitoneal NF [5,29], metastatic gas gangrene with colonic perforation [5,30], intra-abdominal infection with severe sepsis or septic shock is approximately 30% [31]. The main prognostic factors for these patients include advanced age, poor nutrition, concomitant diseases, i.e. diabetes, vascular and chronic renal insufficiency, advanced septic shock, multiple organ failure, immunosuppressed host and nosocomial infection [6,32]. The clinical picture is characterized by intense abdominal pain, a brown discoloration and bullae of the abdominal skin, gases in the soft tissue, abdominal rigidity, additional RS NF and myonecrosis of the AW in cases of clostridium infection [5,6,33]. Indeed, early detection and radical surgical treatment is essential to minimize the morbidity rate and to save life [5,6,23].

The causative triggers for the development of Fournier's gangrene are urogenital, anorectal and cutaneous disorders [1,6,34]. Fournier's gangrene usually begins with pain and itching of the perineum and scrotal skin. In cases originating in the genital area, the infecting bacteria probably pass through Buck's fascia of the penis and spread along the Darto's fascia of the scrotum and penis, Colle's fascia of the perineum, and Scarpa's fascia of the lower AW. The additional necroses of the superficial fascia and fat produces a thin watery malodorous fluid and crepitance (usually associated with polymicrobial infections including *Enterobacteriaceae* and *Clostridiae spp*) are results in more evident signs of necrotizing infection. Patients with SIRS can have high fever, anxiety, altered mental status, leukocitosis, shock and tachypnea. In that particular case, when severe soft tissue infections is already suspected, the usage of the LRNIC scoring system for prediction of NF are very useful for exact diagnosis [2,20]. By the time the progression of clinical signs becomes obvious, the appearance is usually that of a late NF phase, with visible bruising, bullae and cutaneous necrosis due to the extension of the necrotizing process from the deep fascia and horizontal spread [1]. The case history at that moment should suggest the causative microorganisms of infection. Nevertheless, the lack of cutaneous findings early in the course of the disease makes the diagnosis more challenging, and a high suspicion is essential for each clinical sign that appears on the skin and subcutaneous tissue.

The accumulation of gas formation in the soft tissue, which is seen in half of all NF cases, is another cardinal sign of NF diagnosis. It is clearly visible on plain x-ray pictures. More useful clinical findings are visible with ultrasound, CT scan and MRI. We prefer an additional skin puncture with large gauge needles to mobilize gas from subcutaneous spaces. If we do not find any gas bubbles, but the clinical picture presents other relevant clinical signs of NF, we must perform a radical surgical debridement as soon as possible, and prescribe broad-spectrum antibiotics that cover aerobic and anaerobic microbial species [15,24].

Diagnostic imaging modalities

The most important clinical signs of NF are tissue necrosis, putrid discharge, bullae, severe pain, gas formations in soft tissue, rapid spreading through fascial planes and the lack of classical tissue inflammatory signs, i.e. *"dolor, color, rubor, tumor and functio laesa"*. Today, CT and MRI are superior methods compared to sonography, scintigraphy and plain radiography, which also provide useful information about the nature and the extent of necrotizing infection [1,2,35]. Nevertheless, physical examination and a clear understanding of the clinical picture are the most important means in establishing an early diagnosis of any type of NSTI and NF [6,36].

Treatment

Successful treatment of NSTI requires a multidisciplinary approach from the onset and coordination between general practitioners and surgeons for outpatient cases, and between the surgeons and other specialists in hospital facilities. The first and economically most important decision in treating necrotizing infections concerns the need for hospitalization. Most pyodermas and uncomplicated skin and soft tissue infections do not require hospitalization. Complicated necrotizing infections often require admission, especially if fascia or muscle involvement is suspected. If the process is rapidly progressing, signs of systemic toxemia develop, the diagnosis or prognosis is in doubt, exploratory surgery is contemplated or the patient cannot adequately comply with outpatient treatment. These days NSTI and NF still exists as a life threatening soft tissue disease, therefore patient must be promptly admitted into a hospital ICU [6,37] in which appropriate treatment including radical surgical debridement of the entire affected area should be performed. The fluid resuscitation must be ordered immediately upon arrival, to maintain hemodynamic stability and vital functions.

Today, the generally agreed upon algorithm for care is: 1-Resuscitate the patient in shock; 2-Begin with broad spectrum antibiotics which cover polymicrobial infection; 3-Take patient to the operating room for early comprehensive debridement of all dead tissue. Doubt as to the diagnosis can be settled using frozen section histologic analysis. Obtain gram stain and culture from the wound; 4-Further debridement's should be repeated every 24 to 48 hours until the infection is controlled; 5-Antibiotic therapy should be adjusted to adequately cover organisms obtained on initial culture; 6-HBO can be considered in the hemodynamically stable patient, if available (Table 5).

A combination of antibiotics is the key to successful adjuvant therapy, most of our patients having been treated with empirical antimicrobial therapy before we established the early diagnosis of necrotizing infection. In the majority of our cases the wound cultures were collected at the time of initial surgery. Unfortunately, antibiotic therapy alone has little value because tissue hypoxia and ischemia do not permit adequate delivery of antibiotics to the target tissue [6,36]. The polymicrobial infection identified by wound cultures was the dominant causes of NF in our study (Table 1, 4). For that purpose we used a combination of antibiotics that cover a broad spectrum of anaerobes (Clindamycin) and aerobes, gram-positive (Penicillin G or extended spectrum Penicillin, Imipenem and Teicoplanin) and gram-negative organisms (Aminogliycosides, Cephalosporins, or Carbapenems) [36,38]. Our therapeutic regimen usually consisted of Penicillin G, Clindamycin and Gentamicin [36]. In cases when we used Aminoglycosides, renal function with creatinin excretion was additionally monitored. Because of the increasing number of MRSA infections, Daptomycin or Linezolid should be considered as part of the therapeutic regime, until MRSA infection has been excluded. Vancomycin is also in use, but it does not have any effect on exotoxin production [1,2]. For the anaerobes coverage we have provided some other combination of antibiotics like Metronidazole and third generation Cephalosporins [8,25,39]. After gram staining and culture for rapid bacteriologic diagnosis or rapidly frozen biopsy examination have been established, we started with targeted antibiotics. The culture-negative rate in our study was probably not due to the use of empirical antibiotic treatment before the wound culture was available, but it is lower than in other studies [36,40,41]. Unfortunately, contemporary dilemmas about how long to use antibiotics also exist. We recommend continuing with the antibiotic therapy for 3 to 5 days after the systemic signs and symptoms and most local signs of soft tissue infection have resolved. Other authors suggested the same approach [22,25,36,38].

The emergency surgical debridement of all affected tissue is the primary treatment modality for NSTI and NF. It includes prompt and radical surgical debridement, necrectomy and fasciotomy in cases presenting with the compartment syndrome [8,37]. Surgical intervention can be life-saving and must be performed as early as possible. Surgical procedures should be repeated during the next 24 h, 48 h, or longer, depending on the clinical course of the necrotizing infection and vital functions. Numerous studies [5] have shown that the most important variable for the mortality rate is the timing and extent of the first debridement. In the study of Mock et al. [42] the relative risk of death was 7,5 times greater in cases with improper primary debridement, and in the study of Wong et al. [43] it was 9 times greater when primary surgery was delayed more than 24 hours. Incisions are performed parallel to Langer's lines to ensure better surgical wound healing and less scaring [6,36]. We start the incision over the point of maximal fluctuation and then extended in the direction of Langer's lines. The surgery also minimizes the overall tissue loss because it cuts the way the infection spreads in course of facial plan and eliminates the need for amputation of the infected limbs [44]. After the release of pus and fluid by performing incisions which are parallel with Langer's lines we can perform additional perpendicular incisions on the skin [6] to maintain the wound open, and to allow free drainage and to remove additional necrotic tissue. But, skin bridges and flaps generally should be avoided while performing incisions. Every patient who has NSTI and NF needs a regular inspection of the operated wounds during the next 24 hours and later. If there is any concern about the tissue viability, the surgeon must promptly perform a re-operation with additional radical debridement. We maintain that the main reason for the progression of the infection lies in the delay of the first operative debridement, inadequate primary debridement and necrectomy, hemodynamic instability and concomitant illness [36]. The flow of intravascular liquid into third tissue spaces in each presented case was large and therefore hemodynamic resuscitation, nutritional support and enteral feeding in ICU must be started as soon as possible. These measurements also prevented concomitant catabolism [1,2,14,15].

During surgical intervention, the following signs are of greatest importance for the NF diagnosis: grayish necrotic deep fascia, a lack of resistance of normally adherent muscular fascia to blunt finger dissection *("Finger test")*, lack of bleeding from the fascia and the presence of dish-water pus [6,36]. Based on our surgical practice we also recommend an early and very aggressive debridement of all involved tissue that can be easily elevated off of the fascia with gentle pressure or finger spreading. The surgical intervention in which we removed all infected tissue in a single operation, rapidly improved the clinical course of the infection. All deep fascia and muscle should be inspected for potential involvement with streptococcal myositis or clostridium infection. We believe that the mass and the extension of soft tissue that must be initially excised depend on the body region in which the infection appeared. Nevertheless, the extent of debridement should not be needlessly limited because the novel plastic surgical techniques can cover every wound defect size.

Special attention should be paid to the upper and lower extremities, AW with intra-abdominal infection such as secondary peritonitis, and on the CW with persisting sternum infection and mediastinitis [8,11,26]. The extent of debridement is very important on the extremities. In cases with compromised viability and compartment syndrome additional fasciotomies of all fascio-cutaneous spaces should be performed [36]. A suspected case of clostridial myonecrosis requires early surgical exploration and extensive debridement of all involved muscle structures [36]. A tourniquet should be used during the limb surgery to reduce blood loss and offer better examination [36]. The incision proceeds proximally from the infected area in a longitudinal manner, until healthy fascia adherent to the overlying subcutaneous tissue and underlying muscle is encountered. In that moment, the tourniquet should be deflated, the wound checked to confirm tissue viability, and then meticulous hemostatis should be performed [36]. Still, controversy exists regarding how much tissue should be initially excised because the skin may often appear normal. Andreasen et al. [22] investigated the normal-appearing tissue microscopically, and found that soft tissue had extensive vascular micro-thromboses as well as vasculitis. Their finding indicated that this tissue, which has a normal external appearance, has a high risk of full thickness necrosis [22]. Poor prognostic indicators for limb amputation very often include old age, peripheral vascular disease and diabetes [36,44,45]. Amputation must be obligatory considered if the extent of infection includes a large joint and most muscle groups or if the infection is rapidly spreading towards the torso [36,46].

Postoperative wound management consists of serial dressing changes, until the wound becomes free of recurrent or progressive skin and soft tissue necrosis. The wound is washed and dressed with occlusive, adsorptive bandages with antiseptic two or three times a day [36]. We recommend daily antibiotic dressings such as 1% povidone iodine solution or 1% Silver sulfadiazine cream (Dermazin). Articoat and hydrofiber dressing like Aquacel Ag is also a useful method for the control of the infection, during the procedures of secondary wound defect closure [36,47]. After the initial surgery, the wound must be carefully examined in general anesthesia every 24 h, to assess the tissue viability and necrotizing infection progress [36,44]. Serial debridement must be performed more times (median range in our study was four times) because the necrotizing infection is rarely eradicated after a single debridement [36].

Perineal, perianal, or scrotal infections require special consideration (Figure 1). In the presence of a pressure sore, perineal abscess or paraplegia, necrotizing infection spreads into the scrotum, inguinal region and lower AW. In some particular cases, it is necessary to perform a diverting colostomy, cystostomy, or both to facilitate the formation of granulation tissues and wound hygiene, and to protect the flaps or skin grafts healing process. Surgical management includes wide tissue incision, radical debridement with orchiectomy and drainage of all involved areas [13]. The wound is abundantly washed with hydrogen peroxide, saline and 1% povidone iodine solution. Finally, it is dressed with occlusive and adsorptive bandages with antiseptic, and changed twice daily. After the wound stabilizes and fresh granulations form, we perform secondary soft tissue defect reconstructions.

NF of the AW and RS, even today, presents a challenging surgical issue. Skin incision must be performed in the longitudinal direction along the muscle-fascial layers of the inner AW until healthy fascia adherent to the overlying subcutaneous tissue and muscle is encountered. It is not indicated to perform two, three or more parallel incisions or any perpendicular incisions, because the bridges of skin and skin islands will usually not survive. Postoperative wound management on the AW consists of serial dressing changes during the next 24 h to 48 h, until the wound is free of recurrent or ongoing infection. When infection progresses across the deep fascial plane of the AW or a necrotic area on the skin appears, aggressive surgical debridement should be repeated. In our case with NF of the AW and RS we usually performed two to five debridement procedures to stabilize the wound conditions. The primary defect on the AW is usually large and it is repaired with advancement flaps using an abdominoplasty technique,

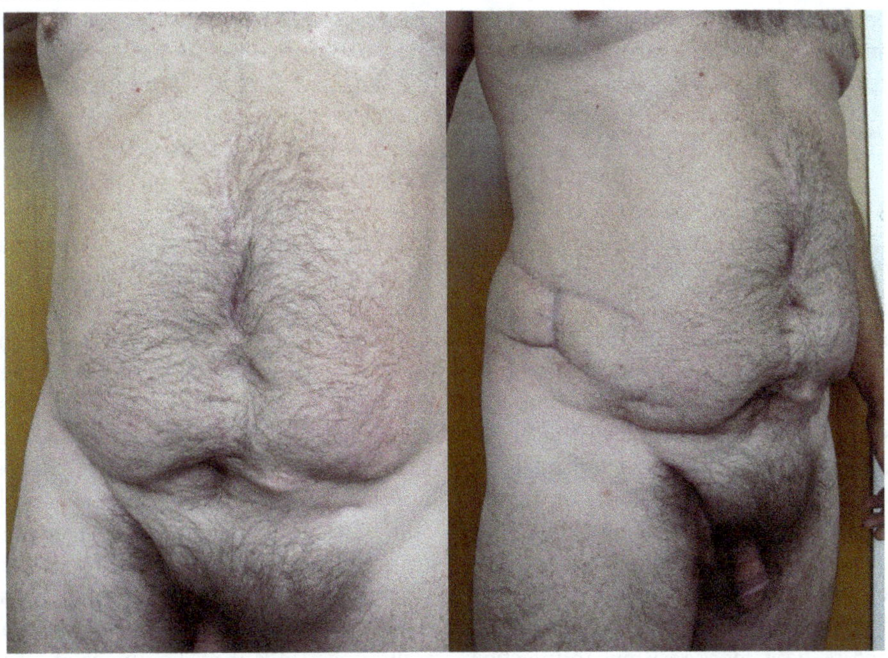

Figure 1 **Postoperative view of Fournier's gangrene and necrotizing fasciitis of the abdominal wall with closed divergent colostomy.**

biological mesh or skin grafts [48]. These days, after the primary surgery of NF we can also use the topical negative pressure therapy (TNP) [49], artificial skin (Integra) [50], synthetic prosthetics [51] and bio-prosthetic (biologic) mesh [52,53]. In our particular case with caecum perforation during inguinal hernia repair, fecal peritonitis and septic shock were present. We performed explorative laparotomy via midline incision and found diffuse peritonitis, ischemia of small bowel and right colon, and NF of the RS. Published reports point out that ultrasound, native abdominal x-ray films or CT scanning are very useful preoperative diagnostic methods for bowel perforation with diffuse peritonitis, but the exact condition is always discovered intraoperatively [15,23]. We decided to apply a combination of antimicrobial therapy that covers aerobes and anaerobes. After we received the results of microbiological analysis, we ordered antibiotics for each causative organism. During the first operation we performed an extensive surgical debridement of the RS, right hemicolectomy, diverting colostomy on the left colon and multiple drainages of the infected intra-abdominal fluid collections. There is still controversy about the optimal surgical management of colonic perforation complicated with peritonitis. Hartmann's resection has been considered the procedure of choice in cases with diffuse peritonitis and remains a safe technique for colectomy in a perforated colon, especially in elderly patients with multiple comorbidities [30,31]. More recently, some have suggested that primary resection with anastomosis is a modern approach, even in the presence of diffuse peritonitis [30]. After the wound is stabilized with fresh granulation tissue, we could perform a second reconstruction of the AW defects, primarily with advanced flaps and skin grafts. The diverting colostomy was closed in a third operation.

HBO therapy

The use of HBO as an adjuvant therapy for NSTI is based on animal and human studies, and continues to be the subject of scientific analysis [45]. Several studies have shown decreased morbidity and mortality when HBO is used postoperatively as adjuvant therapy [26,36,45]. However, HBO should not interfere with or delay the repeated surgical debridement. The newest data indicate that oxygen administration in the perioperative period may reduce the risk of wound infection [36,54]. The reason for this is that the ability of neutrophil leucocytes to kill bacteria depends on the oxygen availability and formation of free oxygen radicals. HBO additionally increases oxygen diffusion into soft tissue and facilitates the synthesis of collagen and angiogenesis [54]. Better perfused tissue is more resistant to infection (especially from anaerobic spp.) [55] and exotoxin excretion by *Clostridium* spp. [56,57]. We have determined the effect of HBO therapy on short term complications of complex war wounds to the upper and lower extremities that included cases with NSTI and NF in patients who were and patients who were not treated according to the North Atlantic Treaty Organization (NATO) emergency war surgery recommendations [36]. We found that HBO therapy significantly reduced the time to wound stabilization and fresh granulation production, as well as the occurrence of wound complications (deep soft tissue infection, osteomyelitis, skin graft lyses and flap necrosis) in patients with Gustilo type III extremity war wounds. Also we have gained additional experience with the use of HBO therapy for severe life-threatening infections such as clostridial myonecrosis and other aerobic and anaerobic NSTI. Regardless of the type of surgical strategy applied, the HBO therapy should never delay the emergency of the surgical intervention, including the treatment of *Clostridium perfrigens* causing gas gangrene [36,54,57].

Reconstructive surgery

The reconstruction of skin defects either on the extremities and torso, or on the abdominal or chest wall, should be performed using several different techniques and surgical materials on each patient. As is often seen, a complete loss of skin or dermal structures needs a complex, multilayer reconstruction especially in functional areas of the body and on the extremities. Novel concepts of layer-specific reconstruction include biologic meshes, which are an alternative to flap and skin graft surgery, especially in abdominal and chest wall reconstructions [58-61]. After the wound stabilizes and fresh granulation tissue without any signs of acute infection we perform staging reconstructions using simple to complex reconstructive methods. The main contributing factor for reconstructive method-selection was the extent and the localization of the defect and the patient's condition [51-53].

Topical negative pressure therapy has been reported to remove exudates, cover wounds securely, stimulate angiogenesis [6,49] and reduce bacterial contamination [50]. It also reduces the surface area of the wound, improves the rate of granulation tissue formation, reduces the number of surgical excision procedures needed, as well as enables better healing performance of skin grafts and biologic meshes. The cost benefit of that novel therapy is evident, but the complications of TNP still exist and include damage to surrounding tissue due to pressure effects, pain during dressing changes and discomfort because of very bulky dressing [52]. Newer data recommend the use of TNP in the acute traumatic military settings [58]. Leininger at all used TNP in the deployed military settings (at R3 stage of-NATO medical care) where they treated all Iraqi casualties with TNP dressing after their first debridement (77 cases) [59]. They reported that infection rates dropped from 81% to 0% after using the TNP management strategy. Our experience has shown the use of this wound management technique to remove exudates, improve the patient comfort, reduce the wound size and the time for wound stabilization, to allow the formation of fresh granulation tissue, and better healing of skin grafts and flaps [36].

Reconstructive options on the extremities start as simple and advance towards the more complex as needed for a given defect. The reconstructive ladder is a useful way to systematically plan the closure of any wound on the extremities [36]. The reconstructive ladder begins with healing by secondary intention as the base level, and advance with primary closure, skin grafting, local flaps, regional flaps and free tissue transfer. The final methods for extremity reconstruction are the use of TNP and perforator flaps (Table 1) [50-53].

NF after abdominal surgery or spreading infections from the perineum or the lower extremities is extremely serious with great defects and carries a high morbidity and mortality rate (Figure 2). The goals of the reconstructive surgery in the management of complex AW defects (AWD) is to restore the structural and functional continuity of the muscle-fascial system, provide stable coverage and achieve local wound closure [60]. The size of the wound defect after NF of the abdominal wall typically depends on the type of infection and the way it spreads. For reconstructive purposes, AWD can be divided into midline or lateral, and to the upper, middle, or lower third of the abdomen. The most useful method for ventral hernia repair with AWD is the use of *"Component separation technique"* by Ramirez and coworkers [61]. They used muscle-fascial components of the AW in continuity with their vascular and nerve supply to restore ventral defects. Midline partial defects of the skin and deep structures can be repaired in several ways. Firstly, we can use primary closure and skin grafts. The next option is a synthetic mesh [51], which cannot be used on the infected field. It comes in various sizes and shapes at low cost. Biological meshes [52] are resistant to infection, allow natural remodeling, potential stretching, are expensive and are of limited size. Further options include the component separation technique, free, local or distant flaps, TNP therapy, and tissue expansion [60]. A combination of all these techniques is also possible. The reconstruction of the structural components of the AW is an important issue, but even more important is the restoration of the AW function. Midline complete defects can be repaired in similar fashion, because the defects include both skin and fascia, which often require component separation technique, biologic mesh, the local flaps with or without tissue expansion. Lateral defects are more often repaired using direct closures, skin grafts, local advancement flaps, distant flaps, or TNP therapy [60].

Conclusion

Necrotizing infections refer to rapidly spreading infections, usually located in the fascial planes of soft tissue

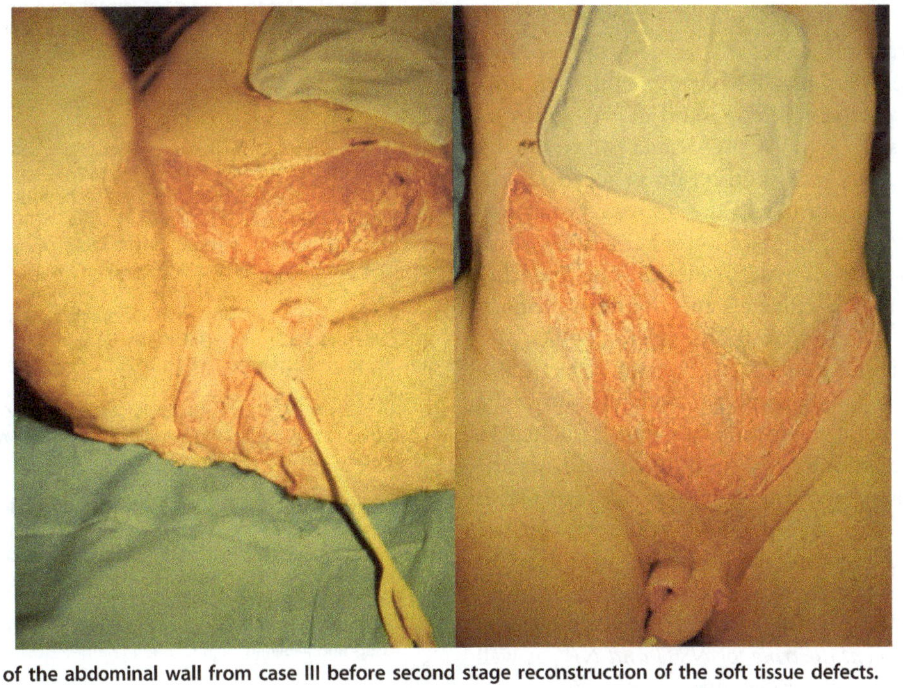

Figure 2 A view of the abdominal wall from case III before second stage reconstruction of the soft tissue defects.

areas, that result in extensive tissue necrosis, severe sepsis, wide spread organ failure and death. The early diagnosis and management of NF is essential since delayed disease recognition and lack of effective treatment modalities increase the mortality of NF [1].

In everyday surgical practice infections that are life threatening conditions and which require early recognition and aggressive surgical debridement along with broad spectrum antibiotics therapy, are rare. When NF becomes a rapidly progressing necrosis of the subcutaneous fat and fascia, it develops into a life threatening disease that needs prompt recognition, extensive debridement, immediate antibiotic therapy and intensive care treatment. Early and aggressive surgery is mandatory for establishing the right diagnosis as well as for removing as much infected tissue as possible in a single operation. The diagnosis remains primarily clinical, but diagnostic adjuncts such as LRINEC scoring system can be useful for early and precise diagnosis [5].

Different types of microorganisms can cause NF. As seen in our clinical study, the majority of cases begin with an existing infection, most frequently on the extremities, in the perineum or on the AW.

As previously stressed, the treatment modalities of NF in different patient groups are very heterogeneous, but the most important factor of mortality is the time of operative intervention, as well as the number of co-morbidities [36]. Patients with DM appear to be particularly at risk, representing over 70% of cases in one large review [46]. The other co-morbidities include obesity, alcohol abuse, immune-deficiency, chronic renal failure, liver cirrhosis, hypertension, peripheral vascular disease and age above 60 years [1,2].

In cases where the diagnosis is uncertain, repeated clinical assessment and multiple vectors approach integrating a range of diagnostic modalities will optimize the final diagnosis [1]. Many physicians today are not familiar enough with NSTI and NF to proceed rapidly with an accurate diagnosis and the necessary management [36]. The majority of cases today are treated on an outpatient basis or in outpatient clinics. On the other hand, each untreated necrotizing infection or a misdiagnosed case has a poor prognosis and severe course.

In highly suspicious cases of necrotizing infections a multidisciplinary team approach is mandatory, involving the GP doctor, general and plastic surgeons, radiologists, microbiologists, physiotherapists and nutritionists. In the majority of clinical cases, surgeons have a high responsibility level for timely and appropriate surgical treatment and therefore the final outcome. Thus, early surgical debridement, combined with broad spectrum antibiotics, intensive care therapy and adjuvant HBO therapy should become part of the *"Treatment doctrine for NSTI and NF"*, as well as for the treatment of clostridial myonecrosis [36].

Patient Consent

Written informed consent was obtained from the patients for publication of this case report and accompanying images. A copy of the written consent is available for review by the Editor-in-Chief of this journal.

Abbreviations

AB: antibiotics; ATA: atmospheres absolute pressure; AW: abdominal wall AWD: abdominal wall defect; CRP: C-reactive protein; CW: chest wall; DM-Diabetes mellitus; GP: General practitioner; HBOT: Hyperbaric oxygen therapy; ICU: Intensive care unit; LRINEC: laboratory risk indictor for necrotizing fasciitis; MODS: multiple organ dysfunction syndrome; MRSA: meticillin resistant *Staphylococcus aureus*; NF: Necrotizing fasciitis; NSTIs: Necrotizing soft tissue infections; PMNs: Polymorphonuclear neutrophils; RS: retroperitineal space; SG: skin graft; SIRS: systemic inflammatory response syndrome; SSTIs: Skin and soft tissue infections; TNP: Topical negative pressure.

Author details

[1]Division of Plastic Surgery and Burns, University Hospital Centre Split, Croatia. [2]Department of Surgery, University Hospital Dubrava, Zagreb, Croatia. [3]Department of Surgery, University Hospital Centre Split, Croatia. [4]Department of Urology, University Hospital Centre Split, Croatia. [5]Department of Orthopedic Surgery, University Hospital Dubrava, Zagreb, Croatia. [6]Deparment of Neurosurgery, University Hospital Dubrava, Zagreb, Croatia.

Authors' contributions

All authors participated in the design of the paper, conceived the paper, and participated in drafting and critical revision for important intellectual content. All authors read and approved the final form of this manuscript.

Competing interests

The authors declare that they have no competing interests.

References

1. Morgan MS: **Diagnosis and management of necrotizing fasciitis: A multiparametric approach.** *J Hosp Infect* 2010, **75**:249-257.
2. Levine EG, Manders SM: **Life-threatening necrotizing fasciitis.** *Clin in Dermat* 2005, **23**:144-147.
3. Tang S, Ho PL, Tang VW, Fung KK: **Necrotizing fasciitis of a limb.** *J Bone Joint Surg* 2001, **3(5)**:709-714.
4. Urschel JD, Takita H, Antkowiak JG: **Necrotizing soft tissue infections of the chest wall.** *Ann Thorac Surg* 1997, **64**:276-279.
5. Sarani B, Strong M, Pascual J, Schwab CW: **Necrotizing fasciitis: Current concept and review of the literature.** *J Am Coll Surg* 2009, **208(2)**:279-288.
6. Marron CD: **Superficial sepsis, cutaneous abscess and necrotizing fasciitis. Emergency surgery.**Edited by: Brooks A, Mahoney PF, Cotton BA, Tai N. Blacwell Publisching; , 1 2010:115-123.
7. Endorf FW, Cancio LC, Klein MB: **Necrotizing soft tissue infections: Clinical guidelines.** *J Burn Care Resurch* 2009, **30(5)**:769-775.
8. Maynor M: **Necrotizing fasciitis 2009.**1-20[http://emedicine.medscape.com/].
9. Angoules AG, Kontakis G, Drakoulakis E, Vrentzos G, Granik MS, Giannoudis PV: **Necrotizing fasciitis of upper and lower limb: A systemic review.** *Injury* 2009, **38(Suppl 5)**:SI26.
10. Wong CH, Chang HC, Pasupathy S, Khin LW, Tan JL, Low CO: **Necrotizing fasciitis: Clinical presentation, microbiology, and determinants of mortality.** *JBJS Am* 2003, **85**:1454-1460.
11. Vlajčić Z, Žic R, Stanec Z, Stanec S: **Algorithm for classification and treatment of poststernotomy wound infection.** *Scan J Plast Reconst Surg Hand Surg* 2007, **41(3)**:114-119.
12. McCormac PM: **Use of prosthetic materials in chest wall reconstruction. Assets and liabilities.** *Surg Clin North Am* 1989, **69(5)**:965-971.

13. Azize Klc, Ylmaz Ali KLc: **Fournier's gangrene: Etiology, treatment, and complications.** *Ann Plast Surg* 2001, **147(5)**:523-527.
14. Sartelli M: **A focus on intra-abdominal infections.** *World J Emerg Surg* 2010, 5:9.
15. Sartelli M, Viale P, Koike K, Pea F, Tumietto F, Van Goor H, Guercioni G, Nespoli A, Trana C, Catena F, Ansaloni L, Leppaniemi A, Biffi W, Moore FA, Poggetti R, Pinna AD, Moore E: **WSES consensus conference: Guidelines for first-line management of intra-abdominal infections.** *World J Emerg Surg* 2011, **6**:2.
16. Pryor JP, Piotrowski E, Seltzer CW, Gracias VH: **Early diagnosis of retroperitineal necrotizing fasciitis.** *Crit Care Med* 2001, **29(5)**:1071-1073.
17. Elliott DC, Kufera JA, Myers RA: **Necrotizing soft tissue infections. Risk factors for morality and strategies for management.** *Ann Surg* 1996, **224**:672-683.
18. Green JR, Dafoe DC, Raffin TA: **Necrotizing fasciitis.** *Chest* 1996, **110(1)**:219-228.
19. Bair MJ, Chi H, Wang Ws, Hsiao Yc, Chaing RA, Chang KY: **Necrotizing fasciitis in southeast Taiwan: Clinical features, microbiology, and prognosis.** *Infect Dis* 2009, **13(2)**:255-260.
20. Wong CH, Khin LW, Heng Ks, Tan KC, Low CO: **LRINEC (Laboratory Risk Indicator for Necrotizing Fasciitis) score: A tool for distinguishing necrotizing fasciitis from other soft infections.** *Crit Care Med* 2004, **32**:1535-1541.
21. Yilmazlar T, Ozturk E, Asloy A, Ozgue H: **Necrotizing soft tissue infections: APACHE II score, dissemination, and survival.** *World J Surg* 2007, **31**:1858-1862.
22. Andreasen TJ, Green SD, Childers BJ: **Massive infectious soft tissue injury: Diagnosis and management of necrotizing fasciitis and purpura fulminosa.** *Plast Reconst Surg* 2001, **107(4)**:1025-1035.
23. Menichetti F, Sganga G: **Definition and classification of intra-abdominal infection.** *J Chemother* 2009, **21(Suppl 1)**:3-4.
24. Taviloglu K, Yanar H: **Necrotizing fasciitis: Strategies for diagnosis and management.** *World J Emerg Surg* 2007, **2**:19.
25. DiNubile MJ, Lipsky BA: **Complicated infections of skin and skin structures: When the infection is more than skin deep.** *J Antimicrob Chemother* 2004, **53(Suppl 2)**:37-50.
26. Cheung PJ, Fung B, tang WM, IP WY: **A review of necrotizing fasciitis in the extremities.** *Hong Kong Med J* 2009, **15(1)**:44-52.
27. Olafson EJ, Zeni T, Wilkes DS: **A 46 years old man with excruciating shoulder pain.** *Chest* 2005, **127(3)**:1039-1044.
28. Kologlu MB, Yildiz RV, Alper B, Yagmurly A, Ciftci E, Gockora IH, Emiroglu M, Dindur H: **Necrotizing fasciitis in children: Diagnostic and therapeutic aspects.** *J Pediat Surg* 2007, **42**:1892-1897.
29. Keskinen P, Leppaniemi A, Pettila V, Piilonen A, Kemppainen E: **Intra-abdominal pressure in severe acute pancreatitis.** *World J Emerg Surg* 2007, **2**:2.
30. Powell JM, Sasapu KK, Macklin C: **Metastatic gas gangrene and colonic perforation: A case report.** *World J Emerg Surg* 2008, **3**:15.
31. Mulier S, Penninck x, Verwaest C, Filez L, Aerts R, Lauwers S, Lauwers P: **Factor affecting mortality in generalized postoperative peritonitis: Multivariate analysis in 96 patients.** *World J Surg* 2003, **27**:379-84.
32. Montravers P, Gauzit R, Muller C, Marmuse JP, Fichelle A, Desmonts JM: **Emergence of antibiotic resistant bacteria in cases of peritonitis after intra abdominal surgery affects the efficacy of empirical antimicrobial therapy.** *Clin Infect Dis* 1996, **23**:486-494.
33. Varos D, Pissiotis C, Georgantas D, Katsaragakis S, Antoniou S, Papadimitriou J: **Role of early and extensive surgery in the treatment of severe necrotizing soft tissue infection.** *Br J Surg* 1993, **80**:1190-11.
34. Ullah S, Khan M, Asad Ullah Jan M: **Fournier's gangrene: A dreadful disease.** *Surgeon* 2009, **7(3)**:138-142.
35. Sharif HS, Clark Dc, Aabed MY, Aideyan OA, Haddad MC, Mattsson TA: **MR imaging of thoracic and abdominal wall infections: Comparison with other imaging procedures.** *Am J Roetgenol* 1990, **154(5)**:989-995.
36. Roje Z, Roje Ž, Eterović D, Družijanić N, Petričević A, Roje T, Čapkun V: **Influence of adjuvant hyperbaric oxygen therapy on short-term complications during surgical reconstruction of upper and lower extremity war injury: A retrospective cohort study.** *Croat Med J* 2008, **49**:224-232.
37. Brandt MM, Corpron CA, Wahl WL: **Necrotizing soft tissue infections: A surgical disease.** *Am J Surg* 2000, **66**:967-970.
38. Naqvi GA, Malik SA, Jan W: **Necrotizing fasciitis of the lower extremity: A case report and current concept of diagnoses and management.** *Scan J Trauma Resusc Emerg Med* 2009, **17**:28.
39. Anaya A, Dellinger EP: **Necrotizing soft tissue infections: Diagnoses and management.** *Clin Infect Dis* 2007, **44**:705-710.
40. Hsiao CT, Weng HH, Yuan YD, Chen CT, Chen IC: **Predictors of mortality in patients with necrotizing fasciitis.** *Am J Emerg Med* 2008, **26**:170-175.
41. Dryden MS: **Skin and soft tissue infections: Microbiology and epidemiology.** *Inter J Antimicrob Agent* 2009, **34(S1)**:52-57.
42. Mok MY, Wong SY, Chan TM: **Necrotizing fasciitis in rheumatic diseases.** *Lupus* 2006, **15**:380-383.
43. Wong CH, How-Chong C, Shanker P: **Necrotizing fasciitis: clinical presentation, microbiology, and determinants of mortality.** *J Bone Joint Surg Am* 2003, **85**:1454-1460.
44. Wong KC, Shih CH: **Necrotizing fasciitis of the extremities.** *J Trauma* 1992, **32(2)**:179-182.
45. Jallali N, Withey S, Butter PE: **Hyperbaric oxygen therapy.** *Am J Surg* 2005, **189**:462-466.
46. Gurlek A, Firat C, Ozturk AE, Alaybeyoglu N, Fazir A, Aslan S: **Management of necrotizing fasciitis in diabetic patients.** *J Diabet and Its Comp* 2007, **21**:265-271.
47. Saffle JR: **Closure of the excided burn wound: Temporary skin substitutes.** *In Clin Plast Surg* 2009, **36(4)**:627-643.
48. Brafa A, Grimaldi L, Brandi C, Nisi G, Calabro M, Campa SA, Aniello CD: **Abdominoplasty as a reconstructive surgical treatment of necrotizing fasciitis of the abdominal wall.** *J Plast Reconst Aesth Surg* 2009, **62**: e136-e139.
49. De Geus HRH, Klooster V, Lakoski S: **Vacuum assisted closure in the treatment of large skin defects due to necrotizing fasciitis.** *Intensive Care Med* 2005, **31**:601-609.
50. Muangman P, Engrav LH, Heimbach DM: **Complex wound management utilizing an artificial dermal matrix.** *Ann Plast Surg* 2006, **57**:199-202.
51. Grevious MA, Cohen M, Pierre JF, Herrmann GE: **The use of prosthetics in abdominal wall reconstruction.** *Clin Plast Surg* 2006, **33(2)**:181-197.
52. Butler CE: **The role of bioprosthetics in abdominal wall reconstruction.** *Clin Plast Surg* 2005, **33(2)**:199-211.
53. Campanelli G, Catena F, Ansaloni L: **Prosthetic abdominal wall hernia repair in emergency surgery: From polypropylene to biological meshes.** *World J Emerg Surg* 2008, **3**:33.
54. Mortensen CR: **Hyperbaric oxygen therapy.** *Curr Anaest & Crit Care* 2008, **19**:333-337.
55. Wong CH, Yam AKT, Tan ABH, Song C: **Approach to debridement in necrotizing fasciitis.** *Am J Surg* 2008, **196**:e19-e24.
56. Karhonen K: **Hyperbaric oxygen therapy in acute necrotizing infection. With a special reference to the effects on tissue gas tensions.** *Ann Chir Gynecol* 2009, **89**:7-36.
57. Kaye D: **Effects of hyperbaric oxygen on Clostridia in vitro and in vivo.** *Proc Soc Exp Biol Med* 1987, **124**:360-366.
58. Fries CSA, Jeffery SLA, Kay AR: **Topical negative pressure and military wounds-A review of the evidence.** *Injury, Int J care Injured* 2011, **42**:436-440.
59. Leininger BE, Rasmussen TE, Smith DL: **Experience with wound VAC and delay primary closure of contaminated soft tissue injuries in Iraq.** *J Trauma* 2006, **61(5)**:1207-1211.
60. Mathes SJ, Steinwald PM, Foster RD, Hoffman WY, Anthony JP: **Complex abdominal wall reconstruction: A comparison of flap and mesh closure.** *Ann Surg* 2000, **232(4)**:586-596.
61. Ramirez OM, Ruas E, Dellon AL: **"Component separation" method for closure of abdominal wall defect: An anatomic and clinical study.** *Plast Reconst Surg* 1990, **86(3)**:519-526.

Cost of care and antibiotic prescribing attitudes for community-acquired complicated intra-abdominal infections in Italy

Lidia Dalfino[1*], Francesco Bruno[1], Sergio Colizza[2], Ercole Concia[3], Andrea Novelli[4], Fabrizio Rebecchi[5], Federico Spandonaro[6] and Cristina Alato[6]

Abstract

Introduction: Complicated intra-abdominal infections (cIAIs) are a common cause of morbidity worldwide, and in spite of improvements in patient care, therapeutic failure still occurs, impacting in-hospital resource consumption. This study aimed to assess the costs associated with the treatment of community-acquired cIAIs, from the Italian National Health Service perspective.

Methods: This retrospective study analyzed the charts of patients who were discharged from four Italian university hospitals between January 1 and December 31, 2009 with a primary diagnosis of community-acquired cIAIs. Patient characteristics, diagnosis, surgical procedure, antibiotic therapy, and length of hospital stay were all recorded and the cost of total hospital care was estimated. Costs were calculated in Euros at 2009 values.

Results: The records of 260 patients (mean age 48.9 years; 57% males) were analyzed. The average cost of care for a patient hospitalized due to cIAI was €4385 (95% CI 3650–5120), with an average daily cost of €419 (95% CI 378–440). Antibiotic therapy represented just under half (44.3%) of hospitalization costs. The strongest predictor of the increase in hospital costs was clinical failure: patients who clinically failed received an average of 8.2 additional days of antibiotic therapy and spent 11 more days in hospital compared with patients who responded to first-line therapy (both $p < 0.05$ vs. patients who were successfully treated). Furthermore, they incurred €5592 in additional hospitalization costs (2.88 times the cost associated with clinical success) with 53% (€2973) of the additional costs attributable to antibiotic therapy. Overall, antibiotic appropriateness rate was 78.8% ($n = 205$), and was significantly higher in patients receiving combination therapy compared with those treated with monotherapy (97.3% vs. 64.6%).

Conclusion: The results of this study suggest that hospitals need to be aware of the clinical and economic consequences of antibiotic therapy of cIAIs and to reduce overall resource use and costs by improving the rate of success with appropriate initial empiric therapy.

Keywords: Antibiotics, Community-acquired intra-abdominal infections, Cost of care, Direct costs, Hospitalization

* Correspondence: lidia.dalfino@yahoo.com
[1]Anesthesia and Intensive Care Unit - Emergency and Organ Transplantation Department, University of Bari, Policlinico of Bari, P.zza G. Cesare 11, 70124 Bari, Italy
Full list of author information is available at the end of the article

Introduction

Intra-abdominal infections (IAIs), encompassing a wide spectrum of pathological conditions from uncomplicated appendicitis to fecal peritonitis, are a common cause of morbidity worldwide. IAIs are defined as complicated (cIAIs) when infection extends beyond the affected hollow viscus into the peritoneal space, causing either localized or diffuse peritonitis [1]. In spite of improvements in patient care, therapeutic failure still occurs in patients with community-acquired (CA) cIAIs [2-5], highly impacting in-hospital resource consumption [2,5,6]. In early European series, patients with community-acquired cIAIs who clinically failed had significantly longer length of hospital stay and incurred significantly higher inpatient charges than those who were treated successfully [2,6]. More recently, the economic rebound of clinical failure has been investigated in a large US multi-institutional database of 6056 patients with cIAIs, showing an additional 4.6 days spent in hospital and inpatient charges of $6368 when clinical failure occurred [5].

The clinical outcome of patients with cIAIs is heavily influenced by prompt surgical source control and timely effective antimicrobial treatment [7,8]. Current guidelines recommend a wide range of first-line single or multiple antimicrobial regimens based on patient characteristics (comorbidities, immunosuppression, and previous antibiotic exposure), expected involved pathogens (inferred by source and origin, community or hospital-acquired, of infection) and local resistance epidemiology [1,5].

Most recent guidelines also consider the antibiotic treatment of cIAIs from a microbiological point of view, particularly in terms of pathogens producing ESBLs (Extended Spectrum Beta-Lactamases). For community-acquired extrabiliary cIAIs, empirical antimicrobial therapy can be divided into categories: treatment for critically ill and non-critically ill patients, and treatment for both groups according to the presence or absence of risk factors for ESBL-producing pathogens. In non-critically ill patients, amoxicillin-clavulanate or ciprofloxacin-metronidazole are possible options, but in the presence of risk factors for ESBL these are not sufficient, and other drugs such as tigecycline and ertapenem are useful. In critically ill patients without risk factors for ESBL, piperacillin-tazobactam is an option, but in the presence of ESBL risk factors carbapenems like imipenem and meropenem are more appropriate [9].

Of note, knowledge of antibiotic drugs costs is suggested as additional criteria supporting clinical decision-making [1,5,9]. In fact, in some US and European studies, a significant influence of empiric antibiotic therapy choice on economic outcome of cIAIs has emerged [3,6,7,10]. However, the wide inter-country variability of antimicrobial prescribing attitudes and of health care and reimbursement systems organization could differently impact on cost estimates. Therefore, due to this limited generalizability of data, referring to pharmacoeconomic analyses from other countries could be misleading.

To the best of our knowledge, a costs analysis of cIAIs hospital care has never been performed in Italy, although IAIs have been ranked as the second most common infectious reason for hospitalization, after respiratory infections [11]. To address this issue, this study aimed to assess the costs associated with the treatment of community-acquired cIAIs, from the Italian National Health Service (i.e. the third payer) perspective.

Methods

Study design

This one-year, multicentre, retrospective, incidence-based observational study was performed in four Italian (Bari, Florence, Turin, and Verona) acute-care university hospitals. The study was conducted in accordance with the ethical principles of the Declaration of Helsinki (and subsequent revisions) and to the current norm for observational studies. The protocol was reviewed and approved by each study site's ethical committees. Due to the retrospective study design, informed consent was not deemed necessary.

Patient selection

Patients were identified by searching computerized hospitalization records of each recruiting hospital for a primary discharge diagnoses of one of five International Classification of Diseases 9th revision (ICD-9) codes suggestive of cIAIs (540.1- acute appendicitis with intra-abdominal abscess, 540.0 - acute appendicitis with diffuse peritonitis, 567.2 - other suppurative peritonitis, 567.8-other specified peritonitis, 567.9 - unspecified peritonitis, 567.0 - peritonitis in infectious disease classified elsewhere. Patients were eligible for inclusion if they (1) were hospitalized between January 1 and December 31, 2009; (2) were at least 18 years old at the time of their hospitalization; (3) had a primary discharge diagnosis suggesting any cIAIs; (4) underwent laparotomy, laparoscopy or percutaneous drainage of an intra-abdominal abscess and (5) received intravenous antibiotics.

Patient analysis

A review of each patient's chart was performed, and relevant parameters were recorded in standardized individual electronic case report forms. These included: patient age, gender, comorbidities (diabetes mellitus, obesity or others), patient lifestyle factors (smoking, alcoholism), known risk factors for antibiotic failure [1,9] (cancer, liver cirrhosis, acute liver failure, renal failure, end stage renal failure, anemia, leukopenia, coagulopathy, immunosuppression, or others), primary and secondary discharge diagnoses, primary surgical procedure and unplanned additional surgeries (if any), laboratory, instrumental and microbiology tests (number, type and results), antibiotic therapy type, dose, and duration, switch to second-line antibiotic drugs and reasons for the switch (clinical failure, antibiotic resistance, adverse event, unspecified), illness severity markers (use of artificial nutrition, antifungal drugs, immune globulins, central venous catheter, renal replacement therapies, mechanical ventilation), medical specialists' consultancies (type and frequency), length of hospital stay, and discharge status (alive/dead). Hospital ward of admission, in-hospital transfers (to other wards or to the intensive care unit [ICU]), and place of discharge (home, other hospitals or long-term care facilities) were also recorded.

Definitions

Primary surgical procedures were categorized according to the source of infection as surgical operations on upper gastrointestinal (GI) tract (biliary or gastro-duodenal tract, and small intestine), gall-bladder, appendix, lower GI tract (colon-rectum), peritoneal abscesses drainage, or others.

Clinical success was defined as patient recovery with either first line empiric antibiotic therapy or a step-down from initial therapy (transition wide/narrow spectrum or intravenous/oral).

Clinical failure was defined as a switch to second-line antibiotic treatment, need for unscheduled additional abdominal surgeries, or patient death [2-4,6,7].

First-line empiric antibiotic therapy was defined as a regimen started at the time of surgical intervention, before the availability of any culture data.

Switch to second-line antibiotic therapy was defined as the addition of one or more parenteral antibiotics to the initial antibiotic regimen or as a complete or partial switch of the initial antibiotic regimen to another parenteral antibiotic regimen.

Unscheduled additional abdominal surgeries were taken into account if they occurred 2 or more days after the primary surgical procedure and were related to poor primary source control. Secondary procedures were not considered in the analysis when there was a mention of other reasons (i.e. technical issues or hemorrhage) that might have led to re-operation.

First-line empiric antibiotic therapy was defined as *appropriate* if all isolated bacteria were sensitive to at least one of the antibiotics administered in patients with documented positive intra-abdominal swabs or blood cultures. Alternatively, in patients with negative or no cultures, empiric therapy was deemed as appropriate when the selected regimen covered enteric gram-negative aerobic and anaerobic bacteria and drug dosing was adequate, according to current guidelines [1]. Antibiotic regimens not fulfilling the above criteria were defined as *inappropriate.*

Leucocytosis was defined by a white blood cell (WBC) count $>12{,}000/mm^3$. *Leukopenia* was defined as a WBC count $<4000/mm^3$.

Cost analysis

A estimate of the cost of antibiotics was performed by multiplying the number of antibiotic days by the unit price of that antibiotic and by the number of per day doses. The overall cost of antibiotic treatment for each patient was the sum of costs calculated for all parenteral antibiotics received by the patient during the hospitalization period. The unit price of antibiotics was based on official ex-factory prices per unit in Italy [12]. Laboratory tests, instrumental tests, and specialists' consultancies utilization were directly recorded and their costs were assessed by referring to fees for providers of specialist services recognized by the Italian National Health Service (I-NHS). Costs related to primary surgical procedures were not included in analysis, as we assume they were independent of the adopted antibiotic therapy.

Other direct costs, including personnel, ordinary maintenance and hotel costs, were indirectly estimated by using Diagnosis-Related Group's tariffs per admission provided to hospitals by the I-NHS. Specifically, this estimate was based on the acknowledged over-threshold per hospital day tariff, which is the per day cost to hospitals for length of stay prolonged over an *a priori* defined threshold (i.e. a tariff applicable to length of stay statistically considered as outliers), assuming that by subtracting the average costs of specialist services provided from this tariff, an acceptable proxy of the general cost sustained for patient management could be obtained.

Costs were expressed in Euro values at the time they were incurred (year 2009 values).

Statistical analysis

Sample size derived from the number of cIAIs patients meeting inclusion criteria, admitted at the four recruiting centers from January 1 to December 31, 2009.

Continuous data are expressed as means ± standard deviation or 95% confidence intervals (CIs), and categorical data as number of events and percentages. Univariate statistical analysis was performed by student t-test or chi-squared test, as appropriate, to compare baseline characteristics and outcomes of clinical success and failure groups.

Due to the retrospective design of the study, a regression model by means of a backward stepwise model selection approach was employed to investigate the independent hospital charges predictors, in order to control for confounding factors and obtain the exact contribution of each parameter to the outcome variable. The model takes into account patient status and controls for type of primary surgical procedure, unplanned additional surgeries, and antibiotic therapy switches. Considered variables were dummy. In order to avoid co-linearity between variables, a Pearson correlation was performed. Covariates in the model were: patient age and gender, one or more high risk factors, primary surgical procedure, surgical approach, antibiotic monotherapy/combination therapy, clinical success/failure, one or more therapeutic failure risk factors, unplanned additional surgeries, more than one additional surgery.

Statistical analyses were performed by using SPSS statistical software version 15.1 (SPSS Inc., Chicago, IL, USA). A P value <0.05 was considered statistically significant.

Results

Patient characteristics

A total of 260 patients (mean age 48.9 years; 57% males) met the study entrance criteria. On hospital arrival, 250 (96.2%) patients were admitted to surgical wards, 8 (3.1%) to medical wards, and 2 (0.7%) to the ICU. The majority of patients (62.3%) were affected by complicated appendicitis. Patients were surgically approached by laparoscopy in slightly more than half of cases, and by laparotomy in the majority of the others (Table 1).

One-hundred forty-four (55.4%) patients received first-line empiric antibiotic therapy as a monotherapy drug regimen, with the most frequent being ampicillin-sulbactam or amoxicillin-clavulanate (37.5%), and piperacillin-tazobactam (18.05%; Figure 1). In the remaining 116 (44.6%) patients, who received combination antibiotic therapy, the most common treatments were amoxicillin-clavulanate or ampicillin-sulbactam (31.9%), fluoroquinolones (19.8%), or piperacillin-tazobactam (13.8%), all in combination with metronidazole (Figure 2).

Of the 48 microbiologically evaluable patients (18.4% of the total patient population), 23 (47.9%) intra-operative abdominal site cultures (21 peritoneal swabs, and 2 intra-operative biopsies), 12 (25.0%) abdominal drainage fluid cultures, 11 (22.9%) blood cultures and 2 (4.2%) surgical wound swabs were performed. Among 34 (70.8%) documented positive cultures, the most frequent isolated pathogen was *Escherichia coli* (58.8%), followed by *Klebsiella pneumoniae* (14.7%).

Due to the low representation of the microbiological evaluable population, antibiotic therapy appropriateness was inferred by covered antimicrobial spectrum and dosing adequacy of starting empiric regimens, as detailed in the methods section. Overall, antibiotic appropriateness rate was 78.8% (n = 205), and was significantly higher in patients receiving combination therapy compared with those treated with monotherapy (97.3% vs. 64.6%). Clinical success chances with appropriate antibiotic therapy

Table 1 Demographic and clinical characteristics

Characteristic	Patients (n = 260)
Mean ± SD age, years	48.9 ± 20
Males, n (%)	149 (57.3)
Comorbidities, n (%)	
Diabetes mellitus	12 (4.6)
Obesity	12 (4.6)
Lifestyle factors, n (%)	
Smoking	27 (10.4)
Alcoholism	0 (0)
Therapeutic failure risk factors, n (%)	
Age > 65 years	63 (24.2)
Cancer	16 (6.2)
Anemia	16 (6.2)
Liver cirrhosis	1 (0.4)
Renal failure	1 (0.4)
Acute liver failure	0 (0)
End stage renal failure	2 (0.8)
Coagulopathy	2 (0.8)
Immunosuppression	2 (0.8)
Leukopenia	0 (0)
Primary surgical intervention site, n (%)	
Appendix	162 (62.3)
Lower GI tract	51 (19.6)
Upper GI tract	13 (5.0)
Gall-bladder	14 (5.4)
Peritoneal abscess	16 (6.1)
Explorative laparotomy/laparoscopy	4 (1.5)
Surgical approach, n (%)	
Laparoscopy	135 (51.9)
Laparotomy	116 (44.6)
Percutaneous	9 (3.5)
Illness severity markers, n (%)	
Parenteral nutrition	52 (20.0)
Central venous catheter	44 (16.9)
Antifungal drugs	28 (10.8)
Enteral nutrition	22 (8.4)
Invasive mechanical ventilation	20 (7.7)
Immune globulins	0 (0)
Renal replacement therapies	0 (0)
ICU transfer, n (%)	24 (9.2)
Mean ± SD length of hospital stay, days	10.4 ± 13
Mortality rate, n (%)	6 (2.3)

GI, gastrointestinal; ICU, intensive care unit; SD, standard deviation.

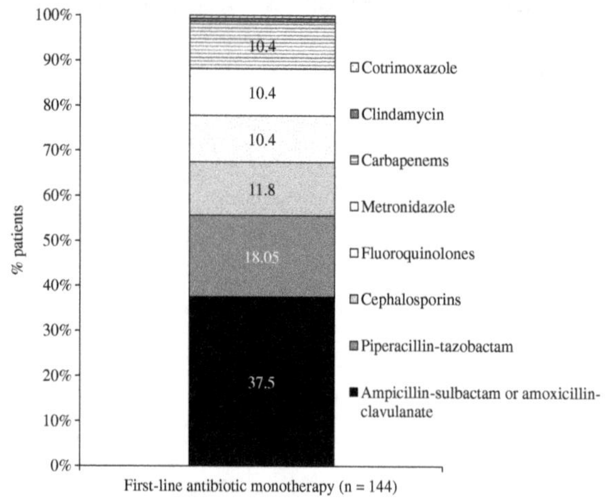

Figure 1 Antibiotics administered to patients who received monotherapy for first-line treatment of complicated intra-abdominal infections. Cephalosporins included: cefazolin, ceftizoxime, cefotaxime, and ceftriaxone; fluoroquinolones included: ciprofloxacin and levofloxacin; carbapenems included imipenem and meropenem; aminoglycosides included: amikacin, gentamicin and tobramycin.

were 78.5% (n = 161) and 34.5% (n = 19) with inappropriate therapy.

In total, 194 (74.6%) patients responded to antibiotic treatment and experienced clinical success (clinical success group), while 66 (25.4%) patients did not respond to

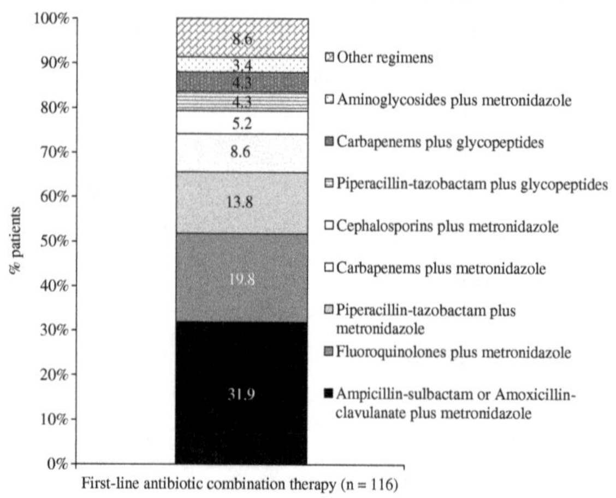

Figure 2 Antibiotic regimens administered to patients who received combination therapy for the first-line treatment of complicated intra-abdominal infections. Cephalosporins included: cefazolin, ceftizoxime, cefotaxime, and ceftriaxone; fluoroquinolones included: ciprofloxacin and levofloxacin; carbapenems included imipenem and meropenem; aminoglycosides included: amikacin, gentamicin and tobramycin. Other regimens included: aminoglycosides plus ampicillin/sulbactam or piperacillin/tazobactam, or imipenem (n = 4), fluoroquinolones plus amoxicillin/clavulanate, cephalosporins, tygecicline or piperacillin/tazobactam (n = 5), fluoroquinolones plus clindamycin (n = 1).

antibiotic therapy (clinical failure group). Ninety-six per cent (95.8%) of patients were discharged to home, 1.5% to long-term care facilities, 0.4% to another hospital, and 2.3% died in hospital.

In-hospital charges

The average cost of care for a patient hospitalized due to cIAI was €4385 (95% CI 3650–5120), with an average daily cost of €419 (95% CI 378–440). Antibiotic therapy cost by itself represented just under half (44.3%) of hospitalization costs. Clinical failure was the strongest independent predictor of hospitalization costs increases in multivariable regression analysis, followed by unscheduled additional abdominal surgeries, combination antibiotic therapy administration, patient comorbidities and illness severity markers ($R^2 = 0.47$) (Table 2).

The critical influence of clinical outcome on hospitalization costs prompted us to investigate clinical characteristics and economic outcome of patients stratified into clinical failure and success groups (Table 3). Compared with the clinical success group, patients in the clinical failure group were older and were more likely to have cancer. More patients in the clinical failure group had undergone lower GI tract surgical procedures, were surgically approached by laparotomy, and had markers indicative of severe disease and required ICU transfer (Table 3). Moreover, they more frequently received antibiotic monotherapy (69.7% vs. 52.1%). Specifically, patients who failed therapy were more like to have received metronidazole monotherapy (21.4% vs. 3.03%) and were less likely to have received the combination of fluoroquinolones plus metronidazole (4.7% vs. 22.6%) as their first-line antibiotic therapy.

The majority of patients who experienced clinical failure (99.6%) switched to second-line antibiotic therapy, 12 (18.2%) underwent unscheduled additional surgeries and 6 (9.1%) died. Second-line antibiotic therapy included switching to entirely different antibiotics in 63.6% of cases and addition of one or more drugs to the initial antibiotic regimen in 36.3% of cases. Reasons for switching therapy were clinical ineffectiveness in 63.6% of patients, microbiologic resistance in 9% and was unreported in 24.2% of patients. Second-line regimens involved meropenem (25.7%), ertapenem (21.2%), tygecicline (19.6%) and glycopeptides (10.6%).

In-hospital charges by therapeutic outcome

Patients who failed antibiotic therapy received an average of 8.2 additional days of antibiotic therapy and spent 11 more days in hospital compared with patients who responded to first-line therapy (both $p < 0.05$ vs. clinical success group). Furthermore, they incurred €5592 in additional hospitalization costs (2.88 times the cost associated with clinical success) with 53% (€2973) of the additional

Table 2 Independent predictors of hospitalization costs associated with complicated intra-abdominal infection

	Not standardized coefficients		Standardized coefficients	t	*P* value	Cost variation (%)
	B	Standard error	Beta			
Constant	3,733.00	793.44		4.705	0.000	
Clinical failure	3,817.85	681.02	0.275	5.606	0.000	+87.04
Unscheduled secondary surgeries	4,558.00	1,059.75	0.226	4.301	0.000	+104
Antibiotic combination therapy	2,264.09	580.05	0.186	3.903	0.000	+51.6
Comorbidities	2,177.45	742.28	0.14	2.933	0.004	+49.6
Therapeutic failure risk factors	1,755.84	675.91	0.137	2.598	0.010	+40
Appendectomy	−3,481.79	698.81	−0.279	−4.982	0.000	−79.4
Cholecystectomy	−2,920.24	1,339.50	−0.109	−2.180	0.030	−66.6
Female gender	−1,043.09	572.92	−0.085	−1.821	0.070	−23.8

costs attributable to antibiotic therapy (Figure 3). All of the other contributors to hospitalization costs were significantly higher in the clinical failure group (Figure 3).

A significant cost difference was still found when average costs per hospital-day were computed, amounting to €386 (95% CI 350–421) for patients experiencing clinical success, and €476 (95% CI 414–539) for patients who failed first-line therapy. Antibiotic cost by itself still was a great contributor to total per day inpatient charges, in both success and failure groups (40% and 48.5%, respectively), being significantly higher in patients who failed starting therapy (€249 vs. €153).

Due to the high contribution of antibiotic therapy to hospitalization costs, daily charges limited to antibiotic therapy course duration have been estimated (Figure 4), and were significantly higher for patients who clinically failed, as compared to those who succeeded (€502 vs. €186). This significant extra cost per antibiotic day in clinical failure cases was confirmed for both single and multiple drug antibiotic regimens (Figure 4).

Discussion

To our knowledge, this is the first multicenter study investigating the economic outcome of hospitalized cIAIs in Italy. This study clearly shows that starting empirical antibiotic therapy has a large impact on the cost of care of community-acquired cIAIs. In this large sample of hospitalized adult patients with community-acquired cIAIs, clinical failure was the strongest independent predictor of increases in hospitalization costs. Compared with patients who are treated successfully, patients who failed therapy received antibiotic therapy for more than one additional week, spent 11 more days in hospital, and incurred a mean €5600 more in hospital charges. Antibiotic therapy was the leading contributor to inpatient charges, and multiple drug regimens was an independent predictor of increases in costs.

Various European and US studies have investigated the clinical outcomes associated with the treatment of community-acquired cIAIs and have shown a clinical failure rate of 17%–35% [2-5], which is consistent with the 25% failure rate observed in our study. However, very few studies have addressed the issue of the economic burden of cIAIs.

Early European series have shown that hospitalization costs are 1.2–1.5 times higher in patients who have failed treatment compared with patients who were treated successfully [2,6]. The present study confirms and substantiates these findings, demonstrating that the costs associated with failing first-line antibiotic therapy is associated with a 2.8-fold increase in hospitalization costs compared with patients who have had clinical success. Importantly, clinical failure was the strongest independent contributor to inpatient hospitalization charges, leading to an increase in costs of 87% after adjusting for comorbidities, therapeutic failure risk factors, type of primary surgical procedure and unscheduled additional surgeries.

The cost of antibiotic therapy explained over 50% of total hospitalization charges, confirming previous studies that have shown that antibiotics contribute 70% of extra costs associated with cIAIs [6]. This large proportion of clinical failure costs deriving from antibiotic therapy most probably arises from the overlap existing between the failure of antibiotic therapy and clinical failure. Although clinical failure, a widely employed measure of drug effectiveness [2-4,6,7], is a composite of three different outcomes (antibiotic therapy switch, re-operation or death), in most instances it is driven by failure of first-line antibiotic therapy. In our study virtually all patients who clinically failed required second-line antibiotic therapy, while re-operation or death involved only a few patients (17.7% and 9.1%, respectively). This is consistent with the results of previous studies which have shown that the majority of costs associated with clinical failure are due to antibiotic therapy [2,7].

Table 3 Demographic and clinical characteristics of patients stratified by clinical outcome

Characteristic	Clinical success group (n = 194)	Clinical failure group (n = 66)	*P* value
Mean ± SD age, years	46.4 ± 19	56.2 ± 21	<0.05
Males, n (%)	113 (58.2)	36 (54.5)	NS
Comorbidities, n (%)			
Diabetes mellitus	7 (3.6)	5 (7.5)	NS
Obesity	9 (4.6)	3 (4.5)	NS
Lifestyle factors, n (%)			
Smoking	22 (11.3)	5 (7.5)	NS
Alcoholism	0 (0)	0 (0)	NS
Therapeutic failure risk factors, n (%)			
Age > 65 years	38 (19.5)	25 (37.8)	<0.05
Cancer	8 (4.1)	8 (12.1)	<0.05
Anemia	6 (3.1)	10 (15.2)	<0.05
Liver cirrhosis	1 (0.5)	0 (0)	NS
Renal failure	1 (0.5)	1 (1.5)	NS
End stage renal failure	2 (1.0)	0 (0)	NS
Coagulopathy	2 (1.0)	0 (0)	NS
Immunosuppression	1 (0.5)	1 (1.5)	NS
Primary surgical intervention site, n (%)			
Appendix	132 (68.0)	30 (45.4)	<0.05
Lower GI tract	23 (11.8)	28 (42.4)	<0.05
Upper GI tract	10 (5.1)	3 (4.5)	NS
Gall-bladder	13 (6.7)	1 (1.5)	NS
Peritoneal abscess	13 (6.7)	3 (4.5)	NS
Other	3 (1.5)	1 (1.5)	NS
Surgical approach, n (%)			
Laparoscopy	111 (57.2)	24 (36.3)	<0.05
Laparotomy	76 (39.2)	40 (60.6)	<0.05
Percutaneous	7 (3.6)	2 (3.0)	NS
Antibiotic treatment, n (%)			
Monotherapy	101 (52.1)	46 (69.7)	<0.05
Combination therapy	93 (47.9)	20 (30.3)	<0.05
Illness severity markers, n (%)			
Parenteral nutrition	27 (13.9)	25 (37.8)	<0.05
Central venous catheter	16 (8.2)	24 (36.3)	<0.05
Antifungal drugs	12 (6.2)	16 (24.2)	<0.05
Enteral nutrition	10 (5.2)	12 (18.2)	<0.05
Invasive mechanical ventilation	6 (3.1)	14 (21.2)	<0.05
ICU admission, n (%)	6 (3.1)	18 (27.3)	<0.05
Mortality rate, n (%)	0 (0)	6 (9.1)	NS

GI, gastrointestinal; ICU, intensive care unit; NS, not significant; SD, standard deviation.

In most cases, clinical failure with antibiotic therapy is driven by unsuitable drug choice [3,4,6]. In the present study, although only "presumed" basing on drug spectrum of coverage adequacy [1], appropriate antibiotic therapy was associated with a 78% chance of clinical success, compared with a 34% chance of clinical success associated with inappropriate therapy. Therefore, the role of antibiotic failure and inappropriateness of drug choice having a large influence on the occurrence of clinical failure could be inferred, as previously demonstrated [3,7,10].

As expected, the appropriateness of empiric antibiotic therapy was more frequently reached with wide spectrum combination therapy. We found that multiple-drug empiric regimens were appropriate in 97% of cases compared with roughly 65% of single drug regimens. Moreover, patients who achieved clinical success were more likely to have received antibiotic combination therapy than those patients who failed antibiotic therapy, confirming previous findings [7]. On the other hand, the costs per day of antibiotic combination regimens were significantly higher than the costs of antibiotic monotherapy, regardless of therapeutic outcome. Importantly, combination therapy was a strong independent predictor of increases in inpatient charges, causing approximately a 50% increase of mean hospitalization costs. Thus, the benefit/cost ratio underpinning the correct management of community-acquired cIAIs seems to be difficult to balance.

Multiple antibiotic regimens aim to expand antimicrobial spectrum and to overcome increased bacterial resistance in community-acquired cIAIs [13,14]. Recently, newly introduced wide spectrum agents, such as ertapenem and tygecicline, have been recommended [8] for use as first-line empiric antibiotic monotherapy regimens in stable, noncritically ill cIAIs patients with extended-spectrum beta-lactamase producing pathogens risk factors, factors that are becoming more frequently involved in community-acquired cIAIs [13,14]. Interestingly, these were also among the most frequent second-line choices in our failing patients, underlying the cost/benefit advantage of such recommendation.

As previously reported [2,6,7], patients who were less healthy due to an increased age, comorbidities or those with known treatment failure risk factors, were significantly more likely to fail antibiotic therapy. These same features independently increased hospitalization costs. Therefore, illness severity must be strongly considered when choosing starting empirical antibiotic therapy, due to its influence on clinical and economic outcomes of patients with cIAIs.

The low rate of intra-operative microbiology tests performed in the present study is worrisome. As choosing antibiotics for the treatment of cIAIs is an empiric decision, local epidemiology knowledge is of outmost importance.

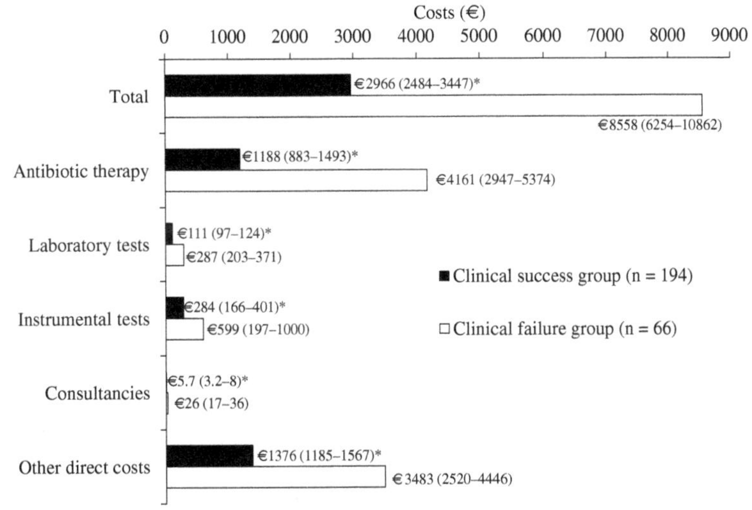

Figure 3 Total hospitalization costs per patient, stratified by therapeutic outcome. Other direct costs category includes personnel, ordinary maintenance and hotel costs. *p < 0.05 vs. clinical failure group.

By increasing the chance of appropriate treatment [1], it could improve outcome and decrease resource utilization in patients subsequently hospitalized in the same institution for the same condition. Thus, we recommend that the consistent taking of swab samples by Italian surgeons is implemented.

As with any retrospective analysis, this study has several limitations. Due to complexities associated with the collection of data, summary measures of illness and comorbidities severity, potentially associated with clinical failure, longer length of hospital stay, and higher inpatient costs were not covered and could not be used in the multivariate model. We were also unable to assess the appropriateness of antibiotic therapy in light of culture results and patient clinical risk profile [1,9] and, therefore, the clinical failure variable, rather than antibiotic appropriateness, was used in the multivariable analysis of independent cost predictors. Finally, being a multicenter study, dissimilarity in standard of care among participating sites cannot be excluded.

Despite these limitations, for the first time we assessed patterns of starting antibiotic therapy, resource utilization and actual costs of caring for inpatients with community-acquired cIAIs in Italian hospitals. The results of this study suggest that hospitals need to be aware of the clinical and economic consequences of antibiotic therapy and to reduce overall resource use and costs by improving the rate of success with appropriate initial empiric therapy.

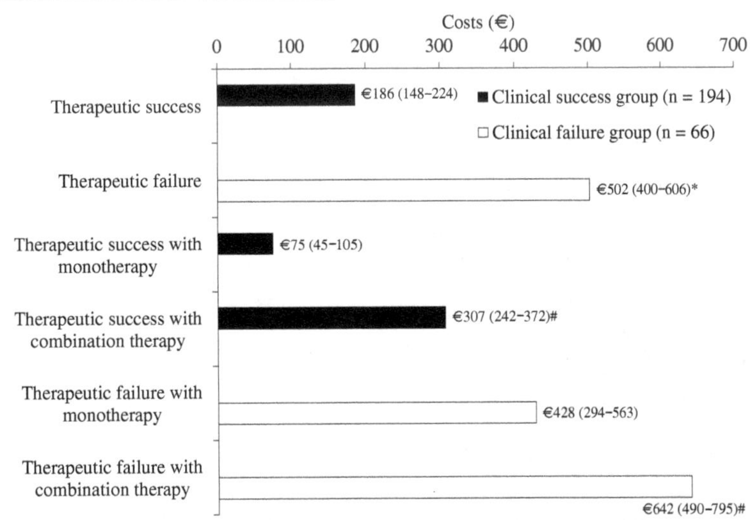

Figure 4 Hospitalization costs per day of antibiotic therapy in patients stratified by therapeutic outcome and antibiotic regimens. *p < 0.05 vs. clinical failure group; #p < 0.05 vs. antibiotic monotherapy group.

Considering the prospective reimbursement system of the Italian NHS, there may be a relevant cost saving at the same reimbursement rate for hospitals, by reducing antibiotic costs of cIAIs. Mandatory peritoneal swab sampling, allowing for local epidemiology driven empiric antibiotic therapy, should be strongly encouraged for each cIAIs patient.

Abbreviations

CI: Confidence interval; cIAIs: Complicated intra-abdominal infections; GI: Gastrointestinal; IAIs: Intra-abdominal infections; ICU: Intensive care unit; WBC: White blood cell.

Competing interests

The authors LD, FB, EC, FR and CA declare that they have no competing interests. SC has received funds from Pfizer. FS has received research and educational grants from Abbott, Bayer, Biogen Idec, Biomarine, BMS, Boehringer-Ingelheim, Celgene, Daiichi Sankyo, Eli Lilly, Genzyme, GlaxoSmithKline, Janssen Cilag, Johnson & Johnson, Medtronic, MSD, Novartis, Novo Nordisk, Obi, Pfizer, Roche, Sanofi Pasteur Servier, Sigma Tau, Stroder, Teva. AN has received funds to support the research and donations from Pfizer, MSD and honorary from Astra Zeneca, MSD, Pfizer, Valeas and Zambon.

Authors' contributions

LD and CA carried out acquisition and interpretation of data, and drafted the manuscript; FB, SC, EC, AN, FR, and FS provided to conception and design of the study, and to manuscript revision; FS and CA performed the statistical analysis. All authors read and approved the final manuscript.

Acknowledgements

The authors would like to thank Simone Boniface of Springer Healthcare Communications, who edited the manuscript for English and styled for submission. This medical writing assistance was funded by Pfizer.

Author details

[1]Anesthesia and Intensive Care Unit - Emergency and Organ Transplantation Department, University of Bari, Policlinico of Bari, P.zza G. Cesare 11, 70124 Bari, Italy. [2]Department of General Surgery, Fatebenefratelli-Isola Tiberina, Rome, Italy. [3]Clinical Infectious Disease, Department of Pathology, University of Verona, Verona, Italy. [4]Department of Health Sciences, Clinical Pharmacology and Oncology Section, University of Florence, Florence, Italy. [5]Digestive, Colorectal, Oncologic and Minimally Invasive Surgery, Department of Surgical Sciences, University of Turin, Turin, Italy. [6]CEIS, University of Rome Tor Vergata, Rome, Italy.

References

1. Solomkin JS, Mazuski JE, Bradley JS, Rodvold KA, Goldstein EJ, Baron EJ, O'Neill PJ, Chow AW, Dellinger EP, Eachempati SR, Gorbach S, Hilfiker M, May AK, Nathens AB, Sawyer RG, Bartlett JG: **Diagnosis and management of complicated intra-abdominal infection in adults and children: guidelines by the Surgical Infection Society and the Infectious Diseases Society of America.** *Clin Infect Dis* 2010, **50**:133–164.
2. Cattan P, Yin DD, Sarfati E, Lyu R, De Zelicourt M, Fagnani F: **Cost of care for inpatients with community-acquired intra-abdominal infections.** *Eur J Clin Microbiol Infect Dis* 2002, **21**:787–793.
3. Krobot K, Yin D, Zhang Q, Sen S, Altendorf-Hofmann A, Scheele J, Sendt W: **Effect of inappropriate initial empiric antibiotic therapy on outcome of patients with community-acquired intra-abdominal infections requiring surgery.** *Eur J Clin Microbiol Infect Dis* 2004, **23**:682–687.
4. Tellado JM, Sen SS, Caloto MT, Kumar RN, Nocea G: **Consequences of inappropriate initial empiric parenteral antibiotic therapy among patients with community-acquired intra-abdominal infections in Spain.** *Scand J Infect Dis* 2007, **39**:947–955.
5. Wong PF, Gilliam AD, Kumar S, Shenfine J, O'Dair GN, Leaper DJ: **Antibiotic regimens for secondary peritonitis of gastrointestinal origin in adults.** *Cochrane Database Sys Rev* 2005, **18**:CD004539.
6. Sturkenboom MC, Goettsch WG, Picelli G, In't Veld B, Yin DD, De Jong RB, Go PM, Herings RM: **Inappropriate initial treatment of secondary intra-abdominal infections leads to increased risk of clinical failure and costs.** *Br J Clin Pharmacol* 2005, **60**:438–443.
7. Edelsberg J, Berger A, Schell S, Mallick R, Kuznik A, Oster G: **Economic consequences of failure of initial antibiotic therapy in hospitalized adults with complicated intra-abdominal infections.** *Surg Infect* 2008, **9**:335–347.
8. Sartelli M, Catena F, Ansaloni L, Leppaniemi A, Taviloglu K, van Goor H, Viale P, Lazzareschi DV, Coccolini F, Corbella D, de Werra C, Marrelli D, Colizza S, Scibè R, Alis H, Torer N, Navarro S, Sakakushev B, Massalou D, Augustin G, Catani M, Kauhanen S, Pletinckx P, Kenig J, Di Saverio S, Jovine E, Guercioni G, Skrovina M, Diaz-Nieto R, Ferrero A, *et al*: **Complicated intra-abdominal infections in Europe: a comprehensive review of the CIAO study.** *World J Emerg Surg* 2012, **7**:36.
9. Sartelli M, Viale P, Catena F, Ansaloni L, Moore E, Malangoni M, Moore FA, Velmahos G, Coimbra R, Ivatury R, Peitzman A, Koike K, Leppaniemi A, Biffl W, Burlew CC, Balogh ZJ, Boffard K, Bendinelli C, Gupta S, Kluger Y, Agresta F, Di Saverio S, Wani I, Escalona A, Ordonez C, Fraga GP, Junior GA, Bala M, Cui Y, Marwah S, *et al*: **2013 WSES guidelines for management of intra-abdominal infections.** *World J Emerg Surg* 2013, **8**:3.
10. Wilson SE, Turpin RS, Hu XH, Sullivan E, Mansley EC, Ma L: **Does initial choice of antimicrobial therapy affect length of stay for patients with complicated intra-abdominal infections?** *Am Surg* 2005, **71**:816–820.
11. De Lalla F, Eandi M: **Indagine sull'uso di antibiotici nel trattamento delle infezioni delle basse vie respiratorie negli ospedali italiani: considerazioni farmacoeconomiche.** *G Ital Chemioter* 1998, **45**:59–87.
12. Agenzia Italiana del Farmaco (AIFA): **Italian Pharmaceutical Formulary.** 2009. http://www.agenziafarmaco.gov.it/wscs_render_attachment_by_id/111.84470.1172743348645ce4c.pdf?id=111.81951.1172658490314 [accessed 26/02/2011].
13. Hawser SP, Bouchillon SK, Hoban DJ, Badal RE: **In vitro susceptibilities of aerobic and facultative anaerobic Gram-negative bacilli from patients with intra-abdominal infections worldwide from 2005–2007: results from the SMART study.** *Int J Antimicrob Agents* 2009, **34**:585–588.
14. Hawser SP, Bouchillon SK, Hoban DJ, Badal RE, Canton R, Baquero F: **Incidence and antimicrobial susceptibility of Escherichia coli and Klebsiella pneumoniae with extended-spectrum beta-lactamases in community- and hospital-associated intra-abdominal infections in Europe: results of the 2008 Study for Monitoring Antimicrobial Resistance Trends (SMART).** *Antimicrob Agents Chemother* 2010, **54**:3043–3046.

16

A review on gastric diverticulum

Farhan Rashid[1,2*], Ahmed Aber[2] and Syed Y Iftikhar[1]

Abstract

The gastric fundal diverticulae are rare. They can present with variable symptoms. We are enclosing a literature review on gastric fundal diverticulum. Lessons have emerged which may help in the management of this rare condition in future.

Introduction

Gastric diverticulum (GD) is an outpouching of the gastric wall. GDs are rare and they are commonly detected incidentally during routine diagnostic testing. Prevalence ranges from 0.04% in contrast study radiographs and 0.01% - 0. 11% at oesophagogastrodeudenum (OGD) [1,2]. The incidence of gastric diverticulum is equally distributed between males and females and typically may present in the fifth and sixth decades. However it is worth mentioning that it may present in patients as young as 9 years old [3].

The lack of exact pathogonomic symptoms and the vague long history of presenting complaints that can range from dyspepsia to major upper gastrointestinal (GI) bleed make this condition a diagnostic challenge.

We conducted a literature search using the "Pubmed" search engine. The following terms "gastric diverticulum" and "Stomach diverticulum" were used to identify the appropriate papers.

In this review, our emphasis is to highlight on the presentation, the pathophysiology, investigations and different management options for this condition.

Presentation of gastric diverticulum

Symptoms of GD vary and can imitate those of other common disorders. It is important to note that most GD are asymptomatic but may present with a vague sensation of fullness or discomfort in the upper abdomen. Presenting complaint might also be the result of a major complication of GD. This includes acute upper gastrointestinal bleed or perforation [1,2] (Table 1).

* Correspondence: farhan_rashid@hotmail.com
[1]Department of Upper GI Surgery, Royal Derby Hospital, Graduate Entry Medical School, Derby, University of Nottingham, UK
Full list of author information is available at the end of the article

Patho-physiology

GD in general is a rare condition; It is found in 0.02% (6/29 900) of autopsy studies and in 0.04% (165/380 000) of upper gastrointestional studies [1,3,4]. Meeroff *et al* reported a prevalence of 0.1-2.6% in an autopsy series [4].

Seventy-five percent of true gastric diverticula were located in the posterior wall of the fundus of the stomach, 2 cm below the oesophagastric junction and 3 cm from the lesser curve. False diverticula were either traction or pulsion and associated with inflammation, other diseases, or both. Diverticula were usually less than 4 cm in size (range, 3 cm to 11 cm) [5,6].

In the literature review we did identify a proposed hypothesis explaining the pathophysiology of this condition. This hypothesis classifies GD cases into congenital and acquired types, with congenital types being more common [5-8]. Based on a review of embryogenesis it had been suggested how a gastric diverticulum can be located within the retroperitoneal space in an attempt to explain the commonest type to GD.

In the period between the 20th and 50th day of gestation, the stomach is transformed from a fusiform swelling of the foregut into its adult form. At this time, there is a 90° rotation of the stomach, which carries with it the duodenum, the pancreas, and the dorsal mesentery. The posterior body wall and dorsal mesentery then fuse encapsulating the pancreas within the retroperitoneum and establishing its adult form [9].

A diverticulum of the posterior wall of the gastric fundus hypothetically could herniate through an area of dorsal mesentery before its fusion with the left posterior body wall. Initially, the diverticulum would lie superior to the pancreas. With further extension, the diverticulum could project posterior to the pancreas.

Table 1 GD presenting symptoms, diagnostic investigations and management

Symptoms	Investigation	Management	Refs
Incidental finding on CT scan	Upper GI contrast study/CT with oral contrast	None	18, 19
Upper GI bleed	OGD	OGD & Adrenaline injection	22, 23
Upper abdominal pain, reflux, bloating	CT with contrast & OGD	Laparoscopic surgical resection	1,5, 29, 30, 31
Upper abdominal pain and anorexia	OGD	PPI	5, 9
Upper abdominal pain	Upper GI contrast study	Exploratory laparotomy plus diverticulectomy	5

Acquired gastric diverticula in contrast are pseudodiverticula, less common and typically located in the antrum. They usually present with a background history of other gastrointestinal pathology, such as peptic ulcer disease, malignancy, pancreatitis, or gastric outlet obstruction. Gastric diverticula had been reported following surgical procedures on the stomach, including Roux-en-Y gastric bypass [4,10,11].

Investigations

Accurate diagnosis is essential given the risk for severe complications, including bleeding and perforation, as well as the association with ectopic mucosa and potential for malignant transformation [12]. The condition can be diagnosed by radiological or endoscopic examinations.

This is usually accomplished with upper gastrointestinal contrast radiographic study (UGI) or oesophagogastroduodenoscopy (OGD). These are the most reliable diagnostic tests but reports in the literature confirm that they can give false negative results [13,14]; especially for a diverticulum with a narrow neck that precludes entry of the contrast or scope. It is stated that the GD is best identified during UGI study using a right, anterior oblique view with the patient in a supine, slightly left lateral decubitus and Trendelenburg position [13-16]. In a large review, Palmer [13] reported that 14 of 262 (5%) GDs are missed during UGI study. Other reports support the use of OGD [10,17] for diagnosis. Distension of the diverticulum by the scope may mimic the patient's symptoms and this maneuver may indicate which patients would benefit from resection [10]. Other reports suggest that computer tomography scanning may be effective; however, the accuracy of this imaging modality is not widely accepted because of the possible misdiagnosis [18,19].

Management

There is no specific treatment plan for an asymptomatic diverticulum [9,20]. The appropriate management for a symptomatic GD depends mainly on the severity of the presenting complaints.

Medical and non surgical therapy

Protein pump inhibitors therapy for few weeks is reported to resolve the symptoms in proven cases of GD [9]. However it is important to note that this does not resolve the underlying pathology and some studies report that patients presented again with refractory symptoms of dyspepsia and worsening epigastric pain that did not settle with either protein pump inhibitors or histamine receptor blockers [21].

There are also reports in the literature of successful endoscopic management of cases of gastric diverticulum that presented with active upper GI bleed. None of these studies reported any further complications that warranted further surgical management [22,23].

Surgical management

Surgical resection is recommended when the diverticulum is large, symptomatic or complicated by bleeding, perforation or malignancy. Both open and laparoscopic resection yield good results. Palmer noted that 6 of 9 patients with symptoms caused by gastric diverticulum who underwent open surgery experienced excellent outcomes [24].

Laparoscopic resection of gastric diverticulum was first described by Fine in 1998 [25]. Since then several cases using the laparoscopic surgical approach have been reported [1,26-32]. All of these cases were successfully managed by laparoscopy, with primary resection of the true gastric diverticulum.

The laparoscopic approach has been described by different authors. The most favourable approach that provides the necessary exposure is by placing the ports in a similar fashion to laparoscopic Nissen fundoplication. This includes a midline port, right upper quadrant, and 2 left upper quadrant ports. The laparoscopic dissection has been performed by either releasing the gastrocolic/gastrosplenic ligament or by mobilizing the short gastric vessels, thus gaining exposure of the superior posterior wall of the stomach. The latter is the most frequently used approach [24,25,27,28]. Because all diverticula were true and located in the gastric fundus, the most direct approach was by taking down of the short gastric vessels. Simple resection of the diverticulum with a laparoscopic cutting stapler was reported to be successful [32]

Recent experience of dealing with gastric fundal diverticulum

A 46 year old male patient, with a 10 year history of GORD, presented with abdominal discomfort and haemoptysis.

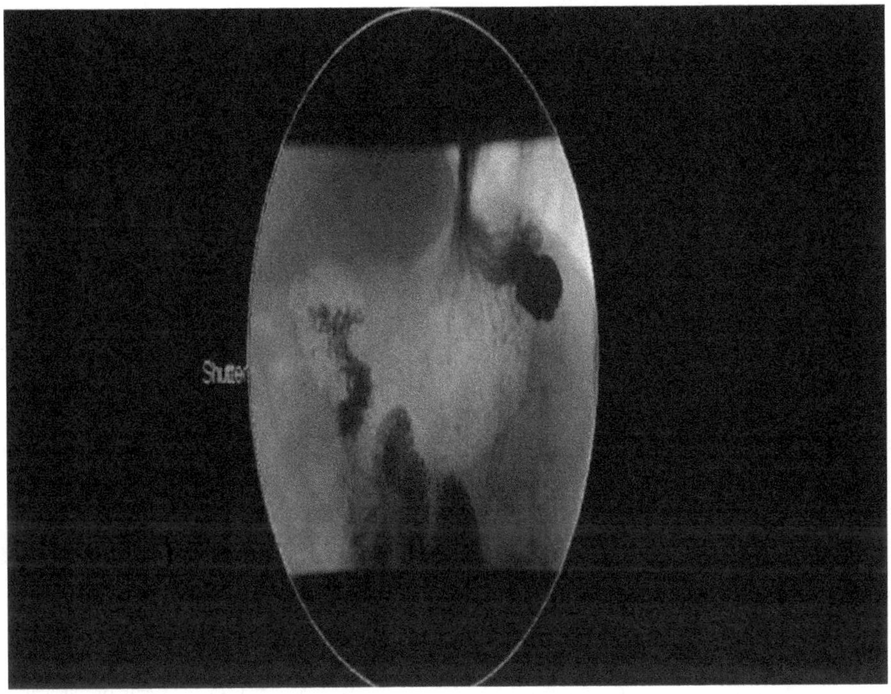

Figure 1 Barium swallow study.

He had also felt nausea and belching with some foul smell. On examination, his abdomen was soft and non tender. He denied any weight loss and was systemically well. All investigations looking for a respiratory cause for his haemoptysis were normal. OGD revealed a gastric fundal pathology, and a small hiatus hernia. The pathology was confirmed with a barium swallow study (Figure 1).

The computed tomography (CT) scan has shown a posterior gastric fundal diverticulum (Figure 2), containing calcified material and measuring approximately 30

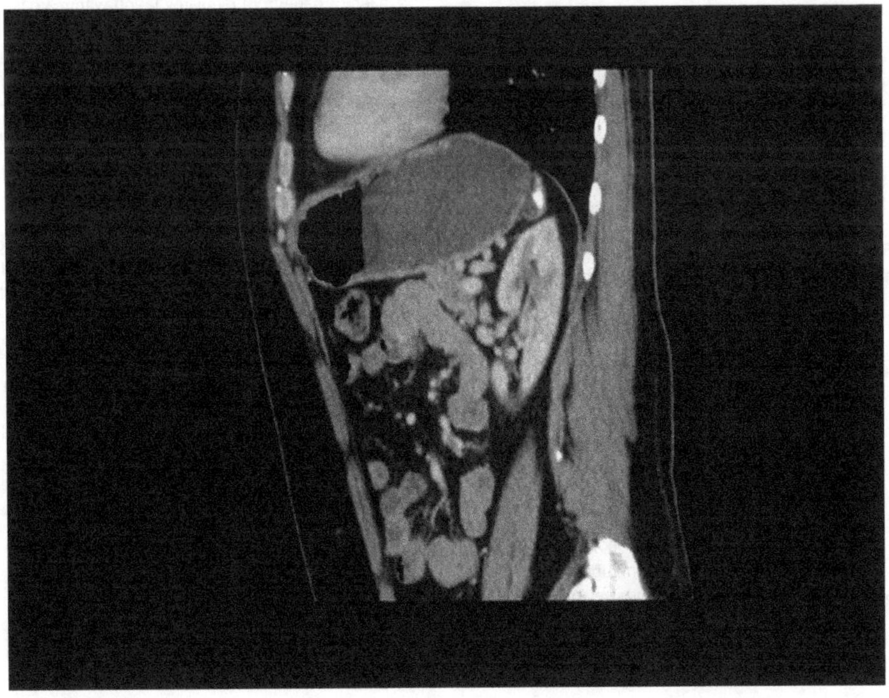

Figure 2 Computed tomography.

mm in diameter. The patient underwent laparoscopic excision of gastric fundal diverticulum and had an uneventful recovery from the operation. The histology of the diverticulum confirmed the normal lining of the stomach. The patient remained asymptomatic on further follow up after 1 year.

Conclusion

A high clinical index of suspicion is needed to diagnose and effectively manage patients with gastric diverticulum. This condition typically present with a long history of vague symptoms such as upper abdominal pain and dyspepsia. It does not always resolve with PPIs and can even be missed on OGD or CT scanning. A focused investigation to look for this particular condition is needed to identify it and subsequently manage it.

We particularly recommend that keep a high index of suspicion in mind especially in patients with a long history of upper abdominal pain and dyspepsia that does not resolve with PPIs and with an insignificant OGD. Although the literature does not describe a standarised approach for the management of this condition, however, we consider laparoscopic repair to be a safe and suitable procedure for this in symptomatic patients who have not responded to medical therapy.

Consent

Written informed consent was obtained from the patient for publication of this case report and accompanying images. A copy of the written consent is available for review by the Editor-in-Chief of this journal

Author details

[1]Department of Upper GI Surgery, Royal Derby Hospital, Graduate Entry Medical School, Derby, University of Nottingham, UK. [2]Department of Surgery, Luton and Dunstable Hospital, Luton, UK.

Authors' contributions

FR and AA performed the literature search, extracted the data and wrote the manuscript. SY helped with radiological images and performed the operation. FR, AA and SYI all helped in writing different subsections of the review. All authors contributed to the manuscript, and all read and approved the final version

Competing interests

The authors declare that they have no competing interests.

References

1. Gockel I, Thomschke D, Lorenz D: **Gastrointestinal: Gastric diverticula.** *J Gastroenterol Hepatol* 2004, **19**:227.
2. Schiller AH, Roggendorf B, Delker-Wegener S, *et al*: **Laparoscopic resection of gastric diverticula: two case reports.** *Zentralbl Chir* 2007, **132**:251e5.
3. Donkervoort SC, Baak LC, Blaauwgeers JL, *et al*: **Laparoscopic resection of a symptomatic gastric diverticulum: a minimally invasive solution.** *JSLS* 2006, **10**:525-7.
4. Meeroff M, Gollan JR, Meeroff JC: **Gastric Diverticulum.** *Am J Gastroeneterol* 1967, **47**:189-203.
5. Rodeberg DA, Zaheer S, Moir CR, Ishitani MB: **Gastric diverticulum: a series of four pediatric patients.** *J Pediatr Gastroenterol Nutr* 2002, **34**:564-567.
6. Wolters VM, Nikkels PG, Van Der Zee DC, *et al*: **A gastric diverticulum containing pancreatic tissue and presenting as congenital double pylorus: case report and review of the literature.** *J Pediatr Gastroenterol Nutr* 2001, **33**:89-91.
7. Cotea E, Vasilescu A, Dimofte G, *et al*: **Gastric diverticula on the greater curvature.** *J Chir Iasi* 2007, **3**:269-273.
8. Love L, Meyers MA, Churchill RJ, Reynes CJ, Monceda R, Gibson D: **Computed tomography of extraperitoneal spaces.** *AJR* 1981, **136**:781-789.
9. Mohan P, Ananthavadivelu , Venkataraman J: **Gastric Diverticulum.** *CMAJ* 2010, **182(5)**:226.
10. Anaise D, Brand DL, Smith NL, Soroff HS: **Pitfalls in the diagnosis and treatment of a symptomatic gastric diverticulum.** *Gastrointestinal Endoscopy* 1984, **30**:28-30.
11. Schweiger F, Noonan J: **An unusual case of gastric diverticulosis.** *Am J Gastroenterol* 1991, **86**:1817-9.
12. Fork FT, Toth E, Lindstrom C: **Early gastric cancer in a fundic diverticulum.** *Endoscopy* 1998, **30(1)**:S2.
13. Palmer ED: **Collective review: gastric diverticula.** *Int Abstr Surg* 1951, **92**:417-428.
14. Seltzer M, Koch A: **A huge gastric diverticulum.** *Dig Dis* 1971, **16**:167-170.
15. Bothen N, Eklof O: **Diverticula and duplications (enterogenous cysts) of the stomach and duodenum.** *Am J Roentgenol, Radium Ther Nucl Med* 1966, **96**:375-381.
16. Eras P, Bernbaum S: **Gastric diverticula: congenital and acquired.** *Am J Gastroenterol* 1972, **57**:120-132.
17. Velanovich V: **Gastric diverticulum.** *Surg Endosc* 1994, **8**:1338-9.
18. Kodera R, Otsuka F, Inagaki K, *et al*: **Gastric diverticulum simulating left adrenal incidentaloma in a hypertensive patient.** *Endocrine Journal* 2007, **54(6)**:969-974.
19. Araki A, Shinohara M, Yamakawa J, *et al*: **Gastric diverticulum preoperatively diagnosed as one of two left adrenal adenomas.** *Int J Urol* 2006, **13**:64-66.
20. Harford W, Jeyarajah R: **Diverticula of the pharynx, esophagus, stomach, and small intestine.** In *Sleisenger & Fordtran's gastrointestinal and liver disease.*. 8 edition. Edited by: Feldman M, Friedman L, Brandt L, et al. Philadelphia (PA): Saunders; 2006:465-77.
21. MaCauley M, Bollard E: **Gastric Diverticulum: A rare cause of refractory epigastric pain.** *The American Journal of Medicine* 2010, **123**:5-6.
22. Zakary N, Langenberg DR, Alshumrany M, Schoeman M: **Acute haemorrhage from dieulafoy lesion within a gastric diverticulum managed endoscopically.** *J Gastroenterol Hepatol* 2009, **24**:1891.
23. Chen J, Su W, Chang C, Lin H: **Bleeding from gastric diverticulum.** *J Gastroenterol Hepatol* 2008, **23**:336.
24. Palmer ED: **Gastric Diverticulosis.** *Am Fam Phys* 1973, **7(3)**:114-117.
25. Fine A: **Laparoscopic resection of a large proximal gastric diverticulum.** *Gastrointest Endosc* 1998, **48(1)**:93-95.
26. Kim SH, Lee SW, Choe WJ, Choe SC, Kim SJ, Koo BH: **Laparoscopic resection of gastric diverticulum.** *J Laparoendosc Adv Surg Tech* 1999, **9(1)**:87-91.
27. Vogt DM, Curet MJ, Zucker KA: **Laparoscopic management of gastric diverticula.** *J Laparoendosc Adv Surg Tech A* 1999, **9(5)**:405-410.
28. Alberts MS, Fenoglio M: **Laparoscopic management of a gastric diverticulum.** *Surg Endosc* 2001, **15(10)**:1227-1228.
29. MaCauley M, Bollard E: **Gastric Diverticulum: A rare cause of refractory epigastric pain.** *The American Journal of Medicine* 2010, **123**:5-6.
30. Hewa TL, Zhang Z, Rozelle C, Terry A: **Gastric antral diverticulum with heterotopic pancreas in a teenage patient.** *JPGN* 2011, **53(5)**:471.
31. McKay R: **Laproscopic resection of a gastric diverticulum: a case report.** *JSLS* 2005, **9**:225-228.
32. Rashid F, Singh R, Cole A, Iftikhar SY: *Troublesome belching with fetor odour. Gut* 2010, **59(3)**:310-324.

17

Management of intra-abdominal infections: recommendations by the WSES 2016 consensus conference

Massimo Sartelli[1*], Fausto Catena[2], Fikri M. Abu-Zidan[3], Luca Ansaloni[4], Walter L. Biffl[5], Marja A. Boermeester[6], Marco Ceresoli[3], Osvaldo Chiara[7], Federico Coccolini[3], Jan J. De Waele[8], Salomone Di Saverio[9], Christian Eckmann[10], Gustavo P. Fraga[11], Maddalena Giannella[12], Massimo Girardis[13], Ewen A. Griffiths[14], Jeffry Kashuk[15], Andrew W. Kirkpatrick[16], Vladimir Khokha[17], Yoram Kluger[18], Francesco M. Labricciosa[19], Ari Leppaniemi[20], Ronald V. Maier[21], Addison K. May[22], Mark Malangoni[23], Ignacio Martin-Loeches[24], John Mazuski[25], Philippe Montravers[26], Andrew Peitzman[27], Bruno M. Pereira[11], Tarcisio Reis[28], Boris Sakakushev[29], Gabriele Sganga[30], Kjetil Soreide[31], Michael Sugrue[32], Jan Ulrych[33], Jean-Louis Vincent[34], Pierluigi Viale[12] and Ernest E. Moore[35]

Abstract

This paper reports on the consensus conference on the management of intra-abdominal infections (IAIs) which was held on July 23, 2016, in Dublin, Ireland, as a part of the annual World Society of Emergency Surgery (WSES) meeting. This document covers all aspects of the management of IAIs. The Grading of Recommendations Assessment, Development and Evaluation recommendation is used, and this document represents the executive summary of the consensus conference findings.

Keywords: Intra-abdominal infections, Sepsis, Peritonitis, Antibiotics

Background

Intra-abdominal infections (IAIs) are an important cause of morbidity and mortality [1]. Early clinical diagnosis, adequate source control to stop ongoing contamination, appropriate antimicrobial therapy dictated by patient and infection risk factors, and prompt resuscitation in critically ill patients are the cornerstones in the management of IAIs. However, several critical controversies can be debated in the management of these patients. Application of management principles to the individual patient is crucial to optimize outcome. In order to clarify these major controversies in the management of IAI, many of the world's leading experts met in Dublin, Ireland, on July 23, 2016, for a specialist multidisciplinary consensus conference under the auspices of the World Society of Emergency Surgery (WSES) and with the support of the World Society of Abdominal Compartment Syndrome (WSACS). This document represents the executive summary of this consensus conference.

Methodology

In constituting the expert panel, the WSES committee invited many of the world's leading experts in the management of IAIs. It was a multidisciplinary expert panel including general and specialist surgeons, emergency and acute care surgeons, infectious disease specialists, and intensivists. The expert panel reviewed the scientific evidence and composed statements which addressed a set of predefined questions.

The statements were formulated and graded according to the Grading of Recommendations Assessment, Development and Evaluation (GRADE) hierarchy of evidence from Guyatt and colleagues [1], summarized in Table 1.

During the WSES annual conference which was held in Dublin, the statements were debated and approved by the committee jury panel. This document represents the executive summary of the final recommendations

* Correspondence: massimo.sartelli@gmail.com
[1]Department of Surgery, Macerata Hospital, Macerata, Italy
Full list of author information is available at the end of the article

Table 1 Grading of Recommendations Assessment, Development and Evaluation (GRADE) hierarchy of evidence from Guyatt and colleagues [1]

Grade of recommendation	Clarity of risk/benefit	Quality of supporting evidence	Implications
1A			
Strong recommendation, high-quality evidence	Benefits clearly outweigh risk and burdens, or vice versa	RCTs without important limitations or overwhelming evidence from observational studies	Strong recommendation, applies to most patients in most circumstances without reservation
1B			
Strong recommendation, moderate-quality evidence	Benefits clearly outweigh risk and burdens, or vice versa	RCTs with important limitations (inconsistent results, methodological flaws, indirect analyses or imprecise conclusions) or exceptionally strong evidence from observational studies	Strong recommendation, applies to most patients in most circumstances without reservation
1C			
Strong recommendation, low-quality or very low-quality evidence	Benefits clearly outweigh risk and burdens, or vice versa	Observational studies or case series	Strong recommendation but subject to change when higher quality evidence becomes available
2A			
Weak recommendation, high-quality evidence	Benefits closely balanced with risks and burden	RCTs without important limitations or overwhelming evidence from observational studies	Weak recommendation, best action may differ depending on the patient, treatment circumstances, or social values
2B			
Weak recommendation, moderate-quality evidence	Benefits closely balanced with risks and burden	RCTs with important limitations (inconsistent results, methodological flaws, indirect or imprecise) or exceptionally strong evidence from observational studies	Weak recommendation, best action may differ depending on the patient, treatment circumstances, or social values
2C			
Weak recommendation, Low-quality or very low-quality evidence	Uncertainty in the estimates of benefits, risks, and burden; benefits, risk, and burden may be closely balanced	Observational studies or case series	Very weak recommendation; alternative treatments may be equally reasonable and merit consideration

approved by the consensus conference. The document was reviewed and approved by both the expert and jury panels.

What is the most appropriate classification for intra-abdominal infections?

Statement 1

The term "intra-abdominal infections" describes a wide heterogeneity of clinical conditions. The anatomical extent of infection, the presumed pathogens involved, risk factors for major resistance patterns, and the patient's clinical condition should be assessed independently so as to classify patients (Recommendation 1 C).

A complete classification that includes the origin of source of infection, the anatomical extent of infection, the presumed pathogens involved and risk factors for major resistance patterns, and the patient's clinical condition does not exist.

A simple and universally accepted classification divides IAIs into complicated and uncomplicated [2]. In the event of uncomplicated IAIs, the infection only involves a single organ and does not extend to the peritoneum. When the focus of infection is controlled by surgical excision, post-operative antibiotic therapy is not necessary [3–5]. In the event of complicated IAIs (cIAIs), the infectious process proceeds beyond the organ into the peritoneum, causing either localized or diffuse peritonitis.

Treatment of patients with cIAIs involves generally both source control, antibiotic therapy, and potentially novel therapies targeted at modulating or ameliorating the host inflammatory response. Antibiotics can prevent local and hematogenous spread and can reduce late complications [6].

This classification has been questioned by some authors because it often has incited confusion by mixing elements of anatomical barrier disruption and severity of disease expression [7].

Peritonitis is an inflammation of the peritoneum. Depending on the underlying pathology, it can be infectious or sterile. Infectious peritonitis is classified into primary peritonitis, secondary peritonitis, and tertiary peritonitis [2]. Primary peritonitis is a diffuse bacterial infection (usually caused by a single organism) without loss of integrity of the gastrointestinal tract, typically seen in cirrhotic patients with ascites or in patients with a peritoneal dialysis catheter. It has a low incidence on surgical wards and is usually managed without any surgical intervention. Secondary peritonitis, the most common form of peritonitis, is an acute peritoneal infection resulting from loss of integrity of the gastrointestinal tract. Tertiary peritonitis is a recurrent infection of the peritoneal cavity that occurs >48 h after apparently successful and adequate surgical source control of secondary peritonitis. It is more common among critically ill or immunocompromised patients and may be often associated with multidrug-resistant organisms (MDROs). It is typically associated with high morbidity and mortality. Tertiary peritonitis has been accepted as a distinct entity. However, it represents an evolution and complication of secondary peritonitis [8–10]. The term "ongoing peritonitis" [11] or "persistent peritonitis" [12] may better indicate that it is not a different disease to secondary peritonitis, but rather represents secondary peritonitis lasting longer and harboring other (selected and more resistant) pathogens.

The term "healthcare-associated infection" (HCAI) is a new term for infections acquired during the course of receiving healthcare. It includes not only hospital-acquired infections but also infections in patients living in nursing facilities, having recent hospitalization within 90 days, and using aggressive medical therapies (intravenous therapy, wound dressing) at home and invasive therapies (hemodialysis, chemotherapy, radiotherapy) in outpatient clinics within 30 days of the index infection [13]. In the setting of IAIs, there is relatively little data regarding the concept of healthcare-associated infections as opposed to hospital-acquired or nosocomial infections.

Differentiating community-acquired intra-abdominal infections (CA-IAIs) from hospital-acquired intra-abdominal infections (HA-IAIs) is useful to define the presumed resistance patterns and identify patients with increased likelihood of infection caused by MDROs.

Among patients with HA-IAIs, those with post-operative peritonitis may be associated with increased mortality due to underlying patient comorbidity, atypical presentation due to non-specific clinical signs, and risk factors for acquiring MDROs and *Candida* spp. infections [14–16].

Grading of the clinical severity of patients with cIAIs has been well described by the sepsis definitions [17]. The data from WISS study showed that mortality was significantly affected by sepsis status when divided into four categories. Mortality rates increase in patients developing organ dysfunction and septic shock. Mortality by sepsis status was as follows: no sepsis 1.2%, sepsis only 4.4%, severe sepsis 27.8%, and septic shock 67.8% [18].

Recently, the third International Consensus Definitions for Sepsis and Septic Shock (Sepsis-3) were published [19], replacing previous classifications [20, 21]. Sepsis is now defined as a life-threatening organ dysfunction caused by a dysregulated host response to infection. Organ dysfunction can be represented by an increase in the Sequential [sepsis-related] Organ Failure Assessment (SOFA) score of 2 points or more. Septic shock should be defined as a subset of sepsis and should be clinically identified by a vasopressor requirement to maintain a mean arterial pressure of 65 mmHg or greater and serum lactate level greater than 2 mmol/L in the absence of hypovolemia.

Designing a classification which is accepted worldwide may be important to stratify patients according to the risk for antimicrobial therapy failure. A new classification would permit uniform regimens for patients having cIAIs and increase the comparability of studies carried out at different centers.

What are the optimal methods in diagnosing IAI that balances benefits and risks?

Statement 2

Early clinical evaluation is essential for diagnosing IAIs. It helps to optimize diagnostic testing and can result in earlier implementation of a proper management plan (Recommendation 1C).

Statement 3

A step-up approach for diagnosis should be used and tailored to the clinical setting, resources, patient's age beginning with clinical and laboratory examination and progressing to imaging examinations (Recommendation 1C).

Diagnosis of complicated IAIs is mainly clinical. Early detection and treatment is essential to minimize complications of IAIs [22, 23].

Patients with IAIs typically present with rapid-onset abdominal pain and signs of local and systemic inflammation (pain, tenderness, fever, tachycardia, and/or tachypnea). Hypotension and hypoperfusion signs such as oliguria, acute alteration of mental status, and lactic acidosis are indicative of ongoing organ failure.

Physical evaluation may limit the differential diagnosis to direct decisions regarding a proper management plan including the need for appropriate diagnostic testing, the need for initiation of antimicrobial therapy, and whether emergent intervention is required [22].

The value of physical findings in the diagnostic work-up for IAIs has been studied in relation to acute appendicitis where signs and symptoms are helpful in diagnosing or excluding appendicitis [24].

The presence of a positive psoas sign, fever, or migratory pain to the right lower quadrant suggests an increased likelihood of appendicitis. Conversely, the presence of vomiting before pain makes appendicitis unlikely [25].

Ultrasound (US) and computed tomography (CT) have been used over the last two decades to complete the clinical assessment of patients with IAIs. Although CT has higher sensitivity and specificity [26], concerns about radiation exposure have recently prompted reappraisal of the roles of sonography [27] including performance by surgeons [28].

Proposals of staged algorithms using a step-up approach with CT performed after an inconclusive or negative US have been proposed in the setting of acute appendicitis and acute diverticulitis [29–32].

Magnetic resonance imaging (MRI) is not routinely available in most hospitals in the emergency setting. It has been proposed to be used in pregnant patients with abdominal pain when US is inconclusive [33]. Recently, a systematic review and meta-analysis of diagnostic performance of MRI for evaluation of acute appendicitis was published [34]. A total of 30 studies that comprised 2665 patients were reviewed. The sensitivity and specificity of MRI for the diagnosis of acute appendicitis was 94% (95% CI, 87–98%) and 96% (95% CI, 95–97%), respectively.

Laparoscopy is gaining wider acceptance in emergency surgery [35]. When imaging has been unhelpful, diagnostic laparoscopy may be used to identify the causative pathology of acute abdominal pain followed by definitive laparoscopic treatment. The accuracy of diagnostic laparoscopy is very high reporting definitive diagnosis rates between 86 and 100% in unselected patients [36, 37].

Which patients are at high risk of failure?

Statement 4

Patient factors are essential when addressing treatment outcome, as advanced age, associated comorbidity, pre-existing disease, and physiologic status greatly influence outcomes (e.g., mortality) (Recommendation 2 C).

Statement 5

Disease factors are essential to consider when addressing risk for treatment failure. (Recommendation 2 C).

Statement 6

While age alone is not decisive for outcome it should be recognized that patients with an accumulated number of risk factors, including advanced age, high disease severity and presenting in sepsis or septic shock, have a very high risk of death. Palliative care should be actively discussed when conditions indicate that operative treatment is futile (Recommendation 2 C).

Defining the patient with IAIs at high risk for failure is difficult. First, it depends on the definition of failure as an outcome; is this mortality? failure of surgical source control? failure of antibiotic control? Various studies use variable definitions of outcome.

Second, "high risk" may be attributed to the patient's underlying condition(s), such as age, comorbidity or the disease severity status on presentation. In addition, a "low-risk" patient may be converted to "high risk" if the care provider loses the "window of opportunity" to diagnose, resuscitate, and start timely treatment. Thus, there are numerous situations that must be taken into account when addressing high-risk patients and treatment failure.

In general, high-risk IAI is attributed to patient factors (advanced age, immunosuppression, malignant disease, and pre-existing medical comorbidities) or disease factors, represented by high-risk scores (such as ASA, APACHE, SOFA scores), delay in intervention (usually >24 h), inability to obtain source control, and an IAI that is healthcare associated (rather than community acquired) [38].

While age alone is not decisive for outcome, it should be recognized that elderly patients are at high risk for adverse outcomes, including death [39]. Core to the associated poor outcomes is the reduced physiological reserve and limited response to any minor or major stressor that comes with age [40] and which is summarized in the concept of "frailty" [41]. While frailty can be readily defined [41, 42], it is difficult to measure in the emergency setting, although attempted by several recent approximated measures [43–46]. In particular, patients with IAIs and pre-existing malignant disease have a particular high risk for a poor outcome [47, 48].

Disease severity on presentation is strongly associated with risk of failure or poor outcome, including death. The risk is in large part disease-dependent (e.g., lower with appendicitis than for perforated gastroduodenal ulcer); thus, the use of one generic risk score may not be sufficient. For all IAIs, the presence of sepsis or septic shock is a generic prognostic feature and defines a disease process that has become systemic, rather than a localized disease process. Several disease specific scores exist for various organ-related IAIs (appendicitis, diverticulitis, perforated ulcers) [49–52], for which none have good accuracy, prediction ability, nor validity and generalizability.

Pre-admission functional status should be considered [53]; compared to an independent status, nursing home residents have a several-fold increased risk for adverse outcomes, including death.

Patients with an accumulated number of risk factors, including very high age and high disease severity and presenting in sepsis or septic shock, have an excessively high risk of death. The appropriateness of advanced, particularly invasive treatment versus palliative measures should be actively discussed [54, 55].

Are prognostic scores useful in clinical practice?

Statement 7

Prognostic scoring systems for complicated IAIs may be useful in clinical practise, especially for audit and research. Scoring systems can be broadly divided into two groups: general organ failure severity (ICU) scores and peritonitis-specific (Surgical) scores. The Sequential Organ Failure Assessment (SOFA) score allows physicians to follow the evolving disease process in critically ill patients in ICU (Recommendation 2 A).

However, although these scores may help guide clinical care, their use in individual patients is much less predictive.

Early prognostic evaluation of cIAIs is important to assess the severity and the prognosis of the disease. It would be valuable to have accurate prognostic scores in IAIs for a variety of reasons which include (1) prediction of prognosis and (2) selection of treatment options/help guide management strategies and allow (3) comparative audit and (4) research, i.e., stratification in clinical trials.

Scoring systems can be broadly divided into two groups:

1. General Organ Failure Severity (ICU) scores
2. Peritonitis-Specific (Surgical) scores

General Organ Failure Severity (ICU) scores

These scores are used in the ICU and can allow continuous assessment of medical and surgical patients. Over the past years, many scoring models have been developed to describe the severity of illness of intensive care patients or to predict the outcome of intensive care treatment. Some require computer-aided calculations and the input of complex variables, whereas others are more simple. The majority of scores assess various organ systems for the presence of dysfunction (respiratory, hemodynamic, renal, neurological, biochemical, coagulation) and are used in sepsis and other general causes of multiorgan failure.

Severity of illness scoring systems such as the full APACHE II or the Simplified Acute Physiology Score (SAPS) are based on the parameters of the first 24 h of ICU stay and may be applicable also in patients with peritonitis [56]. The SOFA score is a simple and objective severity score that allows both calculation of the number and the severity of organ dysfunction in six organ systems (respiratory, coagulation, liver, cardiovascular, renal, and neurologic) [57]. The SOFA scoring system also tracks the time course of a patient's condition during the entire ICU stay. Regular, repeated scoring enables patient condition and disease progression to be monitored and better understood. It allows physicians to follow the evolving disease process in critically ill patients [58].

Peritonitis-Specific (Surgical) scores

These scores are calculated as a one off at the time of surgery and often include intra-operative features of the extent of contamination. Surgical scores can be disease specific; for example, the left-sided colonic Peritonitis Severity Score (PSS) [59]. There are also many scoring systems for perforations of gastroduodenal ulcers, including the Boey Score, Jabalpur Index, Hacettepe Score, and PULP Score [52, 60, 61]. Prognostic scores which can be universally used in a variety of etiologies, include the P-POSSUM, Mannheim Peritonitis Index (MPI), Peritonitis Index Altona (PIA) [62], and WSES complicated IAI score from the WISS study [18]. The MPI score is easy to calculate, even during surgery. It is calculated using simple factors such as degree of peritonitis, age, sex, time from perforation to operation, origin of sepsis, kind of exudates (clear, purulent, or fecal) [63]. Billing et al. demonstrated the reliability of MPI in 2003 patients from seven centers in Europe showing that it is an easy and reliable means of risk evaluation and classification for patients with peritonitis [63].

The WISS study is a multicenter prospective study of 4533 patients published in 2015 [18] specifically to validate the WISS score, which was built on the previous work of the CIAO and CIAOW studies. The WSES/WISS score, estimated at the admission of the patients, includes factors for (1) clinical condition on admission, (2) setting of acquisition, (3) delay in source control, and (4) risk factors including age and immunosuppression. Scores can range from 0 to ≥18. A score above 5.5 was the best predictor of mortality with a sensitivity of 89.2% and specificity of 83.5% (a positive likelihood ratio of 5.4).

However, while all these scores are useful tools for research studies, they are not sufficiently accurate to predict individual patient prognosis. Although it is hoped that these scores may help guide management decisions in the future, at the present time, they are principally used for comparative surgical audit and research tools.

What is the utility of source control? When should source control be undertaken? Is source control necessary in all patients with cIAI? What approaches should be utilized for source control?

Statement 8

Most patients with cIAIs and sepsis/septic shock should undergo an urgent source control procedure; source control can be delayed in less severely-ill patients when the circumstances are appropriate (Recommendation 2 C).

Source control encompasses all the measures undertaken to eliminate the source of infection and to control ongoing contamination. Timing and adequacy of source control are currently the most important issues in the management of IAIs because inadequate and late operation may have a negative effect on outcome [64–69]. The optimal timing of source control has not been rigorously investigated. SIS/IDSA guidelines suggest that source control should be performed as soon as possible in patients with diffuse peritonitis but that intervention could be delayed for logistical reasons as long as 24 h in patients with a localized infection if appropriate antimicrobial therapy is given and careful clinical monitoring is provided [22].

In a review by De Waele, source control was considered an essential element in the management of sepsis and should be considered and performed early after the diagnosis is established in most if not all patients [70]. The 2016 Surviving Sepsis Campaign guidelines suggest that a specific anatomic diagnosis of infection requiring emergent source control should be identified or excluded as rapidly as possible in patients with sepsis or septic shock [71].

Sotto et al. in 2002 found in a retrospective study that time between diagnosis and operation was associated with mortality [72]. In this study, the period between diagnosis and surgery ($P = 0.04$) was predictive of death within 30 days after diagnosis of peritonitis emphasizing the importance of prompt surgical treatment. In another retrospective review of 129 patients [73] with non-traumatic severe intra-abdominal infections, multivariate analysis identified that an operating room latency of 60 h or longer ($P = 0.01$) was a predictor of need for relaparotomy.

Statement 9

Highly selected patients with perforated diverticulitis (including those with an abscess <4 cm in diameter), a peri-appendiceal mass, or a perforated peptic ulcer can be managed without definitive source control if responding satisfactorily to antimicrobial therapy and other supportive measures. (Recommendation 1 B).

An operative intervention remains the most viable therapeutic strategy for managing intra-abdominal sepsis. Surgical source control entails resection or suture of a diseased or perforated viscus (e.g., diverticular perforation, gastroduodenal perforation), removal of the infected organ (e.g., appendix, gallbladder), debridement of necrotic tissue, resection of ischemic bowel, and repair/resection of traumatic perforations with primary anastomosis or exteriorization of the bowel.

However, some data indicate highly selected patients can be managed without definitive source control if responding satisfactorily to antimicrobial therapy alone.

In addition, well-localized fluid collections of appropriate density and consistency (i.e., lack of extensive loculations) may be drained percutaneously with acceptable morbidity and mortality [74–78].

Approximately 15–20% of patients admitted with acute diverticulitis have an abscess on CT scan [79]. These abscesses may be initially treated by intravenous antibiotics alone with or without percutaneous drainage, depending on the size of the abscess. A maximum diameter of 3–6 cm has been generally accepted as a reasonable limit for treatment with antimicrobial therapy alone without drainage [80, 81].

Although the absolute prevalence of perforated diverticulitis complicated by generalized peritonitis is low, it has a significant post-operative mortality, regardless of selected surgical strategy. However, CT findings of distant free air (a known predictor of failure of non-operative treatment) does not necessarily obligate a surgical approach. Dharmarajan et al. [82] described a high success rate for non-operative management in patients with acute diverticulitis and a pneumoperitoneum, excluding those with hemodynamic instability.

Sallinen et al. [83] reported results of non-operative management in patients with CT verified extra-luminal air. This study showed that non-operative treatment was feasible therapy only for hemodynamically stable patients with CT findings of pericolic extra-luminal air or only a small amount of distant intraperitoneal air in the absence of clinical diffuse peritonitis or fluid in the fossa of Douglas. A large amount of distant intraperitoneal air or distant retroperitoneal air even in the absence of clinical generalized peritonitis was associated with a high failure rate (57–60%) of non-operative management.

Recent WSES guidelines for management of acute left colonic diverticulitis [84] state that patients with CT findings of distant air without diffuse fluid may be treated by conservative treatment in selected cases; however, a risk of treatment failure and need for emergency surgery exists.

Antibiotics alone may be used to treat patients with early, non-perforated appendicitis, although there is a significant risk of subsequent recurrence [85].

In patients with complicated appendicitis, presenting with abscess or phlegmon, the optimal management strategy has been somewhat controversial. Several studies have found that non-operative treatment for a peri-appendiceal abscesses or masses results in fewer complications and shorter overall hospitalization [86–88].

In 2010, a meta-analysis [89] was published comparing conservative treatment (i.e., antibiotic therapy with or without percutaneous abscess drainage) to appendectomy for the treatment of complicated appendicitis (cases exhibiting abscess or phlegmon). Seventeen studies (16 non-randomized/retrospective and one non-randomized/prospective) reported clinical data for 1572 patients of whom 847 patients received conservative treatment and 725 underwent acute appendectomy. Conservative treatment was associated with significantly fewer complications, wound infections, abdominal/pelvic abscesses, ileus, bowel obstruction, and additional follow-up surgeries. No significant differences were found in the overall length of hospitalization or in the duration of intravenous antibiotic infusion. Overall, clinical data supports the utility of conservative management rather than appendectomy in selected patients presenting with a peri-appendiceal abscess or phlegmon.

Although the widespread clinical use of H_2 receptor antagonists, proton-pump inhibitors (PPI), and antibiotic therapy directed against *Helicobacter pylori* has greatly reduced surgical treatment of peptic ulcer disease in recent years, complications, especially perforation, are still frequently seen. Non-operative management of perforated peptic ulcer (PPU) may be an option, although urgent repair of perforation is still the standard approach for PPU in many clinical centers. Several studies have indicated that patients with PPU can be successfully treated non-operatively [90–93]. Non-operative management includes the use of nasogastric drainage, supportive care (IV fluids and nutrition), intravenous antibiotics, intravenous PPI, and radiological drainage of intra-abdominal collections.

The 2013 WSES guidelines for management of IAIs [94] state that in selected cases (age <70 years, no shock, no peritonitis, lack of spillage of the water-soluble contrast medium on gastroduodenogram), non-operative management is an option. However, if no improvement of the patient's condition is observed within 24 h, surgical therapy is indicated.

What are the indications for laparoscopic approach to IAIs?

Laparoscopic procedures have become widely accepted by the medical community as a primary means of diagnosing and treating IAIs. On the basis of the anatomical source of infection and the attending surgeon's experience, laparoscopy may be recommended for the treatment of many IAIs [95].

Statement 10

Laparoscopic appendectomy represents the first choice for most patients with acute appendicitis where appropriate resources and skills are available (Recommendation 1 A).

Recent WSES guidelines for diagnosis and treatment of acute appendicitis stated that laparoscopic appendectomy (LA) is the first choice where laparoscopic equipment and skills are available [96]. In the Sauerland et al. review, wound infections were less likely after LA than after open appendectomy (OA) (OR 0.43; CI 0.34–0.54); however, the incidence of intra-abdominal abscesses was increased (OR 1.87; CI 1.19–2.93) [97]. Despite evidence showing that LA is safe in pregnancy, advantages are minor (less pain, less infections, less early deliveries) if compared to the risk of fetal loss. Recent data from reviews of comparative studies [98] (599 LA versus. 2816 OA) showed an increased fetal loss for LA, without significant advantages. A population-based analysis on 859 pregnant women [99] with appendicitis confirmed a better outcome for those treated surgically versus non-operative management, while it found no difference in maternal complications between LA and OA. The role of antibiotic treatment instead of surgical removal for acute early uncomplicated appendicitis is currently unknown.

Statement 11

There is no evidence of any significant advantages between laparoscopic and open repair of perforated peptic ulcer (PPU). However, laparoscopy has less postoperative pain and shorter hospital stay (Recommendation 1 A).

Aside from reduced post-operative analgesic demands, the post-operative outcome of the laparoscopic approach does not differ significantly from that of open surgery. In all reported studies, patients presented with small ulcers and received simple sutures, while many also received an omental patch. There were no studies reporting emergency laparoscopic resection or laparoscopic repair of large ulcers.

A systematic review was published in 2013 [100] including randomized clinical trials comparing laparoscopic surgery versus open surgery for the repair of perforated peptic ulcer using any mechanical method of closure (suture, omental patch, or fibrin sealant).

The authors concluded that laparoscopic surgery results are not clinically different from those of open surgery, but there is clearly a selection bias in the studies performed to date and there is a need of more randomized controlled trials with a larger number of patients.

Statement 12

Early laparoscopic cholecystectomy is safe and feasible in acute cholecystitis and should be the preferred choice in absence of contraindications to pneumoperitoneum, even in high risk patients, where appropriate resources and skills are available (Recommendation 1A).

Recent 2016 WSES guidelines for the management of acute calculous cholecystitis (AAC) [101] stated that cholecystectomy is the gold standard for treatment of ACC. Laparoscopic approach should initially be attempted except in cases of absolute anesthesiology contraindications or septic shock. Many prospective trials have demonstrated that the laparoscopic cholecystectomy is a safe and effective treatment for ACC [102–106]. A recently published meta-analysis demonstrated that laparoscopic cholecystectomy in ACC [107] is the preferred approach having lower mortality and morbidity, significantly shorter post-operative hospital stay, and reduced rate of pneumonia and wound infections, compared with the open technique. Conversion rate ranged from 8 to 35%.

Statement 13

Laparoscopic lavage is not recommended in Hinchey IV diverticulitis because it can not achieve adequate source control. Laparoscopic lavage is safe and not inferior to sigmoid resection in case of Hinchey III but it is not considered the preferred choice, given the lack of evidence of major benefits (Recommendation 1A).

Statement 14

Laparoscopic sigmoid resection is feasible and safe in selected patients, hemodynamically stable, without significant comorbidities and with onset of peritonitis <12-24 hours, only if specific advanced laparoscopic colorectal expertise is available (Recommendation 2 C).

A conservative approach using laparoscopic peritoneal lavage and drainage has been debated in recent years as an alternative to colonic resection. Great debate is still open on this topic, mainly due to the discrepancy and sometime disappointing results of the latest prospective trials such as SCANDIV, Ladies, and DILALA trials [108–110].

A recent meta-analysis showed that laparoscopic lavage is a safe procedure in terms of mortality but is associated with a higher intra-abdominal abscess and re-operation rate during the index admission. No definitive high-level conclusions could be drawn by the available literature at this moment, and further evidence is needed to better define the role of laparoscopic lavage in the management of acute perforated diverticulitis with purulent peritonitis [111].

Recent WSES guidelines for the management of acute diverticulitis in the emergency setting [84] stated that considering the conflicting results laparoscopic lavage as treatment for patients with perforated diverticulitis, Hinchey III disease, may be feasible even if it cannot be considered the treatment of choice.

Laparoscopic sigmoidectomy for diverticulitis has initially been confined to the elective setting. However, laparoscopic sigmoidectomy may be feasible for diverticular peritonitis in the emergency setting also in early cases of type IV diverticulitis. In 2016, a systematic review on laparoscopic sigmoidectomy for diverticulitis in the emergency setting was published [112]. The review included only a small number of patients from four case series and one cohort study (total of 104 patients). High-quality prospective or randomized studies are needed to demonstrate benefits of acute laparoscopic sigmoidectomy compared with open sigmoidectomy for perforated diverticulitis.

Which is the best relaparotomy strategy?

Statement 15

Planned relaparotomy is not recommended as a general strategy in patients with secondary peritonitis (Recommendation 1A).

Some patients are prone to persisting IAIs regardless of eradication of the source of infection and timely relaparotomy provides the only surgical option that significantly improves outcome. In these cases, single operation may not be sufficient to achieve source control; thus, relaparotomy may become necessary [113, 114]. In 2007, van Ruler and the Dutch peritonitis group [115] published a randomized, clinical trial addressing two aspects of closed abdominal management, comparing an on-demand versus planned relaparotomy strategy in patients with severe peritonitis who had the fascia formally closed after the initial laparotomy.

In this trial, a total of 232 patients with severe IAIs (116 on-demand and 116 planned) were randomized. In planned relaparotomy group, relaparotomies were performed every 36 to 48 h after the index laparotomy to inspect, drain, lavage, and perform other necessary abdominal interventions for residual peritonitis or new infectious focus. In on-demand relaparotomy group, relaparotomies were only performed in patients with clinical deterioration or lack of clinical improvement with a likely intra-abdominal cause. Patients in the on-demand relaparotomy group did not have a significantly lower rate of adverse outcomes compared with patients in the planned relaparotomy group but did have a substantial reduction in relaparotomies, health-care utilization, and medical costs. Patients in the on-demand group had shorter median ICU stays (7 versus 11 days; $P = 0.001$) and shorter median hospital stays (27 versus 35 days; $P = 0.008$). Direct medical costs per patient were reduced by 23% using the on-demand strategy.

When and how do you perform a damage control surgery strategy in patients with severe cIAIs?

Statement 16

There is insufficient evidence to advocate damage control surgery as general strategy in patients with secondary peritonitis (Recommendation 1 C).

In order to value current evidence on damage control surgery for abdominal surgical emergencies a PubMed/MEDLINE literature review was recently published by Weber et al. [116]. Minimal evidence exists to validate the benefits of damage control surgery in general surgical abdominal emergencies. The evidence over the past decade is limited to 16 studies including a total of 455 patients, of which the majority are retrospective case series. Damage control surgery has been performed for a wide range of indications, but most frequently for uncontrolled bleeding during elective surgery, hemorrhage from complicated gastroduodenal ulcer disease, generalized peritonitis, acute mesenteric ischaemia, and other sources of intra-abdominal sepsis.

The concept of damage control surgery has been accepted by emergency surgeons and may be a logical extension from pathophysiological principles in trauma to hemorrhage and sepsis as life-saving tactic in emergency surgery performed on physiologically deranged patients. However, the benefits of this strategy are not clear from the literature.

Statement 17

Damage control surgery may be an option in selected significantly physiologically deranged patients with ongoing sepsis (Recommendation 2 C).

Damage control surgery was initially developed in the 1980s by Stone et al. [117] and detailed by Burch et al. in the early 1990s [118]. Damage control surgery strategy was defined as the abbreviated laparotomy for trauma patients with the initial control of surgical bleeding by simple operative techniques such as packing as life-saving techniques. The patient was taken to the ICU where subsequent resuscitation corrected hypothermia, acidosis, and coagulopathy [118]. In severe abdominal sepsis, damage control surgery using an open abdomen strategy may allow early draining of any residual infection and control any persistent source of infection, preventing abdominal compartment syndrome and deferring definitive intervention and anastomosis until the patient is hemodynamically stable and thus better able to heal [119]. The concept of damage control surgery may be easily adapted in patients with advanced sepsis and can incorporate the principles of the Surviving Sepsis Campaign (SSC) [71]. Even if little evidence exists, damage control surgery is employed in a wide range of abdominal emergencies and may be an increasingly recognized life-saving strategy in emergency surgery performed on physiologically deranged patients [119]. However, the role of the OA in the management of severe peritonitis is still being debated [120]. Robledo et al. compared open versus closed abdomen procedures in 40 patients with severe secondary peritonitis. They found no significant difference in mortality rates (55% open versus 30% closed). Nevertheless, the relative risk and odds ratio for death in the closed versus open group (1.83 and 2.85, respectively) led to termination of the study at the first interim analysis. However, in that study, the temporary abdominal closure was accomplished by a sandwich technique with non-absorbable mesh sutured to the fascia. Current clinical guidelines suggest that open abdomen technique should not be used routinely but should be individualized for each patient with abdominal sepsis [121, 122]. However, the benefits of this strategy are not yet clear from the literature.

Statement 18

Temporary abdominal closure using negative pressure therapy (NPT) can be useful to decrease the time to definitive abdominal closure (Recommendation 1 B). Prolonged NPT may increase the risk of enteric fistulae.

Following re-exploration, the goal is early and definitive closure of the abdomen, in order to reduce the complications associated with an open abdomen, such as entero-atmospheric fistulas, fascial retraction with loss of abdominal wall domain, and development of massive incisional hernias. Early definitive closure is the basis for preventing or reducing the risk of these complications [123, 124] and should be the goal when the patient's physiological condition allows. The literature suggests a bimodal distribution of primary closure rates. Early closure depends on post-operative intensive care management, and delayed closure depends on the choice of the temporary abdominal closure technique [125]. The first mode is to close within 4–7 days and achieve a high rate of primary closure, the second mode has a delay (20–40 days) having lower overall closure rate [125]. If a surgeon is unable to close the abdomen early, the use of a progressive closure device may be necessary. A systematic review and meta-analysis of the open abdomen and temporary abdominal closure techniques in non-trauma patients was recently published [126]. The search identified 74 studies comprising 4358 patients of whom 3461 (79%) had peritonitis. The best results achieved for delayed fascial closure and reduced the risk of entero-atmospheric fistula were shown for NPT with continuous (mesh-mediated) fascial traction. However, authors stated that the overall quality of the available evidence was poor and that uniform recommendations cannot be made.

To determine whether active negative pressure peritoneal therapy (NPPT) with the ABThera temporary abdominal closure device reduces systemic inflammation after abbreviated laparotomy, a single-center, randomized controlled trial was performed by Kirkpatrick [127]. Forty-five adults with abdominal injury (46.7%) or intra-abdominal sepsis (52.3%) were randomly allocated to the ABThera ($n = 23$) or Barker's vacuum pack ($n = 22$). The cumulative incidence of primary fascial closure at 90 days was similar between groups. However, the 90-day mortality was less in the ABThera group. Given this potential survival benefit, further well-powered multicenter trials should be conducted to confirm these provocative findings.

When and how do you perform the peritoneal specimens?

Statement 19

Intraperitoneal specimens for microbiological evaluation from the site of infection are always recommended for patients with HA-IAIs or with CA-IAIs at risk for resistant pathogens (previous antimicrobial

therapy) and in critically ill patients (Recommendation 1 B).

Statement 20

Intraperitoneal specimens should be collected in every re-operation (Recommendation 1 C).

Statement 21

Appropriate intraperitoneal specimen is peritoneal fluid/tissue collected from the site of infection (Recommendation 1 C).

Statement 22

Sufficient abdominal fluid/tissue volume (usually at least 1–2 mL of fluid) should be collected and transported to the microbiology laboratory using a transport system that properly handles and preserves the samples to avoid damage or compromise their integrity (Recommendation 1 C).

Statement 23

At the laboratory the intraperitoneal specimen should undergo Gram stain, aerobic and anaerobic culture, and antibiotic susceptibility testing (Recommendation 1 C).

Initial antibiotic therapy for IAIs is empirical in nature because microbiological data (culture and susceptibility results) may require >24 h before they are available for a more detailed analysis. IAIs are often polymicrobial in etiology. In polymicrobial infections, first the particular bacterial strains have to be isolated and identified from intraperitoneal specimen and after that the antibiotic susceptibility test can be performed. Isolation and identification of bacterial strains take more time, and results of antibiotic susceptibility are usually only available after 48 h and later.

However, the results direct expansion of antimicrobial regimen if it is too narrow and to perform a de-escalation if it is too broad [128, 129], particularly in critically ill patients where de-escalation strategy is one of the cornerstones of antimicrobial stewardship programs [129]. A lack of impact on patient outcomes by bacteriological cultures has been documented in patients with community-acquired IAIs, especially in appendicitis [130, 131]. Microbiological identification in CA-IAIs rarely influences the individual patient management. However, routine bacteriological culture and antibiotic susceptibility test in patients with CA-IAIs help to detect epidemiological changes in the resistance patterns of microbial pathogens associated with CA-IAIs. The results of microbiological testing may have great importance for the choice of therapeutic strategy of every patient at risk for antimicrobial resistance [132]. The recommended initial antibiotic regimen for risk patients should be determined according to regional epidemiological data and resistance profile.

The major pathogens involved in CA-IAIs are likely to be due to a patient's own flora and are generally predictable and include *Enterobacteriaceae* (predominantly *Escherichia coli* and *Klebsiella* spp.), viridans group streptococci, and anaerobes (especially *Bacteroides fragilis*). In addition, *Enterococcus* spp. are frequently isolated Gram-positive organisms in CA-IAIs with reported percentages of 7.7–16.5% [133].

In 2012, the Dutch Peritonitis Study Group analyzing all patients from the RELAP trial found that the presence of Gram-positive cocci, predominantly *Enterococcus* spp., was associated with worse outcome, although in secondary peritonitis, microbial profiles did not predict ongoing abdominal infection after initial emergency laparotomy [134].

The main current resistance problem is represented by Extended-spectrum beta-lactamases (ESBLs) producing *Enterobacteriaceae*, which are frequently found in CA-IAIs [135]. Specific risk factors for ESBLs phenotype among infecting pathogens includes recent exposure to antibiotics (particularly beta-lactams or fluoroquinolones) within 90 days of IAIs or known colonization with ESBL-producing *Enterobacteriaceae*. In all HA-IAIs, causative pathogens are less predictable; thus, peri-operative cultures are routinely indicated [136, 137].

In a recent retrospective study, data from 242 patients with secondary peritonitis (88 community acquired, 154 post-operative cases) treated in ICU were obtained. Enterococci were isolated in 47.1% of all patients, followed by *E. coli* (42.6%), and other *Enterobacteriaceae* (33.1%), anaerobes (29.8%), and *Candida* spp. (28.9%). The susceptibility rates and spectrum adequacy rate were lower in post-operative than in community-acquired cases. The spectrum adequacy rate of the most common regimen used for secondary peritonitis in the study center, cefotaxime plus metronidazole, was significantly different for community-acquired and post-operative peritonitis episodes, mainly for cases with polymicrobial positive cultures [138].

Recently, Montravers et al. who evaluated the dynamic change of microbial flora in persistent peritonitis [12] observed a progressive shift of peritoneal flora with the number of reoperations. The proportion of patients harboring MDRO strains increased from 41% at index surgery to 49% at the first, 54% at the second ($P = 0.037$), and 76% at the third re-operation ($P = 0.003$ versus index surgery). Intraperitoneal specimens should be collected in every re-operation and re-intervention.

Appropriate intraperitoneal specimen is peritoneal fluid or pus that is collected from the site of infection. For specimen collection, intraperitoneal fluid, pus, or tissue should be collected in airless sterile syringe with combi-stopper or in sterile test tube. Intraperitoneal specimen can be directly inoculated into appropriate aerobic and anaerobic transport media. Peritoneal swab and fluid from drain tubes are not recommended routinely. Sufficient fluid volume (usually at least 1–2 mL of fluid or tissue) must be collected, and then transported to the microbiology laboratory using a transport system that properly handles and preserves the samples to avoid damage or compromising their integrity [132].

At the laboratory, the intraperitoneal specimen should be examined under a microscope using Gram stain, aerobic and anaerobic culture should be established, and antibiotic susceptibility test should be performed. Received peritoneal fluid or pus may be examined under the microscope immediately because Gram stains may be of value in detecting Gram-positive cocci or yeast. In the event of positive finding of Gram-positive cocci or yeast, the additional empiric anti-cocci or anti-fungi therapy should be considered before definitive culture results are available.

When a microorganism is identified in clinical cultures, antimicrobial susceptibility testing (AST) should always be performed to guide antibiotic therapy.

Results are reported as the minimal inhibitory concentration (MIC), which is the lowest concentration of drug that inhibits the growth of the organism. Reports typically contain a quantitative result in μg/mL and a qualitative interpretation. The interpretation usually categorizes each result as susceptible (S), intermediate (I), and resistant (R) basing on breakpoints established by either the Clinical or Laboratory Standards Institute (CLSI) in the USA or the European Committee for Antimicrobial Susceptibility Testing (EUCAST) in Europe [132].

What are the principles of antimicrobial therapy?

Statement 24

Empirical antimicrobial therapy should be based on local epidemiology, individual patient risk factors for difficult to treat pathogens, clinical severity of infection, and infection source (Recommendation 1 C).

The principles of empiric antibiotic treatment should be defined according to the most frequently isolated microbes, always taking into consideration the local trend of antibiotic resistance.

In this era of prevalent drug-resistant microorganisms, the threat of resistance is a source of major concern that cannot be ignored [139].

In the past 20 years, the incidence of IAIs caused by MDROs has risen dramatically [132].

Quinolone resistance, prevalence of ESBL-producing bacteria, prevalence and mechanisms of carbapenem resistance in the local environment and the place of recent traveling should be always taken into account when an antimicrobial therapy is administered empirically.

Generally, the most important factors in predicting the presence of resistant pathogens in IAIs is acquisition in a healthcare setting (particularly if the patient becomes infected in the ICU or has been hospitalized for more than 1 week), corticosteroid use, organ transplantation, baseline pulmonary or hepatic disease, and previous antimicrobial therapy [136].

Previous antimicrobial therapy is one of the most important risk factors for resistant pathogens [15].

In order to determine risk factors for presence of MDROs in post-operative peritonitis (PP), Augustin et al. reviewed data of 100 patients hospitalized in the ICU for PP. According to logistic regression analysis, the use of broad-spectrum antibiotic between initial intervention and re-operation was the only significant risk factor for emergence of MDROs [15]. For patients with severe sepsis or septic shock, early and properly administered empirical antimicrobial therapy can have a significant impact on the outcome, independent of the anatomical site of infection. Riché et al. [140] in a prospective observational study involving 180 consecutive patients with secondary generalized peritonitis demonstrated a significantly higher mortality rate for patients in septic shock (35 and 8% for patients with and without shock, respectively). Clinical severity should be assessed with the sepsis score criteria or the new proposed criteria for definition of sepsis [19].

Inappropriate therapy in critically ill patients may have a strong negative impact on outcome. An ineffective or inadequate antimicrobial regimen is one of the variables more strongly associated with unfavorable outcomes in critically ill patients. Broad empiric antimicrobial therapy should be started as soon as possible in patients with organ dysfunction (sepsis) and septic shock [141–145].

International guidelines for the management of sepsis and septic shock (the Surviving Sepsis Campaign) recommend intravenously administered antibiotics as soon as possible and in any case within the first hour of onset of sepsis and the use of broad-spectrum agents with adequate penetration of the presumed site of infection [71].

Finally, selection of empirical therapy should take into account the infection source because etiological distribution varies according to the source site, with a prevalence of Gram positive and Candida in the high gastrointestinal tract and a progressive increase of anaerobes and Gram negative towards the lower gastrointestinal tracts.

The epidemiology of intra-abdominal flora in critically ill patients with secondary and tertiary abdominal sepsis was studied by de Ruiter et al. [146]. A 5-year prospective observational cohort study was performed in patients admitted to the ICU with abdominal sepsis syndrome, defined as a perforation of the digestive tract and inflammatory response with organ failure. Abdominal fluid was taken for microbial culture from 221 of the 239 patients admitted with abdominal sepsis. Aerobic Gram-negative bacteria (AGNB) were found in 53% of the cultures of the abdominal fluid taken at the time of operation, of which 45% were *E. coli*; in 36% of patients, more than one AGNB was found. The incidence of AGNB was the highest in colorectal perforations (68.6%) and perforated appendicitis (77.8%) and the lowest in gastroduodenal perforations (20.5%). Gram-positive bacteria were found in 42.5% of the abdominal fluid cultures and most frequently in colorectal perforations (50.0%). Candida was found in 19.9% of patients, with 59.1% of these cultures being *Candida albicans.* The incidence of *Candida* was 41.0% in gastroduodenal perforations and 11.8% in colorectal perforation. Anaerobic bacteria were cultured in 77.8% of patients with perforated appendicitis. Over time, the prevalence of AGNB in abdominal fluid decreased from 117 patients (52.9%) in the first culture to one patient (6.7%) in week 4 (efficacy 87%). The prevalence of Gram-positive bacteria increased from 42.5 to 86.7% in a 4-week period.

Statement 25

The correct dose and correct administration of antimicrobials should include: 1) loading dose when indicated, especially in critically ill patients; 2) extended or prolonged infusion for beta-lactam antibiotics; 3) peritoneal distribution (Recommendation 2 C).

To ensure timely and effective administration of antimicrobial therapy in patients with severe infection, clinicians must consider also the pharmacokinetic/pharmacodynamics properties of the employed antibiotics.

The "dilution effect," also known as the "third spacing phenomenon," is very important for hydrophilic agents. Higher than standard loading doses (LD) of hydrophilic agents such as beta-lactams should be administered to ensure optimal exposure at the infection site, maintaining a therapeutic threshold that considers the effects of renal function [94].

In patients with sepsis and septic shock, missing of LD results in an under exposure to hydrophilic antibiotics that may be critical for patients [147, 148].

Once appropriate initial loading is administered, daily reassessment of the antimicrobial regimen is warranted because pathophysiological changes may significantly affect drug availability [132].

The mechanisms of action of antibiotics should also be taken into account in establishing the maintenance dose. Some antibiotics, including beta-lactam antibiotics, exhibit time-dependent activity and exert optimal bactericidal activity when drug concentrations are maintained above the Minimum Inhibitory Concentration (MIC), whereas high peak concentrations are not beneficial. As a consequence, the more prolonged the time during which the drug levels are above the MIC value, the greater is the chance of clinical cure. In fact, prolonged or continuous infusions of beta-lactams have been proposed in order to maximize the time that the drug concentration exceeds the MIC.

However, the results obtained from clinical studies on the continuous or extended infusion of beta-lactams, including two blinded multicenter RCTs, were not conclusive [149, 150]. The first RCT, of 60 patients, showed that continuous infusion (CI) was associated with higher clinical cure, while the second one, of 432 patients, did not find significant differences in the clinical cure of patients receiving CI or intermittent administration of beta-lactams. This difference could be partially explained by the enrollment of patients on renal replacement therapy in the second RCT.

In addition, these results may not be generalizable to patients with high severity of illness and infections caused by less susceptible pathogens with high MIC for which the greatest potential for a clinically relevant benefit may be predicted by pharmacokinetic/pharmacodynamic theory. This has been supported by some retrospective studies [151, 152]. Prolonged or continuous infusions of beta-lactams should therefore be considered for the treatment of critically ill patients with HAI-IAIs.

Conversely, for antibiotics with concentration dependent activity, such as aminoglycosides, the use of a higher dose at extended interval (i.e., once daily) is strongly recommended [153].

The use of therapeutic drug monitoring (TDM) has been associated with higher clinical success and lower rate of toxicity. It is recommended mainly, but not only, for drugs with a narrow ratio between efficacy and toxicity, such as glycopeptides and aminoglycosides [154].

Antimicrobials typically need to reach a site of action outside the plasma passing through the capillary membranes. Disease- and drug-related factors contribute to differential tissue distribution [155]. Concentration gradient between the plasma and the peritoneal space may be of high relevance in case of multidrug-resistant bacteria. It has been studied for some antibiotics and has shown large variability in drug availability. Data suggest that increased doses of ceftazidime, meropenem, and imipenem are required to reach adequate concentrations in patients with severe intra-abdominal infections [156–158]. In contrast, plasma and peritoneal concentrations of cefepime and cefotaxime seem to be quite similar and an increase in the doses is probably not required [159, 160]. The same concept can be applied for tigecycline with lipophilic characteristics that are minimally impacted by severe intra-abdominal infections [161].

Statement 26

The patient should be reassessed when the results of microbiological testing are available. Antimicrobial de-escalation or withdrawal should be considered (Recommendation 1C).

The results of microbiological testing may have great importance for the choice of therapeutic strategy of every patient, in particular in the adaptation of targeted antimicrobial treatment.

They provide an opportunity to expand antimicrobial regimen if the initial choice was too narrow but also allow de-escalation of antimicrobial therapy if the empirical regimen was too broad.

Antibiotic de-escalation has been associated with lower mortality rates in ICU patients and is now considered a key practice for antimicrobial stewardship purposes [129].

Recently, Montravers et al. [128] valued the characteristics and outcomes of anti-infective de-escalation during healthcare-associated IAIs. They demonstrated that de-escalation is a feasible option in patients with polymicrobial infections such as HAI-IAIs. However, MDR non-fermenting Gram-negative organisms limit its implementation in the setting of IAIs.

Statement 27

In the settings with a high incidence of ESBL-producing Enterobacteriaceae, the extended use of cephalosporins should be discouraged and should be limited to pathogen-directed therapy because of its selective pressure resulting in emergence of resistance (Recommendation 1C).

In the past, cephalosporins have often been used in the treatment of IAIs. In light of the increasing prevalence of ESBL-producing *Enterobacteriaceae* and MRSA due to selection pressures related to overuse of cephalosporins, the routine use of these antibiotics should be strongly discouraged [162].

Ceftolozane/tazobactam [162, 163] and ceftazidime/avibactam [164, 165] are two new cephalosporins/beta-lactamase inhibitor combinations approved for IAIs.

By adding beta-lactamase inhibitor (tazobactam or avibactam), ceftozolane and ceftazidime have a strong activity against Gram-negative MDROs including ESBL-producing Enterobacteriaceae.

These new agents should be combined with metronidazole for complicated IAIs due to limited activity against some *Bacteroides spp*. These antibiotics will be valuable for treating infections caused by Gram-negative MDROs in order to preserve carbapenems. Notably, ceftazidime/avibactam has demonstrated consistent activity against *Klebsiella pneumoniae* carbapenemases (KPCs) producers and ceftolozane/tazobactam against multiresistant *Pseudomonas*.

Cautious clinical use is advised, until their precise roles are further defined as empirical treatment.

Statement 28

Extended use of fluoroquinolones (FQ) should be discouraged because of its selective pressure (mainly ESBLs producing Entrobacteriaceae and MRSA). They should be generally used in patients with allergy to beta-lactams (Recommendation 1C).

FQ have been the most commonly used regimen for complicated IAIs in recent years.

Except for moxifloxacin, FQ have a moderate activity against anaerobes and have been used in combination with metronidazole in the empiric treatment of IAIs. In recent years, resistance of *E. coli* to FQ has risen over time [166].

The worldwide increase in FQ resistance among *E. coli* and other *Enterobacteriaceae* has limited the non-stratified use of FQ for empirical treatment of IAIs, particularly in critically ill patients and those with HAI-IAIs.

Ciprofloxacin, in combination with metronidazole, should be administered only in patients with mild infection and without risk factors for difficult to treat pathogens (DTTPs). In these patients, moxifloxacin monotherapy could be an option [167, 168].

What is the impact of the antimicrobial resistance in IAIs. How do you treat it?

Statement 29

For patients with CA-IAIs, agents with a narrower spectrum of activity should be suggested. However, according to local ecology anti-ESBL-producer coverage may be warranted. By contrast, for patients with HA-IAIs, antimicrobial regimens with broader spectra of activity are preferred (Recommendation 1B).

Hospital-acquired IAIs are associated with an increased likelihood of pathogens with reduced susceptibility to standard antibiotic regimens. In particular, the group of patients with IAIs suffering from resistant bacteria frequently comprises the entire group of post-operative and tertiary peritonitis. According to local bacterial ecology, resistant pathogens can be frequently isolated even in community-acquired secondary peritonitis [170].

In the context of IAIs, the main resistance problem is posed by ESBL-producing *Enterobacteriaceae*, which are alarmingly prevalent in nosocomial infections and frequently observed in community-acquired infections [169–171]. A Carbapenem-sparing regimen is preferred.

The Study for Monitoring Antimicrobial Resistance Trends (SMART) program monitors the activity of antibiotics against aerobic Gram-negative IAIs.

The prevalence of ESBLs in patients with IAIs has increased over time in Asia, Europe, Latin America, the Middle East, North America, and the South Pacific. In contrast, the trend for ESBLs in intra-abdominal infection isolates from Africa has surprisingly, statistically decreased over time [172].

KPC producers are rapidly emerging as a major source of multidrug-resistant infections worldwide. The recent emergence of carbapenem resistance among *Enterobacteriaceae* poses a considerable threat to hospitalized patients [173]. Inappropriate use of carbapenems should be avoided to reduce their selective pressure and association with the increase in carbapenem-resistant *Enterobacteriaceae* (CRE) [174].

Statement 30

Carbapenem sparing treatment should be recommended particularly in the settings where there is a high incidence of carbapenem resistant K. pneumoniae (Recommendation 1B).

The available therapeutic options for the multiresistant Gram-negative bacteria are limited.

In recent years, clinicians have become dependent on carbapenems for treating ESBL infections. This emphasizes the importance of carbapenem-preserving antimicrobial stewardship [162].

The role of β-lactam/β-lactamase inhibitor (BLBLI) combinations towards ESBLs has been debated and controversial even if recent reports suggest their use in ESBL infections [175, 176].

Although tigecycline does not feature in vitro activity against *P. aeruginosa* or certain *Enterobacteriaceae* (*Proteus* spp., *Serratia* spp., *Morganella morganii*, *Providencia stuartii*), it is still an option for complicated IAIs because of its favorable in vitro activity against anaerobic organisms, enterococci, several ESBLs, and some strains of carbapenemase-producing *Enterobacteriaceae* [177, 178]. Because of poor plasma concentrations, tigecycline performs poorly in bacteremic patients, with a much higher risk of failing to clear bacteremia [179]. Tigecycline should not be considered as first-line therapy in patients with healthcare-associated pneumonia and bacteremia.

The recent challenges in the management of Gram-negative MDROs infections, especially in critically ill patients, have revived the clinical use of polymyxins [180–182] and fosfomycin [183]. There are still open questions about the need of combination therapy and the role of carbapenems, administered at high doses and by extended infusions, in the treatment of infections with carbapenem-resistant entetobacteriaceae.

Ceftolozane/tazobactam and ceftazidime/avibactam have recently been approved in some national agencies for the treatment of IAIs [162–165]. Ceftolozone/tazobactam is a new antibiotic that has been approved for treatment of cIAIs (in combination with metronidazole) including infection by ESBLs and *P. aeruginosa* and associated with metronidazole may be valuable for treating infections caused by Gram-negative MDROs in order to preserve carbapenems [162, 163]. It may be useful as empirical therapy to preserve the use of carbapenems in critical patients with risk factors for ESBL isolation or as targeted therapy in patients with isolation of an ESBL-producing *enterobacteriaceae* or *P. aeruginosa* MDR. It should be considered that in some countries, the production of metallo-β-lactamases enzymes, that are not inactivated by ceftolozane/tazobactam, may be one of the mechanisms for carbapenem resistance in *P. aeruginosa.*

Statement 31

Antimicrobial resistance among enterococcal isolates (ampicillin, gentamcin or vancomycin resistance) is mostly found in nosocomial (postoperative or tertiary) peritonitis. In Vancomycin-resistant Enterococcus (VRE), treatment with linezolid (monomicrobial infection) or tigecycline (polymicrobial infection) is appropriate (Recommendation 1 B).

Among Gram-positive bacteria, Enterococci play a significant role in IAIs. Although they are found in community-acquired infections, they were far more prevalent in hospital-acquired infections [184]. In the CIAOW Study [169], Enterococci (*E. faecalis and E. faecium*) were the most prevalent bacteria among all the aerobic Gram-positive bacteria isolated in the intra-operative samples, representing 15.9% of all aerobic isolates. Although Enterococci were also present in community-acquired infections, they were more prevalent in HA-IAIs (22.3% in HA-IAIs versus 13.9% in CA-IAIs). Some studies have demonstrated poor outcomes among patients with documented enterococcal infections [185–188], particularly in those with post-operative IAIs where Enterococci coverage should always be considered. Empirical coverage of Enterococci is not generally recommended for patients with CA-IAIs. The acquisition of glycopeptide resistance by enterococci has seriously affected the treatment and control of these organisms. Many factors can increase the risk of vancomycin-resistant Enterococcus (VRE) infection. These include previous antibiotic therapy, prolonged hospitalization, hospitalization in an intensive care unit, severe illness or underlying pathology, invasive procedures, gastrointestinal surgery, organ transplantation, and close proximity to other VRE-positive patients [189].

The majority of vancomicyn-resistant enterococcus infections have been attributed to *E. faecium,* though glycopeptide resistance occurs in *E. faecalis* and other *Enterococcus* spp. as well [189].

Options for treating vancomicyn-resistant enterococcus infections are linezolid or tigeciclyine [178, 190].

What is the impact of intra-abdominal candidiasis? When and how do you treat intra-abdominal candidiasis?

Statement 32

The presence of Candida spp. in the peritoneal samples is a factor of poor prognosis (Recommendation 1C).

The epidemiological role of *Candida* spp. in IAI has not yet been conclusively defined.

Colonizing strains of *C. albicans* are normally present in small or moderate numbers and they are only regarded as part of the resident gastrointestinal microflora [191].

However, isolation of *Candida* spp. in samples from IAIs is associated with poor outcomes [192].

In community-acquired infections, the role of *Candida* spp. in the prognosis is difficult to demonstrate. In healthcare-associated (mainly post-operative) peritonitis, intra-abdominal candidiasis is associated with increased mortality.

In an observational study, Montravers et al. [193] showed that isolation of *Candida* spp. was an independent risk factor of mortality in nosocomial peritonitis patients. However, antifungal treatment did not improve survival.

Several criteria have been considered as factors of poor prognosis for patients with Candida isolation in peritoneal fluid.

In a retrospective review of a prospective surgical ICU database of patients, Dupont et al. [194] demonstrated that four variables were independently associated with mortality in polymicrobial peritonitis with Candida isolation in peritoneal fluid in critically ill patients. These were (1) APACHE II (Acute Physiology and Chronic Health Evaluation II) score on admission of at least 17, (2) respiratory failure on admission, (3) upper gastrointestinal tract origin of peritonitis, and (4) results of direct examination of peritoneal fluid that were positive for Candida.

Data from 13 hospitals in Italy, Spain, Brazil, and Greece over a 3-year period (2011–2013) including patients from ICU, medical, and surgical wards with intra-abdominal candidiasis was published in 2015 [195]. A total of 481 patients were included in the study. Of these, 27% were hospitalized in ICU. The mean age was 63 years, and 57% of patients were male. Multivariate logistic analysis regression showed that age, increments in 1-point APACHE II scores, secondary peritonitis, septic shock, and non-adequate abdominal source control were significantly associated with mortality. In patients with septic shock, absence of source control resulted in mortality rates above 60% irrespective of administration of an adequate antifungal therapy.

Moreover, a prospective observational study involving 180 consecutive patients with secondary generalized peritonitis (community-acquired and post-operative) at a single center was published by Riché et al. [140]. Septic shock complicating intra-abdominal candidiasis was associated with high mortality rates. Yeast in the peritoneal fluid of post-operative peritonitis were an independent risk factor for death in patients with septic shock.

Statement 33

Two situations justify an empirical antifungal therapy: patients with septic shock in community-acquired infections or patients with post-operative infections (Recommendation 2 C).

No study has specifically evaluated the efficacy of antifungal therapy in IAIs. In recent randomized trials focusing on antifungal therapy of invasive candidiasis, the proportion of patients with a diagnosis of abdominal candidiasis was low [196, 197]. The need for an early adequate systemic antifungal therapy in candida peritonitis is based on the assumption that delayed antifungal therapy initiation is associated to poorer outcome, particularly among those with candidaemia [198–200]. However, a deleterious impact of delayed systemic antifungal therapy initiation has never been demonstrated in candida intra-abdominal infection.

Two situations justify an empirical antifungal therapy: patients with septic shock in community-acquired infections or patients with post-operative infections where the presence of yeast is associated with a poor prognosis.

The EUCAST guidelines consider *Candida glabrata* resistant to azole agents [201]. These organisms were observed in 22% of all intra-abdominal candidiasis in Montravers et al.'s prospective study. This was a non-interventional study in 271 adult ICU patients with proven invasive *Candida* infection who received systemic antifungal therapy [193]. As a consequence, an echinocandin should probably be used as empirical antifungal therapy in critically ill patients having CA-IAIs or HAI-IAIs. First-line fluconazole therapy is preferable in the other cases. The optimal duration of definitive treatment is not established. The IDSA guidelines did not provide any recommendations for duration of therapy [202]. For severe bacterial healthcare-associated IAIs, a duration of antibacterial therapy between 7 and 15 days is recommended [203]. Based on the high rates of recurrence and relapse in candida IAIs, longer duration has been recommended by experts (around 2 to 3 weeks) [195]. De-escalation of empirical antifungal therapy is a safe procedure as illustrated recently in two studies. In a recent study, 835 non-neutropenic adults were recruited in the multicenter prospective observational AmarCAND2 study. Patients receiving systemic antifungal therapy for a documented or suspected invasive candidiasis in the ICU and who were still alive 5 days after antifungal initiation were selected [204]. Among the 647 studied patients, early de-escalation at day 5 after antifungal initiation occurred in 142 patients (22%). Early systemic antifungal therapy (SAT) de-escalation was the sole factor not associated with increased 28-day mortality (RR 1.12, 95% CI 0.76–1.66). In non-neutropenic critically ill adult patients with documented or suspected invasive candidiasis, SAT de-escalation within 5 days was not related to increased day 28 mortality but was associated with decreased SAT consumption. These results suggest, for the first time, that SAT de-escalation may be safe in these patients. In a recent study by Montravers et al. [126] on 206 patients with HCAI-IAIs, de-escalation was performed in 53% of the cases including antifungal agents in 49% of the cases having antifungal therapy. De-escalation was not a risk factor for mortality.

What is the optimal duration of antimicrobial therapy?

Statement 34

In the setting of uncomplicated acute cholecystitis and acute appendicitis post-operative antimicrobial therapy is not necessary (Recommendation 1A).

In the event of uncomplicated IAIs, the infection involves a single organ and does not extend to the peritoneum. When the source of infection is treated effectively by surgical excision, post-operative antimicrobial therapy is not necessary, as demonstrated in managing uncomplicated acute appendicitis or cholecystitis [3–5].

Statement 35

In patients with IAIs, when patients are not severely ill and when source control is complete, a short course (3–5 days) of post-operative therapy is suggested (Recommendation 1A).

Recently, a prospective study on appropriate duration of antimicrobial therapy was published [6]. The study randomized 518 patients with IAIs and adequate source control to receive antibiotics until 2 days after the resolution of fever, leukocytosis, and ileus, with a maximum of 10 days of therapy (control group), or to receive a fixed course of antibiotics (experimental group) for 4 ± 1 calendar days.

In patients with intra-abdominal infections who had undergone an adequate source control procedure, the outcomes after fixed-duration antibiotic therapy (approximately 4 days) were similar to those after a longer course of antibiotics (approximately 8 days) that extended until after the resolution of physiological abnormalities. In this study, most patients were not severely ill.

Statement 36

In patients with ongoing or persistent IAIs, the decision to continue, revise, or stop antimicrobial therapy should be made on the basis of clinician judgment and laboratory information (Recommendation 1 A).

The high mortality associated with abdominal sepsis requires clinicians to maintain a high index of clinical suspicion of treatment failure and the early diagnosis of ongoing infections. These patients should always be monitored carefully including the potential use of inflammatory response markers.

The most studied biomarkers in clinical settings are the acute phase proteins (CRP) and procalcitonin (PCT) [205, 206].

Recently, PCT has been suggested as a novel biomarker that may be useful in guiding therapeutic decision making in the management of sepsis. It may be a helpful tool to determine the timing and appropriateness of escalation of antimicrobial therapy in sepsis. A systematic review and meta-analysis on PCT-guided therapy in ICU patients with severe sepsis and septic shock was published in 2013 [207]. Seven randomized studies comprising a total of 1075 patients with severe sepsis or septic shock were included in the meta-analysis. Both hospital mortality and 28-day mortality were not different between PCT-guided therapy and standard treatment groups. However, duration of antimicrobial therapy was significantly reduced in those using PCT-guided therapy. In 2015, a review on PCT-guided antibiotic therapy for septic patients in the surgical ICU confirmed the benefits of using procalcitonin including cost-effectiveness and timing of termination of antibiotics [208].

However, these results were not confirmed in a prospective study in the setting of patients having only IAIs [209]. In this study including 101 consecutive patients with peri-operative septic shock secondary to intra-abdominal infection, PCT decrease to 0.5 ng/mL lacked sensitivity to predict the treatment response. In addition, a decrease of at least 80% from the peak level failed to accurately predict treatment response. PCT may become a valuable weapon for predicting treatment response. However, its role has not been defined in cIAIs and should always be correlated with clinician judgment.

Which interventions improve antibiotic prescribing practices for patients with IAIs?

Interventions to improve antibiotic prescribing practices for patients with IAIs should be directed at two different levels:

1. Patient level—which includes clinical severity, epidemiological exposures, PK/PD factors, comorbidities, prior antibiotic exposure, prior infection, or colonization with MDROs and infection source
2. Hospital level—including presence of in-hospital antimicrobial stewardship programs, availability of local guidelines and updated microbiological data, infection control policy, educational activities, and structural resources (like computer-assisted order entry)

Significant data supports the importance of antibiotic prescribing practices for patients with IAIs, in critically ill and non-critically ill patients and in community and hospital-acquired infections. Prescribing practices may influence the outcome and cost of treatment as well as the risk of superinfection and resistant pathogens in the individual patient and the broader environment. Components of antibiotic prescribing practices that may influence outcome and the risk of developing superinfection and antibiotic resistant infections include (a) adequacy of empiric antibiotic therapy, (b) the time to initial antibiotic therapy, (c) appropriate pharmacokinetic dosing, (d) de-escalation of antibiotic therapy, (e) length of treatment, and (f) avoidance of unnecessary antibiotic therapy.

Statement 37

Multifaceted interventions are more likely to improve antibiotic prescribing practices than simple, passive interventions. Didactic educational programs alone are generally ineffective. (Recommendation 1B).

Most studies of the implementation of guidelines and prescribing practices, including for IAIs, have involved multifaceted interventions [210–214]. A longitudinal study of a multifaceted program that included locally developed, unit-specific protocols, computer-assisted order entry, and ICU-based pharmacist facilitation in both a trauma and a surgical ICU, demonstrated compliance with protocols and a sustained reduction in multidrug-resistant pathogens [212]. Popovski et al. performed a before-and-after study that examined multifaceted interventions to optimize antibiotic use for IAIs [214]. Interventions included (1) adapting published guidelines based on local susceptibility data with stratification of infection type, (2) creation of educational tools, and (3) educational programs involving multidisciplinary groups. Antibiotic selection was significantly altered, and the change persisted for greater than 2 years. However, no change was noted in the length of treatment. The difficulty of altering prolonged antibiotic therapy is highlighted by a recent randomized, controlled trial of a short, fixed duration of antibiotic therapy for IAIs versus treatment until the resolution of fever, leukocytosis, and ileus in which both the control and treatment groups had substantial non-compliance with significant extended antibiotic therapy (24 and 18%, respectively) [6].

Statement 38

As a single intervention, implementation of locally adapted, interdisciplinary evidence based guidelines that incorporate risk stratification (severity and CA-IAIs versus HA-IAIs) and local resistance data most consistently improves components of AB prescribing for IAI (Recommendation 1 B).

As an individual component of change, the creation of locally adapted evidence-based guidelines incorporating local historical culture data with the involvement of an interdisciplinary team is strongly supported in the literature [210, 213, 214]. The presence of pre-existing locally developed antibiotic protocols was independently associated with improved time to antibiotic treatment and with survival in a 1-month prospective observational trial of 41 French ICUs [215]. An intra-abdominal source of infection accounted for 21% of all infection episodes receiving new antibiotic therapy. Several studies have demonstrated the ability to achieve a high percentage of adequate empiric coverage for IAIs employing this approach (Leone 89%, Raymond 100%, Barie 94%) [216–218].

Statement 39

Computer-assisted order entry, non-physician healthcare provider facilitation, and therapeutic drug monitoring can improve components of antibiotic prescribing practices, if resources are available (Recommendation 2 B).

Computerized decision support programs and computer-assisted implementation methods have been found to be useful in many studies of antibiotic therapy [219–221]. In one cluster randomized trial of three hospitals from Israel, Germany, and Italy, a computerized decision support system significantly increased the rate of appropriate empirical antibiotic treatment of infections, with an adjusted odd ratio of 1.48 [222]. Computer-based advisors and decision support have also been used to improve antibiotic dosing in various populations.

Though seldom examined in isolation, non-physician healthcare providers, most commonly pharmacists and nurses, have facilitated guideline implementation and compliance in most randomized trials and before-and-after studies [223–225].

Which are the determinants of outcome of patients with cIAIs in ICU?

Statement 40

The lack of source control and antibiotic adequacy are the only modifiable risk factors for mortality in patients with cIAIs admitted to the ICU. Organ dysfunction is associated with worse outcomes (Recommendation 1 B).

Patients with cIAIs present with varying severity of illness and may require ICU care in the pre or post-operative periods which may be associated with a high mortality rate.

Although cIAIs are the second most frequent infection in the ICU, outcomes after ICU admission and risk factors have been sparsely studied.

De Waele et al. performed a systematic review of the literature to identify factors independently associated with outcome in patients admitted to the ICU because of cIAIs. Studies were included in the analysis if they include ICU patients with cIAIs and reported the impact of any clinical treatment or microbiological factor on outcome. Thirty-two studies, published between

1999 and 2014, were retrieved and eight were selected for inclusion in this analysis. In total, 3967 patients were analyzed in these eight studies, three studies were single-center studies, and three included fewer than 200 patients. Two studies did not consider any surgical characteristic for analysis; source control adequacy was evaluated to some extent in six but details such as source control timing were only assessed in two. Half of the studies did not consider antibiotic adequacy as a variable; and timing of antibiotic therapy was not assessed in any study. Five studies considered microbiological characteristics as potential factors that may impact outcome. Reported mortality included either ICU mortality or hospital mortality (three each), and 30-day and 4-month mortality. Risk factors associated with mortality could be categorized into three major classes: (1) patient comorbidity, (2) treatment, and (3) severity of illness. All studies reported severity of illness (variable expressed, either scoring systems, organ dysfunction, or need for organ support) as a risk factor for outcome; Acute Kidney Injury (AKI) was cited specifically in five studies. Patient characteristics included age (three studies), gender (one study), and infection source (two studies). Comorbidities that were associated with outcome included cirrhosis (three studies) and hematological cancer (one study). Lack of source control was reported as independently associated with poor outcome in three studies; inadequate antibiotic therapy in one.

Which treatment duration is adequate for critically ill patients with complicated intra-abdominal infection? Which are the major determinants of antibiotic choice in patients with complicated intra-abdominal infection (cIAI)?

Statement 41

If the patient is critically ill the treatment duration can be deferred until after a multi-disciplinary careful evaluation (Recommendation 1B).

Inadequate source control and inappropriate antibiotics are key determinants of mortality in patients having intra-abdominal sepsis and associated bacteremia.

In order to describe characteristics of critically ill patients with secondary blood stream infection (BSI) of intra-abdominal origin and identify predictors of mortality, a retrospective, single-center study that evaluated patients admitted between January 2005 and January 2011 was recently published [67]. Logistic regression analysis revealed inadequate source control ($P = 0.002$) and inappropriate antibiotics ($P = 0.016$) to be independently associated with mortality. In non-critically ill patients with adequate source control procedure after cIAI, the duration of the antimicrobial therapy was well defined [6]. However, for critically ill patients, an individualized approach is always mandatory. Appropriate antibiotic therapy, is a cornerstone for the success.

Statement 42

Principal determinants of antibiotic choice in critically ill patients are based on three parameters: 1) Severity of illness, 2) local ecology, and 3) risk factors of the host. Previous antibiotic use is associated with a higher development of multidrug resistant organisms (MDROs). Broad-spectrum antibiotic therapy, including combination of different antibiotic classes should be recommended in patients with septic shock, settings with high rates of MDRO, and previous antibiotic administration (Recommendation 1B).

Abdominal sepsis is a common indication for admission to the ICU. In 2014, the EPIC II study [226], including 13,796 adult patients from 1265 ICUs in 75 countries, demonstrated ICU mortality was higher in patients with abdominal infections compared to those with other infections (29.4 vs. 24.4%, $P < 0.001$). In patients with septic shock, early appropriate empiric antimicrobial therapy has a significant impact on the outcome, independent of the site of infection [227]. Prompt institution of antimicrobial therapy that is active against the causative pathogen(s) is crucial in the treatment of patients with severe infection and sepsis. In fact, the Surviving Sepsis Campaign strongly recommends initiating antibiotic therapy within the first hour of recognition of severe sepsis, after suitable cultures have been obtained. In a retrospective analysis of a large dataset collected prospectively for the Surviving Sepsis Campaign, Ferrer et al. [228] demonstrated that delay in first antibiotic administration was associated with increased in-hospital mortality in patients with severe sepsis and septic shock.

An antimicrobial policy of de-escalation therapy consisting of the initial use of wide-spectrum antimicrobials followed by a reassessment of treatment when culture results are available should be a principle of antimicrobial stewardship in critically ill patients [229]. Studies have reported conflicting effects on outcomes with de-escalation in various groups of critically ill patients.

To assess the safety and the impact on in-hospital and 90-day mortality of antibiotic de-escalation in patients admitted to the ICU with severe sepsis or septic shock, a prospective study was published in 2014 [230].

By multivariate analysis, factors independently associated with in-hospital mortality were septic shock, elevated SOFA score the day of culture results, and inadequate empirical antimicrobial therapy. In contrast, de-escalation therapy was a protective factor. However, in 2014, a multicenter randomized trial investigating a strategy based on de-escalation of antibiotics resulted in prolonged duration of ICU stay but did not affect the mortality rate [231].

Recently, Montravers et al. demonstrated that de-escalation is a feasible option in patients with polymicrobial infections such as healthcare-associated IAIs [128]. In a context of a dedicated "antibiotic stewardship" program, de-escalation should be encouraged, whenever possible, to optimize antibiotic use [232].

Emphasis on MDRO epidemiology is needed to better understand current strategies of prevention and management of critically ill patients in ICUs [233].

A rational use of antibiotics is important in order to prevent the emergence of multidrug-resistant bacteria, especially in ICUs. In critically ill patients, positive cultures may actually represent contamination. Antibiotic stewardship for critically ill patients may be translated into the implementation of specific guidelines, which were largely promoted by the Surviving Sepsis Campaign, targeted to optimizing choice, dosage, and duration of antibiotics in order to improve outcomes and reduce the development of resistance [234, 235].

What is the best management of patients with abdominal sepsis?

Statement 43

Early identification of sepsis and prompt administration of intravenous fluids and vasopressors are always mandatory. Restoring a mean systemic arterial pressure of 65 to 70 mm Hg is a good initial goal during the hemodynamic support of patients with sepsis (Recommendation 1 A).

The definition of sepsis (Sepsis-3) [19] has returned to the traditional views that sepsis is characterized by organ dysfunction attributed to an infection. Patients with at least two of three clinical abnormalities including Glasgow coma score of 14 or less, systolic blood pressure of 100 mmHg or less, and respiratory rate 22/min or greater may have poor outcome typical of sepsis. Importantly, qSOFA does not define sepsis but provides simple bedside criteria to screen adult patients with suspected infection. Sepsis is now defined as a life-threatening organ dysfunction caused by a dysregulated host response to infection. It can be clinically represented by an increase in the SOFA score of 2 points or more [19]. Norepinephrine is now the first-line vasopressor agent which is used to correct hypotension in the event of septic shock. It is more efficacious than dopamine and is more effective for reversing hypotension in patients with septic shock [71, 236–238]. Septic shock is defined as a subset of sepsis in which particularly profound circulatory, cellular, and metabolic abnormalities who are associated with higher risk of mortality than with sepsis alone. Patients with septic shock can be clinically identified by requirement for vasopressors to maintain a mean arterial pressure of 65 mmHg or greater and serum lactate level less than 2 mmol/L (>18 mg/dL) in the absence of hypovolemia [19]. Under this terminology, "severe sepsis" becomes superfluous. Sepsis should generally warrant greater levels of monitoring and interventions.

In patients with sepsis, the 2016 SCC guidelines suggest that initial hemodynamic resuscitation should be achieved within 3 h [71].

Fluid therapy is needed to improve microvascular blood flow through an increased cardiac output as an essential part of the treatment of sepsis. A fluid challenge should incorporate four determinant elements [236]: (1) crystalloid solutions should be the first choice because they are well tolerated and cheap; (2) fluids should be infused rapidly to induce a quick response but not so fast that an artificial stress response develops; (3) the goal should be an increase in systemic arterial pressure; and (4) avoidance of pulmonary edema which is the most serious complication of fluid infusion through appropriate monitoring that is necessary to prevent edema occurrence.

Hypotension is the most common indicator of inadequate perfusion. Restoring a mean arterial pressure of 65 to 70 mmHg is a good initial goal during hemodynamic support of patients with sepsis [239].

Statement 44

Fluid overload should be avoided in patients with generalized peritonitis, (Recommendation 1C).

In patients with generalized peritonitis, fluid resuscitation should avoid fluid overload, which may aggravate gut edema and lead to increased intra-abdominal pressure (IAP) [239].

The systemic inflammatory response syndrome, increased vascular permeability, and aggressive crystalloid resuscitation predispose to fluid sequestration and collection in the peritoneum. Patients with advanced sepsis commonly develop bowel edema. These changes along with an associated forced closure of the abdominal wall may result in increased IAP ultimately leading to intra-abdominal hypertension (IAH) [238]. Elevated IAP may reduce both regional and global perfusion resulting in significant organ failure. An uncontrolled IAH, with an IAP exceeding 20 mmHg, and new organ failure onset leads to abdominal compartment syndrome (ACS). ACS is a potentially lethal complication affecting splanchnic, cardiovascular, pulmonary, renal, and central nervous systems [117, 240].

What are the role of the adjunctive therapies in sepsis?

Statement 45

There is currently insufficient evidence supporting the use of any adjunctive therapy in patients with septic shock due to intra-abdominal infection (No Recommendation).

Although source control, antimicrobial therapy, and supportive therapies remain the cornerstone of treatment, especially in the early phase of sepsis, the identification of adjunctive therapies may play an important role in patients with ongoing sepsis.

In septic patients, mortality is higher when both pro- and anti-inflammatory cytokine levels are high [241, 242]. The rationale of using extracorporeal blood purification in patients with septic shock is to modulate the immune response. Blood purification for sepsis has consisted of various techniques: high-volume hemofiltration, high-adsorption hemofiltration, high cut-off membrane hemofiltration, plasma exchange, and hybrid systems [243].

A systematic review and meta-analysis of randomized trials to determine the association between various blood purification techniques and all-cause mortality in humans with sepsis was published in 2013 [244]. Ten single-center and six multicenter studies were identified. Ten trials reported patients with either severe sepsis or septic shock, while five trials reported only patients with a diagnosis of sepsis. One trial included patients with sepsis, severe sepsis, or septic shock. The blood purification techniques used included hemoperfusion (ten trials), hemofiltration (four trials), and plasma exchange (two trials).

Overall, blood purification decreased mortality compared with no blood purification. However, these results were driven mainly by hemoperfusion. Pooling of all trials of blood purification for treatment of sepsis was no longer associated with lower mortality after excluding trials using polymyxin B hemoperfusion. PMB-HP has been debated in recent years [245-246]. PMB-HP represents a promising strategy, but the Franch, prospective, multicenter, randomized controlled trial (ABDOMIX group) enrolling 243 patients with septic shock within 12 hours after emergency surgery for peritonitis related to organ perforation [247] failed to demonstrate a benefit. More recently the EUPRATHES (evaluating Polymyxin B Hemoperfusion in a randomized controlled study of adults treated for endotoxemia and septic shock) trial of PMB-HP in patients with septic shock and confirmed endotoxemia also failed to show an improved survival [248].

The use of intravenous immunoglobulin for treating patients with surgical sepsis is controversial. It is based on a potential benefit related to neutralization of endotoxin and various bacterial products. Intravenous immunoglobulin provides antibodies that can neutralize circulating exotoxins produced by organisms and may modulate the systemic inflammatory response induced by cytokine stimulation [249].

In order to evaluate the effects of intravenous immunoglobulin (IVIG) as adjunctive therapy in patients with bacterial sepsis or septic shock on mortality, bacteriological failure rates, and duration of stay in hospital, a Cochrane review was published in 2013 [250]. Forty-three RCTs comparing IVIG (monoclonal or polyclonal) with placebo or no intervention in patients of any age with bacterial sepsis or septic shock were reviewed. Subgroup analysis of ten polyclonal IVIG trials ($n = 1430$) and seven trials on IgM-enriched polyclonal IVIG ($n = 528$) showed significant reductions in mortality in adults with sepsis compared to placebo or no intervention. Pooled analysis of polyclonal and monoclonal IVIG was not done due to clinical heterogeneity. Polyclonal IVIG reduced mortality among adults with sepsis however this benefit was not seen in trials with low risk of bias.

A review of the mechanisms of action and meta-analysis of the clinical effectiveness was recently published [251]. The meta-analysis of 18 RCTs indicated that the use of IVIG reduces the mortality risk of septic patients. Low study quality, heterogeneous dosing regimens and type of Ig preparations, and different control interventions (placebo or albumin) are thought to have probably influenced results. Thus, the study showed that the use of IVIG therapy in adult septic patients may have a rationale and seems to be associated with a reduced mortality. However, the available evidence is not clearly sufficient to support the widespread use of IVIG in the treatment of sepsis.

A meta-analysis of randomized controlled studies published in 2007 compared IVIG preparations [252]. The meta-analysis demonstrated a strong trend in favor of an immunoglobulin preparation enriched with IgA and IgM (IgGAM) compared with preparations containing only IgG. 2016 Surviving Sepsis Campaign guidelines do not support the use of IVIG therapy [71].

Which inflammatory mediators are involved in intra-abdominal sepsis? Are they useful markers in clinical practice?

Statement 46

Inflammatory biomarkers require further controlled studies before their measurement guides clinical care of critically ill/injured patients (No recommendation).

Inflammatory and protein mediators (cytokine, chemokine, acute phase proteins) play an important, but still not completely understood, role in the morbidity and mortality of abdominal sepsis.

Their potential utility includes function as (1) diagnostic/prognostic biomarkers, (2) therapeutic targets, and (3) elucidation of the pathogenic mechanisms of sepsis or injury-related organ dysfunction.

However, there is no consensus on the clinical use of mediators in diagnosing or managing intra-abdominal sepsis or injury. A MEDLINE, PubMed, EMBASE, and the Cochrane Library review on inflammatory mediators in abdominal sepsis was published in 2015 [253].

Serum PCT and C-reactive protein (CRP) appear to be useful to rule out infection or monitor therapy. There have been 33 studies exploring CRP as a marker for abdominal infection or complications after surgery. Kinetic studies demonstrated CRP levels elevate on post-operative day (POD) 1, peak from POD2 to POD3, and decline by POD5 provided that there is no complication or infection. Four reports suggest a persistent threshold of greater than 100 mg/L might indicate abscess/septic complications [254–257]; other studies have refuted this conclusion, leaving uncertainty for clinical utility [258–262].

Twelve trials including two randomized controlled studies evaluated the role of PCT as an indicator to diagnose infection, predict outcomes, or guide treatment of abdominal sepsis.

In some studies, persistent high levels of PCT were associated with infection and or increased septic mortality in patients with sepsis [263, 264], while other studies have not confirmed PCT as an accurate marker for sepsis or to predict a patient's response to the initial treatment [201, 265].

The role of IL-6 as a marker to diagnose sepsis or predict outcomes has also been studied. However, its role remains uncertain and a wide range of cut-off values had been used (from 12 to 2760 pg/mL). Some studies considered IL-6 an indicator for sepsis or for predicting outcome and mortality [266–268]. However, other studies do not support the use of IL-6 as a valid sepsis biomarker [269, 270].

Recent studies have reported endogenous DAMPs (mtDNA, HMGB1) released as a consequence of tissue injury or infection to be promising biomarkers [271, 272]; however, the evidence supporting their role is still limited and their use undefined.

Statement 47

Consideration should be given to draining ascites in the critically ill patient treated for peritonitis, especially if the ascites is associated with IAH (Recommendation 1C).

It has been found that increased levels of both systemic and peritoneal cytokines are associated with post-operative complications, which may discriminate survivors from those who died [273, 274].

These data suggest that measurement of peritoneal cytokines could be a potentially important method to determine and follow the patient's inflammatory reaction.

Although data from research with animal models [275] having inflammatory bowel disease [265, 276] are suggestive, direct evidence does not yet exist to prove that effectively draining this peritoneal fluid makes a difference to complications or survival.

Severe IAH has been shown to significantly reduce perfusion to the intestinal mucosa, which ultimately increases intestinal permeability and results in systemic endotoxemia aggravating the sepsis cascade. Damaged gut is a continual source of inflammation and MODS, referred to as the "Motor of MSOF" [277–282], by inducing the production of cytokines and other biomediators. The release of endotoxin induces production of cytokines, including interleukin (IL)-6, IL-1B, IL-8, tumor necrosis factor-α (TNF-α), and other mediators and movement of these mediators into the systemic circulation may be largely modulated by the mesenteric lymphatic channels, as demonstrated in animal models [283].

In clinical practice, the accumulation of intraperitoneal mediators can be removed by either percutaneous drainage and negative pressure therapy with an open abdomen. Percutaneous drainage is recommended to treat IAH if it is possible to do safely, as it may obviate the need for decompressive laparotomy [119, 284]. If percutaneous drainage is not safely possible, NPPT may be another appropriate option.

A single-center RCT published in 2015 conducted on critically ill and injured patients with an average APACHE score above 22 in critically ill and an ISS over 23 in the injured compared commercial NPPT system with the Barkers VAC PAC in a randomized fashion [125]. Although this study did not find a difference in actual peritoneal fluid drainage or in the behavior of the high level mediators examined (IL-1β, IL-8, IL-10, or IL-12, p70, or TNFα), there was a survival difference in favor of the commercial system. However, it is possible that patient heterogeneity in the complex setting of mixed critical care populations can alone explain the findings, and thus, further studies are required.

Conclusions

In the Appendix, all the recommendations from the "Dublin WSES 2016 Intra-Abdominal Infections Consensus Conference" are listed.

Appendix

Classification, diagnosis, and risk factors

Statement 1

The term "intra-abdominal infections" describes a wide heterogeneity of clinical conditions. The anatomical extent of infection, the presumed pathogens involved, risk factors for major resistance patterns, and the patient's clinical condition should be assessed independently so as to classify patients (*Recommendation 1 C*).

Statement 2

Early clinical evaluation is essential for diagnosing IAIs. It helps to optimize diagnostic testing and can result in earlier implementation of a proper management plan (Recommendation 1C).

Statement 3

A step-up approach for diagnosis should be used and tailored to the clinical setting, resources, patient's age beginning with clinical and laboratory examination and progressing to imaging examinations (Recommendation 1C).

Statement 4

Patient factors are essential when addressing treatment outcome, as advanced age, associated comorbidity, pre-existing disease, and physiologic status greatly influence outcomes (e.g., mortality) (Recommendation 2 C).

Statement 5

Disease factors are essential to consider when addressing risk for treatment failure. (Recommendation 2 C).

Statement 6

While age alone is not decisive for outcome it should be recognized that patients with an accumulated number of risk factors, including advanced age, high disease severity and presenting in sepsis or septic shock, have a very high risk of death. Palliative care should be actively discussed when conditions indicate that operative treatment is futile (Recommendation 2 C).

Statement 7

Prognostic scoring systems for complicated IAIs may be useful in clinical practise, especially for audit and research. Scoring systems can be broadly divided into two groups: general organ failure severity (ICU) scores and peritonitis-specific (Surgical) scores. The Sequential Organ Failure Assessment (SOFA) score allows physicians to follow the evolving disease process in critically ill patients in ICU (Recommendation 2 A).

However, although these scores may help guide clinical care, their use in individual patients is much less predictive.

Source control

Statement 8

Most patients with cIAIs and sepsis/septic shock should undergo an urgent source control procedure; source control can be delayed in less severely-ill patients when the circumstances are appropriate (Recommendation 2 C).

Statement 9

Highly selected patients with perforated diverticulitis (including those with an abscess <4 cm in diameter), a peri-appendiceal mass, or a perforated peptic ulcer can be managed without definitive source control if responding satisfactorily to antimicrobial therapy and other supportive measures. (Recommendation 1 B).

Statement 10

Laparoscopic appendectomy represents the first choice for most patients with acute appendicitis where appropriate resources and skills are available (Recommendation 1 A).

Statement 11

There is no evidence of any significant advantages between laparoscopic and open repair of perforated peptic ulcer (PPU). However, laparoscopy has less post-operative pain and shorter hospital stay (Recommendation 1 A).

Statement 12

Early laparoscopic cholecystectomy is safe and feasible in acute cholecystitis and should be the preferred choice in absence of contraindications to pneumoperitoneum, even in high risk patients, where appropriate resources and skills are available (Recommendation 1A).

Statement 13

Laparoscopic lavage is not recommended in Hinchey IV diverticulitis because it can not achieve adequate source control. Laparoscopic lavage is safe and not inferior to sigmoid resection in case of Hinchey III but it is not considered the preferred choice, given the lack of evidence of major benefits (Recommendation 1A).

Statement 14

Laparoscopic sigmoid resection is feasible and safe in selected patients, hemodynamically stable, without significant comorbidities and with onset of peritonitis <12-24 hours, only if specific advanced laparoscopic colorectal expertise is available (Recommendation 2 C).

Statement 15

Planned relaparotomy is not recommended as a general strategy in patients with secondary peritonitis (Recommendation 1A).

Statement 16

There is insufficient evidence to advocate damage control surgery as general strategy in patients with secondary peritonitis (Recommendation 1C).

Statement 17

Damage control surgery may be an option in selected significantly physiologically deranged patients with ongoing sepsis (Recommendation 2C).

Statement 18

Temporary abdominal closure using negative pressure therapy (NPT) can be useful to decrease the time to definitive abdominal closure (Recommendation 1B). Prolonged NPT may increase the risk of enteric fistulae.

Antimicrobial therapy

Statement 19

Intraperitoneal specimens for microbiological evaluation from the site of infection are always recommended for patients with HA-IAIs or with CA-IAIs at risk for resistant pathogens (previous antimicrobial therapy) and in critically ill patients (Recommendation 1 B).

Statement 20

Intraperitoneal specimens should be collected in every re-operation (Recommendation 1 C).

Statement 21

Appropriate intraperitoneal specimen is peritoneal fluid/tissue collected from the site of infection *(Recommendation 1 C).*

Statement 22

Sufficient abdominal fluid/tissue volume (usually at least 1–2 mL of fluid) should be collected and transported to the microbiology laboratory using a transport system that properly handles and *preserves the samples to avoid damage or compromise their integrity (Recommendation 1 C).*

Statement 23

At the laboratory the intraperitoneal specimen should undergo Gram stain, aerobic and anaerobic culture, and antibiotic susceptibility testing (Recommendation 1 C).

Statement 24

Empirical antimicrobial therapy should be based on local epidemiology, individual patient risk factors for difficult to treat pathogens, clinical severity of infection, and infection source (Recommendation 1 C).

Statement 25

The correct dose and correct administration of antimicrobials should include: 1) loading dose when indicated, especially in critically ill patients; 2) extended or prolonged infusion for beta-lactam antibiotics; 3) peritoneal distribution (Recommendation 2 C).

Statement 26

The patient should be reassessed when the results of microbiological testing are available. Antimicrobial deescalation or withdrawal should be considered (Recommendation 1C).

Statement 27

In the settings with a high incidence of ESBL-producing Enterobacteriaceae, the extended use of cephalosporins should be discouraged and should be limited to pathogen-directed therapy because of its selective pressure resulting in emergence of resistance (Recommendation 1C).

Statement 28

Extended use of fluoroquinolones (FQ) should be discouraged because of its selective pressure (mainly ESBLs producing Entrobacteriaceae and MRSA). They should be generally used in patients with allergy to beta-lactams (Recommendation 1C).

Statement 29

For patients with CA-IAIs, agents with a narrower spectrum of activity should be suggested. However, according to local ecology anti-ESBL-producer coverage may be warranted. By contrast, for patients with HA-IAIs, antimicrobial regimens with broader spectra of activity are preferred (Recommendation 1B).

Statement 30

Carbapenem sparing treatment should be recommended particularly in the settings where there is a high incidence of carbapenem resistant K. pneumoniae (Recommendation 1B).

Statement 31

Antimicrobial resistance among enterococcal isolates (ampicillin, gentamcin or vancomycin resistance) is mostly found in nosocomial (postoperative or tertiary) peritonitis. In Vancomycin-resistant Enterococcus (VRE), treatment with linezolid (monomicrobial infection) or tigecycline (polymicrobial infection) is appropriate (Recommendation 1 B).

Statement 32

The presence of Candida spp. in the peritoneal samples is a factor of poor prognosis (Recommendation 1C).

Statement 33

Two situations justify an empirical antifungal therapy: patients with septic shock in community-acquired infections or patients with post-operative infections (Recommendation 2 C).

Statement 34

In the setting of uncomplicated acute cholecystitis and acute appendicitis post-operative antimicrobial therapy is not necessary (Recommendation 1A).

Statement 35

In patients with IAIs, when patients are not severely ill and when source control is complete, a short course (3–5 days) of post-operative therapy is suggested (Recommendation 1A).

Statement 36

In patients with ongoing or persistent IAIs, the decision to continue, revise, or stop antimicrobial therapy should be made on the basis of clinician judgment and laboratory information (Recommendation 1 A).

Statement 37

Multifaceted interventions are more likely to improve antibiotic prescribing practices than simple, passive interventions. Didactic educational programs alone are generally ineffective.

(Recommendation 1B).

Statement 38

As a single intervention, implementation of locally adapted, interdisciplinary evidence based guidelines that incorporate risk stratification (severity and CA-IAIs versus HA-IAIs) and local resistance data most consistently improves components of AB prescribing for IAI (Recommendation 1 B).

Statement 39

Computer-assisted order entry, non-physician health care provider facilitation, and therapeutic drug monitoring can improve components of antibiotic prescribing practices, if resources are available (Recommendation 2 B).

Critically ill patients

Statement 40

The lack of source control and antibiotic adequacy are the only modifiable risk factors for mortality in patients with cIAIs admitted to the ICU. Organ dysfunction is associated with worse outcomes (Recommendation 1 B).

Statement 41

If the patient is critically ill the treatment duration can be deferred until after a multi-disciplinary careful evaluation (Recommendation 1B).

Statement 42

Principal determinants of antibiotic choice in critically ill patients are based on three parameters: 1) Severity of illness, 2) local ecology, and 3) risk factors of the host. Previous antibiotic use is associated with a higher development of multidrug resistant organisms (MDROs). Broad-spectrum antibiotic therapy, including combination of different antibiotic classes should be recommended in patients with septic shock, settings with high rates of MDRO, and previous antibiotic administration (Recommendation 1B).

Statement 43

Early identification of sepsis and prompt administration of intravenous fluids and vasopressors are always mandatory. Restoring a mean systemic arterial pressure of 65 to 70 mm Hg is a good initial goal during the hemodynamic support of patients with sepsis (Recommendation 1 A).

Statement 44

Fluid overload should be avoided in patients with generalized peritonitis, (Recommendation 1C).

Statement 45

There is currently insufficient evidence supporting the use of any adjunctive therapy in patients with septic shock due to intra-abdominal infection (No Recommendation).

Statement 46

Inflammatory biomarkers require further controlled studies before their measurement guides clinical care of critically ill/injured patients (No recommendation).

Statement 47

Consideration should be given to draining ascites in the critically ill patient treated for peritonitis, especially if the ascites is associated with IAH (Recommendation 1C).

Abbreviations

CA-IAIs: Community-acquired intra-abdominal infections; HA-IAIs: Hospital-acquired intra-abdominal infections; HCAI: Healthcare-associated infection; IAIs: Intra-abdominal infections; MDROs: Multidrug-resistant organisms

Acknowledgements

Not applicable.

Funding

None.

Authors' contributions

MS wrote the first draft of the manuscript. All the authors reviewed the manuscript and approved the final draft.

Competing interests

All authors declare that they have no competing interests.

Author details

[1]Department of Surgery, Macerata Hospital, Macerata, Italy. [2]Department of Emergency Surgery, Maggiore Hospital, Parma, Italy. [3]Department of Surgery, College of Medicine and Health Sciences, UAE University, Al-Ain, United Arab Emirates. [4]General Surgery Department, Papa Giovanni XXIII Hospital, Bergamo, Italy. [5]Acute Care Surgery, The Queen's Medical Center, Honolulu, HI, USA. [6]Department of Surgery, Academic Medical Centre, Amsterdam, Netherlands. [7]Emergency Department, Trauma Center, Niguarda Hospital, Milan, Italy. [8]Department of Critical Care Medicine, Ghent University Hospital, Ghent, Belgium. [9]Department of Surgery, Maggiore Hospital, Bologna, Italy. [10]Department of General, Visceral, and Thoracic Surgery, Klinikum Peine, Academic Hospital of Medical University Hannover, Hannover, Germany. [11]Division of Trauma Surgery, Department of Surgery, School of Medical Sciences, University of Campinas, Campinas, Brazil. [12]Infectious Diseases Unit, Department of Medical and Surgical Sciences, Sant'Orsola Hospital, University of Bologna, Bologna, Italy. [13]Intensive Care Unit, University of Modena, Modena, Italy. [14]General and Upper GI Surgery, Queen Elizabeth Hospital, Birmingham, UK. [15]Department of Surgery, Assia Medical Group, Tel Aviv University Sackler School of Medicine, Tel Aviv, Israel. [16]Departments of Surgery, Critical Care Medicine, and the Regional Trauma Service, Foothills Medical Centre, Calgary, AB, Canada. [17]Department of Emergency Surgery, Mozyr City Hospital, Mozyr, Belarus. [18]Department of General Surgery, Division of Surgery, Rambam Health Care Campus, Haifa, Israel. [19]Department of Biomedical Sciences and Public Health, Unit of Hygiene, Preventive Medicine and Public Health, UNIVPM, Ancona, Italy. [20]Abdominal Center, University Hospital Meilahti, Helsinki, Finland. [21]Department of Surgery, University of Washington, Seattle, WA, USA. [22]Departments of Surgery and Anesthesiology, Division of Trauma and Surgical Critical Care, Vanderbilt University Medical Center, Nashville, TN, USA. [23]American Board of Surgery, Philadelphia, PA, USA. [24]Multidisciplinary Intensive Care Research Organization (MICRO), Wellcome Trust-HRB Clinical Research, Department of Clinical Medicine, Trinity Centre for Health Sciences, St James's University Hospital, Dublin, Ireland. [25]Department of Surgery, School of Medicine, Washington University in Saint Louis, St. Louis, MO, USA. [26]Département d'Anesthésie-Réanimation, CHU Bichat Claude-Bernard-HUPNVS, Assistance Publique-Hôpitaux de Paris, University Denis Diderot, Paris, France. [27]Department of Surgery, UPMC, University of Pittsburgh School of Medicine, Pittsburgh, PA, USA. [28]Emergency post-operative Department, Otavio De Freitas Hospital and Osvaldo Cruz Hospital Recife, Recife, Brazil. [29]General Surgery Department, Medical University, University Hospital St George, Plovdiv, Bulgaria. [30]Department of Surgery, Catholic University of Sacred Heart, Rome, Italy. [31]Department of Gastrointestinal Surgery, Stavanger University Hospital, Stavanger, Department of Clinical Medicine, University of Bergen, Bergen, Norway. [32]Letterkenny University Hospital and Donegal Clinical Research Academy, Letterkenny, Ireland. [33]1st Department of Surgery, Department of Abdominal, Thoracic Surgery and Traumatology, General University Hospital, Praha, Czech Republic. [34]Department of Intensive Care, Erasme Hospital, Université libre de Bruxelles, Brussels, Belgium. [35]Department of Surgery, University of Colorado, Denver, CO, USA.

References

1. Guyatt G, Gutterman D, Baumann MH, Addrizzo-Harris D, Hylek EM, Phillips B, et al. Grading strength of recommendations and quality of evidence in clinical guidelines: report from an American College of Chest Physicians task force. Chest. 2006;129:174–81.
2. Menichetti F, Sganga G. Definition and classification of intra-abdominal infections. J Chemother. 2009;21 Suppl 1:3–4.
3. Andersen BR, Kallehave FL, Andersen HK. Antibiotics versus placebo for prevention of postoperative infection after appendicectomy. Cochrane Database Syst Rev. 2005;3:CD001439.
4. Mazeh H, Mizrahi I, Dior U, Simanovsky N, Shapiro M, Freund HR, et al. Role of antibiotic therapy in mild acute calculus cholecystitis: a prospective randomized controlled trial. World J Surg. 2012;36:1750–9.
5. Regimbeau JM, Fuks D, Pautrat K, Mauvais F, Haccart V, Msika S, et al. Effect of postoperative antibiotic administration on postoperative infection following cholecystectomy for acute calculous cholecystitis: a randomized clinical trial. JAMA. 2014;312:145–54.
6. Sawyer RG, Claridge JA, Nathens AB, Rotstein OD, Duane TM, Evans HL, et al. Trial of short-course antimicrobial therapy for intraabdominal infection. N Engl J Med. 2015;372:1996–2005.

7. Blot S, De Waele JJ, Vogelaers D. Essentials for selecting antimicrobial therapy for intra-abdominal infections. Drugs. 2012;72:e17–32.
8. Gupta S, Kaushik R. Peritonitis—the Eastern experience. World J Emerg Surg. 2006;1:13.
9. Mishra SP, Tiwary SK, Mishra M, Gupta SK. An introduction of tertiary peritonitis. J Emerg Trauma Shock. 2014;7:121–3.
10. Reemst PH, van Goor H, Goris RJ. SIRS, MODS and tertiary peritonitis. Eur J Surg Suppl. 1996;576:47–8.
11. Lamme B, Mahler CW, van Ruler O, Gouma DJ, Reitsma JB, Boermeester MA. Clinical predictors of ongoing infection in secondary peritonitis: systematic review. World J Surg. 2006;30:2170–81.
12. Montravers P, Dufour G, Guglielminotti J, Desmard M, Muller C, Houissa H, et al. Dynamic changes of microbial flora and therapeutic consequences in persistent peritonitis. Crit Care. 2015;19:70.
13. Cardoso T, Almeida M, Friedman ND, Aragão I, Costa-Pereira A, Sarmento E, et al. Classification of healthcare-associated infection: a systematic review 10 years after the first proposal. BMC Med. 2014;12:40.
14. Seguin P, Fédun Y, Laviolle B, Nesseler N, Donnio PY, Mallédant Y. Risk factors for multidrug-resistant bacteria in patients with post-operative peritonitis requiring intensive care. J Antimicrob Chemother. 2010;65:342–6.
15. Augustin P, Kermarrec N, Muller-Serieys C, Lasocki S, Chosidow D, Marmuse JP, et al. Risk factors for multi drug resistant bacteria and optimization of empirical antibiotic therapy in postoperative peritonitis. Crit Care. 2010;14:R20.
16. Lee DS, Ryu JA, Chung CR, Yang J, Jeon K, Suh GY, et al. Risk factors for acquisition of multidrug-resistant bacteria in patients with anastomotic leakage after colorectal cancer surgery. Int J Colorectal Dis. 2015;30:497–504.
17. Esteban A, Frutos-Vivar F, Ferguson ND, Peñuelas O, Lorente JA, Gordo F, et al. Sepsis incidence and outcome: contrasting the intensive care unit with the hospital ward. Crit Care Med. 2007;35:1284–9.
18. Sartelli M, Abu-Zidan FM, Catena F, Griffiths EA, Di Saverio S, Coimbra R, et al. Global validation of the WSES Sepsis Severity Score for patients with complicated intraabdominal infections: a prospective multicenter study (WISS Study). World J Emerg Surg. 2015;10:61.
19. Singer M, Deutschman CS, Seymour CW, Shankar-Hari M, Annane D, Bauer M, et al. The Third International Consensus Definitions for Sepsis and Septic Shock (Sepsis-3). JAMA. 2016;315:801–10.
20. Bone RC, Balk RA, Cerra FB, Dellinger RP, Fein AM, Knaus WA, et al. Definitions for sepsis and organ failure and guidelines for the use of innovative therapies in sepsis. The ACCP/SCCM Consensus Conference Committee. American College of Chest Physicians/Society of Critical Care Medicine. Chest. 1992;101:1644–55.
21. Levy MM, Fink MP, Marshall JC, Abraham E, Angus D, Cook D, et al. 2001 SCCM/ESICM/ACCP/ATS/SIS International Sepsis Definitions Conference. Crit Care Med. 2003;31:1250–6.
22. Solomkin JS, Mazuski JE, Bradley JS, Rodvold KA, Goldstein EJ, Baron EJ, et al. Diagnosis and management of complicated intra-abdominal infection in adults and children: guidelines by the Surgical Infection Society and the Infectious Diseases Society of America. Surg Infect (Larchmt). 2010;11:79–109.
23. Montravers P, Dupont H, Leone M, Constantin JM, Mertes PM, Société française d'anesthésie et de réanimation (Sfar), et al. Guidelines for management of intra-abdominal infections. Anaesth Crit Care Pain Med. 2015;34:117–30.
24. Sandell E, Berg M, Sandblom G, Sundman J, Fränneby U, Boström L, et al. Surgical decision-making in acute appendicitis. BMC Surg. 2015;15:69.
25. Wagner JM, McKinney WP, Carpenter JL. Does this patient have appendicitis? JAMA. 1996;276:1589–94.
26. Doria AS, Moineddin R, Kellenberger CJ, Epelman M, Beyene J, Schuh S, et al. US or CT for diagnosis of appendicitis in children and adults? A meta-analysis Radiology. 2006;241:83–94.
27. Laméris W, van Randen A, van Es HW, van Heesewijk JP, van Ramshorst B, Bouma WH, et al. Imaging strategies for detection of urgent conditions in patients with acute abdominal pain: diagnostic accuracy study. BMJ. 2009;338:b2431.
28. Carroll PJ, Gibson D, El-Faedy O, Dunne C, Coffey C, Hannigan A, et al. Surgeon-performed ultrasound at the bedside for the detection of appendicitis and gallstones: systematic review and meta-analysis. Am J Surg. 2013;205:102–8.
29. Toorenvliet BR, Wiersma F, Bakker RF, Merkus JW, Breslau PJ, Hamming JF. Routine ultrasound and limited computed tomography for the diagnosis of acute appendicitis. World J Surg. 2010;34:2278–85.
30. Andeweg CS, Wegdam JA, Groenewoud J, van der Wilt GJ, van Goor H, Bleichrodt RP. Toward an evidence-based step-up approach in diagnosing diverticulitis. Scand J Gastroenterol. 2014;49:775–84.
31. Shah BR, Stewart J, Jeffrey RB, Olcott EW. Value of short-interval computed tomography when sonography fails to visualize the appendix and shows otherwise normal findings. J Ultrasound Med. 2014;33:1589–95.
32. Koo HS, Kim HC, Yang DM, Kim SW, Park SJ, Ryu JK. Does computed tomography have any additional value after sonography in patients with suspected acute appendicitis? J Ultrasound Med. 2013;32:1397–403.
33. Burke LM, Bashir MR, Miller FH, Siegelman ES, Brown M, Alobaidy M, et al. Magnetic resonance imaging of acute appendicitis in pregnancy: a 5-year multiinstitutional study. Am J Obstet Gynecol. 2015;213:693.e1–6.
34. Duke E, Kalb B, Arif-Tiwari H, Daye ZJ, Gilbertson-Dahdal D, Keim SM, et al. A systematic review and meta-analysis of diagnostic performance of MRI for evaluation of acute appendicitis. AJR Am J Roentgenol. 2016;206:508–17.
35. Stefanidis D, Richardson WS, Chang L, Earle DB, Fanelli RD. The role of diagnostic laparoscopy for acute abdominal conditions: an evidence-based review. Surg Endosc. 2009;23:16–23.
36. Golash V, Willson PD. Early laparoscopy as a routine procedure in the management of acute abdominal pain: a review of 1,320 patients. Surg Endosc. 2005;19:882–5.
37. Gaitán HG, Reveiz L, Farquhar C, Elias VM. Laparoscopy for the management of acute lower abdominal pain in women of childbearing age. Cochrane Database Syst Rev. 2014;5:CD007683.
38. Shirah GR, O'Neill PJ. Intra-abdominal infections. Surg Clin North Am. 2014; 94:1319–33.
39. Desserud KF, Veen T, Soreide K. Emergency general surgery in the geriatric patient. Br J Surg. 2016;103:e52–61.
40. Aunan JR, Watson MM, Hagland HR, Søreide K. Molecular and biological hallmarks of ageing. Br J Surg. 2016;103:e29–46.
41. Clegg A, Young J, Iliffe S, Rikkert MO, Rockwood K. Frailty in elderly people. Lancet. 2013;381:752–62.
42. Robinson TN, Walston JD, Brummel NE, Deiner S, Brown 4th CH, Kennedy M, et al. Frailty for surgeons: review of a National Institute on aging conference on frailty for specialists. J Am Coll Surg. 2015;221:1083–92.
43. Kenig J, Zychiewicz B, Olszewska U, Barczynski M, Nowak W. Six screening instruments for frailty in older patients qualified for emergency abdominal surgery. Arch Gerontol Geriatr. 2015;61:437–42.
44. Joseph B, Zangbar B, Pandit V, Fain M, Mohler MJ, Kulvatunyou N, et al. Emergency general surgery in the elderly: too old or too frail? J Am Coll Surg. 2016;222:805–13.
45. Farhat JS, Velanovich V, Falvo AJ, Horst HM, Swartz A, Patton Jr JH, et al. Are the frail destined to fail? Frailty Index as predictor of surgical morbidity and mortality in the elderly. J Trauma Acute Care Surg. 2012;72:1526–30.
46. Orouji Jokar T, Ibraheem K, Rhee P, Kulavatunyou N, Haider A, Phelan HA, et al. Emergency general surgery specific frailty index: a validation study. J Trauma Acute Care Surg. 2016;81:254–60.
47. Torres VB, Azevedo LC, Silva UV, Caruso P, Torelly AP, Silva E, et al. Sepsis-associated outcomes in critically ill patients with malignancies. Ann Am Thorac Soc. 2015;12:1185–92.
48. Kristjansson SR, Farinella E, Gaskell S, Audisio RA. Surgical risk and post-operative complications in older unfit cancer patients. Cancer Treat Rev. 2009;35:499–502.
49. Thorsen K, Soreide JA, Soreide K. What is the best predictor of mortality in perforated peptic ulcer disease? A population-based, multivariable regression analysis including three clinical scoring systems. J Gastrointest Surg. 2014;18:1261–8.
50. Boermeester MA, Humes DJ, Velmahos GC, Søreide K. Contemporary review of risk-stratified management in acute uncomplicated and complicated diverticulitis. World J Surg. 2016;40:2537–45.
51. Neri A, Marrelli D, Scheiterle M, Di Mare G, Sforza S, Roviello F. Re-evaluation of Mannheim prognostic index in perforative peritonitis: prognostic role of advanced age. A prospective cohort study. Int J Surg. 2015;13:54–9.
52. Thorsen K, Soreide JA, Soreide K. Scoring systems for outcome prediction in patients with perforated peptic ulcer. Scand J Trauma Resusc Emerg Med. 2013;21:25.
53. Finlayson E, Wang L, Landefeld CS, Dudley RA. Major abdominal surgery in nursing home residents: a national study. Ann Surg. 2011;254:921–6.

54. Al-Temimi MH, Griffee M, Enniss TM, Preston R, Vargo D, Overton S, et al. When is death inevitable after emergency laparotomy? Analysis of the American College of Surgeons National Surgical Quality Improvement Program database. J Am Coll Surg. 2012;215:503–11.
55. Soreide K, Desserud KF. Emergency surgery in the elderly: the balance between function, frailty, fatality and futility. Scand J Trauma Resusc Emerg Med. 2015;23:10.
56. Das K, Ozdogan M, Karateke F, Uzun AS, Sozen S, Ozdas S. Comparison of APACHE II, P-POSSUM and SAPS II scoring systems in patients underwent planned laparotomies due to secondary peritonitis. Ann Ital Chir. 2014;85:16–21.
57. Vincent JL, Moreno R, Takala J, Willatts S, De Mendonça A, Bruining H, et al. The SOFA (Sepsis-related Organ Failure Assessment) score to describe organ dysfunction/failure. On behalf of the Working Group on Sepsis-Related Problems of the European Society of Intensive Care Medicine. Intensive Care Med. 1996;22:707–10.
58. Vincent JL, de Mendonça A, Cantraine F, Moreno R, Takala J, Suter PM, et al. Use of the SOFA score to assess the incidence of organ dysfunction/failure in intensive care units: results of a multicenter, prospective study. Working group on "sepsis-related problems" of the European Society of Intensive Care Medicine. Crit Care Med. 1998;26:1793–800.
59. Biondo S, Ramos E, Fraccalvieri D, Kreisler E, Ragué JM, Jaurrieta E. Comparative study of left colonic Peritonitis Severity Score and Mannheim Peritonitis Index. Br J Surg. 2006;93:616–22.
60. Rix TE, Bates T. Pre-operative risk scores for the prediction of outcome in elderly people who require emergency surgery. World J Emerg Surg. 2007;2:16.
61. Møller MH, Engebjerg MC, Adamsen S, Bendix J, Thomsen RW. The Peptic Ulcer Perforation (PULP) score: a predictor of mortality following peptic ulcer perforation. A cohort study. Acta Anaesthesiol Scand. 2012;56:655–62.
62. Kologlu M, Elker D, Altun H, Sayek I. Validation of MPI and PIA II in two different groups of patients with secondary peritonitis. Hepatogastroenterology. 2001;48:147–51.
63. Billing A, Fröhlich D, Schildberg FW. Prediction of outcome using the Mannheim peritonitis index in 2003 patients. Br J Surg. 1994;81:209–13.
64. Billing A, Fröhlich D, Mialkowskyj O, Stokstad P, Schildberg FW. Treatment of peritonitis with staged lavage: prognostic criteria and course of treatment. Langenbecks Arch Chir. 1992;377:305–13.
65. Wacha H, Hau T, Dittmer R, Ohmann C. Risk factors associated with intraabdominal infections: a prospective multicenter study. Peritonitis Study Group. Langenbecks Arch Surg. 1999;384:24–32.
66. Schneider CP, Seyboth C, Vilsmaier M, Küchenhoff H, Hofner B, Jauch KW, et al. Prognostic factors in critically ill patients suffering from secondary peritonitis: a retrospective, observational, survival time analysis. World J Surg. 2009;33:34–43.
67. Tellor B, Skrupky LP, Symons W, High E, Micek ST, Mazuski JE. Inadequate source control and inappropriate antibiotics are key determinants of mortality in patients with intra-abdominal sepsis and associated bacteremia. Surg Infect (Larchmt). 2015;16:785–93.
68. Grunau G, Heemken R, Hau T. Predictors of outcome in patients with postoperative intra-abdominal infection. Eur J Surg. 1996;162:619–25.
69. Mulier S, Penninckx F, Verwaest C, Filez L, Aerts R, Fieuws S, et al. Factors affecting mortality in generalized postoperative peritonitis: multivariate analysis in 96 patients. World J Surg. 2003;27:379–84.
70. De Waele JJ. Early source control in sepsis. Langenbecks Arch Surg. 2010; 395:489–94.
71. Rhodes A, Evans LE, Alhazzani W, Levy MM, Antonelli M, Ferrer R, et al. Surviving sepsis campaign: international guidelines for management of sepsis and septic shock: 2016. Intensive Care Med. 2017 Jan 18.
72. Sotto A, Lefrant JY, Fabbro-Peray P, Muller L, Tafuri J, Navarro F, et al. Evaluation of antimicrobial therapy management of 120 consecutive patients with secondary peritonitis. J Antimicrob Chemother. 2002;50:569–76.
73. Kim JJ, Liang MK, Subramanian A, Balentine CJ, Sansgiry S, Awad SS. Predictors of relaparotomy after nontrauma emergency general surgery with initial fascial closure. Am J Surg. 2011;202:549–52.
74. Betsch A, Wiskirchen J, Trübenbach J, Manncke KH, Belka C, Claussen CD, et al. CT-guided percutaneous drainage of intra-abdominal abscesses: APACHE III score stratification of 1-year results. Eur Radiol. 2002;12:2883–9.
75. Bufalari A, Giustozzi G, Moggi L. Postoperative intraabdominal abscesses: percutaneous versus surgical treatment. Acta Chir Belg. 1996;96:197–200.
76. Theisen J, Bartels H, Weiss W, Berger H, Stein HJ, Siewert JR. Current concepts of percutaneous abscess drainage in postoperative retention. J Gastrointest Surg. 2005;9:280–3.
77. Andersen JC, Bundgaard L, Elbrønd H, Laurberg S, Walker LR, Støvring J, Danish Surgical Society. Danish national guidelines for treatment of diverticular disease. Dan Med J. 2012;59:C4453.
78. Ambrosetti P, Chautems R, Soravia C, Peiris-Waser N, Terrier F. Long-term outcome of mesocolic and pelvic diverticular abscesses of the left colon: a prospective study of 73 cases. Dis Colon Rectum. 2005;48:787–91.
79. Brandt D, Gervaz P, Durmishi Y, Platon A, Morel P, Poletti PA. Percutaneous CT scan guided drainage versus antibiotherapy alone for Hinchey II diverticulitis: a case–control study. Dis Colon Rectum. 2006;49:1533–8.
80. Siewert B, Tye G, Kruskal J, Sosna J, Opelka F, Raptopoulos V, et al. Impact of CT-guided drainage in the treatment of diverticular abscesses: size matters. Am J Roentgenol. 2006;186:680–6.
81. Singh B, May K, Coltart I, Moore NR, Cunningham C. The long-term results of percutaneous drainage of diverticular abscess. Ann R Coll Surg Engl. 2008;90:297–301.
82. Dharmarajan S, Hunt SR, Birnbaum EH, Fleshman JW, Mutch MG. The efficacy of nonoperative management of acute complicated diverticulitis. Dis Colon Rectum. 2011;54:663–71.
83. Sallinen VJ, Mentula PJ, Leppäniemi AK. Nonoperative management of perforated diverticulitis with extraluminal air is safe and effective in selected patients. Dis Colon Rectum. 2014;57:875–81.
84. Sartelli M, Catena F, Ansaloni L, Coccolini F, Griffiths EA, Abu-Zidan FM, et al. WSES Guidelines for the management of acute left sided colonic diverticulitis in the emergency setting. World J Emerg Surg. 2016;11:37.
85. Sallinen V, Akl EA, You JJ, Agarwal A, Shoucair S, Vandvik PO, et al. Meta-analysis of antibiotics versus appendicectomy for non-perforated acute appendicitis. Br J Surg. 2016;103:656–67.
86. Oliak D, Yamini D, Udani VM, Lewis RJ, Arnell T, Vargas H, et al. Initial nonoperative management for periappendiceal abscess. Dis Colon Rectum. 2001;44:936–41.
87. Brown CV, Abrishami M, Muller M, Velmahos GC. Appendiceal abscess: immediate operation or percutaneous drainage? Am Surg. 2003;69:829–32.
88. Kim JK, Ryoo S, Oh HK, Kim JS, Shin R, Choe EK, et al. Management of appendicitis presenting with abscess or mass. J Korean Soc Coloproctol. 2010;26:413–9.
89. Simillis C, Symeonides P, Shorthouse AJ, Tekkis PP. A meta-analysis comparing conservative treatment versus acute appendectomy for complicated appendicitis (abscess or phlegmon). Surgery. 2010;147:818–29.
90. Cao F, Li J, Li A, Fang Y, Wang YJ, Li F. Nonoperative management for perforated peptic ulcer: who can benefit? Asian J Surg. 2014;37:148–53.
91. Crofts TJ, Park KG, Steele RJ, Chung SS, Li AK. A randomized trial of nonoperative treatment for perforated peptic ulcer. N Engl J Med. 1989;320:970–3.
92. Marshall C, Ramaswamy P, Bergin FG, Rosenberg IL, Leaper DJ. Evaluation of a protocol for the non-operative management of perforated peptic ulcer. Br J Surg. 1999;86:131–4.
93. Gul YA, Shine MF, Lennon F. Non-operative management of perforated duodenal ulcer. Ir J Med Sci. 1999;168:254–6.
94. Sartelli M, Viale P, Catena F, Ansaloni L, Moore E, Malangoni M, et al. 2013 WSES guidelines for management of intra-abdominal infections. World J Emerg Surg. 2013;8:3.
95. Coccolini F, Tranà C, Sartelli M, Catena F, Di Saverio S, Manfredi R, et al. Laparoscopic management of intra-abdominal infections: systematic review of the literature. World J Gastrointest Surg. 2015;7:160–9.
96. Di Saverio S, Birindelli A, Kelly MD, Catena F, Weber DG, Sartelli M, et al. WSES Jerusalem guidelines for diagnosis and treatment of acute appendicitis. World J Emerg Surg. 2016;11:34.
97. Sauerland S, Jaschinski T, Neugebauer EA. Laparoscopic versus open surgery for suspected appendicitis. Cochrane Database Syst Rev. 2010;10:CD001546.
98. Wilasrusmee C, Sukrat B, McEvoy M, Attia J, Thakkinstian A. Systematic review and meta-analysis of safety of laparoscopic versus open appendicectomy for suspected appendicitis in pregnancy. Br J Surg. 2012;99:1470–8.
99. Cheng HT, Wang YC, Lo HC, Su LT, Soh KS, Tzeng CW, et al. Laparoscopic appendectomy versus open appendectomy in pregnancy: a population-

based analysis of maternal outcome. Surg Endosc. 2015;29:1394–9.
100. Sanabria A, Villegas MI, Morales Uribe CH. Laparoscopic repair for perforated peptic ulcer disease. Cochrane Database Syst Rev. 2013;2:CD004778.
101. Ansaloni L, Pisano M, Coccolini F, Peitzmann AB, Fingerhut A, Catena F, et al. 2016 WSES guidelines on acute calculous cholecystitis. World J Emerg Surg. 2016;11:25.
102. Kiviluoto T, Sirén J, Luukkonen P, Kivilaakso E. Randomised trial of laparoscopic versus open cholecystectomy for acute and gangrenous cholecystitis. Lancet. 1998;351:321–5.
103. Johansson M, Thune A, Nelvin L, Stiernstam M, Westman B, Lundell L. Randomized clinical trial of open versus laparoscopic cholecystectomy in the treatment of acute cholecystitis. Br J Surg. 2005;92:44–9.
104. Kum CK, Goh PMY, Isaac JR, Tekant Y, Ngoi SS. Laparoscopic cholecystectomy for acute cholecystitis. Br J Surg. 1994;81:1651–4.
105. Pessaux P, Regenet N, Tuech JJ, Rouge C, Bergamaschi R, Arnaud JP. Laparoscopic versus open cholecystectomy: a prospective comparative study in the elderly with acute cholecystitis. Surg Laparosc Endosc Percutan Tech. 2001;11:252–5.
106. Lujan JA, Parrilla P, Robles R, Marin P, Torralba JA, Garcia-Ayllon J. Laparoscopic cholecystectomy vs open cholecystectomy in the treatment of acute cholecystitis: a prospective study. Arch Surg. 1998;133:173–5.
107. Coccolini F, Catena F, Pisano M, Gheza F, Fagiuoli S, Di Saverio S, et al. Open versus laparoscopic cholecystectomy in acute cholecystitis. Systematic review and meta-analysis. Int J Surg. 2015;18:196–204.
108. Angenete E, Thornell A, Burcharth J, Pommergaard HC, Skullman S, Bisgaard T, et al. Laparoscopic lavage is feasible and safe for the treatment of perforated diverticulitis with purulent peritonitis: the first results from the randomized controlled trial DILALA. Ann Surg. 2016;263:117–22.
109. Schultz JK, Yaqub S, Wallon C, Blecic L, Forsmo HM, Folkesson J, et al. Laparoscopic lavage vs primary resection for acute perforated diverticulitis: the SCANDIV randomized clinical trial. JAMA. 2015;314:1364–75.
110. Vennix S, Musters GD, Mulder IM, Swank HA, Consten EC, Belgers EH, et al. Laparoscopic peritoneal lavage or sigmoidectòmy for perforated diverticulitis with purulent peritonitis: a multicentre, parallel-group, randomised, open-label trial. Lancet. 2015;386:1269–77.
111. Ceresoli M, Coccolini F, Montori G, Catena F, Sartelli M, Ansaloni L. Laparoscopic lavage versus resection in perforated diverticulitis with purulent peritonitis: a meta-analysis of randomized controlled trials. World J Emerg Surg. 2016;11:42.
112. Vennix S, Boersema GS, Buskens CJ, Menon AG, Tanis PJ, Lange JF, et al. Emergency laparoscopic sigmoidectomy for perforated diverticulitis with generalised peritonitis: a systematic review. Dig Surg. 2016;33:1–7.
113. Koperna T, Schulz F. Relaparotomy in peritonitis: prognosis and treatment of patients with persisting intraabdominal infection. World J Surg. 2000;24:32–7.
114. Van Ruler O, Lamme B, de Vos R, Obertop H, Reitsma JB, Boermeester MA. Decision making for relaparotomy in secondary peritonitis. Dig Surg. 2008;25:339–46.
115. Van Ruler O, Mahler CW, Boer KR, Reuland EA, Gooszen HG, Opmeer BC, et al. Comparison of on-demand vs planned relaparotomy strategy in patients with severe peritonitis: a randomized trial. JAMA. 2007;298:865–72.
116. Weber DG, Bendinelli C, Balogh ZJ. Damage control surgery for abdominal emergencies. Br J Surg. 2014;101:e109–18.
117. Stone HH, Strom PR, Mullins RJ. Management of the major coagulopathy with onset during laparotomy. Ann Surg. 1983;197:532–5.
118. Burch JM, Ortiz VB, Richardson RJ, Martin RR, Mattox KL, Jordan Jr GL. Abbreviated laparotomy and planned reoperation for critically injured patients. Ann Surg. 1992;215:476–83.
119. Sartelli M, Abu-Zidan FM, Ansaloni L, Bala M, Beltrán MA, Biffl WL, et al. The role of the open abdomen procedure in managing severe abdominal sepsis: WSES position paper. World J Emerg Surg. 2015;10:35.
120. Robledo FA, Luque-de-León E, Suárez R, Sánchez P, de-la-Fuente M, Vargas A, et al. Open versus closed management of the abdomen in the surgical treatment of severe secondary peritonitis: a randomized clinical trial. Surg Infect (Larchmt). 2007;8:63–72.
121. Kirkpatrick AW, Roberts DJ, De Waele J, Jaeschke R, Malbrain ML, De Keulenaer B, Pediatric Guidelines Sub-Committee for the World Society of the Abdominal Compartment Syndrome, et al. Intra-abdominal hypertension and the abdominal compartment syndrome: updated consensus definitions and clinical practice guidelines from the World Society of the Abdominal Compartment Syndrome. Intensive Care Med. 2013;39:1190–206.
122. Bleszynski MS, Chan T, Buczkowski AK. Open abdomen with negative pressure device vs primary abdominal closure for the management of surgical abdominal sepsis: a retrospective review. Am J Surg. 2016;211:926–32.
123. Demetriades D, Salim A. Management of the open abdomen. Surg Clin North Am. 2014;94:131–53.
124. Regner JL, Kobayashi L, Coimbra R. Surgical strategies for management of the open abdomen. World J Surg. 2012;36:497–510.
125. Godat L, Kobayashi L, Costantini T, Coimbra R. Abdominal damage control surgery and reconstruction: world society of emergency surgery position paper. World J Emerg Surg. 2013;8.
126. Atema JJ, Gans SL, Boermeester MA. Systematic review and meta-analysis of the open abdomen and temporary abdominal closure techniques in non-trauma patients. World J Surg. 2015;39:912–25.
127. Kirkpatrick AW, Roberts DJ, Faris PD, Ball CG, Kubes P, Tiruta C, et al. Active negative pressure peritoneal therapy after abbreviated laparotomy: the intraperitoneal vacuum randomized controlled trial. Ann Surg. 2015;262:38–46.
128. Montravers P, Augustin P, Grall N, Desmard M, Allou N, Marmuse JP, et al. Characteristics and outcomes of anti-infective de-escalation during health care-associated intra-abdominal infections. Crit Care. 2016;20:83.
129. Tabah A, Cotta MO, Garnacho-Montero J, Schouten J, Roberts JA, Lipman J, et al. A systematic review of the definitions, determinants, and clinical outcomes of antimicrobial de-escalation in the intensive care unit. Clin Infect Dis. 2016;62:1009–17.
130. Gladman MA, Knowles CH, Gladman LJ, Payne JG. Intra-operative culture in appendicitis: traditional practice challenged. Ann R Coll Surg Engl. 2004;86:196–201.
131. Davies HO, Alkhamesi NA, Dawson PM. Peritoneal fluid culture in appendicitis: review in changing times. Int J Surg. 2010;8:426–9.
132. Sartelli M, Weber DG, Ruppé E, Bassetti M, Wright BJ, Ansaloni L, et al. Antimicrobials: a global alliance for optimizing their rational use in intra-abdominal infections (AGORA). World J Emerg Surg. 2016;11:33.
133. Jeon HG, Ju HU, Kim GY, Jeong J, Kim MH, Jun JB. Bacteriology and changes in antibiotic susceptibility in adults with community-acquired perforated appendicitis. PLoS One. 2014;9:e111144.
134. Van Ruler O, Kiewiet JJ, Van Ketel RJ, Boermeester MA, Dutch Peritonitis Study Group. Initial microbial spectrum in severe secondary peritonitis and relevance for treatment. Eur J Clin Microbiol Infect Dis. 2012;31:671–82.
135. Al-Hasan MN, Eckel-Passow JE, Baddour LM. Impact of healthcare-associated acquisition on community-onset Gram-negative bloodstream infection: a population-based study. Eur J Clin Microbiol Infect Dis. 2012;31:1163–71.
136. Swenson BR, Metzger R, Hedrick TL, McElearney ST, Evans HL, Smith RL, et al. Choosing antibiotics for intra-abdominal infections: what do we mean by "high risk"? Surg Infect (Larchmt). 2009;10:29–39.
137. Chong YP, Bae IG, Lee SR, Chung JW, Jun JB, Choo EJ, et al. Clinical and economic consequences of failure of initial antibiotic therapy for patients with community-onset complicated intra-abdominal infections. PLoS One. 2015;10:e0119956.
138. Steinbach CL, Töpper C, Adam T, Kees MG. Spectrum adequacy of antibiotic regimens for secondary peritonitis: a retrospective analysis in intermediate and intensive care unit patients. Ann Clin Microbiol Antimicrob. 2015;14:48.
139. McDonald LC. Trends in antimicrobial resistance in health care-associated pathogens and effect on treatment. Clin Infect Dis. 2006;42 Suppl 2:S65–71.
140. Riché FC, Dray X, Laisné MJ, Matéo J, Raskine L, Sanson-Le Pors MJ, et al. Factors associated with septic shock and mortality in generalized peritonitis: comparison between community-acquired and postoperative peritonitis. Crit Care. 2009;13:R99.
141. Shani V, Muchtar E, Kariv G, Robenshtok E, Leibovici L. Systematic review and meta-analysis of the efficacy of appropriate empiric antibiotic therapy for sepsis. Antimicrob Agents Chemother. 2010;54:4851–63.
142. Ferrer R, Artigas A, Suarez D, Palencia E, Levy MM, Arenzana A, Edusepsis Study Group, et al. Effectiveness of treatments for severe sepsis: a prospective, multicenter, observational study. Am J Respir Crit Care Med. 2009;180:861–6.
143. Castellanos-Ortega A, Suberviola B, García-Astudillo LA, Holanda MS, Ortiz F, Llorca J, et al. Impact of the Surviving Sepsis Campaign protocols on hospital

length of stay and mortality in septic shock patients: results of a three-year follow-up quasi-experimental study. Crit Care Med. 2010;38:1036–43.
144. Puskarich MA, Trzeciak S, Shapiro NI, Arnold RC, Horton JM, Studnek JR, et al. Association between timing of antibiotic administration and mortality from septic shock in patients treated with a quantitative resuscitation protocol. Crit Care Med. 2011;39:2066–71.
145. Dellinger RP, Levy MM, Rhodes A, Annane D, Gerlach H, Opal SM, et al. Surviving Sepsis Campaign: international guidelines for management of severe sepsis and septic shock, 2012. Intensive Care Med. 2013;39:165–228.
146. de Ruiter J, Weel J, Manusama E, Kingma WP, Van der Voort PH. The epidemiology of intra-abdominal flora in critically ill patients with secondary and tertiary abdominal sepsis. Infection. 2009;37:522–7.
147. Taccone FS, Laterre PF, Dugernier T, Spapen H, Delattre I, Wittebole X, et al. Insufficient β-lactam concentrations in the early phase of severe sepsis and septic shock. Crit Care. 2010;14:R126.
148. Plachouras D, Karvanen M, Friberg LE, Papadomichelakis E, Antoniadou A, Tsangaris I, et al. Population pharmacokinetic analysis of colistin methanesulfonate and colistin after intravenous administration in critically ill patients with infections caused by gram-negative bacteria. Antimicrob Agents Chemother. 2009;53:3430–6.
149. Dulhunty JM, Roberts JA, Davis JS, Webb SA, Bellomo R, Gomersall C, et al. Continuous infusion of beta-lactam antibiotics in severe sepsis: a multicenter double-blind, randomized controlled trial. Clin Infect Dis. 2013;56:236–44.
150. Dulhunty JM, Roberts JA, Davis JS, Webb SA, Bellomo R, Gomersall C, et al. A multicenter randomized trial of continuous versus intermittent beta-lactam infusion in severe sepsis. Am J Respir Crit Care Med. 2015;192:1298–305.
151. Lodise Jr TP, Lomaestro B, Drusano GL. Piperacillin-tazobactam for Pseudomonas aeruginosa infection: clinical implications of an extended-infusion dosing strategy. Clin Infect Dis. 2007;44:357–63.
152. Lorente L, Jiménez A, Martín MM, Iribarren JL, Jiménez JJ, Mora ML. Clinical cure of ventilator-associated pneumonia treated with piperacillin/tazobactam administered by continuous or intermittent infusion. Int J Antimicrob Agents. 2009;33:464–8.
153. Freeman CD, Nicolau DP, Belliveau PP, Nightingale CH. Once-daily dosing of aminoglycosides: review and recommendations for clinical practice. J Antimicrob Chemother. 1997;39:677–86.
154. Schuts EC, Hulscher ME, Mouton JW, Verduin CM, Stuart JW, Overdiek HW, et al. Current evidence on hospital antimicrobial stewardship objectives: a systematic review and meta-analysis. Lancet Infect Dis. 2016;16:847–56.
155. Klevens RM, Morrison MA, Nadle J, Petit S, Gershman K, Ray S, et al. Invasive methicillin-resistant Staphylococcus aureus infections in the United States. JAMA. 2007;298:1763–71.
156. Buijk SL, Gyssens IC, Mouton JW, Van Vliet A, Verbrugh HA, Bruining HA. Pharmacokinetics of ceftazidime in serum and peritoneal exudate during continuous versus intermittent administration to patients with severe intra-abdominal infections. J Antimicrob Chemother. 2002;49:121–8.
157. Dahyot-Fizelier C, Lefeuvre S, Laksiri L, Marchand S, Sawchuk RJ, Couet W, et al. Kinetics of imipenem distribution into the peritoneal fluid of patients with severe peritonitis studied by microdialysis. Clin Pharmacokinet. 2010;49:323–34.
158. Karjagin J, Lefeuvre S, Oselin K, Kipper K, Marchand S, Tikkerberi A, et al. Pharmacokinetics of meropenem determined by microdialysis in the peritoneal fluid of patients with severe peritonitis associated with septic shock. Clin Pharmacol Ther. 2008;83:452–9.
159. Seguin P, Verdier MC, Chanavaz C, Engrand C, Laviolle B, Donnio PY, et al. Plasma and peritoneal concentration following continuous infusion of cefotaxime in patients with secondary peritonitis. J Antimicrob Chemother. 2009;63:564–7.
160. Ikawa K, Morikawa N, Hayato S, Ikeda K, Ohge H, Sueda T. Pharmacokinetic and pharmacodynamic profiling of cefepime in plasma and peritoneal fluid of abdominal surgery patients. Int J Antimicrob Agents. 2007;30:270–3.
161. Scheetz MH, Reddy P, Nicolau DP, Noskin GA, Postelnick MJ, Stosor V, et al. Peritoneal fluid penetration of tigecycline. Ann Pharmacother. 2006;40:2064–7.
162. Eckmann C, Solomkin J. Ceftolozane/tazobactam for the treatment of complicated intra-abdominal infections. Expert Opin Pharmacother. 2015;16:271–80.
163. Solomkin J, Hershberger E, Miller B, Popejoy M, Friedland I, Steenbergen J, et al. Ceftolozane/tazobactam plus metronidazole for complicated intra-abdominal infections in an era of multidrug resistance: results from a randomized, double-blind, phase 3 trial (ASPECT-cIAI). Clin Infect Dis. 2015;60:1462–71.
164. Mawal Y, Critchley IA, Riccobene TA, Talley AK. Ceftazidime-avibactam for the treatment of complicated urinary tract infections and complicated intra-abdominal infections. Expert Rev Clin Pharmacol. 2015;8:691–707.
165. Mazuski JE, Gasink LB, Armstrong J, Broadhurst H, Stone GG, Rank D, et al. Efficacy and safety of ceftazidime-avibactam plus metronidazole versus meropenem in the treatment of complicated intra-abdominal infection–results from a randomized, controlled, double-blind, phase 3 program. Clin Infect Dis. 2016;62:1380–9.
166. Ortega M, Marco F, Soriano A, Almela M, Martínez JA, Muñoz A, et al. Analysis of 4758 Escherichia coli bacteraemia episodes: predictive factors for isolation of an antibiotic-resistant strain and their impact on the outcome. J Antimicrob Chemother. 2009;63:568–74.
167. Goldstein EJ, Solomkin JS, Citron DM, Alder JD. Clinical efficacy and correlation of clinical outcomes with in vitro susceptibility for anaerobic bacteria in patients with complicated intra-abdominal infections treated with moxifloxacin. Clin Infect Dis. 2011;53:1074–80.
168. Chen CW, Ming CC, Ma CJ, Shan YS, Yeh YS, Wang JY. Prospective, randomized, study of ampicillin-sulbactam versus moxifloxacin monotherapy for the treatment of community-acquired complicated intra-abdominal infections. Surg Infect (Larchmt). 2013;14:389–96.
169. Sartelli M, Catena F, Ansaloni L, Coccolini F, Corbella D, Moore EE, et al. Complicated intra-abdominal infections worldwide: the definitive data of the CIAOW study. World J Emerg Surg. 2014;9:37.
170. Zalacain M, Biedenbach DJ, Badal RE, Young K, Motyl M, Sahm DF. Pathogen prevalence and antimicrobial susceptibility among enterobacteriaceae causing hospital-associated intra-abdominal infections in adults in the United States (2012–2013). Clin Ther. 2016;38:1510–21.
171. Ben-Ami R, Rodriguez-Bano J, Arsian H, Pitout JD, Quentin C, Calbo ES, et al. A multinational survey of risk factors for infection with extended-spectrum β-lactamase-producing Enterobacteriaceae in non-hospitalized patients. Clin Infect Dis. 2009;49:682–90.
172. Morrissey I, Hackel M, Badal R, Bouchillon S, Hawser S, Biedenbach D. A review of ten years of the study for monitoring antimicrobial resistance trends (SMART) from 2002 to 2011. Pharmaceuticals (Basel). 2013;6:1335–46.
173. Patel N, Harrington S, Dihmess A, Woo B, Masoud R, Martis P, et al. Clinical epidemiology of carbapenem-intermediate or -resistant Enterobacteriaceae. J Antimicrob Chemother. 2011;66:1600–8.
174. Lepper PM, Grusa E, Reichl H, Högel J, Trautmann M. Consumption of imipenem correlates with beta-lactam resistance in Pseudomonas aeruginosa. Antimicrob Agents Chemother. 2002;46:2920–5.
175. Perez F, Bonomo RA. Can we really use ß-lactam/ß-lactam inhibitor combinations for the treatment of infections caused by extended-spectrum ß-lactamase-producing bacteria? Clin Infect Dis. 2012;54:175–7.
176. Gutiérrez-Gutiérrez B, Pérez-Galera S, Salamanca E, de Cueto M, Calbo E, Almirante B, et al. A multinational, preregistered cohort study of β-Lactam/β-lactamase inhibitor combinations for treatment of bloodstream infections due to extended-spectrum-β-lactamase-producing Enterobacteriaceae. Antimicrob Agents Chemother. 2016;60:4159–69.
177. Montravers P, Dupont H, Bedos JP, Bret P, Tigecycline Group. Tigecycline use in critically ill patients: a multicentre prospective observational study in the intensive care setting. Intensive Care Med. 2014;40:988–97.
178. Eckmann C, Montravers P, Bassetti M, Bodmann KF, Heizmann WR, Sánchez García M, et al. Efficacy of tigecycline for the treatment of complicated intra-abdominal infections in real-life clinical practice from five European observational studies. J Antimicrob Chemother. 2013;68 Suppl 2:ii25–35.
179. McGovern PC, Wible M, El-Tahtawy A, Biswas P, Meyer RD. All-cause mortality imbalance in the tigecycline phase 3 and 4 clinical trials. Int J Antimicrob Agents. 2013;41:463–7.
180. Falagas ME, Rafailidis PI. Re-emergence of colistin in today's world of multidrug-resistant organisms: personal perspectives. Expert Opin Investig Drugs. 2008;17:973–81.
181. Falagas ME, Kasiakou SK, Kofteridis DP, Roditakis G, Samonis G. Effectiveness and nephrotoxicity of intravenous colistin for treatment of patients with infections due to polymyxin-only-susceptible (POS) gram-negative bacteria. Eur J Clin Microbiol Infect Dis. 2006;25:596–9.
182. Ruiz J, Núñez ML, Pérez J, Simarro E, Martínez-Campos L, Gómez J. Evolution of resistance among clinical isolates of Acinetobacter over a 6-year period. Eur J Clin Microbiol Infect Dis. 1999;18:292–5.

183. Pontikis K, Karaiskos I, Bastani S, Dimopoulos G, Kalogirou M, Katsiari M, et al. Outcomes of critically ill intensive care unit patients treated with fosfomycin for infections due to pandrug-resistant and extensively drug-resistant carbapenemase-producing Gram-negative bacteria. Int J Antimicrob Agents. 2014;43:52–9.
184. Montravers P, Lepape A, Dubreuil L, Gauzit R, Pean Y, Benchimol D, et al. Clinical and microbiological profiles of community-acquired and nosocomial intra-abdominal infections: results of the French prospective, observational EBIIA study. J Antimicrob Chemother. 2009;63:785–94.
185. Sitges-Serra A, Lopez MJ, Girvent M, Almirall S, Sancho JJ. Postoperative enterococcal infection after treatment of complicated intra-abdominal sepsis. Br J Surg. 2002;89:361–7.
186. Burnett RJ, Haverstock DC, Dellinger EP, Reinhart HH, Bohnen JM, Rotstein OD, et al. Definition of the role of enterococcus in intraabdominal infection: analysis of a prospective randomized trial. Surgery. 1995;118:716–21.
187. Dupont H, Friggeri A, Touzeau J, Airapetian N, Tinturier F, Lobjoie E, et al. Enterococci increase the morbidity and mortality associated with severe intra-abdominal infections in elderly patients hospitalized in the intensive care unit. J Antimicrob Chemother. 2011;66:2379–85.
188. Kaffarnik MF, Urban M, Hopt UT, Utzolino S. Impact of enterococcus on immunocompetent and immunosuppressed patients with perforation of the small or large bowel. Technol Health Care. 2012;20:37–48.
189. Noskin GA. Vancomycin-resistant Enterococci: clinical, microbiologic, and epidemiologic features. J Lab Clin Med. 1997;130:14–20.
190. Birmingham MC, Rayner CR, Meagher AK, Flavin SM, Batts DH, Schentag JJ. Linezolid for the treatment of multidrug-resistant, gram-positive infections: experience from a compassionate-use program. Clin Infect Dis. 2003;36:159–68.
191. Knoke M. Gastrointestinal microecology of humans and Candida. Mycoses. 1999;42 Suppl 1:30–4.
192. Montravers P, Dupont H, Gauzit R, Veber B, Auboyer C, Blin P, et al. Candida as a risk factor for mortality in peritonitis. Crit Care Med. 2006;34:646–52.
193. Montravers P, Mira JP, Gangneux JP, Leroy O, Lortholary O, AmarCand study group. A multicentre study of antifungal strategies and outcome of Candida spp. peritonitis in intensive-care units. Clin Microbiol Infect. 2011;17:1061–7.
194. Dupont H, Paugam-Burtz C, Muller-Serieys C, Fierobe L, Chosidow D, Marmuse JP, et al. Predictive factors of mortality due to polymicrobial peritonitis with Candida isolation in peritoneal fluid in critically ill patients. Arch Surg. 2002;137:1341–6.
195. Bassetti M, Righi E, Ansaldi F, Merelli M, Scarparo C, Antonelli M, et al. A multicenter multinational study of abdominal candidiasis: epidemiology, outcomes and predictors of mortality. Intensive Care Med. 2015;41:1601–10.
196. Pappas PG, Rotstein CM, Betts RF, Nucci M, Talwar D, De Waele JJ, et al. Micafungin versus caspofungin for treatment of candidemia and other forms of invasive candidiasis. Clin Infect Dis. 2007;45:883–93.
197. Kuse ER, Chetchotisakd P, da Cunha CA, Ruhnke M, Barrios C, Raghunadharao D, et al. Micafungin versus liposomal amphotericin B for candidaemia and invasive candidosis: a phase III randomised double-blind trial. Lancet. 2007;369:1519–27.
198. Lortholary O, Renaudat C, Sitbon K, Madec Y, Denoeud-Ndam L, Wolff M, et al. Worrisome trends in incidence and mortality of candidemia in intensive care units (Paris area, 2002–2010). Intensive Care Med. 2014;40:1303–12.
199. Kollef M, Micek S, Hampton N, Doherty JA, Kumar A. Septic shock attributed to Candida infection: importance of empiric therapy and source control. Clin Infect Dis. 2012;54:1739–46.
200. Garey KW, Rege M, Pai MP, Mingo DE, Suda KJ, Turpin RS, et al. Time to initiation of fluconazole therapy impacts mortality in patients with candidemia: a multi-institutional study. Clin Infect Dis. 2006;43:25–31.
201. EUCAST Clinical breakpoints (Bacterial v 6.0 and Fungal v 8.0): http://www.eucast.org/clinical_breakpoints. Accessed 05 Feb 2017.
202. Pappas PG, Kauffman CA, Andes DR, Clancy CJ, Marr KA, Ostrosky-Zeichner L, et al. Executive summary: clinical practice guideline for the management of Candidiasis: 2016 update by the Infectious Diseases Society of America. Clin Infect Dis. 2016;62:409–17.
203. Blot S, De Waele JJ. Critical issues in the clinical management of complicated intra-abdominal infections. Drugs. 2005;65:1611–20.
204. Bailly S, Leroy O, Montravers P, Constantin JM, Dupont H, Guillemot D, et al. Antifungal de-escalation was not associated with adverse outcome in critically ill patients treated for invasive candidiasis: post hoc analyses of the AmarCAND2 study data. Intensive Care Med. 2015;41:1931–40.
205. Clyne B, Olshaker JS. The C-reactive protein. J Emerg Med. 1999;17:1019–25.
206. Sridharan P, Chamberlain RS. The efficacy of procalcitonin as a biomarker in the management of sepsis: slaying dragons or tilting at windmills? Surg Infect (Larchmt). 2013;14:489–511.
207. Prkno A, Wacker C, Brunkhorst FM, Schlattmann P. Procalcitonin-guided therapy in intensive care unit patients with severe sepsis and septic shock—a systematic review and meta-analysis. Crit Care. 2013;17:R291.
208. Carr JA. Procalcitonin-guided antibiotic therapy for septic patients in the surgical intensive care unit. J Intensive Care. 2015;3:36.
209. Jung B, Molinari N, Nasri M, Hajjej Z, Chanques G, Jean-Pierre H, et al. Procalcitonin biomarker kinetics fails to predict treatment response in perioperative abdominal infection with septic shock. Crit Care. 2013;17:R255.
210. Gross PA, Pujat D. Implementing practice guidelines for appropriate antimicrobial usage: a systematic review. Med Care. 2001;39:II55–69.
211. Davey P, Brown E, Charani E, Fenelon L, Gould IM, Holmes A, et al. Interventions to improve antibiotic prescribing practices for hospital inpatients. Cochrane Database Syst Rev. 2013;4:CD003543.
212. Dortch MJ, Fleming SB, Kauffmann RM, Dossett LA, Talbot TR, May AK. Infection reduction strategies including antibiotic stewardship protocols in surgical and trauma intensive care units are associated with reduced resistant gram-negative healthcare-associated infections. Surg Infect (Larchmt). 2011;12:15–25.
213. Dubrovskaya Y, Papadopoulos J, Scipione MR, Altshuler J, Phillips M, Mehta SA. Antibiotic stewardship for intra-abdominal infections: early impact on antimicrobial use and patient outcomes. Infect Control Hosp Epidemiol. 2012;33:427–9.
214. Popovski Z, Mercuri M, Main C, Sne N, Walsh K, Sung M, et al. Multifaceted intervention to optimize antibiotic use for intra-abdominal infections. J Antimicrob Chemother. 2015;70:1226–9.
215. Montravers P, Dupont H, Gauzit R, Veber B, Bedos JP, Lepape A, et al. Strategies of initiation and streamlining of antibiotic therapy in 41 French intensive care units. Crit Care. 2011;15:R17.
216. Leone M, Bourgoin A, Cambon S, Dubuc M, Albanèse J, Martin C. Empirical antimicrobial therapy of septic shock patients: adequacy and impact on the outcome. Crit Care Med. 2003;31:462–7.
217. Raymond DP, Pelletier SJ, Crabtree TD, Gleason TG, Hamm LL, Pruett TL, et al. Impact of a rotating empiric antibiotic schedule on infectious mortality in an intensive care unit. Crit Care Med. 2001;29:1101–8.
218. Barie PS, Hydo LJ, Shou J, Larone DH, Eachempati SR. Influence of antibiotic therapy on mortality of critical surgical illness caused or complicated by infection. Surg Infect (Larchmt). 2005;6:41–54.
219. Kullar R, Goff DA, Schulz LT, Fox BC, Rose WE. The "epic" challenge of optimizing antimicrobial stewardship: the role of electronic medical records and technology. Clin Infect Dis. 2013;57:1005–13.
220. Leibovici L, Gitelman V, Yehezkelli Y, Poznanski O, Milo G, Paul M, et al. Improving empirical antibiotic treatment: prospective, nonintervention testing of a decision support system. J Intern Med. 1997;242:395–400.
221. Paul M, Andreassen S, Tacconelli E, Nielsen AD, Almanasreh N, Frank U, et al. Improving empirical antibiotic treatment using TREAT, a computerized decision support system: cluster randomized trial. J Antimicrob Chemother. 2006;58:1238–45.
222. Pestotnik SL, Classen DC, Evans RS, Burke JP. Implementing antibiotic practice guidelines through computer-assisted decision support: clinical and financial outcomes. Ann Intern Med. 1996;124:884–90.
223. Halm EA, Atlas SJ, Borowsky LH, Benzer TI, Singer DE. Change in physician knowledge and attitudes after implementation of a pneumonia practice guideline. J Gen Intern Med. 1999;14:688–94.
224. Marrie TJ, Lau CY, Wheeler SL, Wong CJ, Vandervoort MK, Feagan BG. A controlled trial of a critical pathway for treatment of community-acquired pneumonia. CAPITAL Study Investigators. Community-Acquired Pneumonia Intervention Trial Assessing Levofloxacin. JAMA. 2000;283:749–55.
225. Weingarten SR, Riedinger MS, Hobson P, Noah MS, Johnson B, Giugliano G, et al. Evaluation of a pneumonia practice guideline in an interventional trial. Am J Respir Crit Care Med. 1996;153:1110–5.
226. De Waele J, Lipman J, Sakr Y, Marshall JC, Vanhems P, Barrera Groba C, et al. Abdominal infections in the intensive care unit: characteristics, treatment and determinants of outcome. BMC Infect Dis. 2014;14:420.
227. Barie PS, Hydo LJ, Shou J, Larone DH, Eachempati SR. Duration of hypotension before initiation of effective antimicrobial therapy is the critical determinant of

survival in human septic shock. Crit Care Med. 2006;34:1589–96.
228. Ferrer R, Martin-Loeches I, Phillips G, Osborn TM, Townsend S, Dellinger RP, et al. Empiric antibiotic treatment reduces mortality in severe sepsis and septic shock from the first hour: results from a guideline-based performance improvement program. Crit Care Med. 2014;42:1749–55.
229. Garnacho-Montero J, Escoresca-Ortega A, Fernández-Delgado E. Antibiotic de-escalation in the ICU: how is it best done? Curr Opin Infect Dis. 2015;28:193–8.
230. Garnacho-Montero J, Gutiérrez-Pizarraya A, Escoresca-Ortega A, Corcia-Palomo Y, Fernández-Delgado E, Herrera-Melero I, et al. De-escalation of empirical therapy is associated with lower mortality in patients with severe sepsis and septic shock. Intensive Care Med. 2014;40:32–40.
231. Leone M, Bechis C, Baumstarck K, Lefrant JY, Albanèse J, Jaber S, et al. De-escalation versus continuation of empirical antimicrobial treatment in severe sepsis: a multicenter non-blinded randomized noninferiority trial. Intensive Care Med. 2014;40:1399–408.
232. Kaki R, Elligsen M, Walker S, Simor A, Palmay L, Daneman N. Impact of antimicrobial stewardship in critical care: a systematic review. J Antimicrob Chemother. 2011;66:1223–30.
233. Martín-Loeches I, Diaz E, Vallés J. Risks for multidrug-resistant pathogens in the ICU. Curr Opin Crit Care. 2014;20:516–24.
234. Bassetti M, De Waele JJ, Eggimann P, Garnacho-Montero J, Kahlmeter G, Menichetti F, et al. Preventive and therapeutic strategies in critically ill patients with highly resistant bacteria. Intensive Care Med. 2015;41:776–95.
235. Vincent JL, Bassetti M, François B, Karam G, Chastre J, Torres A, et al. Advances in antibiotic therapy in the critically ill. Crit Care. 2016;20:133.
236. Vincent JL, De Backer D. Circulatory shock. N Engl J Med. 2013;369:1726–34.
237. Martin C, Papazian L, Perrin G, Saux P, Gouin F. Norepinephrine or dopamine for the treatment of hyperdynamic septic shock? Chest. 1993;103:1826–31.
238. De Backer D, Aldecoa C, Njimi H, Vincent JL. Dopamine versus norepinephrine in the treatment of septic shock: a meta-analysis. Crit Care Med. 2012;40:725–30.
239. Sartelli M, Catena F, Di Saverio S, Ansaloni L, Malangoni M, Moore EE, et al. Current concept of abdominal sepsis: WSES position paper. World J Emerg Surg. 2014;9:22.
240. Bailey J, Shapiro MJ. Abdominal compartment syndrome. Crit Care. 2000;4:23–9.
241. Kellum JA, Kong L, Fink MP, Weissfeld LA, Yealy DM, Pinsky MR, et al. Understanding the inflammatory cytokine response in pneumonia and sepsis: results of the Genetic and Inflammatory Markers of Sepsis (GenIMS) Study. Arch Intern Med. 2007;167:1655–63.
242. Gogos CA, Drosou E, Bassaris HP, Skoutelis A. Pro- versus anti-inflammatory cytokine profile in patients with severe sepsis: a marker for prognosis and future therapeutic options. J Infect Dis. 2000;181:176–80.
243. Peng Z, Pai P, Han-Min W, Jun Z, Hong-Bao L, Rong L, et al. Evaluation of the effects of pulse high-volume hemofiltration in patients with severe sepsis: a preliminary study. Int J Artif Organs. 2010;33:505–11.
244. Zhou F, Peng Z, Murugan R, Kellum JA. Blood purification and mortality in sepsis: a meta-analysis of randomized trials. Crit Care Med. 2013;41:2209–20.
245. Cruz DN, Perazella MA, Bellomo R, de Cal M, Polanco N, Corradi V, et al. Effectiveness of polymyxin B-immobilized fiber column in sepsis: a systematic review. Crit Care. 2007;11:R47.
246. Cruz DN, Antonelli M, Fumagalli R, Foltran F, Brienza N, Donati A, et al. Early use of polymyxin B hemoperfusion in abdominal septic shock: the EUPHAS randomized controlled trial. JAMA. 2009;301:2445–52.
247. Payen DM, Guilhot J, Launey Y, Lukaszewicz AC, Kaaki M, Veber B, et al. Early use of polymyxin B hemoperfusion in patients with septic shock due to peritonitis: a multicenter randomized control trial. Intensive Care Med. 2015;41:975–84.
248. Klein DJ, Foster D, Schorr CA, Kazempour K, Walker PM, Dellinger RP. The EUPHRATES trial (Evaluating the Use of Polymyxin B Hemoperfusion in a Randomized controlled trial of Adults Treated for Endotoxemia and Septic shock): study protocol for a randomized controlled trial. Trials. 2014;15:218.
249. Rodríguez A, Rello J, Neira J, Maskin B, Ceraso D, Vasta L, et al. Effects of high-dose of intravenous immunoglobulin and antibiotics on survival for severe sepsis undergoing surgery. Shock. 2005;23:298–304.
250. Alejandria MM, Lansang MA, Dans LF, 3rd Mantaring JB. Intravenous immunoglobulin for treating sepsis, severe sepsis and septic shock. Cochrane Database Syst Rev. 2013;9:CD001090.
251. Busani S, Damiani E, Cavazzuti I, Donati A, Girardis M. Intravenous immunoglobulin in septic shock: review of the mechanisms of action and meta-analysis of the clinical effectiveness. Minerva Anestesiol. 2016; 82:559–72.
252. Kreymann KG, de Heer G, Nierhaus A, Kluge S. Use of polyclonal immunoglobulins as adjunctive therapy for sepsis or septic shock. Crit Care Med. 2007;35:2677–85.
253. Xiao Z, Wilson C, Robertson HL, Roberts DJ, Ball CG, Jenne CN, et al. Inflammatory mediators in intra-abdominal sepsis or injury—a scoping review. Crit Care. 2015;19:373.
254. Schentag JJ, O'Keeffe D, Marmion M, Wels PB. C-reactive protein as an indicator of infection relapse in patients with abdominal sepsis. Arch Surg. 1984;119:300–4.
255. Almeida AB, Faria G, Moreira H, Pinto-de-Sousa J, Correia-da-Silva P, Maia JC. Elevated serum C-reactive protein as a predictive factor for anastomotic leakage in colorectal surgery. Int J Surg. 2012;10:87–91.
256. Witczak A, Juralowicz P, Modzelewski B, Gawlik M. C-reactive protein as a marker of postoperative septic complications. Pol Przegl Chir. 2012;84:93–8.
257. Scepanovic MS, Kovacevic B, Cijan V, Antic A, Petrovic Z, Asceric R, et al. C-reactive protein as an early predictor for anastomotic leakage in elective abdominal surgery. Tech coloproctol. 2013;17:541–7.
258. Kaufmann P, Tilz GP, Smolle KH, Demel U, Krejs GJ. Increased plasma concentrations of circulating intercellular adhesion molecule-1 (cICAM-1) in patients with necrotizing pancreatitis. Immunobiology. 1996;195:209–19.
259. Celik IH, Yilmaz Y, Erdeve O, Demirel G, Oguz SS, Uras N, et al. The acute-phase response in differentiating sepsis from inflammation in neonates who require abdominal surgery. Acta Chir Belg. 2012;112:292–6.
260. Tschaikowsky K, Hedwig-Geissing M, Braun GG, Radespiel-Troeger M. Predictive value of procalcitonin, interleukin-6, and C-reactive protein for survival in postoperative patients with severe sepsis. J Crit Care. 2011;26:54–64.
261. Mokart D, Merlin M, Sannini A, Brun JP, Delpero JR, Houvenaeghel G, et al. Procalcitonin, interleukin 6 and systemic inflammatory response syndrome (SIRS): early markers of postoperative sepsis after major surgery. Br J Anaesth. 2005;94:767–73.
262. Reith HB, Mittelkotter U, Wagner R, Thiede A. Procalcitonin (PCT) in patients with abdominal sepsis. Intensive Care Med. 2000;26 Suppl 2:S165–9.
263. Novotny AR, Emmanuel K, Hueser N, Knebel C, Kriner M, Ulm K, et al. Procalcitonin ratio indicates successful surgical treatment of abdominal sepsis. Surgery. 2009;145:20–6.
264. Bezmarevic M, Mirkovic D, Soldatovic I, Stamenkovic D, Mitrovic N, Perisic N, et al. Correlation between procalcitonin and intra-abdominal pressure and their role in prediction of the severity of acute pancreatitis. Pancreatology. 2012;12:337–43.
265. Barbić J, Ivić D, Alkhamis T, Drenjancević D, Ivić J, Harsanji-Drenjancević I, et al. Kinetics of changes in serum concentrations of procalcitonin, interleukin-6, and C- reactive protein after elective abdominal surgery. Can it be used to detect postoperative complications? Coll Antropol. 2013;37:195–201.
266. Ravishankaran P, Shah AM, Bhat R. Correlation of interleukin-6, serum lactate, and C-reactive protein to inflammation, complication, and outcome during the surgical course of patients with acute abdomen. J Interferon Cytokine Res. 2011;31:685–90.
267. Yamamoto T, Umegae S, Matsumoto K, Saniabadi AR. Peritoneal cytokines as early markers of peritonitis following surgery for colorectal carcinoma: a prospective study. Cytokine. 2011;53:239–42.
268. Steppan J, Hofer S, Funke B, Brenner T, Henrich M, Martin E, et al. Sepsis and major abdominal surgery lead to flaking of the endothelial glycocalix. J Surg Res. 2011;165:136–41.
269. Yamamoto T, Umegae S, Kitagawa T, Matsumoto K. Intraperitoneal cytokine productions and their relationship to peritoneal sepsis and systemic inflammatory markers in patients with inflammatory bowel disease. Dis Colon Rectum. 2005;48:1005–15.
270. Sarbinowski R, Arvidsson S, Tylman M, Oresland T, Bengtsson A. Plasma concentration of procalcitonin and systemic inflammatory response syndrome after colorectal surgery. Acta Anaesthesiol Scand. 2005;49:191–6.
271. Manganelli V, Signore M, Pacini I, Misasi R, Tellan G, Garofalo T, et al. Increased HMGB1 expression and release by mononuclear cells following surgical/anesthesia trauma. Crit Care. 2010;14:R197.
272. Albayrak Y, Albayrak A, Celik M, Gelincik I, Demiryilmaz I, Yildirim R, et al. High mobility group box protein-1 (HMGB-1) as a new diagnostic marker in patients

with acute appendicitis. Scand J Trauma Resusc Emerg Med. 2011;19:27.
273. Scheingraber S, Bauerfeind F, Bohme J, Dralle H. Limits of peritoneal cytokine measurements during abdominal lavage treatment for intraabdominal sepsis. Am J Surg. 2001;181:301–8.
274. Jansson K, Redler B, Truedsson L, Magnuson A, Matthiessen P, Andersson M, et al. Intraperitoneal cytokine response after major surgery: higher postoperative intraperitoneal versus systemic cytokine levels suggest the gastrointestinal tract as the major source of the postoperative inflammatory reaction. Am J Surg. 2004;187:372–7.
275. Hendriks T, Bleichrodt RP, Lomme RM, De Man BM, van Goor H, Buyne OR. Peritoneal cytokines predict mortality after surgical treatment of secondary peritonitis in the rat. J Am Coll Surg. 2010;211:263–70.
276. Holzheimer RG, Schein M, Wittmann DH. Inflammatory response in peritoneal exudate and plasma of patients undergoing planned relaparotomy for severe secondary peritonitis. Arch Surg. 1995;130:1314–9.
277. Fink MP, Delude RL. Epithelial barrier dysfunction: a unifying theme to explain the pathogenesis of multiple organ dysfunction at the celllular level. Crit Care Clin. 2005;21:177–96.
278. Mayberry JC, Welker KJ, Goldman RK, Mullins RJ. Mechanism of acute ascities formation after trauma resuscitation. Arch Surg. 2003;138:773–6.
279. Marshall JC, Vincent JL, Fink MP, Cook DJ, Rubenfeld G, Foster D, et al. Measures, markers, and mediators: toward a staging system for clinical sepsis. A report of the Fifth Toronto Sepsis Roundtable, Toronto, Ontario, Canada, October 25–26, 2000. Crit Care Med. 2003;31:1560–7.
280. Johnson D, Mayers I. Multiple organ dysfunction syndrome: a narrative review. Can J Anaesth. 2001;48:502–9.
281. Suliburk J, Helmer K, Moore F, Mercer D. The gut in systemic inflammatory response syndrome and sepsis. Enzyme systems fighting multiple organ failure. Eur Surg Res. 2008;40:184–9.
282. Deitch EA. Role of the gut lymphatic system in multiple organ failure. Curr Opin Crit Care. 2001;7:92–8.
283. Cavriani G, Domingos HV, Soares AL, Trezena AG, Ligeiro-Oliveira AP, Oliveira-Filho RM, et al. Lymphatic system as a path underlying the spread of lung and gut injury after intestinal ischemia/reperfusion in rats. Shock. 2005;23:330–6.
284. Latenser BA, Kowal-Vern A, Kimball D, Chakrin A, Dujovny N. A pilot study comparing percutaneous decompression with decompressive laparotomy for acute abdominal compartment syndrome in thermal injury. J Burn Care Rehabil. 2002;23:190–5.

18

Addition of lactic acid levels improves the accuracy of quick sequential organ failure assessment in predicting mortality in surgical patients with complicated intra-abdominal infections

Yun Tae Jung[1], Jiyeon Jeon[2], Jung Yun Park[1], Myung Jun Kim[1], Seung Hwan Lee[1] and Jae Gil Lee[1*]

Abstract

Background: The quick sequential organ failure assessment (qSOFA) alone has a poor sensitivity for predicting mortality in patients with complicated intra-abdominal infections, and plasma lactate levels have been shown to have a strong association with mortality in critically ill patients. Therefore, this study aimed to compare the performance of qSOFA with a score derived from a combination of qSOFA and serum lactate levels for predicting mortality in surgical patients with complicated intra-abdominal infections.

Methods: This retrospective study was performed at a university hospital. The medical records of 457 patients who presented to the emergency department (ED) between January 2008 and December 2016 and required emergency gastrointestinal surgery for a complicated intra-abdominal infection were reviewed retrospectively. qSOFA criteria, sequential organ failure assessment (SOFA) scores, and plasma lactate levels during their ED stay were collected. We performed area under receiver operating characteristic (AUROC) curve and sensitivity analysis to compare the performance of qSOFA alone with that of a score derived from the use of a combination of the qSOFA and lactate levels for predicting patient mortality.

Results: Fifty patients (10.9%) died during hospitalization. The combined qSOFA and lactate level score was superior to qSOFA alone (AUROC = 0.754 vs. 0.717, $p = 0.039$, respectively) and comparable to the full SOFA score (AUROC = 0.754 vs. 0.795, $p = 0.127$, respectively) in predicting mortality. Sensitivity and specificity of qSOFA alone were 46 and 86%, respectively, and those of the combined score were 72 and 73%, respectively ($p < 0.001$).

Conclusion: A score derived from the qSOFA and serum lactate levels had better predictive performance with higher sensitivity than the qSOFA alone in predicting mortality in patients with complicated intra-abdominal infections and had a comparable predictive performance to that of the full SOFA score.

Keywords: Retrospective studies, Lactate, Intra-abdominal infection, Mortality

* Correspondence: jakii@yuhs.ac
[1]Department of Surgery, Yonsei University College of Medicine, 50-1 Yonsei-ro, Seodaemun-gu, Seoul 03722, Republic of Korea
Full list of author information is available at the end of the article

Background

Sepsis has been a major cause of death for many decades in critically ill patients worldwide [1, 2]. Despite its high morbidity and mortality, there is no diagnostic gold standard test for sepsis. For the past decade, sepsis had been defined as a systemic inflammatory response syndrome (SIRS) by the host to an infection [3]. Owing to advances in our understanding of the pathophysiology of sepsis, a 2016 consensus conference redefined sepsis as "life-threatening organ dysfunction caused by a dysregulated host response to infection" [4].

Based on this new definition, sepsis is now diagnosed when a ≥ 2-point change occurs in the sequential organ failure assessment (SOFA) score because of an infection. However, due to the complex nature of the SOFA score, the 2016 task force introduced quick SOFA (qSOFA) for the rapid identification of patients at a high risk of mortality in the setting where all components of the SOFA score cannot be measured [4]. The qSOFA score includes (1) systolic blood pressure (SBP) ≤ 100 mmHg, (2) respiratory rate (RR) ≥ 22 breaths/min, and (3) an altered mental status (AMS). The total qSOFA score ranges from 0 to 3. Despite its simplicity, qSOFA showed better accuracy than SIRS criteria for predicting patient mortality in non-intensive care unit (ICU) settings in many studies [5–7]. However, others have questioned its utility as a quick screening tool due to its poor sensitivity [8–10].

Because of the limited sensitivity of qSOFA, we performed this study based on three assumptions. First, qSOFA alone has a poor sensitivity for predicting mortality in patients with complicated intra-abdominal infections. Second, plasma lactate levels have been shown to have a strong association with mortality in critically ill patients [11–13]. Therefore, the combination of the qSOFA score with a score based on lactate levels should have a better prognostic performance than qSOFA alone. Finally, the combination score should have a prognostic performance comparable to that of the full SOFA score. The aim of this study was to compare the performance of qSOFA with a combined score derived from qSOFA and serum lactate levels for predicting in-hospital mortality in surgical patients with complicated intra-abdominal infections.

Methods

Study population

We retrospectively reviewed the medical records of 1226 adult patients who underwent emergency gastrointestinal surgery for a complicated intra-abdominal infection from January 2008 to December 2016. Among this population, 511 patients were admitted via the emergency department (ED), but 51 of these patients did not have their plasma lactate level checked. Three patients with infection source inadequately controlled were also excluded because operations with inadequate source control usually end up with critical consequences regardless of their preoperative conditions. Excluding these 54 patients, 457 patients were finally included in the study.

Data collection

Components of the qSOFA and full SOFA scores during the patients' ED stay were collected from the electronic medical record (EMR). The qSOFA score included one point for each of the following: (1) systolic blood pressure ≤ 100 mmHg, (2) respiratory rate ≥ 22 breaths/min, and (3) altered mental status (AMS). The patient's baseline characteristics, initial laboratory values, operation-related data, and clinical outcomes were collected from the EMR. In our ED, the initial mental status of non-traumatic patients is recorded using the alert/verbal/painful/unresponsive (AVPU) responsiveness scale. Therefore, the AVPU scale was used instead of the Glasgow Coma Scale score when calculating the central nervous system component of the full SOFA score [14, 15].

One additional point was added to the patient's qSOFA score when their plasma lactate level was ≥ 2 mmol/L during their ED stay. This newly calculated combined score (qSOFA + lactate score) ranged from 0 to 4. Sensitivity analysis for each criterion was performed at a cutoff value of 2 for the qSOFA score, the qSOFA + lactate score, and the full SOFA score. Plasma lactate levels were included because they have been shown to be useful in predicting mortality in critically ill patients in numerous prior studies [11–13].

This study was approved by the Yonsei University Institutional Review Board (4-2017-0726), and informed consent was waived due to the retrospective design of the study.

Statistical analysis

A Student t test and the Mann-Whitney U test were performed for continuous variables, as appropriate, and presented as the mean ± standard deviation or median (interquartile range [IQR]). Categorical variables were presented as a frequency (%) and compared using the chi-square or Fisher's exact test, as appropriate. Sensitivity analysis, receiver operating characteristic (ROC) curve, and area under ROC curve (AUROC) with 95% confidence intervals (CI) were analyzed for each score. To compare sensitivities and specificities of each score, generalized estimating equations and the weighted least square method were used.

The findings were considered statistically significant when p values were less than 0.05. Statistical analysis was performed using SPSS® Statistics 23.0 (IBM Corp., Armonk, NY), SAS (version 9.4, SAS Inc., Cary, NC, USA), and R package (version 3.1.3, https://www.r-project.org/).

Results

Baseline characteristics

Of the 457 patients, 407 (89.1%) patients survived, and 50 (10.9%) patients died during hospitalization. Non-survivors had a higher average age (68.94 ± 15.27 vs. 62.11 ± 16.19 years, respectively; $p = 0.005$), ASA score ($p = 0.007$), and APACHE II score (28.26 ± 9.08 vs. 20.11 ± 7.86, respectively; $p < 0.001$) (Table 1).

Components of qSOFA, lactate level, and full SOFA score

A SBP ≤ 100 mmHg and a RR ≥ 22 breaths/min were observed in 39.4 and 26.7% of the patients, respectively. Only 3.3% of the patients showed an AMS. The non-survivor group had higher qSOFA, qSOFA + lactate, and full SOFA scores (Table 2).

Predictive performance of qSOFA alone

The SIRS had the lowest predictive performance among the criteria (AUROC = 0.672, 95% CI = 0.599–0.745), though it was better than that of a single plasma lactate level with a cutoff value of 2.0 mmol/L (AUROC = 0.659, 95% CI = 0.581–0.736). The qSOFA score showed a better predictive performance compared to SIRS criteria, but this difference was not statistically significant (AUROC = 0.717, 95% CI = 0.673–0.758 vs. AUROC = 0.672, 95% CI = 0.599–0.745; $p = 0.325$). Furthermore, qSOFA had the lowest sensitivity (46%), though it had the highest specificity (86%) (Table 3).

Predictive performance of the qSOFA + lactate score

When the qSOFA score was combined with one additional point for hyperlactatemia, its predictive performance was significantly improved compared to that seen with the qSOFA alone (AUROC = 0.754, 95% CI = 0.712–0.793 vs. AUROC = 0.717, 95% CI = 0.673–0.758 $p = 0.039$, respectively) (Fig. 1). The qSOFA + lactate score had a higher sensitivity [72% (60–85%) vs. 46% (32–60%), respectively] with little change in specificity [73% (68–77%) vs. 86% (83–90%), respectively] ($p < 0.001$) compared with that of the qSOFA score alone.

Table 1 Baseline characteristics of the study population ($n = 457$)

Variables	Total population	Survivors ($n = 407$)	Non-survivors ($n = 50$)	p value
Age, years	62.86 ± 16.22	62.11 ± 16.19	68.94 ± 15.27	0.005
Sex, n (%) male/female	280 (61.3)/177 (38.7)	253 (62.2)/154 (37.8)	27 (54.0)/23 (46.0)	0.264
Body weight, kg	58.36 ± 11.58	58.38 ± 11.32	58.23 ± 13.69	0.931
BMI, kg/m^2	21.90 ± 3.64	21.83 ± 3.54	22.47 ± 4.42	0.243
ASA score, n (%)				0.007
1	131 (28.7)	120 (29.5)	11 (22.0)	
2	124 (27.1)	114 (28.0)	10 (20.0)	
3	153 (33.5)	137 (33.7)	16 (32.0)	
4	45 (9.8)	34 (8.4)	11 (22.0)	
5	4 (0.9)	2 (0.5)	2 (4.0)	
APACHE II score	21.23 ± 8.50	20.11 ± 7.86	28.26 ± 9.08	< 0.001
Comorbidity, n (%)				
Hypertension	172 (37.6)	145 (35.6)	27 (54.0)	0.011
Diabetes	65 (14.2)	59 (14.5)	6 (12.0)	0.633
CRF	39 (8.5)	36 (8.8)	3 (6.0)	0.787
Malignancy	212 (46.4)	183 (45.0)	29 (58.0)	0.081
Diagnosis, n (%)				0.632
Perforation	382 (83.6)	338 (83.0)	44 (88.0)	
Strangulation	58 (12.7)	54 (13.3)	4 (8.0)	
Ischemia	17 (3.7)	15 (3.7)	2 (4.0)	
Site, n (%)				0.789
Stomach	111 (24.3)	100 (24.6)	11 (22.0)	
Small bowel	163 (35.7)	143 (35.1)	20 (40.0)	
Colorectal	183 (40.0)	164 (40.3)	19 (38.0)	
Laparoscopy/open, n (%)	71 (15.5)/386 (84.5)	69 (17.0)/338 (83.0)	2 (4.0)/48 (96.0)	0.013

BMI body mass index, *ASA* American Society of Anesthesiologists, *APACHE* acute physiology and chronic health evaluation, *CRF* chronic renal failure

Table 2 Distribution of qSOFA criteria, lactate levels, and qSOFA, qSOFA + lactate, and SOFA scores

Variable	Total population	Survivors ($n = 407$)	Non-survivors ($n = 50$)	p value
SBP ≤ 100, n (%)	180 (39.4)	144 (35.4)	36 (72.0)	< 0.001
RR ≥ 22, n (%)	122 (26.7)	98 (24.1)	24 (48.0)	< 0.001
AMS, n (%)	15 (3.3)	11 (2.7)	4 (8.0)	0.070
Lactate, mmol/L	1.7 [1.0–3.1]	1.6 [0.9–2.8]	3.3 [1.775–4.875]	< 0.001
Lactate ≥ 2.0 mmol/L, n (%)	200 (43.8)	164 (40.3)	36 (72.0)	< 0.001
qSOFA, n (%)				< 0.001
0	234 (51.2)	223 (54.8)	11 (22.0)	
1	145 (31.7)	129 (31.7)	16 (32.0)	
2	71 (15.5)	51 (12.5)	20 (40.0)	
3	7 (1.5)	4 (1.0)	3 (6.0)	
qSOFA + lactate score, n (%)				< 0.001
0	163 (35.7)	158 (38.8)	5 (10.0)	
1	147 (32.2)	138 (33.9)	9 (18.0)	
2	86 (18.8)	68 (16.7)	18 (36.0)	
3	54 (11.8)	39 (9.6)	15 (30.0)	
4	7 (1.5)	4 (1.0)	3 (6.0)	
Full SOFA	1 [0–4]	1 [0–3]	5 [3–8.25]	< 0.001

SBP systolic blood pressure, *RR* respiratory rate, *AMS* altered mental status, *qSOFA* quick sequential organ failure assessment, *SOFA* sequential organ failure assessment

Comparison of the qSOFA + lactate score with the full SOFA score

The qSOFA + lactate score had a predictive performance comparable to the full SOFA score (AUROC = 0.754, 95% CI = 0.712–0.793 vs. AUROC = 0.795, 95% CI = 0.755–0.831, respectively; $p = 0.127$) (Fig. 2) (Table 3). The full SOFA score had a higher sensitivity [82% (71–93%) vs. 72% (60–85%)], and a lower specificity [56% (51–61%) vs. 73% (68–77%)], compared to the qSOFA + lactate score, but these differences were not statistically significant ($p = 0.123$) (Table 3).

Discussion

Our study results showed that the qSOFA alone has a poor sensitivity and a modest predictive performance. There are rising concerns on the poor sensitivity of qSOFA, despite its high specificity, and potential delays in identification and resuscitation for patients at a high risk of mortality [16]. The addition of one point for hyperlactatemia (plasma lactate level > 2.0 mmol/L) resulted in improved sensitivity with a slightly decreased specificity. The addition of the use of serum lactate levels to the qSOFA improved the predictive performance significantly, increasing it to a level comparable to

Table 3 Predictive performance for each diagnosis or score

Variable	Sensitivity	Specificity	AUROC
Lactate, %	72 (58–83)	60 (55–64)	0.659 (0.581–0.736)
SIRS, %	98 (89–100)	23 (19–27)	0.672 (0.599–0.745)
qSOFA, %	46 (32–60)	86 (83–90)	0.717 (0.673–0.758)
qSOFA + lactate, %	72 (60–85)	73 (68–77)	0.754 (0.712–0.793)
Full SOFA, %	82 (71–93)	56 (51–61)	0.795 (0.755–0.831)

SIRS systemic inflammatory response syndrome, *qSOFA* quick sequential organ failure assessment, *SOFA* sequential organ failure assessment, *AUROC* area under the receiver operating characteristic curve

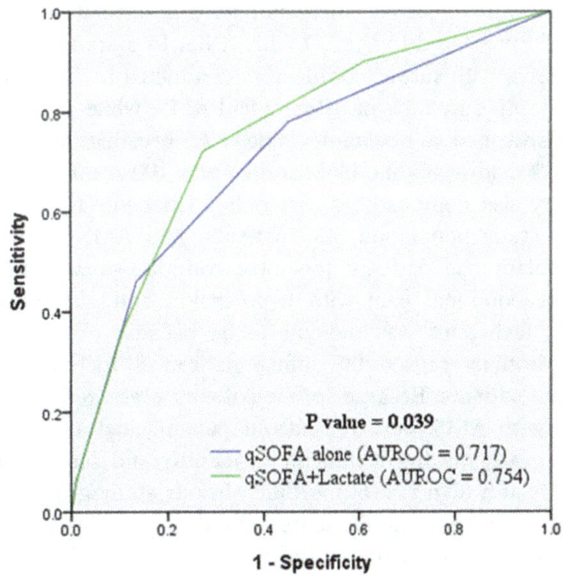

Fig. 1 Receiver operation characteristic curve for patient mortality using qSOFA alone and qSOFA + lactate score. The combined qSOFA and lactate level score has a higher AUROC than qSOFA alone (AUROC = 0.754 vs. 0.717, $p = 0.039$, respectively). AUROC = area under receiver operating curve, qSOFA = quick sequential organ failure assessment, SOFA = sequential organ failure assessment

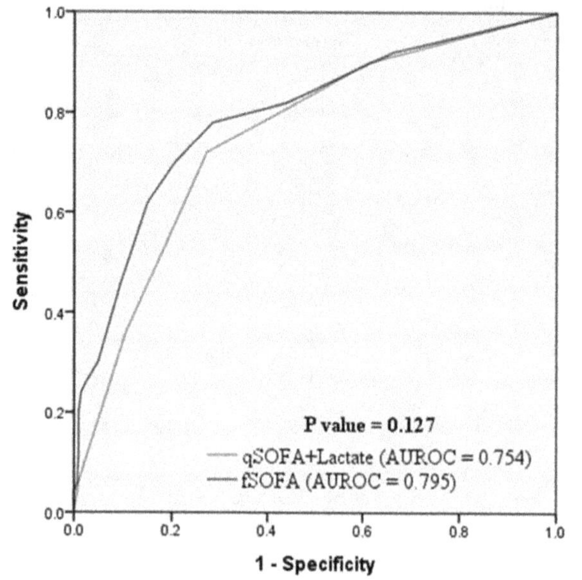

Fig. 2 Receiver operating characteristic curve for patient mortality using qSOFA + lactate and full SOFA scores. The combined qSOFA and lactate level score has a comparable AUROC with full SOFA score (AUROC = 0.754 vs. 0.795, $p = 0.127$, respectively). AUROC = area under receiver operating curve, qSOFA = quick sequential organ failure assessment, SOFA = sequential organ failure assessment

that of the full SOFA. The strengths of the qSOFA include its simplicity, rapidity, and ease of performance for all health care providers without requiring complicated equipment or laboratory results. However, after the qSOFA was introduced, we observed that surgical patients who required emergency gastrointestinal surgery rarely presented to the ED with AMS. In a study of ED patients with suspected infection conducted by Williams et al. [8], only 5.1% of patients had AMS, while 21.1% of patients had a respiratory rate ≥ 22 breaths/min, and 26.8% had a systolic blood pressure ≤ 100 mmHg. Our study also demonstrates that only 15 patients (3.3%) in our study population (457 patients) had AMS. In this population of patients, the most common presentation was abdominal pain with hypotension and tachypnea. The tachypnea was thought to be because of shallow respirations caused by diffuse peritoneal irritation in some patients. Because so few patients presented to the ED with AMS, only 17% of our patients had a qSOFA score ≥ 2, making it difficult to identify and screen patients at a high risk of mortality. In our study group, 27 patients with a qSOFA score < 2 did not survive. Other studies have emphasized the poor sensitivity of qSOFA as a screening test for sepsis [8, 9].

To improve the sensitivity of qSOFA, we analyzed several combination scores including qSOFA and diagnostic markers of inflammation, such as C-reactive protein, white blood cell count, delta neutrophil index, and plasma lactate concentration. As suggested in many studies, plasma lactate concentration is an important predictor of mortality in critically ill patients [11–13]. Plasma lactate concentration alone with a cutoff value of 2 mmol/L did not show a good predictive performance in our study, but when combined with qSOFA, it was the best predictor of in-hospital mortality in our study population.

The rapid point-of-care measurement and accuracy of plasma lactate levels is an important advantage [17]. Singer et al. reported that an early bedside point-of-care (POC) lactate evaluation in the ED was associated with the early administration of intravenous fluid resuscitation and improved mortality in patients with suspected sepsis [18]. The use of plasma lactate levels improves the discriminatory ability of qSOFA without complicating its use as a quick and simple screening method.

The association between full SOFA scores and patient mortality has been confirmed in previous studies [5, 19–21]. However, the calculation of the full SOFA score is time-consuming since many laboratory values and a significant amount of clinical information are needed. Therefore, the use of full SOFA scores is only suited for patients in an ICU environment. The use of the qSOFA + lactate score is a simple and rapid way to screen patients at high risk of mortality in pre-ICU, such as in the ED, or even in pre-hospital settings with a predictive performance comparable with that seen with the full SOFA score. The use of the qSOFA + lactate score will assist clinicians in immediately assessing the risk of mortality in patients with suspected intra-abdominal infection, allowing more rapid resuscitation and control of the infective source and reducing patient mortality.

Strengths and limitations of our study

A strength of this study is that it is the first to be performed solely in the surgical population. Early resuscitative therapy can be delivered to patients with intra-abdominal infection who have a high risk of mortality based on the results of a simple screening using qSOFA and a plasma lactate measurement. This could lead to an improved survival rate for patients who require emergency gastrointestinal surgery for a suspected intra-abdominal infection.

The present study has several limitations. First, surgical patients presenting to the ED are likely to get individualized treatment and do not always follow a tailored protocol. In a study performed by Rivers et al. in 2001 [22], patients requiring emergent surgery were excluded from the study protocol because they had a variety of different infections and had a different degree of urgency for surgical intervention. The diversity of patient characteristics and treatments in our study may have affected the outcome of our study. Second, our study is a retrospective study performed in a single center with a small study population. Due to the retrospective nature of the study, all of our patients had already undergone emergency gastrointestinal surgery. Prospective studies of patients presenting to the ED with suspected intra-abdominal infection, regardless of a consequent emergency gastrointestinal surgery, are needed to clarify the benefits of using the qSOFA + lactate score compared to qSOFA for predicting patient mortality.

Conclusions

The qSOFA score alone has poor sensitivity in screening surgical patients presenting to the ED with a high risk of mortality. Combining the qSOFA score with an additional one point for hyperlactatemia has a better predictive performance with higher sensitivity for patient mortality than that seen with qSOFA alone and comparable to that seen with full SOFA.

Abbreviations

AMS: Altered mental status; AUROC: Area under receiver operating characteristic curve; AVPU: Alert/verbal/painful/unresponsive; CI: Confidence interval; ED: Emergency department; EMR: Electronic medical record; ICU: Intensive care unit; IQR: Interquartile range; POC: Point-of-care; qSOFA: Quick sequential organ failure assessment; ROC: Receiver operating characteristic; RR: Respiratory rate; SBP: Systolic blood pressure; SIRS: Systemic inflammatory response syndrome; SOFA: Sequential organ failure assessment

Acknowledgements

The authors would like to thank HY Kim for assisting with the statistical analyses, and we thank all the coordinators for their valuable help and cooperation.

Funding

Not applicable

Authors' contributions

JGL designed the study. YTJ, JJ, JYP, MJK, and SHL were responsible for the data acquisition. YTJ analyzed and interpreted the data with JGL, JJ, JYP, MJK, and SHL. YTJ wrote the article. All authors read and approved the final manuscript.

Competing interests

The authors declare that they have no competing interests.

Author details

[1]Department of Surgery, Yonsei University College of Medicine, 50-1 Yonsei-ro, Seodaemun-gu, Seoul 03722, Republic of Korea. [2]Yonsei University College of Nursing, 50-1 Yonsei-ro, Seodaemun-gu, Seoul 03722, Republic of Korea.

References

1. Park DW, Chun BC, Kim JM, et al. Epidemiological and clinical characteristics of community-acquired severe sepsis and septic shock: a prospective observational study in 12 university hospitals in Korea. J Korean Med Sci. 2012;27:1308–14.
2. Martin GS, Mannino DM, Eaton S, et al. The epidemiology of sepsis in the United States from 1979 through 2000. N Engl J Med. 2003;348:1546–54.
3. Bone RC, Balk RA, Cerra FB, et al. Definitions for sepsis and organ failure and guidelines for the use of innovative therapies in sepsis. The ACCP/SCCM Consensus Conference Committee. American College of Chest Physicians/ Society of Critical Care Medicine. Chest. 1992;101:1644–55.
4. Singer M, Deutschman CS, Seymour CW, et al. The Third International Consensus Definitions for Sepsis and Septic Shock (Sepsis-3). JAMA. 2016;315:801–10.
5. Seymour CW, Liu VX, Iwashyna TJ, et al. Assessment of clinical criteria for sepsis: for the Third International Consensus Definitions for Sepsis and Septic Shock (Sepsis-3). JAMA. 2016;315:762–74.
6. Finkelsztein EJ, Jones DS, Ma KC, et al. Comparison of qSOFA and SIRS for predicting adverse outcomes of patients with suspicion of sepsis outside the intensive care unit. Crit Care. 2017;21:73.
7. Park HK, Kim WY, Kim MC, et al. Quick sequential organ failure assessment compared to systemic inflammatory response syndrome for predicting sepsis in emergency department. J Crit Care. 2017;42:12–7.
8. Williams JM, Greenslade JH, McKenzie JV, et al. Systemic inflammatory response syndrome, quick sequential organ function assessment, and organ dysfunction: insights from a prospective database of ED patients with infection. Chest. 2017;151:586–96.
9. Dorsett M, Kroll M, Smith CS, et al. qSOFA has poor sensitivity for prehospital identification of severe sepsis and septic shock. Prehosp Emerg Care. 2017;21(4):489–97.
10. Askim A, Moser F, Gustad LT, et al. Poor performance of quick-SOFA (qSOFA) score in predicting severe sepsis and mortality—a prospective study of patients admitted with infection to the emergency department. Scand J Trauma Resusc Emerg Med. 2017;25:56.
11. Bou Chebl R, El Khuri C, Shami A, et al. Serum lactate is an independent predictor of hospital mortality in critically ill patients in the emergency department: a retrospective study. Scand J Trauma Resusc Emerg Med. 2017;25:69.
12. Freire Jorge P, Wieringa N, de Felice E, et al. The association of early combined lactate and glucose levels with subsequent renal and liver dysfunction and hospital mortality in critically ill patients. Crit Care. 2017;21:218.
13. Lokhandwala S, Andersen LW, Nair S, et al. Absolute lactate value vs relative reduction as a predictor of mortality in severe sepsis and septic shock. J Crit Care. 2017;37:179–84.
14. Kelly CA, Upex A, Bateman DN. Comparison of consciousness level assessment in the poisoned patient using the alert/verbal/painful/ unresponsive scale and the Glasgow Coma Scale. Ann Emerg Med. 2004;44:108–13.
15. McNarry AF, Goldhill DR. Simple bedside assessment of level of consciousness: comparison of two simple assessment scales with the Glasgow Coma Scale. Anaesthesia. 2004;59:34–7.
16. Sartelli M, Kluger Y, Ansaloni L, et al. Raising concerns about the Sepsis-3 definitions. World J Emerg Surg. 2018;13:6.
17. Shapiro NI, Fisher C, Donnino M, et al. The feasibility and accuracy of point-of-care lactate measurement in emergency department patients with suspected infection. J Emerg Med. 2010;39:89–94.
18. Singer AJ, Taylor M, LeBlanc D, et al. ED bedside point-of-care lactate in patients with suspected sepsis is associated with reduced time to iv fluids and mortality. Am J Emerg Med. 2014;32:1120–4.
19. Vincent JL, de Mendonca A, Cantraine F, et al. Use of the SOFA score to assess the incidence of organ dysfunction/failure in intensive care units: results of a multicenter, prospective study. Working group on "sepsis-related problems" of the European Society of Intensive Care Medicine. Crit Care Med. 1998;26:1793–800.
20. Rivera-Fernandez R, Nap R, Vazquez-Mata G, et al. Analysis of physiologic alterations in intensive care unit patients and their relationship with mortality. J Crit Care. 2007;22:120–8.
21. Sakr Y, Vincent JL, Ruokonen E, et al. Sepsis and organ system failure are major determinants of post-intensive care unit mortality. J Crit Care. 2008;23:475–83.
22. Rivers E, Nguyen B, Havstad S, et al. Early goal-directed therapy in the treatment of severe sepsis and septic shock. N Engl J Med. 2001;345:1368–77.

Permissions

All chapters in this book were first published in WJES, by BioMed Central; hereby published with permission under the Creative Commons Attribution License or equivalent. Every chapter published in this book has been scrutinized by our experts. Their significance has been extensively debated. The topics covered herein carry significant findings which will fuel the growth of the discipline. They may even be implemented as practical applications or may be referred to as a beginning point for another development.

The contributors of this book come from diverse backgrounds, making this book a truly international effort. This book will bring forth new frontiers with its revolutionizing research information and detailed analysis of the nascent developments around the world.

We would like to thank all the contributing authors for lending their expertise to make the book truly unique. They have played a crucial role in the development of this book. Without their invaluable contributions this book wouldn't have been possible. They have made vital efforts to compile up to date information on the varied aspects of this subject to make this book a valuable addition to the collection of many professionals and students.

This book was conceptualized with the vision of imparting up-to-date information and advanced data in this field. To ensure the same, a matchless editorial board was set up. Every individual on the board went through rigorous rounds of assessment to prove their worth. After which they invested a large part of their time researching and compiling the most relevant data for our readers.

The editorial board has been involved in producing this book since its inception. They have spent rigorous hours researching and exploring the diverse topics which have resulted in the successful publishing of this book. They have passed on their knowledge of decades through this book. To expedite this challenging task, the publisher supported the team at every step. A small team of assistant editors was also appointed to further simplify the editing procedure and attain best results for the readers.

Apart from the editorial board, the designing team has also invested a significant amount of their time in understanding the subject and creating the most relevant covers. They scrutinized every image to scout for the most suitable representation of the subject and create an appropriate cover for the book.

The publishing team has been an ardent support to the editorial, designing and production team. Their endless efforts to recruit the best for this project, has resulted in the accomplishment of this book. They are a veteran in the field of academics and their pool of knowledge is as vast as their experience in printing. Their expertise and guidance has proved useful at every step. Their uncompromising quality standards have made this book an exceptional effort. Their encouragement from time to time has been an inspiration for everyone.

The publisher and the editorial board hope that this book will prove to be a valuable piece of knowledge for researchers, students, practitioners and scholars across the globe.

List of Contributors

Yukako Takami, Toshimori Koh, Minoru Nishio and Noboru Nakagawa
Department of Surgery, Social Insurance Kobe Central Hospital, 2-1-1, Sohyama-cho, Kita-ku, Kobe City 651-1145, Japan

Massimo Sartelli
Department of Surgery, Macerata Hospital, Via Santa Lucia 2, 62100 Macerata, Italy

Fikri M. Abu-Zidan
Department of Surgery, College of Medicine and Health Sciences, UAE University, Al-Ain, United Arab Emirates

Luca Ansaloni
General Surgery I,Papa Giovanni XXIII Hospital, Bergamo, Italy

Miklosh Bala
Trauma and Acute Care Surgery Unit, Hadassah Hebrew University Medical Center, Jerusalem, Israel

Amin Makni, Mohamed Jouini, Montassar Kacem and Zoubeir Ben Safta
Department of Surgery 'A', La Rabta Hospital, Tunis, Tunisia

Chang Sik Shin, Young Nam Roh and Jae Il Kim
Department of Surgery, Ilsan Paik Hospital, Inje University College of Medicine, 170 Juhwaro, Ilsanseogu, Goyangsi, Gyeonggido, Republic of Korea

Massimo Sartelli
Department of Surgery, Macerata Hospital, Macerata, Italy

Fausto Catena
Department of Emergency Surgery, Maggiore Parma Hospital, Parma, Italy

Salomone Di Saverio
Trauma Surgery Unit, Maggiore Hospital, Bologna, Italy

Luca Ansaloni
General Surgery Department, Papa Giovanni XXIII hospital, Bergamo, Italy

Frederick A Moore
Department of Surgery, University of Florida, Gainesville, Florida, USA

Rao Ivatury
Department of Surgery, Virginia Commonwealth University Medical Center, Richmond, VA, USA

Raul Coimbra
Department of Surgery, UC San Diego Health System, San Diego, USA

Ari Leppaniemi
Department of Abdominal Surgery, University Hospital Meilahti, Helsinki, Finland

Carlos A Ordonez
Department of Surgery, Universidad del Valle, Fundacion Valle del Lili, Cali, Colombia

Sanjay Marwah
Department of Surgery, Pt BDS Post-graduate Institute of Medical Sciences, Rohtak, India

Igor Gerych
Department of Surgery 1, Lviv Regional Hospital, Danylo Halytsky Lviv National Medical University, Lviv, Ukraine

Jae Gil Lee
Department of Surgery, Yonsei University College of Medicine, Seoul, Korea

Ossama Zakaria
Division of Pediatric Surgery, Departments of Surgery, Faculty of Medicine, Suez Canal University, Ismailia, Egypt
Sporting Students' Health Insurance Hospital, Alexandria, Egypt

Tamer A Sultan
Department of Surgery Faculty of Medicine, Meoufyia University, Egypt

Tarek H Khalil
Department of Radiology, Faculty of Medicine, Suez Canal University, Ismailia, Egypt

Tamer Wahba
Department of Radiology, Students' Hospital Alexandria University, Egypt

Maru Kim, Sung-Jeep Kim and Hang Joo Cho
Department of Trauma Surgery, College of Medicine, The Catholic University of Korea, Seoul, Republic of Korea

Panu Mentula and Ari Leppäniemi
Meilahti hospital, Department of Abdominal Surgery, University of Helsinki, Haartmaninkatu 4, 00029 Helsinki, HUS, Finland

Massimo Sartelli
Department of Surgery, Macerata Hospital, Via Santa Lucia 2, 62100 Macerata, Italy

Dieter G. Weber
Department of Trauma Surgery, Royal Perth Hospital, Perth, Australia

Etienne Ruppé
Genomic Research Laboratory, Geneva University Hospitals, Geneva, Switzerland

Matteo Bassetti
Infectious Diseases Division, Santa Maria Misericordia University Hospital, Udine, Italy

Hervé Dupont
Département d'Anesthésie-Réanimation, CHU Amiens-Picardie, and INSERM U1088, Université de Picardie Jules Verne, Amiens, France

Soumitra R. Eachempati
Department of Surgery, Division of Burn, Critical Care, and Trauma Surgery (K.P.S., S.R.E.), Weill Cornell Medical College/New York-Presbyterian Hospital, New York, USA

Mushira Abdulaziz Enani
Department of Medicine, Infectious Disease Division, King Fahad Medical City, Riyadh, Saudi Arabia

Valery N. Egiev
Department of Surgery, Pirogov Russian National Research Medical University, Moscow, Russian Federation

Tanya L. Zakrison
Division of Trauma and Surgical Critical Care, DeWitt Daughtry Family Department of Surgry, University of Miami, Miami, FL, USA

Antonio Corcione
Anesthesia and Intensive Care Unit, AORN dei Colli Vincenzo Monaldi Hospital, Naples, Italy

Rita M. Melotti
Anesthesiology and Intensive Care Unit, Sant'Orsola University Hospital, Bologna, Italy

Claudio Viscoli
Infectious Diseases Unit, University of Genoa (DISSAL) and IRCCS San Martino-IST, Genoa, Italy

Massimo Sartelli
Department of Surgery, Macerata Hospital, Macerata, Italy

Pierluigi Viale
Clinic of Infectious Diseases, Department of Internal Medicine Geriatrics and Nephrologic Diseases, St Orsola-Malpighi University Hospital, Bologna, Italy

Fausto Catena
Emergency Surgery, Maggiore Parma Hospital, Parma, Italy

Luca Ansaloni
Department of General Surgery, Ospedali Riuniti, Bergamo, Italy

Sanjay Marwah
Department of Surgery, Pt BDS Post-graduate Institute of Medical Sciences, Rohtak, India

Boris Sakakushev
First Clinic of General Surgery, University Hospital /UMBAL/ St George Plovdiv, Plovdiv, Bulgaria

Victor Kong
Department of Surgery, Edendale Hospital, Pietermaritzburg, Republic of South Africa

Noel Naidoo
Department of Surgery, Port Shepstone Hospital, Kwazulu Natal, South Africa

Helmut A Segovia Lohse
II Catedra de Clinica Quirúrgica, Hospital de Clínicas, San Lorenzo, Paraguay

Alfredo Verni
Department of Surgery, Cutral Co Clinic, Neuquen, Argentina

Tomohisa Shoko
The Shock Trauma and Emergency Medical Center, Matsudo City Hospital, Chiba, Japan

Phillipo L Chalya, Joseph B Mabula, Alphonce B Chandika and Japhet M Gilyoma
Department of Surgery, Weill-Bugando University College of Health Sciences, Mwanza, Tanzania

Mheta Koy, Hyasinta M Jaka and Rodrick Kabangila
Department of Internal Medicine, Weill- Bugando University College of Health Sciences, Mwanza, Tanzania

Mabula D Mchembe
Department of Surgery, Muhimbili University of Health and Allied Sciences, Dar Es Salaam, Tanzania

Luca Sorrentino, Osvaldo Chiara, Fabrizio Sammartano and Stefania Cimbanassi
Trauma Team and Emergency Surgery, Niguarda Trauma Center, Niguarda Ca' Granda Hospital, Piazza Ospedale Maggiore 3, Milan 20162, Italy

Massimiliano Mutignani
Digestive Endoscopy Service, Niguarda Ca' Granda Hospital, Piazza Ospedale Maggiore 3, Milan 20162, Italy

Paolo Brioschi
Intensive Care Unit, Niguarda Trauma Center, Niguarda Ca' Granda Hospital, Piazza Ospedale Maggiore 3, Milan 20162, Italy

Salomone Di Saverio, Marica Galati, Nazareno Smerieri, Michele Masetti, Elio Jovine and Antonio D Pinna
Emergency and Trauma Surgery Unit, Departments of Emergency and Surgery, Maggiore Hospital Trauma Center, Bologna, Italy

Federico Coccolini
General Surgery I, Ospedali Riuniti di Bergamo, Bergamo, Italy

Walter L Biffl
Department of Surgery, Denver Health, University of Colorado Health Sciences Denver, Denver Health Medical Center, 777 Bannock Street, Denver CO 80204, USA

Stefano Mandalà
Department of General and Emergency Surgery, Associated Hospitals "Villa Sofia - Cervello", Palermo, Italy

Johannes Jeekel
Department of Surgery, Erasmus University Medical Center, Rotterdam, The Netherlands

Fausto Catena
Emergency Surgery Unit, Department of General and Multivisceral Transplant Surgery, S Orsola Malpighi University Hospital, Bologna, Italy

Zdravko Roje
Division of Plastic Surgery and Burns, University Hospital Centre Split, Croatia

Željka Roje
Department of Surgery, University Hospital Dubrava, Zagreb, Croatia

Dario Matić
Department of Surgery, University Hospital Centre Split, Croatia

Davor Librenjak
Department of Urology, University Hospital Centre Split, Croatia

Stjepan Dokuzović
Department of Orthopedic Surgery, University Hospital Dubrava, Zagreb, Croatia

Josip Varvodić
Deparment of Neurosurgery, University Hospital Dubrava, Zagreb, Croatia

Lidia Dalfino and Francesco Bruno
Anesthesia and Intensive Care Unit - Emergency and Organ Transplantation Department, University of Bari, Policlinico of Bari, P.zza G. Cesare 11, 70124 Bari, Italy

Sergio Colizza
Department of General Surgery, Fatebenefratelli-Isola Tiberina, Rome, Italy

Ercole Concia
Clinical Infectious Disease, Department of Pathology, University of Verona, Verona, Italy

Andrea Novelli
Department of Health Sciences, Clinical Pharmacology and Oncology Section, University of Florence, Florence, Italy

Fabrizio Rebecchi
Digestive, Colorectal, Oncologic and Minimally Invasive Surgery, Department of Surgical Sciences, University of Turin, Turin, Italy

Federico Spandonaro and Cristina Alato
CEIS, University of Rome Tor Vergata, Rome, Italy

Farhan Rashid and Syed Y Iftikhar
Department of Upper GI Surgery, Royal Derby Hospital, Graduate Entry Medical School, Derby, University of Nottingham, UK

Ahmed Aber
Department of Surgery, Luton and Dunstable Hospital, Luton, UK

Massimo Sartelli
Department of Surgery, Macerata Hospital, Macerata, Italy

Fausto Catena
Department of Emergency Surgery, Maggiore Hospital, Parma, Italy

Fikri M. Abu-Zidan
Department of Surgery, College of Medicine and Health Sciences, UAE University, Al-Ain, United Arab Emirates

Luca Ansaloni
General Surgery Department, Papa Giovanni XXIII Hospital, Bergamo, Italy

Ari Leppaniemi
Abdominal Center, University Hospital Meilahti, Helsinki, Finland

Ronald V. Maier
Department of Surgery, University of Washington, Seattle, WA, USA

Addison K. May
Departments of Surgery and Anesthesiology, Division of Trauma and Surgical Critical Care, Vanderbilt University Medical Center, Nashville, TN, USA

Mark Malangoni
American Board of Surgery, Philadelphia, PA, USA

Kjetil Soreide
Department of Gastrointestinal Surgery, Stavanger University Hospital, Stavanger, Department of Clinical Medicine, University of Bergen, Bergen, Norway

Michael Sugrue
Letterkenny University Hospital and Donegal Clinical Research Academy, Letterkenny, Ireland

Jan Ulrych
1st Department of Surgery, Department of Abdominal, Thoracic Surgery and Traumatology, General University Hospital, Praha, Czech Republic

Jean-Louis Vincent
Department of Intensive Care, Erasme Hospital, Université libre de Bruxelles, Brussels, Belgium

Yun Tae Jung, Jung Yun Park, Myung Jun Kim, Seung Hwan Lee and Jae Gil Lee
Department of Surgery, Yonsei University College of Medicine, 50-1 Yonsei-ro, Seodaemun-gu, Seoul 03722, Republic of Korea

Jiyeon Jeon
Yonsei University College of Nursing, 50-1 Yonsei-ro, Seodaemun-gu, Seoul 03722, Republic of Korea

Index

www.ingramcontent.com/pod-product-compliance
Lightning Source LLC
LaVergne TN
LVHW080734210926
848485LV00003B/553